Clinical Guide to
Paediatrics

The *Clinical Guides* series

Series Editor: Christian Fielder Camm

The *Clinical Guides* are a brand new resource for junior doctors and medical students. They provide practical and concise information on symptoms, common conditions, and day-to-day problems faced in the clinical environment. They are easy to navigate and allow swift access to information as it is needed, with step-by-step guidance on investigations, decision-making and interventions, and how to survive and thrive on clinical rotations and attachments.

Clinical Guide to Paediatrics

Edited by

Rachel Varughese
Specialist Registrar in Paediatrics
Oxford University Hospitals NHS Foundation Trust, UK

and

Anna Mathew
Consultant Paediatrician
University Hospitals Sussex NHS Foundation Trust, Worthing, UK
Chair of MRCPCH Clinical Examinations, RCPCH

Series Editor:

Christian Fielder Camm
Cardiology Specialist Registrar
Royal Berkshire Hospital, Reading, UK

WILEY Blackwell

This edition first published 2022
© 2022 John Wiley & Sons Ltd

The right of Rachel Varughese and Anna Mathew to be identified as the authors of the editorial material in this work has been asserted in accordance with law.

Registered Offices
John Wiley & Sons, Inc., 111 River Street, Hoboken, NJ 07030, USA
John Wiley & Sons Ltd, The Atrium, Southern Gate, Chichester, West Sussex, PO19 8SQ, UK

Editorial Office
9600 Garsington Road, Oxford, OX4 2DQ, UK

For details of our global editorial offices, customer services, and more information about Wiley products visit us at www.wiley.com.

Wiley also publishes its books in a variety of electronic formats and by print-on-demand. Some content that appears in standard print versions of this book may not be available in other formats.

Library of Congress Cataloging-in-Publication Data

Names: Varughese, Rachel, editor. | Mathew, Anna, editor.
Title: Clinical guide to paediatrics / edited by Rachel Varughese and Anna Mathew.
Other titles: Clinical guides series.
Description: First edition. | Hoboken, NJ : Wiley-Blackwell, 2022. | Series: Clinical guides series | Includes bibliographical references and index.
Identifiers: LCCN 2021027295 (print) | LCCN 2021027296 (ebook) | ISBN 9781119539117 (paperback) | ISBN 9781119539124 (adobe pdf) | ISBN 9781119539094 (epub)
Subjects: MESH: Pediatrics
Classification: LCC RJ61 (print) | LCC RJ61 (ebook) | NLM WS 100 | DDC 618.92–dc23
LC record available at https://lccn.loc.gov/2021027295
LC ebook record available at https://lccn.loc.gov/2021027296

Cover image: Wiley
Cover design: © Gettyimages\PIXOLOGICSTUDIO/SCIENCE PHOTO LIBRARY

Set in 8.5/10.5pt Frutiger-Light by Straive, Pondicherry, India

SKYD84FFC78-EDB7-4C46-BD17-744E4765EBD0_062122

Contents

List of Contributors

Abdulhakim Abdurrazaq
Department of Paediatrics, Walsall Manor Hospital, Walsall Healthcare NHS Trust, Walsall, UK

Geetha Anand
Department of Paediatrics, John Radcliffe Hospital, Oxford University Hospitals NHS Foundation Trust, Oxford, UK

Rachel Atherton
Department of Paediatrics, Oxford University Hospitals NHS Foundation Trust, Oxford, UK

Rebecca Brown
Department of Paediatrics, London School of Paediatrics, London, UK

Dannika Buckley
Department of Paediatrics, University Hospitals Sussex NHS Foundation Trust, Worthing, West Sussex, UK

Catarina Pinto Carr
Department of Paediatrics, East Surrey Hospital, Surrey and Sussex Healthcare NHS Trust, UK

Benjamin Carter
Department of Paediatrics, University Hospitals Sussex NHS Foundation Trust, Chichester, UK

Samyami S. Chowdhury
Department of Paediatric Neurology, John Radcliffe Hospital, Oxford University Hospitals NHS Foundation Trust, Oxford, UK

Duana Cook
Department of Paediatrics, University Hospitals Sussex NHS Foundation Trust, Worthing, UK

Eleanor Duckworth
University College Hospital, University College London Hospitals NHS Foundation Trust, London, UK

Gary Foley
Department of Paediatrics, Centre for Genomics and Child Health, London, UK

Emma Hughes
Department of Paediatrics, Great Western Hospitals NHS Foundation Trust, Swindon, UK

Sally-Anne Hulton
Department of Paediatric Nephrology, Birmingham Women's and Children's NHS Foundation Trust, Birmingham, UK

Robin Joseph
Oxford University Hospitals NHS Foundation Trust, Oxford, UK

Umaiyal Kugathasan
University Hospitals Sussex NHS Trust, Brighton, UK

Ilana Levene
National Perinatal Epidemiology Unit, University of Oxford, Oxford, UK

Anna Mathew
Department of Paediatrics, University Hospitals Sussex NHS Foundation Trust, Worthing, UK

Simon Mattus
Department of Paediatrics, Wexham Park Hospital, Frimley Health NHS Foundation Trust, Slough, UK

Katie Mckinnon
Department of Paediatrics, North Middlesex University Hospital, London, UK

Philippa Mikolajski
Department of Paediatrics, Oxford University Hospitals NHS Foundation Trust, Oxford, UK

Lottie Mount
Department of Community Paediatrics, Sussex Community NHS Foundation Trust, Brighton, UK

Maxine Murray
Medica Group, Hastings, UK

Karim Noordally
Department of Paediatrics, Oxford University Hospitals NHS Foundation Trust, Oxford, UK

Emily Operto
Department of Paediatrics, The Royal Brompton Hospital, London, UK

Kate Park
Department of Paediatric Radiology, Oxford University Hospitals NHS Foundation Trust, Oxford, UK

Ashish Patel
Department of Paediatric Nephrology, Birmingham Women's and Children's NHS Foundation Trust, Birmingham, UK

Rebecca Puddifoot
Department of Paediatrics, Wexham Park Hospital, Frimley Health NHS Foundation Trust, Slough, UK

Sithara Ramdas
Department of Paedatrics, Oxford University Hospitals NHS Foundation Trust, Oxford, UK

Helen Ratcliffe

Oxford Vaccine Group, Centre for Clinical Vaccinology and Tropical Medicine, Oxford, UK

Gillian Rivlin

Department of Paediatrics, Oxford University Hospitals NHS Foundation Trust, Oxford, UK

Claire Roome

Department of Paediatrics, Wexham Park Hospital, Frimley Health NHS Foundation Trust, Slough, UK

Tim Sell

Department of Paediatrics, Oxford University Hospitals NHS Foundation Trust, Oxford, UK

Domenico Sirico

Department of Women's and Children's Health, Paediatric Cardiology Unit, Padua University Hospital, Padua, Italy

Andrew L. Smith

Department of Paediatrics, Children's Services, Homerton University Hospital NHS Foundation Trust, London, UK

Nicola J. Smith

Department of Paediatrics, Oxford University NHS Foundation Trust, Oxford, UK

Eleni Louka

Department of Paediatric Haematology, Oxford University Hospitals NHS Foundation Trust, Oxford, UK

Dora Steel

Department of Paediatrics, London School of Paediatrics, London, UK

Caroline Taylor

Department of Paediatrics, Buckinghamshire Healthcare NHS Trust, Aylesbury, UK

Rachel Varughese

Department of Paediatrics, Oxford University Hospitals NHS Foundation Trust, Oxford, UK

Samantha White

Department of Paediatrics, Wexham Park Hospital, NHS Frimley Health Foundation Trust, UK

Jenny Woodruff

Department of Paediatrics, Oxford University Hospitals NHS Foundation Trust, Oxford, UK

Acronyms and Abbreviations

AAT	alpha-1-antitrypsin
ABD	acute behavioural disturbance
ACE	angiotensin-converting enzyme
AChR	acetylcholine receptor
ACS	acute chest syndrome
ACTH	adrenocorticotropic hormone
ADEM	acute demyelinating encephalomyelitis
AED	anti-epileptic drug
AFP	alpha-fetoprotein
AGN	acute glomerulonephritis
AIDS	acquired immunodeficiency syndrome
AIHA	autoimmune haemolytic anaemia
AIS	arterial ischaemic stroke
AKI	acute kidney injury
ALL	acute lymphoblastic leukaemia
ALP	alkaline phosphatase
ALT	alanine aminotransferase
ANA	antinuclear antibody
ANCA	antineutrophil cytoplasmic antibody
APTT	activated partial thromboplastin time
ARB	angiotensin receptor blocker
ARF	acute rheumatic fever
ASA	anterior spinal artery
ASD	atrial septal defect
ASOT	anti-streptolysin O titre
AST	aspartate aminotransferase
AVM	arteriovenous malformation
AVNRT	AV nodal re-entry tachycardia
AVRT	atrioventricular re-entry tachycardia
AVSD	atrioventricular septal defect
BIMDG	British Inherited Metabolic Diseases Group
BiPAP	bilevel positive airway pressure
BMI	Body Mass Index
BNF	British National Formulary
BNP	B-type natriuretic peptide
BP	blood pressure
BPPV	benign paroxysmal positional vertigo
BPVC	benign paroxysmal vertigo of childhood
BSPED	British Society for Paediatric Endocrinology and Diabetes
CAMHS	Child and Adolescent Mental Health Service
CF	cystic fibrosis
CFRD	cystic fibrosis–related diabetes
CFTR	cystic fibrosis transmembrane regulator
CGD	chronic granulomatous disease
CHD	congenital heart disease
CMPA	cow's milk protein allergy
CMV	cytomegalovirus
CNS	central nervous system
COPD	chronic obstructive pulmonary disease
CPAP	continuous positive airway pressure
CPVT	catecholaminergic polymorphic ventricular tachycardia
CRH	corticotropin-releasing hormone
CRP	C-reactive protein
CSF	cerebrospinal fluid
CT	computed tomography
CVST	cerebral venous sinus thrombosis
DAT	direct antiglobulin test
DCM	dilated cardiomyopathy
DDH	developmental dysplasia of the hip
DI	diabetes insipidus
DIC	disseminated intravascular coagulation
DJ	duodenojejunal
DKA	diabetic ketoacidosis
DMSA	dimercaptosuccinic acid
DOT	directly observed therapy
dsDNA	double-stranded DNA
DWI	diffusion-weighted imaging
EBV	Epstein–Barr virus
ECG	electrocardiogram
ECMO	extracorporeal membrane oxygenation
EDS	Ehlers–Danlos syndrome
EEG	electroencephalogram
EM	erythema multiforme
ENT	Ear, Nose and Throat
ERCP	endoscopic retrograde cholangiopancreatography
ESR	erythrocyte sedimentation rate
ETN	erythema toxic neonatorum
FAOD	fatty acid oxidation defect
FBC	full blood count
FFA	free fatty acids
FFP	fresh frozen plasma
FHM	familial hemiplegic migraine
FII	fabricated or induced illness
FVC	forced vital capacity
γ-GT	gamma-glutamyltransferase
G6PD	glucose-6-phosphate dehydrogenase
GAL-1-PUT	galactose-1-phosphate uridyl transferase
GAS	group A *Streptococcus*
GBS	group B *Streptococcus*
GBS	Guillain–Barré syndrome
GCS	Glasgow Coma Scale
GGT	gamma-glutamyltransferase
GI	gastrointestinal
GOR	gastro-oesophageal reflux
GORD	gastro-oesophageal reflux disease
GSD	glycogen storage disorders

GU	genitourinary	LSA	left subclavian artery
HACEK	*Haemophilus, Aggregatibacter, Cardiobacterium, Eikenella, Kingella*	LV	left ventricle
		LVH	left ventricular hypertrophy
HbF	foetal haemoglobin	LVOT	left ventricular outflow tract
HCG	human chorionic gonadotropin	MAHA	microangiopathic haemolytic anaemia
HCM	hypertrophic cardiomyopathy	MAOI	monoamine oxidase inhibitor
HCT	haematocrit	MC&S	microscopy, culture and sensitivity
HDU	high-dependency unit	MCADD	medium-chain acyl-CoA dehydrogenase deficiency
HHFNC	heated humidified high-flow nasal cannula oxygen		
HHS	hyperosmolar hyperglycaemic state	MCHC	mean corpuscular haemoglobin concentration
HHV	human herpesvirus	MCUG	micturating cystourethrogram
Hib	*Haemophilus influenzae* type B	MCV	mean corpuscular volume
HIDA	hepatobiliary iminodiacetic acid	MDT	multi-disciplinary team
HIV	human immunodeficiency virus	MELAS	mitochondrial myopathy, encephalopathy, lactic acidosis and stroke-like episodes
HLA	human leucocyte antigen		
HLH	haemophagocytic lymphohistiocytosis	MEN1	multiple endocrine neoplasia
HNIg	human normal immunoglobulin	MenB	meningococcal group B
HONK	hyperglycaemic hyperosmolar non-ketotic coma	MG	myasthenia gravis
HPV	human papillomavirus	MMR	measles, mumps, rubella
HR	heart rate	MODY	maturity-onset diabetes of the young
HS	hereditary spherocytosis	MRCP	magnetic resonance cholangio pancreatogram
HSP	Henoch–Schönlein purpura	MRSA	methicillin-resistant *Staphyloccocus aureus*
HSV	herpes simplex virus	MSH	melanocyte-stimulating hormone
HUS	haemolytic uraemic syndrome	MSSA	methicillin-sensitive *Staphylococcus aureus*
HVA	homovanillic acid	NAC	N-acetylcysteine
IA	innominate artery	NAI	non-accidental injury
IBCLC	International Board Certified Lactation Consultant	NCSE	non-convulsive status epilepticus
IBD	inflammatory bowel disease	NDM	neonatal diabetes mellitus
IBS	irritable bowel syndrome	NEAD	non-epileptic attack disorder
ICD	implantable cardioverter-defibrillator	NEC	necrotising enterocolitis
ICP	intracranial pressure	NG	nasogastric
IDA	iron-deficiency anaemia	NICE	National Institute for Health and Care Excellence
IEM	inborn errors of metabolism	NJ	nasojejunal
Ig	immunoglobulin	NMS	neuroleptic malignant syndrome
IIH	idiopathic intracranial hypertension	NPA	naso-pharyngeal aspirate
ILCA	International Lactation Consultant Association	NSAIDs	non-steroidal anti-inflammatory drugs
IM	intramuscular	NT-proBNP	N-terminal-pro hormone BNP
INR	international normalised ratio	OGD	oesophago-gastro-duodenoscopy
IOH	initial orthostatic hypotension	OH	orthostatic hypotension
IST	inappropriate sinus tachycardia	OI	osteogenesis imperfecta
ITP	immune thrombocytopenia	ORS	oral rehydration solution
IUGR	intrauterine growth restriction	PA	pulmonary artery
IV	intravenous	PaCO$_2$	partial pressure of carbon dioxide
IVC	inferior vena cava	PAC	premature atrial contraction
IVIg	intravenous immunoglobulin	PAS	Paediatric Appendicitis Score
JIA	juvenile idiopathic arthritis	pCO$_2$	partial pressure of carbon dioxide
JRA	juvenile rheumatoid arthritis	PCR	polymerase chain reaction
JVP	jugular venous pressure	PCV	pneumococcal conjugate vaccine
LA	left atrium	PDA	patent ductus arteriosus
LAIV	live attenuated influenza vaccine	PE	pulmonary embolism
LCCA	left common carotid artery	PEFR	peak expiratory flow rate
LDH	lactate dehydrogenase	PEG-J	percutaneous endoscopic transgastric jejunostomy
LFTs	liver function tests		
LMA	laryngeal mask airway	PEG	percutaneous endoscopic gastrostomy
LMWH	low molecular weight heparin	PH	pulmonary hypertension
LP	lumbar puncture	PICC	peripherally inserted central catheter
LQT	long QT	PICU	paediatric intensive care unit

PLE	protein-losing enteropathy		SSRI	selective serotonin reuptake inhibitor
PNES	psychogenic non-epileptic seizures		SSSS	staphylococcal scalded skin syndrome
PNET	primitive neuroectodermal tumour		STARS	Syncope Trust And Reflex anoxic Seizures
PO	per os (orally)		SUFE	slipped upper femoral epiphysis
POMC	pro-opiomelanocortin		SVC	superior vena cava
POTS	postural orthostatic tachycardia syndrome		SVT	supraventricular tachycardia
PPHN	persistent pulmonary hypertension of the newborn		T1DM	type 1 diabetes mellitus
PPI	proton pump inhibitor		TAPVC	total anomalous pulmonary venous connection
PPS	psychogenic pseudosyncope		TB	tuberculosis
PRES	posterior reversible encephalopathy syndrome		TCA	tricyclic antidepressant
PSRA	post-streptococcal reactive arthritis		TEN	toxic epidermal necrolysis
PT	prothrombin time		TFTs	thyroid function tests
PUJ	pelvi-ureteric junction		TIBC	total iron-binding capacity
PUV	posterior urethral valves		TMJ	temporomandibular joint
PVC	premature ventricular contraction		Tn	troponin
PVL	Panton–Valentine leukocidin		tPA	tissue plasminogen activator
RA	right atrium		TSH	thyroid-stimulating hormone
RAA	renin-angiotensin-aldosterone		TSS	toxic shock syndrome
RAST	radioallergosorbent test		TTP	thrombotic thrombocytopaenic purpura
RBC	red blood cell		U&E	urea and electrolytes
RCPCH	Royal College of Paediatrics and Child Health		UC	ulcerative colitis
RhD	rhesus D		UDP	uridine 5-diphospho-glucuronosyltransferase
RhF	rheumatoid factor		UKDILAS	UK Drugs in Lactation Advisory Service
RIF	right iliac fossa		URTI	upper respiratory tract infection
RIG	rabies immunoglobulin		USS	ultrasound scan
RR	respiratory rate		UTI	urinary tract infection
RSV	respiratory syncytial virus		VBG	venous blood gas
RV	right ventricle		VF	ventricular fibrillation
RVH	right ventricular hypertrophy		VHF	viral haemorrhagic fever
SaO$_2$	oxygen saturation		VMA	vanillylmandelic acid
SBI	serious bacterial illness		VOC	vaso-occlusive crisis
SBR	serum bilirubin		VP	ventriculo-peritoneal
SCD	sickle cell disease		VSD	ventricular septal defect
SIADH	syndrome of inappropriate antidiuretic hormone secretion		VT	ventricular tachycardia
			VUJ	vesico-ureteric junction
SIRS	systemic inflammatory response syndrome		VUR	vesico-ureteric reflux
SJS	Stevens–Johnson syndrome		VWD	von Willebrand disease
SLE	systemic lupus erythematosus		VWF	von Willebrand factor
SNRI	serotonin and noradrenaline reuptake inhibitor		VZV	varicella zoster virus
SOL	space-occupying lesion		WCC	white cell count
SSPE	subacute sclerosing panencephalitis		WHO	World Health Organisation

About the Companion Website

This book is accompanied by a companion website:

www.wiley.com/go/varughese/paediatrics

The website includes:

- Diagnosis to consider
- Additional references
- Guidelines
- Audio podcast script

The website includes Diagnoses to Consider from all the chapters, as well as a large number of self-assessment questions in MCQ and EMQ format. Additionally, there are a number of clinical cases to work through.

How to Use This Book

This book is primarily aimed at those dealing with acute paediatric complaints. It has been designed to focus on developing appropriate differential diagnoses from the vantage point of viewing a patient presenting with a set of signs or symptoms.

Chapters are divided into sections based on the system to which they best refer. Each chapter starts with a diagnostic algorithm, which is presented as a flowchart in order to help readers create a framework for thinking about differentials. Diagnoses are divided into 'dangerous', 'common' and 'diagnoses to consider'. It is appreciated that there is often overlap between a diagnosis that may be 'dangerous' and one that is 'common'.

In each chapter, the dangerous and common diagnoses are considered in more detail, by considering appropriate history questions to ask, examinations to perform and management highlights to consider. Diagnoses to consider should prompt the reader to think about these possible diagnoses, which, although often less common, are important to note. Further details regarding diagnoses to consider are included in the companion website to this book.

In addition, there is a section at the end of the book covering useful tips for common paediatric problems and another section covering management of key emergency conditions for easy reference.

Additional references and guidelines that underpin the book can be found online at: www.wiley.com/go/varughese/paediatrics.

1.1 Wheeze

Duana Cook

Department of Paediatrics, University Hospitals Sussex NHS Foundation Trust, Worthing, UK

CONTENTS

1.1.1 CHAPTER AT A GLANCE

> **Box 1.1.1   Chapter at a Glance**
>
> - Wheeze indicates obstruction to airflow within the respiratory tract
> - Wheeze can be chronic, but any acute wheeze accompanied by increased work of breathing requires rapid assessment and treatment
>
> - Anaphylaxis and severe exacerbations of asthma can be life-threatening emergencies
> - If acute wheeze is suspected, immediate senior help and treatment must be initiated without waiting to undertake a detailed history

1.1.2 DEFINITION

Wheeze is a high-pitched, whistling sound made while breathing, due to partial obstruction or narrowing of the airways.

> **Box 1.1.2   Description of Wheeze**
>
> - **Pitch** High-pitched wheezing suggests obstruction in smaller airways, whereas low-pitched wheezing suggests obstruction of larger airways
>
> - **Position in respiratory cycle.** Wheeze is most commonly expiratory, but biphasic wheeze can be present in significant obstruction
> - **Monophonic or polyphonic wheeze.** This indicates whether one or many airways are affected by the obstruction

---

1.1.3 DIAGNOSTIC ALGORITHM

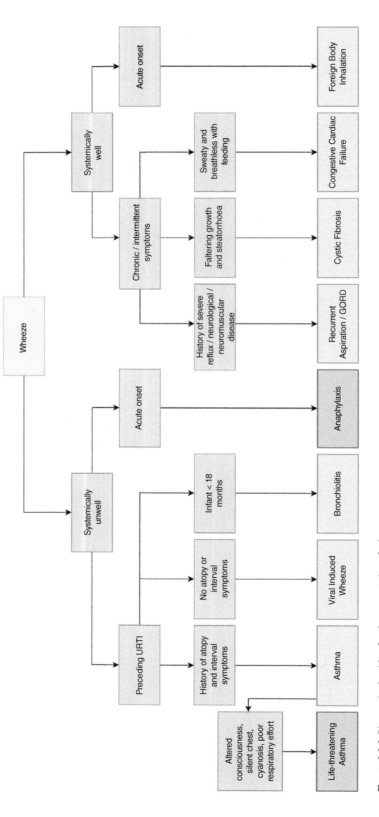

Figure 1.1.1 Diagnostic algorithm for the presentation of wheeze.

1.1.4 DIFFERENTIALS LIST

Dangerous Diagnoses

1. *Asthma (Severe/Life-Threatening)*
- Chronic reversible small airways obstruction caused by airway inflammation and bronchial hyper-reactivity
- In severe episodes the calibre of the airway can become severely compromised, requiring immediate treatment and, if necessary, respiratory support
- Severe exacerbations can result in altered consciousness, agitation and poor respiratory effort, such that the wheeze disappears leaving a 'silent chest'
- In such circumstances there may be limited response to inhaled or nebulised therapy and treatment will need to be escalated swiftly
- Symptoms are frequently triggered by environmental factors or intercurrent illnesses

2. *Anaphylaxis*
- Serious life-threatening immunoglobulin (Ig) E-mediated allergic reaction requiring immediate treatment
- Systemic response is caused by the release of immune and inflammatory mediators from degranulating basophils and mast cells
- Acute airway obstruction and profound hypotension can be rapidly fatal without treatment
- Associated symptoms include angioedema, urticaria and vomiting
- Allergens commonly include medicines, food, immunotherapy or insect stings

Common Diagnoses

1. *Asthma (Mild/Moderate)*
- Chronic reversible small airways obstruction caused by airway inflammation and bronchial hyper-reactivity
- Symptoms are frequently triggered by environmental factors or intercurrent illness, and respond to bronchodilators

2. *Viral-Induced Wheeze*
- Wheeze is caused by inflammation and congestion of the lower respiratory tract
- Generally affects young children <5 years due to small-calibre airways
- Wheeze occurs only with intercurrent viral upper respiratory tract infections and there are no interval symptoms

3. *Bronchiolitis*
- Affects infants under 18 months, predominantly in the winter months
- Respiratory syncytial virus (RSV) accounts for the majority of cases
- Inflammation and congestion of the lower respiratory tract can progress to difficulty in feeding and increased work of breathing
- Severity can vary from mild to life-threatening

4. *Inhalation of Foreign Body*
- Food is the most common foreign body to aspirate, although any small object may be inhaled
- Peak incidence is between 6 months and 4 years old
- Parents may provide a history, e.g. coughing, gagging or choking episode while eating/ playing with small objects
- Foreign body inhalation can be life-threatening, but if presenting with wheeze, complete airway obstruction is unlikely as the foreign body is likely below the carina

Diagnoses to Consider

1. *Cystic Fibrosis*
- The most common inherited life-limiting condition in Caucasians, inherited as autosomal recessive
- Defective cystic fibrosis transmembrane regulator (CFTR) gene located on chromosome 7 causes abnormal ion transport across the epithelium of the respiratory tract and pancreas. This leads to increased viscosity of secretions
- Consider this in a child with a history of faltering growth and recurrent respiratory tract infections

When to consider: in patients with a known family history of cystic fibrosis or repeated chest infections

2. *Recurrent Aspiration ± Gastro-oesophageal Reflux Disease (GORD)*
- Aspiration into the lungs can occur at any age, but it is particularly a problem in some ex-premature infants, those with a genetic predisposition and children with neuro-muscular conditions
- It can lead to lower respiratory tract inflammation and infection

When to consider: in those with known severe GORD, or with risk factors for an unsafe swallow, e.g. neuro-muscular or neurological conditions

3. *Congestive Cardiac Failure*
- A progressive state in which the cardiac output is insufficient to meet systemic demands, resulting in pulmonary oedema
- Congenital cardiac abnormalities and cardiomyopathy can lead to congestive cardiac failure

When to consider: in those with suspected congenital cardiac disease, faltering growth or breathlessness during feeds

1.1.5 KEY HISTORY FEATURES

Dangerous Diagnosis 1

Diagnosis: Asthma (severe/life-threatening)

Questions

1. **Onset of episode and any triggers?** Timing of onset, any known triggers and speed of deterioration are important in determining severity
2. **Recent admission(s) with severe asthma ± high-dependency unit (HDU)/paediatric intensive care unit (PICU) care?** Recent admissions and involvement of intensive care are red flags and should alert the medical team to a possible similar outcome
3. **On polytherapy for the management of asthma?** Background treatment necessitating three or more drugs suggests more severe, difficult-to-control asthma
4. **Has there been treatment provided at home?** An account of the medication already administered will inform ongoing therapy

Dangerous Diagnosis 2

Diagnosis: Anaphylaxis

Questions

1. **Any exposure to known allergens?** Those who have had allergic reactions previously (e.g. to peanuts or latex) may go on to develop more severe reactions with repeated exposure
2. **What was the nature of the onset?** Anaphylaxis usually occurs soon after exposure to an allergen, with rapid progression of symptoms and signs
3. **Any history of asthma, eczema or hay fever?** Allergies are more common in those with atopic conditions, and food allergies are particularly more common in those with eczema
4. **Has there been treatment provided at home?** Those with known severe allergies may have an EpiPen® and antihistamines at home

Common Diagnosis 1

Diagnosis: Asthma (mild/moderate)

Questions

1. **Are there interval symptoms?** Cough and wheeze between asthma exacerbations are known as interval symptoms. Over time it may be possible to identify triggers that set off these symptoms. This suggests a diagnosis of chronic airway inflammation, making asthma rather than viral-induced wheeze the more likely diagnosis
2. **Has the patient ever had wheezy episodes before?** Children with asthma get recurrent episodes of cough, wheeze and breathlessness, even without an infectious trigger
3. **Does the patient (or any first-degree family member) have a history of other atopic conditions?** Atopy is an inherited predisposition to allergen sensitisation and conditions include asthma, eczema and hay fever. Having one atopic condition increases the risk of having another

---

Box 1.1.3   Common Triggers in Asthma
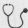

- Upper respiratory tract infections
- Pollution
- Cigarette smoke
- Exercise

- Cold weather
- House dust mite
- Animal dander: dogs or cats
- Aero-allergens: grass or tree pollen

Common Diagnosis 2

Diagnosis: Viral-induced wheeze

Questions

1. **Is the patient under 5 years old?** Viral-induced wheeze usually occurs in those aged under 5 years, due to their small-calibre airways being more susceptible to occlusion by inflammation and congestion
2. **Was there a preceding coryzal illness?** There is usually a preceding coryzal illness reported in the history

3. **Do they experience wheeze when well?** Children with viral-induced wheeze are wheeze free between the episodes of viral upper respiratory tract infections and do not get interval symptoms.

Common Diagnosis 3
Diagnosis: Bronchiolitis

Questions
1. **Is the patient <18 months?** Bronchiolitis occurs mainly in those aged under 18 months, with the majority of those affected being 1–9 months of age
2. **Were there any preceding symptoms?** There is usually a preceding coryzal illness for 2–3 days prior to the onset of difficulty in breathing
3. **Have they had a cough?** Bronchiolitis is associated with a classic wheezy-sounding 'bronchiolitic' cough
4. **Has feeding been affected?** Due to a combination of nasal congestion and difficulty in breathing, infants struggle to maintain their usual feeding pattern. A reduction of more than one-third from baseline is considered significant

Common Diagnosis 4
Diagnosis: Inhalation of foreign body

Questions
1. **Was there a sudden onset?** The patient is likely to have a history of sudden onset of wheeze, associated with choking, coughing or difficulty in breathing
2. **What was the child doing when the problem began?** Parents may give a history of possible aspiration, as the patient may have been playing with small toys or eating prior to the onset of symptoms
3. **How old is the patient?** Inhalation of foreign body is more common in infants and toddlers – peak incidence is between 6 months and 4 years

1.1.6 KEY EXAMINATION FEATURES

Box 1.1.4   Signs of Increased Work of Breathing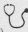

- **Tachypnoea.** An increase in the respiratory rate can be an early sign of respiratory distress
- **Tachycardia.** The heart rate may increase in response to hypoxia
- **Colour changes.** If the patient is significantly hypoxic, you may notice cyanosis around the mouth, the inside of the lips or on the fingernails. They may also appear pale
- **Grunting.** A noise is heard on exhalation, due to breathing against a closed glottis, in an attempt to keep the airways open
- **Recessions.** Tracheal tug and retractions between the

intercostal muscles and under the costal margin (subcostal) indicate an increased respiratory effort
- **Use of accessory muscles.** Sternocleidomastoid contraction and abdominal breathing increase the volume of the thoracic cavity
- **Position.** A 'tripod' position indicates accessory muscle use
- **Head bobbing.** In babies and young infants the head moving up and down is a reflection of accessory muscle use
- **Nasal flaring.** A compensatory increase in upper airway diameter

---

Dangerous Diagnosis 1
Diagnosis: Asthma (severe/life-threatening)

Examination Findings
1. **Signs of increased work of breathing.** Increased work of breathing, prolonged expiratory phase and widespread polyphonic wheeze are common findings in moderate to severe attacks. In severe exacerbations, the patient is unable to complete full sentences in one breath and may be too breathless to eat
2. **Signs of cardiac compromise.** Tachycardia is common with severe attacks, and hypotension can also occur. Pulsus paradoxus (marked reduction in systolic blood pressure during inspiration) can be seen in severe attacks
3. **Signs of neurological compromise due to hypoxia.** Confusion, drowsiness and altered consciousness are signs of neurological compromise, which indicates life-threatening asthma
4. **Silent chest.** In life-threatening cases the chest can be 'silent' as air movement is so poor

Box 1.1.5   Assessing the Severity of an Asthma Exacerbation

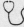

Mild to moderate	Severe	Life-threatening
• SaO$_2$ >92% in air • No clinical features of severe wheeze • May have some increased work of breathing	Any one of: • SaO$_2$ <92% • PEFR 33–50% best or predicted • Too breathless to talk or feed • Heart rate >140 (1–5y) or >125 (5+) • Respiratory rate >40 (1–5y) or >30 (5+) • Use of accessory muscles	SaO$_2$ <92% plus any of: • PEFR <33% best or predicted • Exhaustion • Silent chest • Poor respiratory effort • Agitation • Altered consciousness • Cyanosis

PEFR, peak expiratory flow rate; SaO$_2$, oxygen saturation
Source: Reproduced with permission from British Thoracic Society (2019).
Quick reference guide to the 2019 BTS/SIGN Asthma Guideline. London: BTS.

Dangerous Diagnosis 2
Diagnosis: Anaphylaxis

Examination Findings
1. **Involvement of the skin or mucosal tissue or both.** Exposure of the patient may reveal a widespread urticarial rash (hives), flushing or swelling of the lips, tongue and/or uvula (angioedema)
2. **Signs of increased work of breathing.** The patient may be tachypnoeic and/or hypoxic and have wheeze or stridor
3. **Symptoms and signs of end-organ dysfunction.** Hypotension, syncope or dizziness, weakness, blurred vision and abdominal pain all signal evolving anaphylactic shock

Common Diagnosis 1
Diagnosis: Asthma (mild/moderate)

Examination Findings
1. **Signs of chronic disease in poorly controlled asthma.** In older children with established disease you may find a Harrison's sulcus, a permanent indentation below the 6th rib
2. **Signs of increased work of breathing.** Increased work of breathing, prolonged expiratory phase and widespread polyphonic wheeze are common findings in moderate exacerbations (less noticeable with milder episodes)
3. **Absence of cardiac or neurological compromise.** Children's cardiovascular and neurological statuses remain stable in mild to moderate exacerbations

Common Diagnosis 2
Diagnosis: Viral-induced wheeze

Examination Findings
1. **Signs of viral upper respiratory tract infection.** Coryza, nasal congestion, cough and mild fever may be present
2. **Signs of increased work of breathing.** Variable degrees of respiratory distress may be present. Auscultation reveals widespread bilateral expiratory wheeze, possibly associated with transmitted upper airway noises

Common Diagnosis 3
Diagnosis: Bronchiolitis

Examination Findings
1. **Signs of viral upper respiratory tract infection.** Coryza, nasal congestion and mild fever may all be present, with 'snuffly' breathing
2. **Cough.** A tight, wheezy 'bronchiolitic' cough is classic, and can last for several weeks after the baby is clinically better
3. **Signs of increased work of breathing.** Infants can present with respiratory distress, including head bobbing and nasal flaring. They may have difficulty feeding due to their breathlessness. Younger infants can present with apnoeas
4. **Simultaneous crackles and wheeze.** Widespread fine end-inspiratory crackles and biphasic wheeze are often heard on auscultation

Figure 1.1.2 Changes in chronic obstructive respiratory disease. (A) Harrison's sulcus, as demonstrated by a persistent indentation at the level of the anterior insertion of the diaphragm. (B) Lateral view of a normally inflated lung. (C) Lateral view of a hyperinflated lung with a flattened diaphragm.

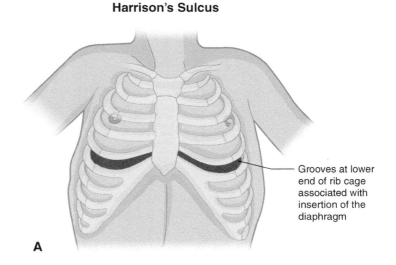

Harrison's Sulcus

Grooves at lower end of rib cage associated with insertion of the diaphragm

A

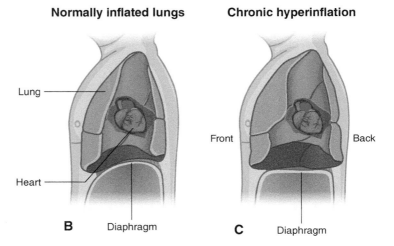

Normally inflated lungs

Chronic hyperinflation

Lung

Front   Back

Heart

B   Diaphragm

C   Diaphragm

Figure 1.1.3 Harrison's sulcus – note the chronic indentation of the lower ribcage. Source: Reproduced with permission from Newell, S.J., and Darling, J.C. (2014). *Paediatrics lecture notes*. Chichester: Wiley Blackwell.

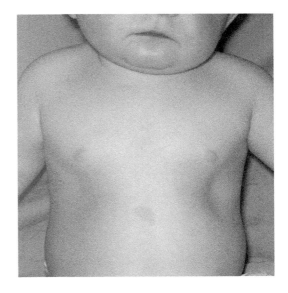

Common Diagnosis 4

Diagnosis: Inhalation of foreign body

Examination Findings

1. **Stridor.** Stridor is suggestive of a foreign body in the larynx or trachea. In this case there is a risk of complete airway obstruction. Although reduced, air entry may be equal bilaterally
2. **Lateralising signs.** Tracheal deviation, asymmetrical chest wall movement, unilateral wheeze and concomitant reduced breath sounds point to a foreign body in a bronchus
3. **Signs of increased work of breathing.** There will be monophonic wheeze with variable degrees of respiratory distress, depending on the location of the foreign body

1.1.7 KEY INVESTIGATIONS

Not all children will require invasive investigations; often diagnoses are made on clinical evidence from history and examination. Consider carefully which investigations are required for which patient.

Bedside

Table 1.1.1 Bedside tests of use in patients presenting with wheeze

Test	When to perform	Potential result
Oxygen saturations	• All children with wheeze • May reveal need for oxygen supplementation	• Sats <94% indicates hypoxia • Sats 92–94% may be tolerated • Sats <92% in asthma indicates a severe attack
Sputum MC&S/ cough swab	• Suspected exacerbation of CF	• Positive culture and sensitivities guide antibiotic choice
NPA	• Suspected bronchiolitis	• Identification of the responsible viral pathogen • Helps with cohorting patients with the same virus
Blood gas (capillary or venous)	• Significant respiratory distress	• ↓ pH and ↑CO_2 indicate respiratory acidosis and guide need for respiratory support
Peak flow (PEFR)	• Children with asthma	• A drop in PEFR will indicate the severity of an asthma exacerbation: <50% and <33% of best PEFR indicate severe and life-threatening episodes, respectively

CF, cystic fibrosis; CO_2, carbon dioxide; MC&S, microscopy, culture and sensitivity; NPA, naso-pharyngeal aspirate; PEFR, peak expiratory flow rate; Sats, saturation.

Blood Tests

Table 1.1.2 Blood tests of use in patients presenting with wheeze

Test	When to perform	Potential result
FBC	Suspected pneumonia in those with: • CF • Suspected aspiration with GORD	• ↑ white cells, particularly neutrophilia, consistent with bacterial infection
CRP	• Suspected pneumonia as above	• ↑ in infection or inflammation
Blood culture	• Suspected pneumonia as above	• Positive cultures confirm bacterial infection • Sensitivities direct antibiotic choice
Total IgE	• Atopic children	• Provides supporting information for atopic status
Allergen-specific RAST	• Anaphylaxis with suspected trigger	• Confirmation of allergy to suspected trigger

CF, cystic fibrosis; CRP, C-reactive protein; FBC, full blood count; GORD, gastro-oesophageal reflux disease; Ig, immunoglobulin; RAST, radioallergosorbent test.

Imaging

Table 1.1.3 Imaging modalities of use in patients presenting with wheeze

Test	When to perform	Potential result
Chest x-ray	Suspected • Foreign body inhalation • Pneumonia due to CF or GORD • Cardiac failure • Uncertain underlying diagnosis • Wheeze refractory to treatment	• Foreign body inhalation: ipsilateral collapse, air trapping • Exacerbation of CF: consolidation • Cardiac failure: enlarged cardiac shadow, pulmonary oligaemia or congestion, fluid in interlobar fissures • Asthma + bronchiolitis: hyperinflation • Bronchiolitis: perihilar bronchial thickening
Echocardiogram	• Suspected cardiac failure	• Identifies causative cardiac lesion • Estimates ventricular function

CF, cystic fibrosis; GORD, gastro-oesophageal reflux disease.

Special

Table 1.1.4 Special tests of use in patients presenting with wheeze

Test	When to perform	Potential result
Sweat test	• Diagnostic test in suspected CF	• >60 mmol/L of chloride is diagnostic of CF
Spirometry	• Those over 5 years old with acute exacerbations of CF • Also used for monitoring chronic asthma	• In CF, the flow volume curve reflects deterioration from baseline and guides treatment options • In asthma, the degree of obstruction reflects overall control
24 hr pH impedance monitoring	• Suspected GORD when resistant to conventional medication	• Reflux index will indicate whether severe gastric reflux exists
Assessment of swallow/ videofluoroscopy	• Suspected recurrent aspirations	• Confirms presence and degree of aspiration

CF, cystic fibrosis; GORD, gastro-oesophageal reflux disease.

Box 1.1.6   How to Measure Peak Expiratory Flow Rate (PEFR)

1. Connect a clean mouthpiece to the meter
2. Ensure the gauge is set to zero
3. Make sure the child is standing or sitting upright
4. Ask them to take as deep a breath in as they can and hold it
5. Ask the child to place the mouthpiece in their mouth and form as tight a seal as possible around it with their lips. Ensure they do not obstruct the gauge with their fingers when holding the meter
6. Then ask them to breathe out as hard as they can
7. Read the meter and record it, and repeat 3 times, taking the best reading

Measurement of Peak Expiratory Flow Rate (PEFR)

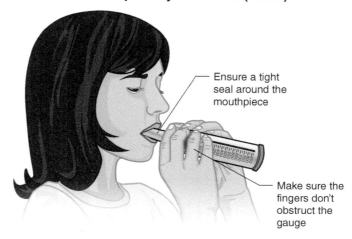

Ensure a tight
seal around the
mouthpiece

Make sure the
fingers don't
obstruct the
gauge

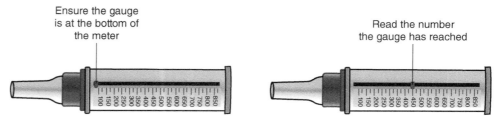

Ensure the gauge
is at the bottom of
the meter

Read the number
the gauge has reached

Figure 1.1.4 A child using a peak flow meter.

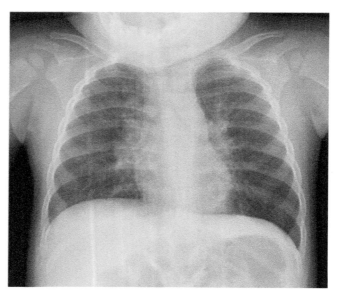

Figure 1.1.5 A chest x-ray is not required for a diagnosis of bronchiolitis, but may be performed in unwell children to exclude other pathologies. This chest x-ray is typical of bronchiolitis, showing perihilar bronchial thickening.

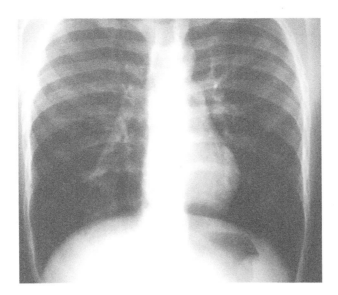

Figure 1.1.6 A chest x-ray showing hyperinflation in acute asthma. Source: Reproduced with permission from Newell, S.J., and Darling, J.C. (2014). *Paediatrics lecture notes*. Chichester: Wiley Blackwell.

1.1.8 KEY MANAGEMENT PRINCIPLES

Diagnosis-specific management strategies are outlined here. It is expected that an 'ABCDE' approach to assessment and management is always undertaken (see Chapter 12.1, *The A to E Assessment*).

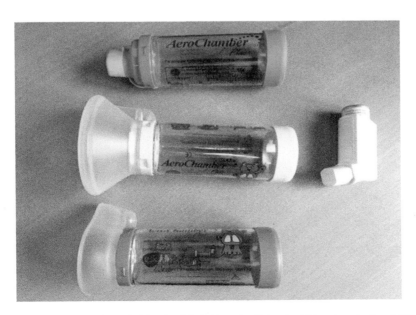

Figure 1.1.7 A spacer is an essential device when administering inhaled bronchodilators in children, in order to maximise delivery of medication to the lungs.

Dangerous Diagnosis 1
Diagnosis: Asthma (severe/life-threatening)

Management Principles
1. **Assess and record asthma severity.** The severity must be clearly recorded and reassessed regularly (see Box 1.1.5). If severe/life-threatening, seek senior help immediately
2. **Frequent reassessment to gauge response to treatment.** Escalate and involve local paediatric intensive care if condition worsens and/or response to treatment is ineffective
3. **Institute management according to local asthma guidelines.** Every unit should have a clear guideline for the management of acute, severe asthma. For general emergency management of severe asthma, see Chapter 13.3, *Acute Asthma Management*.

Dangerous Diagnosis 2
Diagnosis: Anaphylaxis

Management Principle
1. **Follow anaphylaxis protocol.** Anaphylaxis is an emergency with a prescriptive management (see Chapter 13.2, *Anaphylaxis Management*).

Common Diagnosis 1
Diagnosis: Asthma (mild/moderate)

Management Principles
1. **Assess and record asthma severity.** The severity must be clearly recorded and reassessed regularly (see Box 1.1.5). Any features of severe asthma require a reconsideration of management and urgent senior advice
2. **Bronchodilators.** Bronchodilators are the mainstay of management and once symptoms are responsive, they can be 'stretched' in frequency. Frequent reassessment to gauge response to treatment is vital
3. **Oral steroids.** Steroids are used in asthma exacerbations for their anti-inflammatory effect. Prednisolone is most commonly used or can be substituted for dexamethasone

Common Diagnosis 2
Diagnosis: Viral-induced wheeze

Management Principles
Viral-induced wheeze is managed according to the same general principles as acute asthma, although steroids are not routinely indicated:
1. **Oxygen supplementation**
2. **Bronchodilators**
3. **'Stretch' bronchodilators**
4. **Escalate in children with poor response or deterioration**

Common Diagnosis 3
Diagnosis: Bronchiolitis

Management Principles
1. **Oxygen supplementation.** Give oxygen if required to maintain saturations >92%.
2. **Humidified high-flow oxygen.** If work of breathing is significant, then consider respiratory support from heated humidified high-flow nasal cannula oxygen (HHFNC) such as Optiflow™ or Vapotherm®
3. **Feeding support.** In patients who are unable to tolerate adequate oral feeds, give supplementary feeds via nasogastric or orogastric tube. If they do not tolerate this or have impending respiratory failure, then fluids should be given intravenously
4. **Intubation.** Patients with bronchiolitis presenting with frequent apnoea, or severe respiratory distress, may require intubation

Box 1.1.7   Management of Mild to Moderate Asthma Exacerbation

Mild exacerbation	• Salbutamol inhaler via spacer (see doses below) *Reassess in 15 minutes: if improving, reassess in 1 hour. If stable, discharge.* Discharge plan: • Written asthma plan • Plan GP/asthma nurse review within 48 hours
Moderate exacerbation	Burst therapy: • Salbutamol inhaler via spacer (see doses below) *Reassess at 15 minutes: if ongoing wheeze/respiratory distress* • 2 further doses of salbutamol plus ipratropium bromide inhaler after 20 and 40 minutes *Reassess at 15 minutes* • Normal observations: discharge as above • Response suboptimal: admit to ward • Salbutamol inhaler up to 10 puffs 1–4 hourly • Prednisolone *Reassess hourly*
Doses	
Salbutamol 100 μg/dose	1–4 years: 5 puffs >5 years: 10 puffs
Ipratropium bromide 20 μg/dose	1–4 years: 4 puffs >5 years: 8 puffs
Prednisolone*	1–4 years: 10–20 mg for 3 days >5 years: 30–40 mg for 3 days
*or dexamethasone	0.3 mg/kg PO × 1 dose

PO, per os (orally).

Common Diagnosis 4
Diagnosis: Inhalation of foreign body

Management Principles
1. **Encourage cough.** If the child is alert and coughing effectively, this is the mechanism most likely to dislodge the foreign body
2. **Foreign body removal.** If the child is in distress or drowsy, then back blows and chest thrusts may be performed. Seek senior help
3. **Bronchoscopy.** This may be necessary if the above are not successful, the foreign body is in a lower airway or in an unconscious child. Give face mask oxygen and arrange urgent rigid bronchoscopy with a local PICU

1.2 Stridor

Rachel Varughese

Department of Paediatrics, Oxford University Hospitals NHS Foundation Trust, Oxford, UK

CONTENTS

1.2.1 CHAPTER AT A GLANCE

> **Box 1.2.1   Chapter at a Glance**
>
> - Stridor can be life-threatening and dangerous diagnoses need to be excluded
> - With heightened awareness, prompt, effective and time-critical airway support can be provided
> - If in doubt, call for help and avoid upsetting the child, as this could precipitate complete airway obstruction

1.2.2 DEFINITION

Stridor is a harsh, vibratory, often high-pitched sound caused by airflow turbulence in a partially obstructed airway.

Clinical Guide to Paediatrics, First Edition. Edited by Rachel Varughese and Anna Mathew. Series Editor: Christian Fielder Camm.
© 2022 John Wiley & Sons Ltd. Published 2022 by John Wiley & Sons Ltd.
Companion website: www.wiley.com/go/varughese/paediatrics

1.2.3 DIAGNOSTIC ALGORITHM

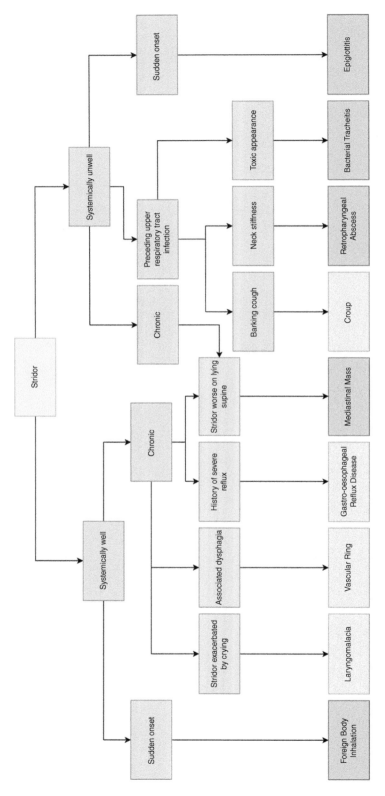

Figure 1.2.1 Diagnostic algorithm for the presentation of stridor.

1.2.4 DIFFERENTIALS LIST

Dangerous Diagnoses

All cases of acute stridor in children are treated as emergency assessments until potentially life-threatening causes have been ruled out.

1. **Epiglottitis**
   - Epiglottitis is a potentially fatal condition caused by inflammation of the epiglottis
   - Progression can be rapid and profound
   - The child is often described as having a 'toxic appearance'
   - Historically, almost exclusively caused by Haemophilus influenzae type B (Hib)
   - Since the introduction of the Hib vaccine, the incidence of epiglottitis has markedly declined
2. **Bacterial Tracheitis**
   - Bacterial tracheitis is an uncommon but life-threatening cause of stridor, produced by inflammation of the trachea
   - Leads to purulent exudate, which can be seen on bronchoscopy
   - Tends to be associated with an antecedent upper respiratory tract infection
   - Staphylococcal and streptococcal species are the most common pathogens
3. **Foreign Body Inhalation**
   - Aspiration of a foreign body is most commonly of food, although any small object may be inhaled
   - Be suspicious of sudden-onset stridor in an otherwise well child
   - Complete airway obstruction can occur

Common Diagnoses

1. **Viral Laryngotracheobronchitis ('Croup')**
   - Commonly known as 'croup', this is a frequent cause of stridor, associated with an antecedent upper respiratory tract infection
   - A 'barking cough' is characteristic
   - Usually due to infection with parainfluenza viruses, commonly affecting children from 6 months to 3 years old
   - Severity can vary from mild to life-threatening
2. **Laryngomalacia**
   - Laryngomalacia is the commonest cause of infantile stridor
   - Caused by soft immature cartilage of the upper larynx, which collapses inwards during the inspiratory phase of respiration

Diagnoses to Consider

1. **Retropharyngeal Abscess**
   - Deep neck infection involving abscess formation between prevertebral fascia and constrictor muscles
   - Most commonly, retropharyngeal abscesses affect children under the age of 5 years (after this, retropharyngeal lymph nodes atrophy)

   When to consider: in a stridulous patient who has a history of fever, particularly with recent tonsillitis or sinusitis, or pain on moving the neck
2. **Gastro-oesophageal Reflux Disease**
   - Recurrent gastro-oesophageal reflux can cause upper airway inflammation and stridor

   When to consider: in those with a history of chronic reflux or with risk factors for an unsafe swallow, e.g. neurological or neuromuscular conditions
3. **Vascular Ring**
   - A vascular ring describes a congenital abnormality of the aorta and major vessels, where the trachea and oesophagus become encircled by vessels

   When to consider: in children under 12 months. Since there is often oesophageal involvement, there may be associated dysphagia
4. **Mediastinal Mass**
   - There are several causes ranging from benign to sinister. Cystic malformations, enlarged thymus, lymphoma, fatty tumours, neurogenic tumours and solid tumours (e.g. cardiac, sarcoma, teratoma) can all present with stridor

   When to consider: in children whose stridor is associated with chest pain, shortness of breath when supine, or dysphagia. Symptoms can be subtle and varied given the variety of underlying causes

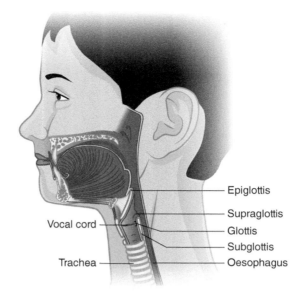

Figure 1.2.2 Anatomical diagram indicating the key structures in the upper airway. A solid understanding of these structures can help identify the pathology underlying stridor.

Box 1.2.2   Post-extubation Injury/Subglottic Stenosis

- Glottic and subglottic swelling can cause stridor
- Post-extubation injury describes mechanical damage and swelling, usually caused by a large endotracheal tube or following prolonged intubation
- Subglottic stenosis is sometimes seen in ex-premature infants following prolonged intubation in the neonatal period

- Symptoms typically appear within 1 hour of extubation in post-extubation injury. In ex-premature infants, symptoms may become more noticeable with an upper respiratory tract infection (URTI), due to inflammation of the airways
- Congenital forms exist, but are rare and tend to be associated with other genetic syndromes

---

1.2.5 KEY HISTORY FEATURES

Dangerous Diagnosis 1
Diagnosis: Epiglottitis

Questions
1. **Has the patient received a full course of *Haemophilus influenzae* B (Hib) vaccine?** In children, infectious aetiology is almost always due to infection with *Haemophilus influenzae* B. It is important to note that infections despite vaccination do still occur
2. **Was the onset sudden with rapid progression of symptoms?** Often, parents will describe their child as having been completely healthy hours before
3. **Are there any other infective symptoms?** There may be a high fever and sore throat, but spontaneous cough is uncommon. Parents may be anxious that the child looks very unwell

Dangerous Diagnosis 2
Diagnosis: Bacterial tracheitis

Questions
1. **Was there any preceding upper respiratory tract infection (URTI)?** Commonly symptoms are preceded by URTI by 2–3 days
2. **Is cough present?** In comparison to epiglottitis, bacterial tracheitis is associated with a productive cough, which may lead to retrosternal pain
3. **Does the child look 'toxic' and systemically unwell?** Deterioration over days with an increasingly high fever, cough, stridor, hoarseness and a toxic appearance helps distinguish this from viral croup

Dangerous Diagnosis 3
Diagnosis: Foreign body inhalation

Questions
1. **How old is the patient?** Peak incidence is between 6 months and 4 years old
2. **What was the child doing before symptoms began?** Parents will often be able to identify a likely object that may have been inhaled, for example if onset was while eating or playing
3. **What was the nature of onset?** There may be a sudden onset of coughing, gagging or choking

Common Diagnosis 1
Diagnosis: Viral laryngotracheobronchitis ('croup')

Questions
1. **Was there any preceding illness?** Typically, croup develops 48 hours into a viral upper respiratory tract illness
2. **Is a barking cough present?** Croup is characterised by a typical 'barking' cough

Common Diagnosis 2
Diagnosis: Laryngomalacia

Questions
1. **Is the child less than 4 weeks old?** Symptoms typically arise within the first 2–4 weeks of life
2. **Is there an intermittent pattern to the onset of stridor?** It may be noticed more when the child is upset, while they are asleep or with concurrent upper respiratory tract infections
3. **Are there associated feeding difficulties?** For example, slow feeding with frequent breaks is common with laryngomalacia

---

Box 1.2.3   The Phases of Stridor

- It is important to consider the 'phase' of stridor. Identifying this early on can help to narrow down your differential diagnosis
- Stridor can be inspiratory, expiratory or biphasic:
- **Inspiratory stridor:** indicates obstruction *at or above* the vocal cords
- **Expiratory stridor:** indicates obstruction *below* the vocal cords
- **Biphasic stridor:** indicates obstruction *at or below* the vocal cords

---

1.2.6 KEY EXAMINATION FEATURES

See also Box 1.1.4 in Chapter 1.1, Signs of Increased Work of Breathing.

Box 1.2.4   Considerations for Examination in All Children with Stridor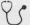

- The priority is not to cause any distress to the child
- Distress risks precipitating complete airway obstruction
- Do not perform any examination of the airway or invasive procedures such as blood taking without experienced senior support
- A limited examination should be undertaken in a position where the child is comfortable
- The majority of assessments can be performed through distant observation

---

Box 1.2.5   Pre-terminal Signs of Respiratory Distress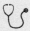

- Exhaustion
- Bradycardia
- Silent chest
- Significant apnoea

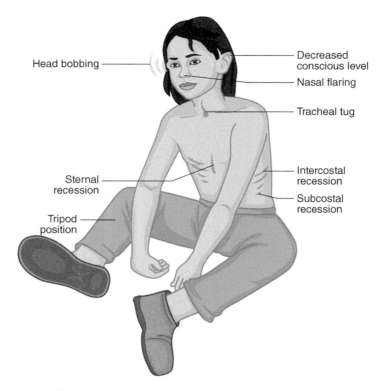

Head bobbing

Decreased
conscious level

Nasal flaring

Tracheal tug

Sternal
recession

Intercostal
recession

Subcostal
recession

Tripod
position

Figure 1.2.3 Signs of increased work of breathing. Recognition of respiratory distress and grade of severity is essential, and informs the need to consider intubation.

Dangerous Diagnosis 1
Diagnosis: Epiglottitis

Examination Findings
1. **Patient position: tripod.** The child may sit leaning forwards, using their arms to support a tripod posture. They may naturally hold their jaw forward to facilitate opening their airway
2. **Toxic appearance.** This signifies how unwell they may look, with a high fever and sweating. They may also hold their mouth open, drooling saliva
3. **Signs of increased work of breathing.** Stridor is inspiratory. Accessory muscle use is common
4. **Altered mental state.** If the patient is severely compromised, there might be cyanosis and fluctuating levels of consciousness, predicting respiratory arrest

Dangerous Diagnosis 2
Diagnosis: Bacterial tracheitis

Examination Findings
1. **Patient most comfortable lying flat.** In contrast to patients with epiglottitis, these patients can usually lie flat
2. **Toxic appearance.** Stridor is biphasic. There may be a high-grade fever with signs of respiratory distress
3. **Voice changes.** A hoarse voice is associated with halitosis and purulent tracheal secretions

Dangerous Diagnosis 3
Diagnosis: Foreign body inhalation

Examination Findings
1. **Coughing, gagging, choking, cyanosis.** All these findings are symptoms suggestive of a foreign body in the larynx. There is a risk of complete airway obstruction
2. **Reduced but equal air entry.** Although air entry will be reduced, bilateral equal air entry suggests a foreign body in the trachea
3. **Lateralising signs.** Asymmetrical chest movement, tracheal deviation and decreased breath sounds unilaterally point to a foreign body below the carina (most commonly the right main bronchus)

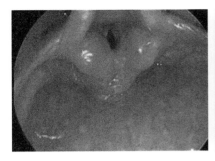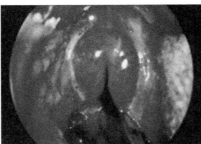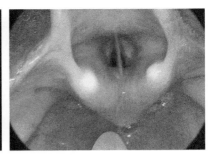

Figure 1.2.4 Laryngoscopy view of (A) normal larynx, (B) epiglottitis and (C) larynx with a foreign body. Source: Reproduced with permission from Advanced Life Support Group (2016). *Advanced paediatric life support: a practical approach to emergencies*, 6th edn. Oxford: Wiley Blackwell.

Common Diagnosis 1
Diagnosis: Viral laryngotracheobronchitis ('croup')

Examination Findings
1. **Features of viral illness.** Low-grade fever, nasal congestion
2. **Signs of respiratory distress.** Nasal flaring, suprasternal recession and accessory muscle use are common

Box 1.2.6   The Modified Westley Clinical Scoring System for Croup

	Score					
	0	**1**	**2**	**3**	**4**	**5**
Inspiratory stridor	Not present	When agitated/active	At rest	–	–	–
Intercostal recession	None	Mild	Moderate	Severe	–	–
Air entry	Normal	Mildly decreased	Severely decreased	–	–	–
Cyanosis	None	–	–	–	With agitation/activity	At rest
Level of consciousness	Normal	–	–	–	–	Altered

Total possible score 0–17:

- <4 – mild croup
- 4–6 – moderate croup (admission, consider high-dependency unit)
- >6 – severe croup (consider tracheal intubation)

Common Diagnosis 2
Diagnosis: Laryngomalacia

Examination Findings
1. **Variable stridor.** This can be biphasic or inspiratory
2. **Patient position.** Classically, stridor worsens when the child is lying flat, or when agitated
3. **Systemically well.** As this is an intermittent problem, children are generally well. There may be signs of faltering growth if feeding difficulties have been particularly prominent

1.2.7 KEY INVESTIGATIONS

Not all children will require invasive investigations. Blood tests should be targeted towards children who present systemically unwell or those with complicated infection.

Bedside

Table 1.2.1 Bedside tests of use in patients presenting with stridor

Test	When to perform	Potential result
Oxygen saturations	• All children with stridor • May reveal a need for oxygen supplementation	• <92% indicates need for supplemental oxygen and consideration for respiratory support
MC&S of tracheal secretions	• Suspected bacterial tracheitis • Difficult to obtain unless during laryngoscopy	• Positive culture confirms bacterial infection • Sensitivities guide antibiotic choice

MC&S, microscopy, culture and sensitivity.

Blood Tests

Table 1.2.2 Blood tests of use in patients presenting with stridor

Test	When to perform	Potential result
FBC	• Suspected bacterial infection • Suspected mediastinal mass	• ↑ White cells, particularly neutrophilia, consistent with bacterial infection • ↑ White cells may also indicate malignancy • ↓ Hb, white blood cells and platelets (pancytopenia) suggest bone marrow failure, concerning for malignancy
CRP	• Suspected bacterial infection	• ↑ in infection or inflammation
Blood film	• Suspected mediastinal mass	• Finding peripheral blasts on the blood film is suggestive of leukaemia
Blood cultures	• Suspected bacterial infection	• Positive cultures confirm bacterial infection • Sensitivities help in antibiotic choice

CRP, C-reactive protein; FBC, full blood count; Hb, haemoglobin.

Imaging

Table 1.2.3 Imaging modalities of use in patients presenting with stridor

Test	When to perform	Potential result
Chest x-ray	Suspected: • Foreign body inhalation • Mediastinal mass • Uncertain underlying diagnosis • Stridor refractory to treatment	• Foreign body inhalation: ipsilateral collapse, air trapping • Mediastinal mass: lymphadenopathy, thymus, cystic malformation • Croup: may see 'steeple sign' (Figure 1.2.6)
Lateral C-spine x-ray	• Useful if considering retropharyngeal mass	• Retropharyngeal mass in inspiratory film confirms abscess
CT neck/chest	• Definitive investigation for retropharyngeal abscess • Useful if considering mediastinal mass	• Helps confirm the diagnosis • Thymus, cysts, vascular malformations, lymphadenopathy and masses can all be assessed

CT, computed tomography.

Special

Table 1.2.4 Special tests of use in patients presenting with stridor

Test	When to perform	Potential result
Flexible endoscopy/ bronchoscopy	• Consider in suspected structural airway anomalies – only once emergency differentials are excluded • Secretions can be sent for MC&S to guide antibiotic rationalisation	• Visualisation of abnormalities, e.g. subglottic stenosis • Positive culture confirms bacterial infection • Sensitivities determine antibiotic choice

MC&S, microscopy, culture and sensitivity.

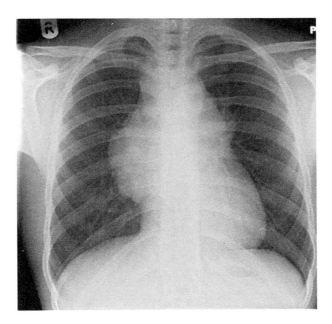

Figure 1.2.5 Chest x-ray of an anterior mediastinal mass.

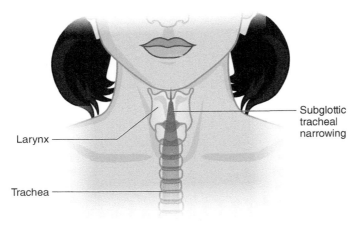

Figure 1.2.6 The 'steeple sign'. The shape of a church steeple is produced by subglottic tracheal narrowing. This sign supports the diagnosis of croup.

1.2.8 KEY MANAGEMENT PRINCIPLES

Diagnosis-specific management strategies are outlined here. It is expected that an 'ABCDE' approach to assessment and management is always undertaken (see Chapter 12.1, *The A to E Assessment*).

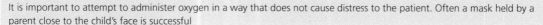

Box 1.2.7 Oxygenation in Stridor	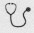

It is important to attempt to administer oxygen in a way that does not cause distress to the patient. Often a mask held by a parent close to the child's face is successful

Dangerous Diagnosis 1
Diagnosis: Epiglottitis

Management Principles
1. **Airway examination.** This is conducted during the process of obtaining a secure airway, and should only be undertaken by senior skilled anaesthetists with support of the Ear, Nose and Throat (ENT) team. Upon laryngoscopy, the glottic opening may be difficult to visualise in severe swelling of the epiglottis and supraglottic tissues
2. **Obtain a secure airway.** This should be conducted by a clinician experienced in difficult airway management, most often a senior anaesthetist. Commonly an inhalational anaesthetic is used with the child in a seated position. An ENT surgeon should ideally be involved as well in case a surgical airway becomes necessary
3. **Vascular access.** Cannulation and blood sampling should be done while the child is under anaesthesia to avoid upsetting them. Fluid resuscitation should then proceed as necessary
4. **Antimicrobials.** Consult local hospital policy for antibiotic protocol in suspected epiglottitis. This will normally involve broad-spectrum, high-dose cephalosporins

Dangerous Diagnosis 2
Diagnosis: Bacterial tracheitis

Management Principles
1. **Airway examination.** As with epiglottitis, this should be performed by an anaesthetist with ENT support. Laryngoscopy may show normal supraglottic structures, purulent exudate and slough beyond the vocal cords. If debris is easily visible, suctioning should be attempted
2. **Obtain a secure airway.** Follow similar principles to epiglottitis
3. **Vascular access.** Cannulation and blood sampling should be done once the airway is secure
4. **Antimicrobials.** Consult local hospital policy for the antibiotic protocol

Dangerous Diagnosis 3
Diagnosis: Foreign body inhalation

Management Principles
1. **Encourage cough.** In an alert, coughing child, principles of basic life support apply. There is no substitute for an effective cough in dislodging a foreign body in an upper airway
2. **Basic life support.** If coughing is ineffective, basic life support must be instigated. This involves giving back blows, followed by either chest thrusts (for infants) or abdominal thrusts (for children). In unconscious children, rescue breaths and chest compressions are indicated
3. **Rigid bronchoscopy.** This will be necessary if the foreign body is in a lower airway or cannot be coughed out. This will likely necessitate tertiary ENT or Respiratory support

Common Diagnosis 1
Diagnosis: Viral laryngotracheobronchitis ('croup')

Management Principles
1. **Nebulised adrenaline.** This is a simple and non-invasive therapy intended to reduce oedema through vasoconstriction of the affected mucosa. Effects are often short-lived and repeated administration may be required, therefore patients should not be discharged immediately after showing clinical response
2. **Steroids.** Dexamethasone is usually the steroid of choice in viral croup. Effects are delayed and longer-acting compared to nebulised adrenaline, with maximum benefit demonstrated after 6 hours

3. **Tracheal intubation.** This will only be required for severe cases. Consider this based on clinical severity, guided by the Westley score (see Box 1.2.6). A gradually increasing leak around the endotracheal tube may signify improvement of sub-glottic oedema

Common Diagnosis 2
Diagnosis: Laryngomalacia

Management Principles
1. **Conservative management.** Normally, no treatment is required. Warn parents of the natural history: stridor may worsen over the first few months of life as inspiratory air flow increases, then usually resolves by 2 years of age. It may become prominent during crying or viral infections
2. **Oxygenation if required.** Some children with laryngomalacia require supplementary oxygen. Children suffering with cyanotic episodes or apnoeas should be evaluated with a sleep study and have closer follow-up
3. **Feeding support.** A small proportion of infants may require dietetic support with feeding

1.3 Difficulty in Breathing

Duana Cook

Department of Paediatrics, University Hospitals Sussex NHS Foundation Trust, Worthing, UK

CONTENTS

1.3.1 CHAPTER AT A GLANCE

Box 1.3.1 Chapter at a Glance

- Difficulty in breathing is one of the most common presenting complaints in paediatric patients
- It has many potential causes, some of which can be serious, so each child with difficulty in breathing should be assessed on an individual basis and treated appropriately

- There is a significant crossover of conditions leading to difficulty in breathing, stridor and wheeze, and this chapter will primarily focus on diagnoses that have not been discussed in Chapters 1.1 and 1.2

1.3.2 DEFINITION

Difficulty in breathing can be objective, with signs of respiratory distress, or subjective, with complaints of 'shortness of breath'.

Clinical Guide to Paediatrics, First Edition. Edited by Rachel Varughese and Anna Mathew. Series Editor: Christian Fielder Camm.
© 2022 John Wiley & Sons Ltd. Published 2022 by John Wiley & Sons Ltd.
Companion website: www.wiley.com/go/varughese/paediatrics

1.3.3 DIAGNOSTIC ALGORITHM

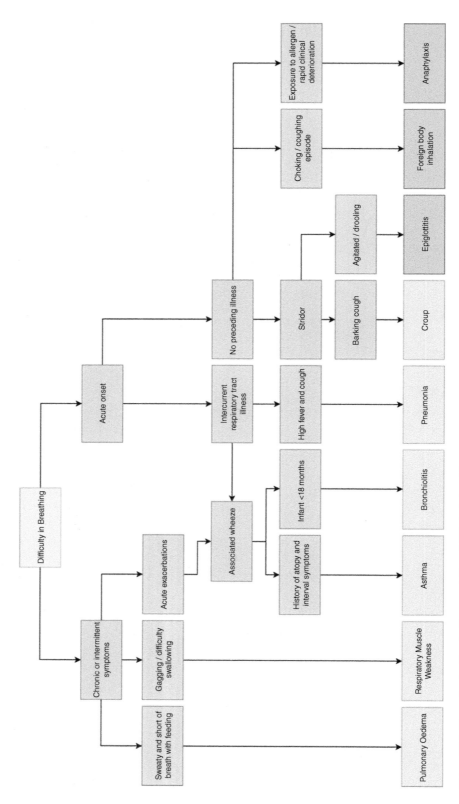

Figure 1.3.1 Diagnostic algorithm for the presentation of difficulty in breathing.

1.3.4 DIFFERENTIALS LIST

Dangerous Diagnoses

1. Epiglottitis
- Epiglottitis is a potentially fatal condition caused by inflammation of the epiglottis
- It is characterised by inspiratory stridor
- The child is often described as having a 'toxic appearance'
- Historically, almost exclusively caused by *Haemophilus influenzae* type B (Hib)
- Since the introduction of the Hib vaccine, the incidence of epiglottitis has markedly declined

2. Foreign Body Inhalation
- Aspiration of a foreign body is most commonly due to food, although any small object may be inhaled
- Peak incidence is between 6 months and 4 years old
- Depending on where the foreign body is lodged, it can cause wheeze or stridor, in addition to difficulty in breathing

3. Anaphylaxis
- Serious life-threatening immunoglobulin (Ig) E-mediated allergic reaction requiring immediate treatment
- Systemic response is caused by the release of immune and inflammatory mediators from degranulating basophils and mast cells
- Acute airway obstruction and profound hypotension can be rapidly fatal without treatment
- Associated symptoms include angio-oedema, urticaria and vomiting
- Allergens commonly include medicines, food, immunotherapy or insect stings

Common Diagnoses

1. Pneumonia
- Infection of the lung with inflammation and interstitial infiltrates
- Typically presents with fever, cough, and difficulty in breathing
- Causative organism can be viral or bacterial
- More common in children aged <5 years

2. Asthma
- Chronic reversible small airways obstruction caused by airway inflammation and bronchial hyper-reactivity
- Symptoms are frequently triggered by environmental factors or intercurrent illness and respond to bronchodilators
- Presents with cough, wheeze and difficulty in breathing
- Severity ranges from mild to life-threatening
- Asthma is covered in detail in Chapter 1.1, and will not be discussed further in this chapter

3. Bronchiolitis
- Affects infants under 18 months, predominantly in the winter months
- Respiratory syncytial virus (RSV) accounts for the majority of cases
- Inflammation and congestion of the lower respiratory tract can progress to difficulty in feeding and increased work of breathing
- Severity ranges from mild to life-threatening
- Bronchiolitis is covered in detail in Chapter 1.1, and will not be discussed further in this chapter

4. Viral Laryngotracheobronchitis ('Croup')
- Commonly known as 'croup', this is a common cause of stridor and difficulty in breathing, associated with an antecedent upper respiratory tract infection
- A 'barking cough' is characteristic
- Usually due to infection with parainfluenza viruses, commonly affecting children from 6 months to 3 years old
- Severity ranges from mild to life-threatening
- Viral laryngotracheobronchitis ('croup') is covered in detail in Chapter 1.2, and will not be discussed further in this chapter

Diagnoses to Consider

1. Pneumothorax
- Presence of air in the pleural space, which can cause lung collapse
- May be idiopathic, secondary to underlying lung pathology or to trauma
- Tall, thin males are particularly at risk of developing spontaneous pneumothorax
- A tension pneumothorax is potentially life-threatening if it is not treated rapidly

When to consider: in tall, thin adolescent males, or with underlying predisposing conditions (Marfan syndrome, asthma, cystic fibrosis, recent trauma or thoracic procedures)

2. **Pulmonary Oedema**
   - Excess fluid in alveolar spaces, leading to impaired gas exchange
   - Congenital cardiac abnormalities can lead to congestive cardiac failure with pulmonary oedema
   - Non-cardiogenic pulmonary oedema may be hepatic or renal in origin

   When to consider: in an infant presenting with faltering growth and breathlessness when feeding, particularly if cardiac, hepatic or renal disorders are suspected

3. **Respiratory Muscle Weakness**
   - Neuromuscular conditions such as Duchenne muscular dystrophy, congenital myopathies and spinal muscle atrophy can cause chest wall weakness
   - Bulbar dysfunction leads to reduced/absent cough and gag reflexes, increasing aspiration risk or, when severe, upper airway obstruction

   When to consider: in those with suspected neuromuscular disease, which may be preceded by difficulty achieving gross motor developmental milestones

Box 1.3.2   Neuromuscular Disease Potentially Causing Respiratory Muscle Weakness   △△

Neuromuscular disease	Inheritance	Types	Onset	Clinical picture
Muscular dystrophy	X-linked recessive, de novo mutation	Duchenne's is the most severe Becker's is the milder variant, presenting later	Between 3 and 6 years	Delayed walking, difficulty rising from sitting/lying (Gower's sign), pelvic and shoulder girdle weakness, pseudohypertrophy of calf muscles Cardiomyopathy and respiratory failure can develop over time
Spinal muscular atrophy	Autosomal recessive	Four main types Type 1 is the most severe	From infancy (type 1) to adulthood (type 4)	Progressively increasing hypotonia and muscle weakness with no cognitive delay Respiratory failure as weakness progresses
Congenital myopathies	Varies, can be autosomal dominant, autosomal recessive, x-linked	Three main types X-linked most severe	From birth	Hypotonia and weakness, variable progression. May be static or slowly progressive Respiratory failure develops in severe disease

4. **Hyperventilation**
   - Psychogenic hyperventilation is a diagnosis of exclusion
   - There is tachypnoea without any associated increased work of breathing
   - It may be induced by fever, toxins or drugs

   When to consider: in children with no associated increased work of breathing who may be able to report a preceding feeling of anxiety, having otherwise been well

Box 1.3.3   Other Conditions Causing Difficulty in Breathing   △△

Diagnosis	When to consider
Allergic rhinitis	Constant rhinitis, allergic salute, throat clearing
Cystic fibrosis	Faltering growth, clubbing, purulent sputum, oily and fluffy stools that float in the pan
Pertussis	Paroxysmal cough with inspiratory 'whoop', unimmunised child or mother
Psychogenic/ habitual cough	Disappears during sleep
Recurrent aspiration	Choking with feeds/chesty after feeds, neuromuscular disease
Tuberculosis	At risk area/community, progressive cough, night sweats, weight loss, haemoptysis

---

Box 1.3.4   Conditions Primarily Presenting with Wheeze or Stridor   △△

Although difficulty in breathing is a universal sign of respiratory pathology, many of the differential diagnoses may present with either wheeze or stridor as their predominant symptom
As such, further discussion of the following diagnoses is confined to their relevant chapters:

- Chapter 1.1, Wheeze: foreign body, anaphylaxis, asthma, bronchiolitis
- Chapter 1.2, Stridor: epiglottitis, foreign body, viral laryngotracheobronchitis

1.3.5 KEY HISTORY FEATURES

Common Diagnosis 1
Diagnosis: Pneumonia

Questions
1. **Have they had a cough?** Cough may be apparent before obvious difficulty in breathing is noted. It frequently starts as a dry cough, but later becomes wet as secretions increase
2. **Has there been a fever?** Fever may occur several times a day and usually responds to antipyretics. Persistent fever might suggest a secondary empyema
3. **Have they complained of pain anywhere?** Children with pneumonia may experience pleuritic chest pain or describe abdominal pain due to diaphragmatic irritation. In non-verbal children this may manifest as distress on coughing
4. **Was there a preceding illness?** Secondary pneumonia can develop days to weeks after an initial viral illness
5. **Is there a background history contributing to this illness?** Children with cystic fibrosis, primary ciliary dyskinesia or immunodeficiency are at higher risk of pneumonia. Children with gastro-oesophageal reflux or neuromuscular disease are at risk of aspiration pneumonia

---

Box 1.3.5   Differential Diagnoses of Cough   △△

Coughing is the action of quickly expelling air from the lungs. This acts to protect the airway, removing secretions and other irritants
Cough is the result of a variety of conditions affecting different parts of the airway

Upper airways	• Upper respiratory tract infection, e.g. common cold, pharyngitis, tonsillitis, sinusitis, croup • Allergy, e.g. allergic rhinitis • Inflammation secondary to gastro-oesophageal reflux disease (GORD)
Lower airways	• Lower respiratory tract infections, e.g. bronchiolitis, pertussis • Asthma • Foreign body inhalation • Congenital abnormality, e.g. trachea-oesophageal fistula • Bronchiectasis – usually secondary to damage to the airway from chronic infection, e.g. in cystic fibrosis or immunodeficiency
Lung parenchyma	• Pneumonia – can be viral or bacterial • Empyema
Non-respiratory	• Psychogenic cough

1.3.6 KEY EXAMINATION FEATURES

See Chapter 1.1, *Wheeze*, Box 1.1.4, *Signs of Increased Work of Breathing*, and Chapter 1.2, *Stridor*, Figure 1.2.3, *Signs of Increased Work of Breathing*.

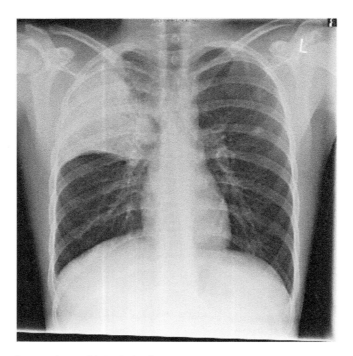

Figure 1.3.2 Right upper lobe collapse and consolidation in focal pneumonia.

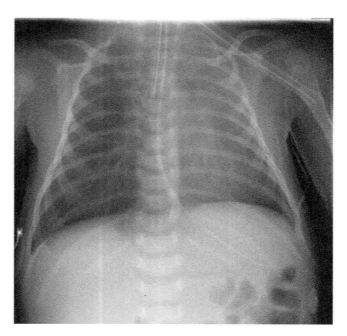

Figure 1.3.3 Left upper lobe collapse due to pneumonia – veil-like opacity over the chest, with raised left hemidiaphragm. Note this patient has a nasogastric tube and endotracheal tube in situ.

Common Diagnosis 1
Diagnosis: Pneumonia

Examination Findings
1. **Fever and cough.** These are the most common presenting symptoms in a child with pneumonia. There might be associated tachycardia
2. **Signs of increased work of breathing.** The child may be tachypnoeic, have intercostal and subcostal recession, nasal flaring and may be grunting
3. **Signs of consolidation.** On the affected side, reduced chest expansion may be noted with dullness to percussion. There may also be decreased air entry and crepitations heard on auscultation. Signs may be bilateral in bronchopneumonia and focal in lobar pneumonia
4. **'Stony' dullness to percussion at lung bases.** This finding is suggestive of an effusion that, in the context of an underlying pneumonia, could be a simple parapneumonic effusion or an empyema

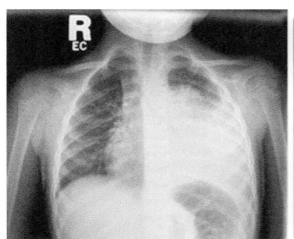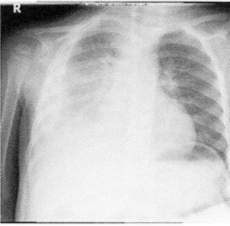

Figure 1.3.4 Two chest x-rays showing pleural effusions, commonly seen as a complication of pneumonia. (A) Pleural effusion in upright patient, with meniscus of fluid. (B) Patient lying supine with fluid tracking up the side of the chest.

Figure 1.3.5 A round pneumonia is usually a paediatric phenomenon, due to immature inter-alveolar connections, leading to limited spread of bacterial infection.

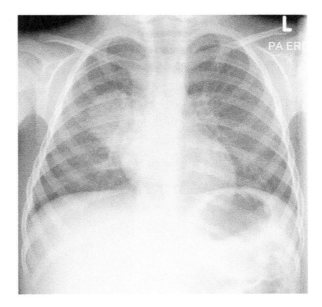

1.3.7 KEY INVESTIGATIONS

Not all children will require invasive investigations. Blood tests should be targeted towards children with suspected severe or complicated infection.

Bedside

Table 1.3.1 Bedside tests of use in patients presenting with difficulty in breathing

Test	When to perform	Potential result
Oxygen saturations	• All children with difficulty in breathing	• <92% indicates need for supplemental oxygen and consideration for respiratory support
NPA	• Suspected bronchiolitis	• Identification of the responsible viral pathogen • Aids with cohorting patients with the same virus
Sputum MC&S	• Older children with suspected pneumonia (difficult to collect in young children)	• Positive culture confirms bacterial infection • Sensitivities guide antibiotic choice
Blood gas	• Significant respiratory distress or oxygen requirement	• ↓ pH and ↑CO_2 indicate respiratory acidosis and guide need for respiratory support
PEFR	• Children with asthma or neuromuscular disease • Provides a comparison to baseline	• A drop in PEFR will indicate the severity of an asthma exacerbation: <50% and <33% of best PEFR indicate severe and life-threatening episodes, respectively

CO_2, carbon dioxide; MC&S, microscopy, culture and sensitivity; NPA, Naso-pharyngeal aspirate; PEFR, peak expiratory flow rate

Blood Tests

Table 1.3.2 Blood tests of use in patients presenting with difficulty in breathing

Test	When to perform	Potential result
FBC CRP Blood culture	Suspected: • Epiglottitis • Complicated pneumonia	• ↑ White cells, particularly neutrophilia, consistent with bacterial infection • ↑ CRP in infection or inflammation • Positive cultures confirm bacterial infection • Sensitivities direct antibiotic choice
U&E	• If on diuretics for pulmonary oedema • If receiving IV fluid maintenance • Complicated pneumonia	• Electrolytes can become deranged with diuretic use • ↓ Na in SIADH as a complication of pneumonia

CRP, C-reactive protein; FBC, full blood count; IV, intravenous; Na, sodium; SIADH, syndrome of inappropriate antidiuretic hormone secretion; U&E, urea and electrolytes

Imaging

Table 1.3.3 Imaging modalities of use in patients presenting with difficulty in breathing

Test	When to perform	Potential result
Chest x-ray	Suspected • Pneumothorax • Foreign body inhalation • Pneumonia • Bronchiolitis • Asthma • Pulmonary oedema Do not delay treatment of a tension pneumothorax waiting for an x-ray	• Pneumothorax: absent lung markings/crisp lung edge • Foreign body inhalation: lung collapse or air trapping • Pneumonia: consolidation • Bronchiolitis: peri-bronchial thickening • Asthma: hyperinflation • Pulmonary oedema: enlarged cardiac shadow, pulmonary oligaemia or congestion, fluid in interlobar fissures
Echocardiogram	• Pulmonary oedema due to suspected cardiac failure	• Identifies causative cardiac lesion • Estimates ventricular function

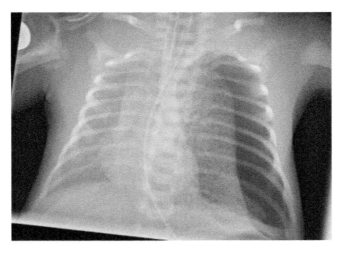

Figure 1.3.6 Left-sided tension pneumothorax with mediastinal shift away

---

Box 1.3.6   Types and Causes of Respiratory Failure

There are two types of respiratory failure:

Type 1 respiratory failure

- **Blood gas:** hypoxaemia, with a low or normal carbon dioxide level
- **Pathophysiology:** caused by damage to the lung tissue, which leads to a ventilation–perfusion mismatch
- **Possible causes:** pneumonia, pulmonary oedema or chronic conditions such as cystic fibrosis

Type 2 respiratory failure

- **Blood gas:** hypoxaemia with a high carbon dioxide level
- **Pathophysiology:** occurs when alveolar ventilation is inadequate to eliminate sufficient carbon dioxide
- **Possible causes:** chest wall deformities or neuromuscular disease causing respiratory muscle weakness

---

Special

Table 1.3.4 Special tests of use in patients presenting with difficulty in breathing

Test	When to perform	Potential result
Spirometry	• Provides a comparison to baseline in children with chronic asthma • Children with neuromuscular respiratory weakness	• Asthma: obstructive pattern – degree of obstruction reflects severity of exacerbation • Neuromuscular respiratory weakness: restrictive pattern

1.3.8 KEY MANAGEMENT PRINCIPLES

Diagnosis-specific management strategies are outlined here. It is expected that an 'ABCDE' approach to assessment and management is always undertaken (see Chapter 12.1, *The A to E Assessment*).

Common Diagnosis 1
Diagnosis: Pneumonia

Management Principles
1. **Oxygen supplementation.** Administer oxygen to maintain saturations >92%
2. **Antibiotics.** For the majority of children with pneumonia, oral antibiotics for 5–7 days will be sufficient, even when severe. For children unable to tolerate or absorb oral medication, or with signs of evolving sepsis, intravenous (IV) antibiotics are indicated. Refer to local guidelines and consider a macrolide if suspicious of atypical pneumonia

3. **Fluid status**. Consider nasogastric (NG) or IV fluids if patient is unable to tolerate oral fluids/feeds and if clinically dehydrated. Due to the risk of 'syndrome of inappropriate antidiuretic hormone secretion' (SIADH), electrolytes should be monitored while on IV fluids, and two-thirds maintenance volume is often chosen

4. **Reassessment and reconsideration.** Most children with pneumonia will respond to treatment after 48 hours of antibiotics. If there is no improvement, antibiotic choice and dose should be reviewed, and consideration should be given to the possibility of a secondary complication such as an empyema

---

Box 1.3.7   When to Consider an x-ray in Suspected Community-Acquired Pneumonia

The British Thoracic Society guidelines on 'Guidelines for the management of community acquired pneumonia in children' suggest the following:

- Children with signs and symptoms of community-acquired pneumonia should not routinely have a chest x-ray
- If symptoms do not respond to 48 hours of treatment with antibiotics or there are atypical symptoms such as a high fever
- for 7 days, an x-ray should be done to rule out secondary complications such as empyema
- Follow-up x-rays should only be done in those with lobar collapse, suspected round pneumonia or unresolving symptoms

---

Box 1.3.8   Common Causes of Pneumonia in Childhood

Age group	Organisms
Newborn	Group B streptococcus, Gram-negative enterococci
Under 5s	Viruses: respiratory syncytial virus, metapneumovirus, adenovirus Bacteria: *Streptococcus pneumoniae*, *Haemophilus influenzae*, *Staphylococcus aureus*
Over 5s	*Mycoplasma pneumoniae*, *Streptococcus pneumoniae*, *Chlamydia pneumoniae*
All ages	*Mycobacterium tuberculosis*

Box 1.3.9   When to Suspect Atypical Pneumonia

- Most commonly caused by *Mycoplasma* in children
- More common in children over the age of 5
- Constitutional symptoms such as low-grade fever, headache and fatigue may be more prominent than respiratory symptoms
- Cough can be a late presenting feature and can be persistent
- *Mycoplasma* can cause wheeze and bilateral chest signs
- X-ray changes can be minimal
- Consider if no response to first-line antibiotics

2.1 Cyanosis

Jenny Woodruff and Rachel Varughese

Department of Paediatrics, Oxford University Hospitals NHS Foundation Trust, Oxford, UK

CONTENTS

2.1.1 CHAPTER AT A GLANCE

Box 2.1.1 Chapter at a Glance

- Cyanosis signifies potentially life-threatening pathology
- Likely causes are dependent on the age of the patient, but it is most commonly due to respiratory or cardiac disease
- Cyanosis can be underappreciated in children with darker skin pigmentation, and examination should always include the mucosal membranes

- Cyanosis can be described as central or peripheral. This chapter will focus on central cyanosis

2.1.2 DEFINITION

Cyanosis is a bluish discoloration of the tissues, resulting from increased (usually >5 g/dL) deoxygenated haemoglobin in the circulation, translating to oxygen saturation <85%.

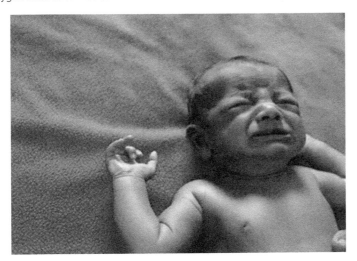

Figure 2.1.1 Central cyanosis in a baby. Source: Reproduced with permission of Shutterstock, https://www.shutterstock.com/image-photo/cyanotic-blue-baby-crying-pain-distress-1684775899.

Clinical Guide to Paediatrics, First Edition. Edited by Rachel Varughese and Anna Mathew. Series Editor: Christian Fielder Camm.
© 2022 John Wiley & Sons Ltd. Published 2022 by John Wiley & Sons Ltd.
Companion website: www.wiley.com/go/varughese/paediatrics

Box 2.1.2 Peripheral Cyanosis

- Patients with peripheral cyanosis have normal arterial oxygen saturation. Cyanosis is only seen in the extremities where blood flow is slower
- Slower blood flow → lengthened time for red cells to unload oxygen to peripheral tissues → increased deoxygenated blood on venous side of capillary beds

Conditions causing peripheral cyanosis:

- **Septic and cardiogenic shock**
  - Peripheral cyanosis is not always benign
  - In sepsis and cardiogenic shock, there is a critical reduction in tissue perfusion, which lengthens transit time for red cells across capillary beds

- **Acrocyanosis and perioral cyanosis**
  - Episodic cyanosis in hands, feet and around the mouth due to venous bed congestion
  - May occur in infants while crying, coughing or vomiting
  - Oxygen saturations and mental state remain normal throughout
- **Cold exposure**
  - Vasoconstriction from cold exposure causes venous stasis, leading to peripheral cyanosis
- **Polycythaemia**
  - Increased red blood cells result in sluggish blood flow

2.1.3 DIAGNOSTIC ALGORITHM

See page 39.

2.1.4 DIFFERENTIALS LIST

All causes of central cyanosis in children are potentially life-threatening.

Dangerous Diagnoses

1. **Cyanotic Congenital Heart Disease**
   - Any congenital cardiac disease that results in deoxygenated blood in the systemic circulation can cause cyanosis
   - There are several mechanisms for cyanotic heart disease:
     - Right-to left shunting across septal defect (usually 'right heart' lesions)
     - Right-to-left shunting across patent ductus arteriosus (usually 'left heart' lesions – may present with circulatory collapse rather than cyanosis, see Chapter 2.2, *Circulatory Collapse*)
     - Outflow tract anomalies
   - Antenatal screening picks up 30–60% of congenital heart defects
   - The vast majority will present in newborn infants
   - Babies with duct-dependent lesions may go unrecognised until the patent ductus arteriosus (PDA) shuts (usually by 48 hours of age, can be up to 21 days)
2. **Pneumothorax**
   - Cyanosis is a consequence of impaired lung inflation due to air trapped within pleural space
   - Spontaneous pneumothorax can be primary (without underlying lung disease, particularly seen in tall, thin males) or secondary (in underlying lung disease)
   - Can follow blunt or penetrating trauma, or birth
   - If following trauma, consider haemothorax as an alternative diagnosis
   - Can occur as a life-threatening complication of severe asthma
   - A tension pneumothorax is life-threatening if it is not treated rapidly
3. **Upper Airway Obstruction**
   - Upper airway obstruction can quickly lead to alveolar hypoventilation and hypoxia
   - Causes include infection (croup, epiglottitis, bacterial tracheitis), foreign body or complications of congenital airway anomalies
   - Stridor is likely to be a prominent feature, along with respiratory distress
   - In the setting of airway obstruction, cyanosis is a sinister sign with risk of rapidly fatal outcome if obstruction is not treated
   - Upper airway obstruction is covered in detail in Chapter 1.2 and will therefore not be discussed in the rest of this chapter
4. **Asthma**
   - Asthma is a disorder of variable bronchoconstriction due to airway hyper-responsiveness
   - Severity ranges from asymptomatic to fatal
   - In acute asthma exacerbation, bronchoconstriction leads to alveolar hypoventilation and hypoxia
   - Asthma is covered in detail in Chapter 1.1 and will therefore not be discussed in the rest of this chapter

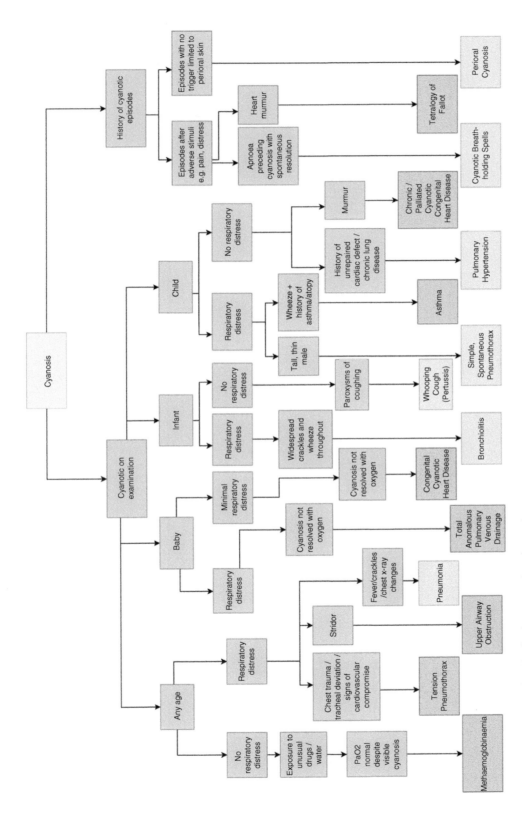

Figure 2.1.2 Diagnostic algorithm for the presentation of cyanosis.

Box 2.1.3   Conditions Causing Right-To-Left Shunting across Septal Defect

Condition	Details
Pulmonary atresia	• Pulmonary valve or artery is underdeveloped, and blood cannot flow from RV to PA • Blood shunted across VSD
Critical pulmonary stenosis	• Pulmonary valve is critically narrowed. Occurs in isolation as well as being part of tetralogy of Fallot (overriding aorta, RVH, pulmonary stenosis and VSD) • Blood shunted across VSD
Tricuspid atresia	• Tricuspid valve does not form, so no blood flows from RA to RV • Blood shunted across ASD
Ebstein anomaly	• Tricuspid valve malformation, usually causing regurgitation • Blood shunted across ASD
TAPVC	• Pulmonary veins do not attach to the left atrium, but connect to the right side (SVC, IVC or RA directly) • Blood mixes in RA and is shunted across ASD

ASD, atrial septal defect; IVC, inferior vena cava; PA, pulmonary artery; RA, right atrium; RV, right ventricle; RVH, right ventricular hypertrophy; SVC, superior vena cava; TAPVC, total anomalous pulmonary venous connection; VSD, ventricular septal defect

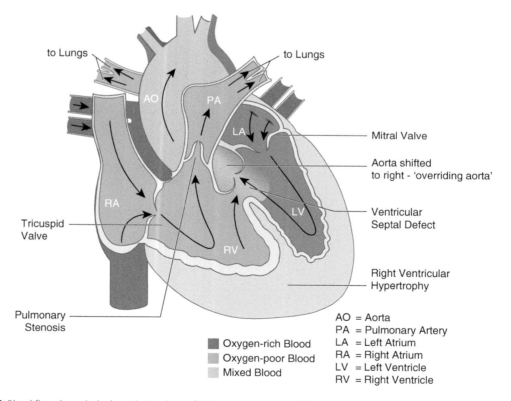

Figure 2.1.3 Blood flow through the heart in Tetralogy of Fallot. There is an overriding aorta, right ventricular hypertrophy, pulmonary stenosis and ventricular septal defect (VSD). Degree of cyanosis is determined by degree of pulmonary stenosis, as this dictates the significance of the right-to-left shunt through the VSD.

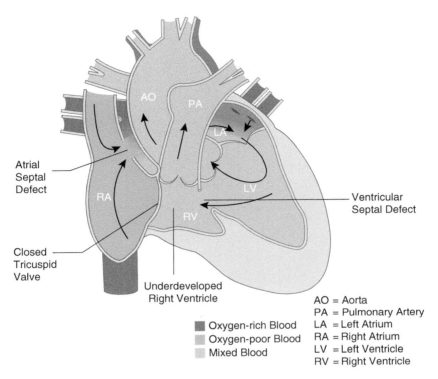

Atrial
Septal
Defect

Ventricular
Septal Defect

Closed
Tricuspid
Valve

Underdeveloped
Right Ventricle

AO = Aorta
PA = Pulmonary Artery
LA = Left Atrium
RA = Right Atrium
LV = Left Ventricle
RV = Right Ventricle

■ Oxygen-rich Blood
■ Oxygen-poor Blood
▨ Mixed Blood

Figure 2.1.4 Blood flow through the heart in tricuspid atresia. Inability of blood to pass from right atrium to right ventricle means deoxygenated blood passes through an atrial septal defect. Mixed blood is then pumped out of the left ventricle. Some also passes to the right ventricle via a ventricular septal defect and is pumped into the pulmonary artery.

Box 2.1.4 Outflow Tract Anomalies

Conditions	Details
Transposition of the great arteries	• Aorta arises from the right ventricle (carrying deoxygenated blood) and the pulmonary artery arises from the left ventricle (taking oxygenated blood back to the lungs) • There is usually some mixing across an atrial septal defect
Truncus arteriosus	• One single vessel arises from the heart, containing the combined output from the left and right ventricles
Double outlet right ventricle	• Both aorta and pulmonary artery arise from the right ventricle • There is usually a large ventricular septal defect to allow mixing of circulations

Common Diagnoses

1. Cyanotic Breath-Holding Spells
- Episodes of cyanosis associated with a classic progression of symptoms
- Initially an adverse stimulus – often pain or distress causing crying – followed by apnoea starting in expiration. There is rapid onset of cyanosis, which may be followed by loss of consciousness with posturing/eye rolling/trembling
- Spells are extremely frightening to parents. Loss of tone can be striking, but episodes are benign
- Episodes usually occur between 6 months and 5 years of age

2. Pneumonia
- Bacterial or viral infection of the pulmonary parenchyma
- Cyanosis results from reduced alveolar gas exchange, due to infective consolidation, which may also be complicated by lung collapse
- Pneumonia is covered in detail in Chapter 1.3 and will not be discussed further in this chapter

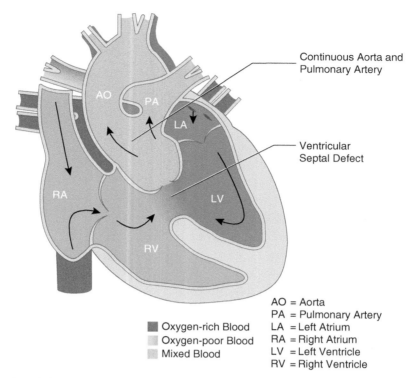

Continuous Aorta and
Pulmonary Artery

Ventricular
Septal Defect

■ Oxygen-rich Blood
■ Oxygen-poor Blood
■ Mixed Blood

AO = Aorta
PA = Pulmonary Artery
LA = Left Atrium
RA = Right Atrium
LV = Left Ventricle
RV = Right Ventricle

Figure 2.1.5 Blood flow through the heart in truncus arteriosus. The single outlet for aorta and pulmonary artery means there is mixing of blood between right and left ventricles.

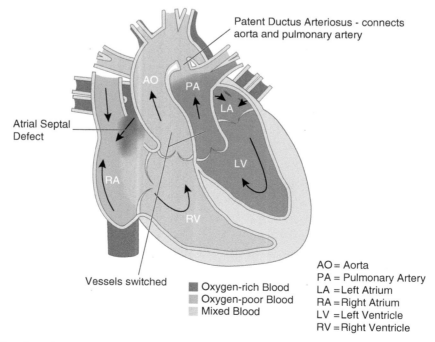

Patent Ductus Arteriosus - connects
aorta and pulmonary artery

Atrial Septal
Defect

Vessels switched

■ Oxygen-rich Blood
■ Oxygen-poor Blood
■ Mixed Blood

AO = Aorta
PA = Pulmonary Artery
LA = Left Atrium
RA = Right Atrium
LV = Left Ventricle
RV = Right Ventricle

Figure 2.1.6 Blood flow through the heart in transposition of the great arteries. Great vessels are switched. Here, mixing of blood takes place via an atrial septal defect and patent ductus arteriosus.

3. Bronchiolitis
- Lower respiratory tract infection affecting small-calibre airways in infants aged 0–18 months
- Typically caused by respiratory syncytial virus (RSV) – the usual course starts with upper respiratory coryzal symptoms, followed by a lower respiratory illness
- Airway oedema and secretions lead to obstruction of small airways and atelectasis
- Wide spectrum of disease, from very mild to critical
- Bronchiolitis is covered in detail in Chapter 1.3 and will not be discussed further in this chapter

Diagnoses to Consider
1. Pulmonary Hypertension
- Pulmonary hypertension (PH) is a state of abnormally high mean pulmonary artery pressure
- In general PH is caused by abnormal pulmonary vasculature, increased pulmonary blood flow, or increased pulmonary venous pressure (usually due to increased left atrial pressure)
- There are a variety of causes, including parenchymal lung disease, cardiac disease, chronic thromboembolism, sickle cell disease and vascular remodelling
- Newborns in the first 24 hours of life may be affected by persistent pulmonary hypertension of the newborn (PPHN)

When to consider: in those with pre-existing cardiac disease, particularly if there is a history of unrepaired cardiac shunts, e.g. a ventricular septal defect (VSD), or in children with chronic respiratory conditions, e.g. bronchopulmonary dysplasia, cystic fibrosis or previous congenital diaphragmatic hernia

---

Box 2.1.5   Persistent Pulmonary Hypertension of the Newborn (PPHN)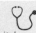

- PPHN is a cause of cyanosis seen only in neonates, usually in the first 24 hours of life
- In normal circumstances after birth, there is a natural fall in pulmonary vascular resistance and increase in systemic vascular resistance as the lungs are inflated
- This fails to happen in PPHN. Persistently high pulmonary vascular pressures cause right-to-left shunting of deoxygenated blood via the ductus arteriosus

Risk factors for PPHN

- Those needing significant resuscitation at birth
- Sepsis
- Parenchymal lung disease: meconium aspiration syndrome, congenital pneumonia, respiratory distress syndrome
- Lung hypoplasia: congenital diaphragmatic hernia, congenital cystic adenomatous malformation (CCAM) or oligohydramnios
- Down syndrome

Management principles

- Pulmonary vasodilation: inhaled nitric oxide
- Inotropes: supporting systemic pressure reduces right-to-left shunt
- Optimise oxygen delivery to tissues: high-frequency oscillatory ventilation if needed
- Extracorporeal membrane oxygenation (ECMO) if unresponsive to other treatments

---

2. Whooping Cough (Pertussis)
- Caused by infection with *Bordetella pertussis*
- Leads to paroxysms of cough that, if severe, cause cyanosis. Classic accompanying features include inspiratory 'whoop' and post-tussive vomiting
- The patient is likely to appear well between coughing spells
- Infants younger than 1 year old are most likely to present with cyanosis and are at greatest risk of morbidity and mortality
- Neonates can present with apnoeas

When to consider: in those in whom parents report paroxysmal coughing spells with resultant vomiting, cyanosis or apnoea. It is particularly important to ask about immunisation history (babies pre-vaccination age should be protected by maternal immunisation during pregnancy)

3. Methaemoglobinaemia
- Cyanosis can be caused by the presence of abnormal haemoglobin that impairs the oxygen-carrying capacity of blood
- In methaemoglobinaemia, the iron is converted from the ferrous (Fe^{2+}) to the ferric (Fe^{3+}) state. Blood may appear chocolate brown
- Rare congenital forms exist, caused by autosomal recessive mutations in the gene for cytochrome b5 reductase enzyme
- Triggers include dapsone, metoclopramide, nitrites (nitric oxide, sodium nitroprusside), and there may be a history of drinking from well water. Anaemia and glucose-6-phosphate dehydrogenase (G6PD) can both exacerbate methaemoglobin toxicity

- Pulse oximetry does not correlate to true tissue hypoxia as the methaemoglobin cannot easily release oxygen to the tissues

When to consider: in children presenting acutely with cyanosis without respiratory distress

Cyanosis can also be seen in specific circumstances for example in neonates with PPHN, (box 2.1.5) children with neurological conditions (box 2.1.6) or after house fires (box 2.1.7).

Box 2.1.6   Neurological Considerations in Cyanosis   △△

- Neurological conditions that result in disordered breathing comprise an important cause of central cyanosis in children
- Common aetiologies include major head trauma, poisoning, brief resolved unexplained events (BRUE) and seizures

- However, any neurological disease that results in altered mental status or weakness can lead to hypoventilation and cyanosis

---

Box 2.1.7   House Fires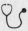

House fires can cause cyanosis in several ways:

- Decreased concentration of ambient oxygen
- Carbon monoxide toxicity – impairs oxygen delivery
- Cyanide poisoning – impairs oxygen utilisation

- Thermal injury – causes upper airway obstruction
- Smoke particles – cause lower airway obstruction

Box 2.1.8   Chronic Cyanosis

- Chronic cyanosis in children is commonly due to two reasons: cystic fibrosis (CF) or severe congenital cardiac lesions
- Around 10% of congenital cardiac lesions are not amenable to full surgical correction, one example being hypoplastic left heart syndrome
- In these cases, surgery is offered to prolong life, resulting ultimately in a Fontan's circulation with passive flow to the pulmonary artery and lungs from the superior vena cava and inferior vena cava
- Children on this surgical pathway have reduced pulmonary blood flow compared to a normal circulation and their saturations in room air would typically be 75–85%

- In CF, hypoxia is the end result of years of reduced sputum clearance and recurrent infections, leading to lung inflammation and ultimately scarring. Children with resting hypoxia in CF would be treated with home oxygen and assessed for lung transplantation
- Pulmonary hypertension also causes chronic hypoxia and can be a complication of cardiac anomalies or of CF, or be idiopathic
- When assessing unwell children with these conditions, look for clubbing and try to find out the child's usual saturation level to assess if they have deteriorated from their baseline

---

2.1.5 KEY HISTORY FEATURES

Box 2.1.9   Timing of Cyanosis

- Most babies are born blue – but in nearly all, the saturations normalise by 10 minutes of age as the baby's circulation undergoes all the changes from foetal to neonatal circulation
- The timing of the cyanosis is important. In some babies, cyanosis continues from birth. In others, cyanosis is noticed at a day or so old – or at a couple of weeks or a few months of age
- If it is from birth it could be due to persistent pulmonary hypertension of the newborn (PPHN), congenital pneumonia, sepsis, meconium aspiration, respiratory distress syndrome (due to surfactant deficiency) or congenital heart disease

- If it happens at a day or two old, or up to 2–3 weeks old, it is most likely to be due either to sepsis or congenital heart disease that is duct dependent, causing cyanosis when the ductus arteriosus shuts
- If cyanosis starts at weeks or a few months old, then it is most likely either due to sepsis or to congenital heart disease, causing heart failure and pulmonary oedema
- The level of respiratory distress is also important. If recessions are mild or absent despite cyanosis, then PPHN or congenital cardiac disease is most likely

Dangerous Diagnosis 1
Diagnosis: Cyanotic congenital heart disease

Questions
1. **Did the baby have any cardiac problems on antenatal scan?** Variable figures are documented, but up to 60% of congenital heart disease cases are detected on antenatal scans. Outflow tract abnormalities and total anomalous pulmonary venous drainage are less likely to be picked up on antenatal scans
2. **Any history of maternal diabetes?** 5% of infants of diabetic mothers are affected by congenital heart disease, compared to the background rate of around 1%. This is particularly raised in those mothers with poor periconceptional glycaemic control
3. **Is there history of maternal medications associated with congenital heart disease?** Several medications are linked to increased risk of cardiac disease. These include sodium valproate, lithium, diazepam and isotretinoin
4. **Any family history of congenital heart disease?** Family history of a first-degree relative with congenital heart disease is a risk factor
5. **Does cyanosis come and go?** Children with tetralogy of Fallot (and other forms of pulmonary stenosis with VSD) may have 'cyanotic spells', otherwise known as 'hypercyanotic episodes', where there is an acute increase in right-to-left shunt across the VSD

Box 2.1.10   Cyanotic Spells in Tetralogy of Fallot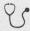

Precipitating factors

- Crying/agitation
- Feeding
- Waking from sleep
- Defecating
- Fever

Clinical pattern of cyanotic spell:

- Crying/irritability/anxiety
- Rapid, deep breathing
- Increased cyanosis
- Reduced murmur intensity (reduced blood flow across pulmonary stenosis)

Older children may instinctively squat as this increases venous return, improving blood flow to the lungs

---

Dangerous Diagnosis 2
Diagnosis: Pneumothorax

Questions
1. **Was there any preceding trauma or possible iatrogenic cause?** Pneumothoraces can be secondary to chest trauma (including birth!). They may be iatrogenic, e.g. secondary to positive pressure ventilation, central venous line insertion or cardiothoracic surgery
2. **Any history of underlying lung disease?** Asthma and cystic fibrosis predispose to spontaneous pneumothorax due to rupture of emphysema-like lung structures known as blebs and bullae
3. **Any history of connective tissue disorder?** Marfan syndrome is associated with spontaneous pneumothorax, reported in 5–12% of patients
4. **Is there pleuritic chest pain?** Children with spontaneous pneumothorax may describe pleuritic chest pain that catches them with a sharp pain on inspiration. They may be reluctant to breathe deeply or cough
5. **Is there shortness of breath?** In pneumothorax significant enough to cause cyanosis, there will be marked shortness of breath

Common Diagnosis 1
Diagnosis: Cyanotic breath-holding spells

Questions
1. **What is the age of the child?** Breath-holding spells are most common between 6 and 24 months of age, but can occur up to 5 years
2. **Are episodes of cyanosis preceded by an upsetting incident?** Episodes occur after painful or distressing events, which may seem very minor (e.g. being denied a certain toy, being told off or falling over)
3. **Are episodes accompanied by breath-holding in expiration?** Crying is followed by apnoea starting in expiration. Rapid onset of cyanosis may be followed by loss of consciousness with posturing/eye rolling/trembling, which can give the appearance of a seizure

4. Is there lethargy consistent with a postictal phase? There should be no postictal phase. It is important to differentiate the episode from a seizure

---

Box 2.1.11   Eisenmenger Syndrome

- Affects teenagers/adults with large unrepaired or undetected heart defects
- Chronic left-to-right shunt (atrial septal defect/ventricular septal defect/atrioventricular septal defect/patent ductus arteriosus) causes high pulmonary vascular resistance and pulmonary hypertension

- When pulmonary pressures exceed systemic pressure, there is a reversal of shunt, and previously acyanotic defects become cyanotic
- Timely repair of these defects is therefore very important

Box 2.1.12   Differentiating Cyanosis Due to Cardiac and Respiratory Causes

	Respiratory cause	Cardiac cause
Examination	Respiratory distress with tachypnoea. May have wheeze or creps. Murmur unlikely	Mild tachypnoea or normal respiratory examination. May have a murmur or weak pulses
Ventilation: $PaCO_2$ on blood gas	Raised	Normal
Chest x-ray	Abnormal	May be normal or abnormal (enlarged cardiac shadow, pulmonary oligaemia or congestion)
ECG and echo	Normal	Abnormal
Response to 100% FiO_2	Large improvement	Minimal improvement

ECG, electrocardiogram; FiO_2, fraction of inspired oxygen; PaCO2, partial pressure of oxygen

---

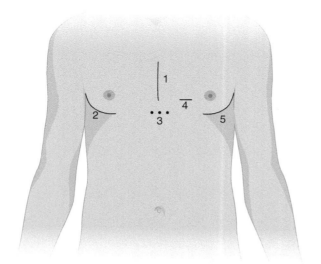

Figure 2.1.7 In the absence of a detailed history, careful examination of thoracic scars provides essential clues to previous cardiac operations. 1. Sternotomy: all complex cardiac surgery; pulmonary artery banding. 2. Right thoracotomy: Blalock–Taussig shunt (a palliative measure to increase pulmonary blood flow in duct-dependent cyanotic heart defects, e.g. critical pulmonary stenosis or pulmonary atresia); pulmonary artery banding; other non-cardiac surgery, such as lobectomy or tracheoesophageal fistula repair. 3. Post-surgical drain scars. 4. Device insertion: pacemaker; implantable cardioverter-defibrillator. 5. Left thoracotomy: Blalock–Taussig shunt; patent ductus arteriosus ligation; pulmonary artery banding; coarctation of aorta repair; other non-cardiac surgery such as lobectomy or tracheoesophageal fistula repair.

2.1.6 KEY EXAMINATION FEATURES

Dangerous Diagnosis 1
Diagnosis: Cyanotic congenital heart disease

Examination Findings
1. **Murmur.** Cyanotic congenital heart disease often gives rise to a murmur, though not always. Types of murmurs vary according to the underlying cardiac lesion
2. **Added heart sounds.** S3 is the sound of rapid ventricular filling (heard in heart failure due to a compliant, dilated left ventricle), which can sometimes be heard in normal children. S4 is the sound of forcible atrial contraction against a ventricle with decreased compliance
3. **Abnormal S2.** In normal circumstances, the pulmonary valve closes after the aortic valve during inspiration. Most cyanotic heart disease causes a single second heart sound, except for total anomalous pulmonary venous connection (TAPVC), where significantly increased right-sided blood flow causes wide fixed splitting
4. **Cyanosis out of proportion to respiratory distress.** Babies with cyanotic congenital heart defects might be profoundly blue. If there is minimal respiratory distress, despite marked cyanosis, consider cardiac disease. (This is not the case in heart failure, left-sided obstructive disease or TAPVC)
5. **Signs of shock.** Babies with duct-dependent lesions presenting due to duct closure may be shocked, with tachycardia, reduced perfusion, hypotension and altered mental status

Dangerous Diagnosis 2
Diagnosis: Pneumothorax

Examination Findings
1. **Respiratory distress.** Tachypnoea and recessions are often present, along with pleuritic chest pain
2. **Reduced breath sounds on the side of the pneumothorax.** Due to the trapped pleural air, transmission of the sound of air entry is reduced. On inspection, expansion of that side of the chest will also be reduced
3. **Hyper-resonance to percussion on the side of the pneumothorax.** This is often difficult to detect in neonates, but is more helpful in older children. Instead, in babies, transillumination of the chest will reveal the pneumothorax
4. **Deviation of trachea and displacement of apex beat.** In tension pneumothorax, there is mediastinal shift away from the pneumothorax

Common Diagnosis 1
Diagnosis: Cyanotic breath-holding spells

Examination Findings
1. **Normal examination in a young child.** Examination will be normal. Peak incidence is between 6 and 24 months old
2. **Facial cyanosis.** If witnessed during an episode, or by video, facial cyanosis is evident after the child stops breathing

2.1.7 KEY INVESTIGATIONS

Bedside

Table 2.1.1 Bedside tests of use in patients presenting with cyanosis

Test	When to perform	Potential result
Oxygen saturation	• All children with cyanosis	• Cyanosis usually visible with sats <80% • Normal sats in the presence of visible cyanosis is suspicious for mild methaemoglobinaemia • Be aware that in severe methaemoglobinaemia, sats may read 85% regardless of the true saturation
Pre- (right hand) and post-ductal (any other limb) saturations	• To look for right-to-left shunt across a PDA	• Saturation >5% lower post-ductal than pre-ductal is suggestive of shunt across PDA due to congenital heart disease or pulmonary hypertension
Hyperoxia test – administer 100% oxygen for 10 minutes	• To differentiate between respiratory or cardiac pathology • Discuss with a senior clinician first as oxygen can quicken PDA closure in duct-dependent lesions	• Respiratory causes should respond to oxygen • The desaturating effect of right-to-left shunts in cyanotic heart disease or pulmonary hypertension cannot be overcome by oxygen
Arterial blood gas	• To assess ventilation in those with respiratory distress	• Type 1 respiratory failure (low/normal $PaCO_2$) or Type 2 (high $PaCO_2$) • Metabolic acidosis in duct-dependent lesion with closing duct, due to poor perfusion • Normal PaO_2 in the presence of cyanosis suspicious for methaemoglobinaemia
ECG	• To look for signs of congenital heart disease • In cyanotic breath-holding spells to rule out long QT interval	• Right axis deviation in most cyanotic heart disease • Reassuringly normal QT interval

ECG, electrocardiogram; PaCO2, partial pressure of oxygen; PDA, patent ductus arteriosus

Blood Tests

Table 2.1.2 Blood tests of use in patients presenting with cyanosis

Test	When to perform	Potential result
FBC	• All children with cyanosis • Visible cyanosis less likely if anaemic • Breath-holding spells improve if anaemia is treated	• ↑ Neutrophils consistent with bacterial infection • ↑ Lymphocytes consistent with pertussis • Anaemia
CRP	• Suspected bacterial infection	• CRP ↑ in infection or inflammation
Blood culture	• Suspected pneumonia with signs of sepsis	• Positive cultures confirm bacterial infection • Sensitivities direct antibiotic choice
U&E	• If on diuretics for cardiac failure • If receiving IV fluid maintenance • Complicated pneumonia	• Electrolytes can become deranged with diuretic use • ↓ Na in SIADH as a complication of pneumonia

CRP, C-reactive protein; FBC, full blood count; IV, intravenous; Na, sodium; SIADH, syndrome of inappropriate antidiuretic hormone secretion; U&E, urea and electrolytes

Imaging

Table 2.1.3 Imaging Modalities of use in patients presenting with cyanosis

Test	When to perform	Potential result
Chest x-ray	• Suspected respiratory or cardiac pathology • Not required if strong clinical evidence of pneumonia or bronchiolitis with minimal oxygen requirement	• Pneumothorax: absent lung markings/crisp lung edge • Pneumonia: consolidation • Bronchiolitis: bronchial wall thickening, hyperinflation • Cardiac failure: enlarged cardiac shadow, pulmonary oligaemia or congestion, fluid in interlobar fissures • Tetralogy of Fallot: boot-shaped heart
Lung ultrasound	• Higher accuracy than chest x-ray for pneumothorax • Increasing use in Accident & Emergency and paediatric intensive care unit	• Lack of lung sliding and B lines is diagnostic of a pneumothorax
Echocardiogram	• Those with suspected congenital heart disease	• Diagnosis of structural heart disease • Estimation of pulmonary arterial pressures in pulmonary hypertension

Special

Table 2.1.4 Special tests of use in patients presenting with cyanosis

Test	When to perform	Potential result
Naso-pharyngeal aspirate	• Suspected bronchiolitis	• Identification of the responsible viral pathogen
Pernasal swab	• Suspected pertussis	• Confirmation of *Bordetella pertussis*
Co-oximetry	• Suspected methaemoglobinaemia, as a modification of standard pulse oximetry	• Estimation of methaemoglobin percentage
Genetic testing	• Suspected congenital methaemoglobinaemia	• Confirms hereditary cause

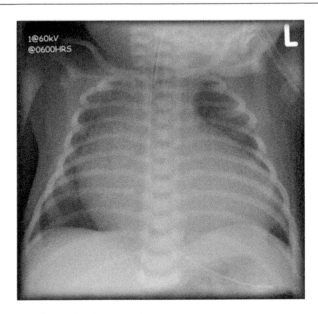

Figure 2.1.8 Cardiomegaly on chest x-ray due to Ebstein's anomaly

2.1.8 KEY MANAGEMENT PRINCIPLES

Diagnosis-specific management strategies are outlined here. It is expected that an 'ABCDE' approach to assessment and management is always undertaken (see Chapter 12.1, *The A to E Assessment*).

Dangerous Diagnosis 1
Diagnosis: Congenital cyanotic heart disease

Management Principles
All children with newly suspected cyanotic heart disease
1. **Arrange urgent echo and paediatric cardiology review.** Further management will depend on the lesion found. Transfer to a unit with cardiac surgery

If suspected duct-dependent lesion presenting on duct closure
2. **Prostaglandin infusion to maintain ductus arteriosus patency.** If there is clinical suspicion, prostaglandin can be started without confirmatory echo. It can be given peripherally initially, but should be moved to central administration as soon as possible, to ensure uninterrupted infusion
3. **Titrate prostaglandin infusion aiming for balance between pulmonary and systemic circulations.** Target saturations between 75 and 85%, partial pressure of carbon dioxide ($PaCO_2$) of 5–6 KPa, palpable femoral pulses and resolving acidosis
4. **Monitor for prostaglandin side effects.** The most common side effects are fever and apnoea, which might require mechanical ventilation

Dangerous Diagnosis 2
Diagnosis: Pneumothorax

Management Principles
1. **Emergency needle thoracocentesis for a tension pneumothorax.** Tension pneumothorax can cause cardiac arrest due to reduced venous return, so immediate treatment is vital. Insert a cannula in the mid-clavicular line, second rib space. Remove needle and secure cannula in position, attaching a three-way tap to allow further aspiration of air if needed. In most children a pink (20G) needle is appropriate, but this should be upsized in a teenager
2. **Chest drain insertion.** Many pneumothoraces, particularly those presenting with cyanosis, will require a chest drain
3. **Conservative management – watch and wait, give oxygen.** Consider this in stable children with a spontaneous pneumothorax. Over 75% of small spontaneous pneumothoraces (≤15% of the hemithorax) will resolve with conservative treatment. Oxygen administration can help resorption of the gas from the pleural space

---

Box 2.1.13   Indications for Chest Drain   △△

Chest drain insertion is indicated for the following categories of pneumothorax in children:

- Tension pneumothorax previously treated with needle thoracocentesis
- Pneumothorax associated with trauma (e.g. crush injury to chest). These are important to treat as they commonly develop into a tension pneumothorax

- Pneumothorax associated with positive pressure ventilation
- Pneumothorax causing hypoxia
- Large pneumothorax (>15% of hemithorax or in adolescents >2 cm lung edge to pleura at level of hilum)

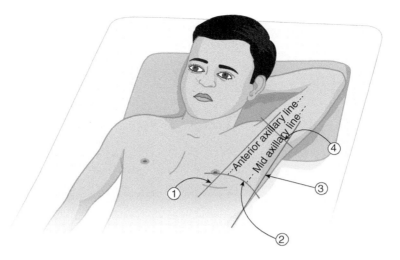

Figure 2.1.9 Safe triangle for chest drain insertion – bordered anteriorly by pectoralis major (1), inferiorly by the 5th rib (2), posteriorly by latissimus dorsi (3) and superiorly by the axilla (4). Insertion should be between the anterior axillary and mid-axillary lines in the 5th intercostal space. The incision should be made on the top edge of the rib to avoid the neurovascular bundle that runs along the inferior edge of each rib.

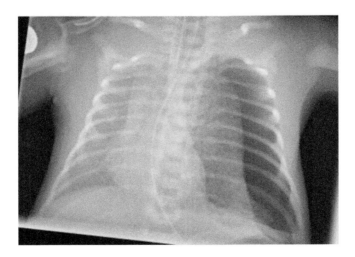

Figure 2.1.10 Left-sided tension pneumothorax with mediastinal shift away.

Common Diagnosis 1
Diagnosis: Cyanotic breath-holding spells

Management Principles
1. **Rule out serious causes of cyanotic spells.** Rule out long QT syndrome by doing an electrocardiogram (ECG; see Chapter 2.3, *Syncope*)
2. **Explain condition and reassure parents.** The episodes are very frightening to witness, and it is important to explain to families that they are not seizures, are not dangerous and do not cause brain damage. The episodes are involuntary and are not a sign of poor parenting or behavioural problems. The episodes will improve with age (they peak around age 2) and generally resolve completely before school age
3. **Test and treat iron-deficiency anaemia.** There is a high rate of anaemia in children having breath-holding spells, and a significant reduction in their frequency with treatment for iron-deficiency anaemia for 3 months

---

Box 2.1.14   Ventilatory Options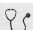

The options for oxygen supplementation and ventilatory support include (from least to most invasive):

1. Low-flow nasal cannulae (2 L/min flow maximum)
2. Headbox oxygen
3. High-flow humidified oxygen (1–2 L/kg/minute flow)
4. Continuous positive airway pressure (CPAP)
5. Bilevel positive airway pressure (BiPAP)
6. Invasive ventilation

2.2 Circulatory Collapse

Rachel Varughese[1] and Abdulhakim Abdurrazaq[2]
[1] *Department of Paediatrics, Oxford University Hospitals NHS Foundation Trust, Oxford, UK*
[2] *Department of Paediatrics, Walsall Manor Hospital, Walsall Healthcare NHS Trust, Walsall, UK*

CONTENTS

2.2.1 CHAPTER AT A GLANCE

> **Box 2.2.1   Chapter at a Glance**
>
> - In circulatory shock, supply does not meet demand
> - There are five main types of shock: hypovolaemic, distributive, cardiogenic, obstructive and dissociative
> - Shock can also be divided into:
>   - Compensated (homeostasis maintains blood pressure)
>   - Uncompensated (blood pressure is compromised)
>   - Irreversible (permanent organ damage and death)
> - As seen in the algorithm in Figure 2.2.1, diagnosis of the underlying condition relies heavily on history and context, since once a child presents with shock, many features are global
> - Any suspicion of shock or impending shock should prompt early discussion with the paediatric intensive care unit (PICU)
> - Management will only be successful by making an ABCDE assessment and treating as problems are revealed
> - Goals are immediate identification of life-threatening conditions, e.g. tension pneumothorax, recognition of impending circulatory compromise and early classification of the type of shock

2.2.2 DEFINITION

Shock is a state of inadequate end-organ and tissue perfusion, resulting from insufficient delivery of oxygen and nutrients to meet the metabolic demands.

Clinical Guide to Paediatrics, First Edition. Edited by Rachel Varughese and Anna Mathew. Series Editor: Christian Fielder Camm.
© 2022 John Wiley & Sons Ltd. Published 2022 by John Wiley & Sons Ltd.
Companion website: www.wiley.com/go/varughese/paediatrics

2.2.3 DIAGNOSTIC ALGORITHM

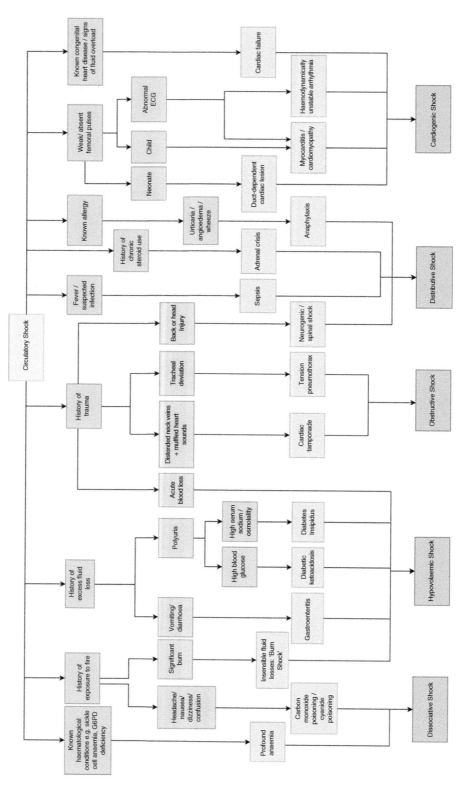

Figure 2.2.1 Diagnostic algorithm for the presentation of circulatory shock.

2.2.4 DIFFERENTIALS LIST

All differential diagnoses are life-threatening. Underlying conditions are numerous, and it is not possible to provide an exhaustive list. Here, shock will be grouped into types, in order to enforce structure in a complex and extensive topic.

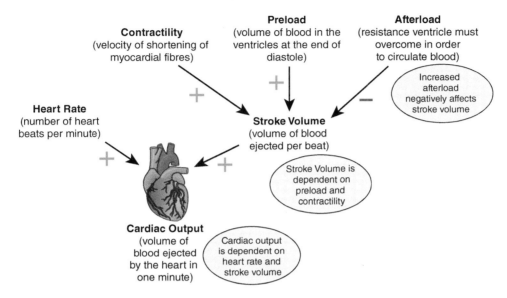

Figure 2.2.2 Relationships between essential cardiovascular states, explaining how cardiac output can be affected by multiple mechanisms. +, positive correlation; –, negative correlation. The relationship between preload and stroke volume is described by the Frank-Starling mechanism. An increase in preload increases stroke volume up to a certain point, after which further increases do not improve stroke volume, but instead lead to increased hydrostatic pressure in the pulmonary capillaries, which causes pulmonary oedema.

Dangerous Diagnoses
1. Hypovolaemic Shock
- Hypovolaemia is the state of reduced intravascular volume
- This causes decrease in preload, decreasing stroke volume
- The resulting impaired cardiac output leads to insufficient delivery of oxygen and nutrients to end organs, leading to shock

---

Box 2.2.2   Causes of Hypovolaemic Shock

- Haemorrhage:
  - Trauma – external, head, chest, pelvis, abdomen, long bones
  - Surgery
  - Gastrointestinal bleeding
  - Obstetric bleeding
- Intravascular volume loss:
  - Gastroenteritis
  - Diabetes insipidus

- Diabetic ketoacidosis
- Sepsis*
- Anaphylaxis*
- Interstitial loss:
  - Burns
  - Nephrotic syndrome
  - Intestinal obstruction
  - Ascites

*sepsis and anaphylaxis are commonly thought of as causes of distributive shock, however, since both conditions cause capillary leak and profound intravascular volume loss, there is also an important hypovolaemic component to consider.

---

2. Distributive Shock
- Shock resulting from decreased systemic vascular resistance
- Blood becomes inappropriately distributed within the vasculature. Also known as vasodilatory shock
- Characterised by peripheral vasodilatation, with venous pooling and inadequate arterial tissue perfusion to meet metabolic demands
- Some causes of distributive shock, such as sepsis and anaphylaxis, also result in volume depletion, due to increased capillary permeability, meaning intravascular volume is lost into the tissues

Box 2.2.3 Causes of Distributive Shock

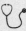

- Sepsis:
  - Vasodilation occurs due to dysregulated immune response to infection, causing systemic cytokine release (known as systemic inflammatory response syndrome – SIRS)
- Anaphylaxis:
  - Vasodilation occurs due to histamine release
- Neurological injury:
  - There is uncontrolled vasodilation resulting from the sudden loss of sympathetic tone (neurogenic shock). There can be profound shock, due to lack of usual sympathetic compensation, e.g. tachycardia, peripheral vasoconstriction
- Non-infectious causes of SIRS:
  - Burns

- Pancreatitis
- Adrenal insufficiency
- Drugs:
  - Nitrates
  - Opioids
  - Adrenergic blockers
- Toxic shock:
  - Distinct from sepsis
  - Here, cytokine release (stimulated by exotoxins of *Staphylococcus-aureus* and group A *Streptococci*) lead to vasodilation and capillary leak

3. Cardiogenic Shock

- Cardiogenic shock is an acute state of circulatory failure due to impairment of myocardial contractility
- Impairment of cardiac contractility leads to insufficient end-organ perfusion
- Rare cause of circulatory collapse in children

Box 2.2.4 Causes of Cardiogenic Shock

- Congenital heart disease + post-operative period after cardiac surgery
- Rhythm disorder:
  - Supraventricular tachycardia (SVT) is the most common arrhythmia in children, although it is frequently well tolerated
- Acquired heart diseases:
  - Myocarditis
  - Chemotherapy toxicity
  - Severe Kawasaki disease (rare)
  - Endocarditis (rare)
  - Rheumatic fever (rare)

- Metabolic
  - Primary, e.g. glycogen storage disease
  - Secondary, e.g. hyperkalaemia, hypercalcaemia
- Cardiomyopathy
  - Divided into dilated, hypertrophic and restrictive
  - Variety of underlying conditions, both congenital and acquired
- Extra-cardiac disease
  - Overlap with other conditions, which contribute to cardiogenic shock by failing to deliver adequate oxygen to the myocardium
  - Examples: sepsis, pulmonary embolism, pneumothorax, cardiac tamponade

Box 2.2.5 Congenital Heart Disease Reliant on Patent Ductus Arteriosus (PDA) Blood Flow

These conditions are not traditionally considered 'cyanotic'. Although they lead to deoxygenated blood in the systemic circulation, they tend to present when the PDA closes, and are known as 'duct dependent'. The result is profoundly poor peripheral perfusion due to cardiogenic shock, and patients often present pale.

Cyanotic lesions are described in Chapter 2.1.

Conditions	Details
Hypoplastic left heart syndrome	• Most of the left-sided structures, including the left ventricle, aorta and valves, are underdeveloped • There is usually a left-to-right shunt at an atrial septal defect, then a right-to-left shunt at a PDA allowing mixed blood into the systemic circulation
Critical aortic stenosis	• In severe left ventricular outflow obstruction, systemic circulation may be entirely reliant on a right-to-left shunt across the PDA
Interrupted aortic arch	• Separation between ascending and descending aorta • There is often a large ventricular septal defect allowing mixing, and then a right-to-left shunt at the PDA, feeding the systemic circulation
Coarctation of the aorta	• Not often cyanotic, but if there is significant pre-ductal aortic narrowing, aortic pressure distally may be low enough to cause a right-to-left shunt across the PDA

4. Obstructive Shock

- Physical obstruction of either pulmonary or systemic blood flow, causing abrupt impairment of cardiac output
- Obstruction of blood flow into the heart means decreased diastolic filling (and decreased preload), therefore reducing cardiac output
- Obstruction of blood flow out of the heart means excessive afterload, also reducing cardiac output

---

Box 2.2.6   Causes of Obstructive Shock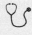

- Congenital:
  - Duct-dependent cardiac lesions once patent ductus arteriosus has closed: hypoplastic left heart, critical aortic stenosis, severe coarctation of the aorta, interrupted aortic arch
- Acquired:
  - Tension pneumothorax – mostly following penetrating thoracic trauma

- Massive pulmonary embolism – rare in children, there is usually a predisposition, e.g. central venous access device, or hypercoagulable state, e.g. sickle cell disease, inherited thrombophilias
- Cardiac tamponade – mostly following penetrating thoracic trauma, but may be secondary to infection, malignancy or following cardiac surgery

---

5. Dissociative Shock

- Oxygen delivery is limited by the oxygen-carrying capacity of the blood, meaning haemoglobin is unable to deliver oxygen to tissues
- There is normal cardiac function, responsive vasculature and normal intravascular filling
- Causes include profound anaemia (sickle cell disease, severe malaria), carbon monoxide poisoning, methaemoglobinaemia and cyanide poisoning

---

Box 2.2.7   Causes of Dissociative Shock

- Anaemia:
  - Reduced oxygen-binding capacity of the blood, due to limited haemoglobin
  - Over time, the oxygen dissociation curve shifts to the right, meaning haemoglobin will have a reduced affinity for oxygen, allowing quicker release at the tissues
- Conditions causing increased oxygen affinity:
  - Increased oxygen affinity (oxygen dissociation curve shifted to the left) means little oxygen is released at the tissues

- Carbon monoxide poisoning
- Methaemoglobinaemia – ferrous iron in haem is converted to ferric form
- Cyanide poisoning:
  - Impairment of oxidative phosphorylation, where oxygen is utilised for energy at a mitochondrial level

---

2.2.5 KEY HISTORY FEATURES

Dangerous Diagnosis 1
Diagnosis: Hypovolaemic shock

Questions
1. **Is there a history of bleeding?** Acute blood loss by trauma might be immediately obvious. It is important to ask about recent surgery, as bleeding might be concealed. A history of coffee-ground vomiting or melaena points towards gastrointestinal bleeding
2. **Has there been reduced intake of fluid, or pathological increased output?** Ask about vomiting or diarrhoea – gastroenteritis is the most common cause of hypovolaemia in children. Decreased intake of fluids may accompany upper and lower respiratory tract infections. Pathological urinary losses are seen in diabetic ketoacidosis and diabetes insipidus
3. **Any recent complaints of abdominal pain?** Acute abdominal pathology, such as intestinal obstruction and peritonitis, can lead to fluid translocation from the intra- to the extravascular fluid compartment
4. **Is there a significant burn?** Insensible losses from burns can cause 'burn shock', due to hypovolaemia

Dangerous Diagnosis 2
Diagnosis: Distributive shock

Questions
1. **Any recent infections or febrile illnesses?** The most prevalent cause of distributive shock is sepsis. There may not be any specific history features – level of suspicion should remain high. Children at high risk, such as those on chemotherapy or with known immunodeficiencies, should be considered septic until proven otherwise
2. **Any known allergies?** Anaphylaxis is a common cause of distributive shock and often (not always) patients will have a known allergy
3. **Any recent trauma to the head or back?** Head or spinal injury affecting the central nervous system can disrupt the autonomic pathways that control vascular tone. Most often, this involves cervical spine trauma
4. **Is there a history of long-term steroid use?** High-dose steroid use (>2.5 mg/m²/day prednisolone or >10 mg/m²/day hydrocortisone or equivalent) causes adrenal suppression. Risks increase the higher the dose and longer the continuous treatment. Children with known adrenal insufficiency, or who are on long-term steroids, should have medic-alert bracelets

Dangerous Diagnosis 3
Diagnosis: Cardiogenic shock

Questions
1. **Any known congenital cardiac disease?** There may be known congenital heart disease, which may have had corrective surgery. If not, ask about antenatal scans – approximately 60% of congenital cardiac abnormalities are identified using antenatal ultrasound scanning
2. **Over what time period were the onset of symptoms?** Babies with underlying chronic heart failure may present with a long history of failure to thrive or breathless, sweaty feeding. Many older children may have complained of intermittent abdominal pain in the past, along with the typical symptoms of anorexia, dyspnoea and fatigue. Myocarditis may be precipitated by a viral prodrome and may have a very acute onset and rapid progression
3. **Any history of palpitations?** Children may report palpitations or awareness of their heartbeat in dysrhythmias

Dangerous Diagnosis 4
Diagnosis: Obstructive shock

Questions
1. **Is there a recent history of chest injury?** Consider tension pneumothorax or cardiac tamponade
2. **Were there antenatal concerns about cardiac anomalies?** Severe congenital cardiac lesions that are not identified antenatally may go undiagnosed at birth in the setting of a patent ductus arteriosus. Lesions such as critical aortic stenosis, coarctation of the aorta and hypoplastic left heart may present with acute obstructive shock when the duct starts to close – usually within a few days of life (can be up to 3 weeks)
3. **Are there risk factors for pulmonary embolism?** Pulmonary embolism (PE) is rare in well children. Always consider PE in those at higher risk: patients with sickle cell disease, coagulation disorders and indwelling central venous catheters

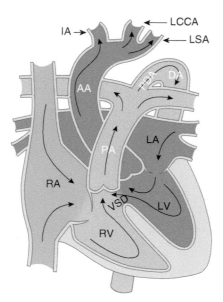

Figure 2.2.3 Blood flow in a duct-dependent circulation in a baby with interrupted aortic arch. AA, ascending aorta; DA, descending aorta; IA, innominate artery; LA, left atrium; LCCA, left common carotid artery; LSA, left subclavian artery; LV, left ventricle; PA, pulmonary artery; PDA, patent ductus arteriosus; RA, right atrium; RV, right ventricle; VSD, ventricular septal defect

Figure 2.2.4 Blood flow through the heart in hypoplastic left heart syndrome. The left ventricle is grossly underdeveloped. Oxygenated blood passes to the right atrium via an atrial septal defect and mixed blood is then pumped out of the pulmonary artery, reaching the systemic circulation via the patent ductus arteriosus (PDA). When the PDA closes, systemic circulation is suddenly compromised, resulting in shock.

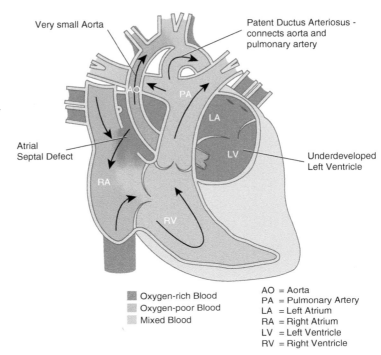

Very small Aorta

Patent Ductus Arteriosus - connects aorta and pulmonary artery

Atrial Septal Defect

Underdeveloped Left Ventricle

◼ Oxygen-rich Blood
◼ Oxygen-poor Blood
◼ Mixed Blood

AO = Aorta
PA = Pulmonary Artery
LA = Left Atrium
RA = Right Atrium
LV = Left Ventricle
RV = Right Ventricle

Dangerous Diagnosis 5
Diagnosis: Dissociative shock

Questions
1. **Are they under 6 months old?** Infants under 6 months are at higher risk of methaemoglobinaemia due to reduced levels of a key enzyme: NADH cytochrome b5 methaemoglobin reductase. This enzyme deficiency may also be inherited
2. **Has there been exposure to nitrates?** This is again about methaemoglobinaemia. Ask about exposure to nitrate-containing drinking water (often from wells). Some medicines also contain nitrates, such as trimethoprim and sulfamethoxazole
3. **Do they have known anaemia or glucose-6-phosphate dehydrogenase (G6PD) deficiency?** Profound anaemia itself is a risk for dissociative shock – made more likely by conditions such as sickle cell anaemia. Patients with G6PD and pyruvate kinase deficiency have impaired production of co-factors for NADH cytochrome b5 methaemoglobin reductase
4. **Have they been exposed to fire? Do other family members report symptoms of carbon monoxide exposure?** Carbon monoxide is produced from incomplete burning of fuels. A history may not be immediately obvious, but domestic appliances and fireplaces can produce carbon monoxide. Every home should be fitted with an alarm. If other family members report headaches, dizziness or nausea that resolves upon leaving the house, carbon monoxide poisoning is a likely possibility

2.2.6 KEY EXAMINATION FEATURES

Box 2.2.8 What Stage of Shock?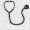

Circulatory shock can be broadly divided into three stages:

- Compensated shock:
  - Normal homeostatic mechanisms compensate for reduced perfusion
  - Heart rate increases
  - Systolic blood pressure maintained
  - Signs of peripheral vasoconstriction become evident
- Decompensated shock:
  - Compensation is not enough to maintain blood pressure and hypotension develops

- Heart rate is significantly elevated
- Signs of poor perfusion to end organs emerge, e.g. confusion, drowsiness, reduced urine output
- Irreversible shock:
  - Progression of end-organ dysfunction leads to irreversible damage
  - Death is imminent without intervention
  - Bradycardia is a very concerning agonal event

Shock is a clinical diagnosis. If suspected, senior help should be sought urgently and assessment conducted by the most experienced clinician available. Diagnosis-specific examination findings vary widely depending on aetiology.

Many examination features are common across different types of shock. Tables 2.2.1–2.2.6 summarise general findings seen in the A to E assessment in patients with circulatory shock.

Table 2.2.1 End-of-bed assessment

	Signs	Interpretation
General appearance	• Unfocused gaze • Weak cry • Decreased responsiveness to painful procedures	• Decreased cerebral perfusion
	• Mottled skin	• Indicates poor perfusion but can be misleading in cold environments

Table 2.2.2 Airway assessment

	Signs	Interpretation
Patency	• Added airway sounds, e.g. snoring, stridor	• Compromised airway

Table 2.2.3 Breathing assessment

	Signs	Interpretation
Respiratory rate	• Tachypnoea	• Common in shock – non-specific • Can be related to underlying pathology or as a compensatory response to metabolic acidosis
Work of breathing	• Severe respiratory distress	• Anaphylaxis • Obstructive shock • Cardiogenic shock
	• Inadequate respiratory effort in the setting of metabolic acidosis	• Tiring – unable to compensate for acidosis
Breath sounds	• Stridor or wheeze	• Anaphylaxis
	• Crackles	• Pneumonia → septic shock • Pulmonary oedema → cardiogenic shock
	• Asymmetry	• Tension pneumothorax • Airway obstruction • If injury, consider haemothorax

Table 2.2.4 Circulation assessment

	Signs	Interpretation
Pulse quality	• Decreased pulse volume	• Peripheral vasoconstriction – compensatory mechanism for shock
	• Bounding pulses	• Distributive shock
Pulse rate	• Tachycardia	• Early compensatory mechanism • May be the only sign in early compensated shock • Tachyarrhythmia
	• Normal/low heart rate (in presence of other signs of shock)	• Cervical or high-thoracic spinal cord injury → neurogenic shock • Consider ingestion of drugs, e.g. beta blockers
	• Bradycardia	• Bradyarrhythmia → cardiogenic shock • Agonal event

(Continued)

Table 2.2.4 (Continued)

	Signs	Interpretation
Capillary refill time	• Capillary refill time >2 seconds	• Peripheral vasoconstriction – compensatory mechanism
	• Capillary refill time <1 second	• Distributive shock ('flash capillary refill')
Blood pressure (manual cuff)	• Normal blood pressure	• Compensated shock
	• Hypotension	• Decompensated shock *Needs rapid identification as likely to deteriorate fast to cardiopulmonary arrest
	• Upper limb BP > lower limb BP	• Coarctation of the aorta • Interrupted aortic arch
	• Pulse pressure abnormal	• Narrow pulse pressure (<30 mmHg): suggests hypovolaemic or cardiogenic shock • Wide pulse pressure (>40 mmHg): suggests distributive
Neck veins	• Distended neck veins	• Cardiac failure • Obstruction to venous return: cardiac tamponade, tension pneumothorax, haemothorax
Heart sounds	• Cardiac murmur or gallop rhythm	• Cardiogenic shock
	• Muffled heart sounds	• Cardiac tamponade

Table 2.2.5 Disability assessment

	Signs	Interpretation
Blood glucose	• High blood sugar • High ketones	• Diabetic ketoacidosis
Glasgow Coma Scale (GCS)	• GCS <14	• Indicates decreased cerebral perfusion
	• GCS <8	• Concern about self-maintenance of airway

Table 2.2.6 Exposure assessment

	Signs	Interpretation
Temperature	• Fever • Hypothermia	• Septic shock • Be aware of iatrogenic hypothermia
Abdomen	• Distension, peritonism	• Acute abdomen, e.g. bowel perforation
	• Hepatomegaly	• Cardiac failure
	• Injury	• Haemorrhagic shock (hypovolaemic) • Remember inflicted injury may have a concealed history
Trauma assessment	• Injury	• Haemorrhagic shock (hypovolaemic) • Neurogenic shock
Skin	• Urticaria/facial oedema	• Anaphylaxis
	• Purpura	• Septic shock
	• Bruises/abrasions	• Trauma • Inflicted injury

Dangerous Diagnosis 1

Diagnosis: Hypovolaemic shock

Examination Findings

1. **Dehydration**. A dehydration assessment is not always accurate. Multiple factors should be taken into account. See the assessment of dehydration in Chapter 12.3, Box 12.3.2.
2. **Narrow pulse pressure.** Narrow pulse pressure (<30 mmHg) is caused by compensatory increased systemic vascular resistance in hypovolaemia

3. **Evidence of injury.** Most often, trauma is obvious from the history. However, this may not always be the case, particularly if there are safeguarding concerns. Besides obvious external injury, some sources of bleeding, such as intra-abdominal, may not be immediately obvious. Suspicious bruises and abrasions elsewhere increase the likelihood of serious non-accidental injury

Dangerous Diagnosis 2
Diagnosis: Distributive shock

Examination Findings
1. **Hypotension.** Hypotension can be particularly profound as a result of intravascular fluid loss due to capillary leak and a reduction in vascular resistance, meaning that compensatory vasoconstriction does not occur
2. **Bounding pulse, warm and flushed peripheries.** Peripheral vasodilation may lead to 'flash' (fast) capillary refill time, with bounding pulses
3. **Wide pulse pressure.** Due to loss of systemic vascular resistance, diastolic blood pressure falls, creating a wide pulse pressure >40 mmHg
4. **Wheeze.** In anaphylaxis, airway compromise accompanies cardiovascular compromise. Urticaria and angioedema may be present, but their absence does not exclude anaphylaxis

Dangerous Diagnosis 3
Diagnosis: Cardiogenic shock

Examination Findings
1. **Tachycardia.** Persistent tachycardia is a compensatory mechanism to deal with reduced cardiac output. Disproportionate tachycardia may indicate an arrhythmia
2. **Dyspnoea.** Pulmonary oedema as a result of cardiac failure may cause subjective breathlessness as well as objective respiratory distress, which can be severe. There will be crackles on auscultation
3. **Jugular vein distension and hepatomegaly.** Distended neck veins are often hard to appreciate in children, but are present in cardiac failure due to poor cardiac contractility. There may also be hepatic congestion causing hepatomegaly
4. **Volume of pulses.** Weak pulses are suggestive of poor cardiac contractility
5. **Gallop rhythm.** An audible third heart sound, associated with rapid ventricular filling
6. **Narrow pulse pressure.** Narrow pulse pressure (<30 mmHg) is caused by compensatory increased systemic vascular resistance

Dangerous Diagnosis 4
Diagnosis: Obstructive shock

Examination Findings
1. **Is there tracheal deviation?** Tracheal deviation is strongly suggestive of a tension pneumothorax or haemothorax
2. **Are there asymmetrical breath sounds?** Asymmetry of breath sounds suggest a pneumothorax or haemothorax. Both cause ipsilateral decreased chest expansion and reduced breath sounds. Percussion note is hyper-resonant in pneumothorax and dull in haemothorax
3. **Jugular vein distension.** Besides cardiac failure, distended neck veins also point to an obstruction to venous return. This could be caused by cardiac tamponade, tension pneumothorax or haemothorax
4. **Muffled heart sounds.** This suggests pericardial fluid, indicative of cardiac tamponade. It is strengthened when pulsus paradoxus (an exaggerated decrease of systolic blood pressure during inspiration) is present
5. **Difference in upper and lower limb pulses/blood pressures.** Decreased pulses and blood pressure in the lower limbs compared to the upper extremities suggest structural heart disease, e.g. interrupted aortic arch, likely presenting following spontaneous ductal closure

Dangerous Diagnosis 5
Diagnosis: Dissociative shock

Examination Findings
1. **Cyanosis.** Reduction in oxygen delivery to tissues leads to hypoxia. Oxygen saturations may be inaccurately estimated by routine monitors and give overestimates in both carbon monoxide poisoning and methaemoglobinaemia
2. **Tachycardia and dyspnoea.** Both occur as compensatory mechanisms to deal with lack of oxygen at a tissue level

2.2.7 KEY INVESTIGATIONS

Stabilisation of 'ABC' always takes precedence over further diagnostic evaluation in any patient with clinical shock. All patients with shock will require the full list of bedside and blood tests listed here.

Bedside

Table 2.2.7 Bedside tests of use in patients presenting with circulatory collapse

Test	Justification	Potential result
Blood glucose (mmol/L)	• Glucose easily correctable	• <2.6 – hypoglycaemia, store depletion • >10 – significant stress • >11 – consider DKA
Blood gas (arterial, capillary or venous)	• Measure of gas exchange, as well as perfusion • Distinguishes between respiratory, metabolic or mixed acidosis/alkalosis	• Acidosis (pH <7.35) most likely • ↑ CO_2 – respiratory acidosis • ↓ CO_2 – respiratory compensation • Lactate >2 indicates poor perfusion
ECG/cardiac monitoring	• Diagnoses arrhythmias	• SVT • Less commonly, VT or bradyarrhythmia

CO_2, carbon dioxide; DKA, diabetic ketoacidosis; ECG, electrocardiogram; SVT, supraventricular tachycardia; VT, ventricular tachycardia

Blood Tests

Table 2.2.8 Blood tests of use in patients presenting with circulatory collapse

Test	Justification	Potential result
FBC	• Hb, platelets and white cell differential point to underlying diagnosis • Hb may underestimate blood loss in acute haemorrhage	• ↓ Hb – chronic anaemia or acute haemorrhage • ↓ Platelets – DIC, acute haemorrhage • ↑ Platelets – sepsis • ↑ Neutrophils - sepsis
U&E, LFTs	• Reduced perfusion may cause end-organ failure	• ↑ Urea and creatinine – acute kidney injury • ↑ Liver enzymes – hepatic injury • ↑ Sodium – diabetes insipidus
Clotting	• DIC can complicate sepsis	• ↑ PT and APTT – DIC, sepsis • ↓ Fibrinogen – DIC, sepsis
Blood culture and sensitivity	• Confirm sepsis • Identify organism • Rationalise antibiotics	• Positive culture confirms bacterial infection • Sensitivities guide antibiotic choice
Crossmatch	• If transfusions predicted, best to give matched blood	• Crossmatched blood for transfusion

APTT, activated partial thromboplastin time; DIC, disseminated intravascular coagulation; FBC, full blood count; Hb, haemoglobin; LFTs, liver function tests; PT, prothrombin time; U&E, urea and electrolytes

Imaging

Table 2.2.9 Imaging modalities of use in patients presenting with circulatory collapse

Test	When to perform	Potential result
Chest x-ray	• Patients with respiratory distress	• Pneumothorax: absent lung markings/crisp lung edge • Haemothorax: opacification with blunted phrenic angles and fluid level • Tension pneumo/haemothorax: mediastinal shift • Pneumonia: consolidation • Cardiac failure: enlarged cardiac shadow, pulmonary oligaemia or congestion, fluid in interlobar fissures

Further imaging, such as computed tomography (CT), can be helpful in identifying spinal injuries and intra-abdominal pathology (e.g. obstruction, perforation, bleed). However, stabilisation is required prior to this.

Special

Table 2.2.10 Special tests of use in patients presenting with circulatory collapse

Test	When to perform	Potential result
Paired urine and serum osmolality	• Suspected diabetes insipidus (DI)	• Raised serum osmolality with decreased urine osmolality points to DI
Bedside echocardiography	• All types of shock, if skilled clinician available for rapid assessment	• Underlying cardiac problems, myocardial performance, distribution of blood flow, vascular tone, cardiac response to interventions
Carbon monoxide pulse oximeter	• Suspected carbon monoxide poisoning • Normal pulse oximeters not reliable if carboxyhaemoglobin present	• Estimation of carboxyhaemoglobin level
B-type natriuretic peptide (BNP) levels	• Suspected cardiogenic shock • Helps to confirm myocardial dysfunction	• High BNP is a poor prognostic factor
Arterial catheter	• Patients who remain critically unwell, in high-dependency or intensive care • Allows invasive measurement of arterial blood pressure	• Accurate continuous measurement

2.2.8 KEY MANAGEMENT PRINCIPLES

Early recognition of shock saves lives. All assessment and management should follow an ABCDE approach with continual reassessment. It is expected that at the first suspicion of circulatory shock, the consultant (or most senior available clinican) is made aware and will be present (see Chapter 12.1, *The A to E Assessment*).

Management is highly variable depending on the underlying cause. Options are briefly outlined here, as comprehensive guidelines for each condition would be too extensive.

Dangerous Diagnosis 1
Diagnosis: Hypovolaemic shock

Management Principles
1. **Fluid resuscitation.** The primary management is intravenous (IV) fluid replacement. Fluid boluses of 20 mL/kg 0.9% sodium chloride should be used and repeated as required. If there is haemorrhagic shock, packed red blood cell transfusion of 10–20mL/kg should be given.
   Diabetic ketoacidosis (DKA) requires thoughtful fluid prescribing. The risk of cerebral oedema must be balanced with dehydration. Always use a protocol and discuss with a consultant if >30 mL/kg fluid bolus is indicated
2. **Limit fluid losses.** If there is vomiting, insert a nasogastric (NG) tube and keep on free drainage. If there is active bleeding, activate the major haemorrhage protocol and give tranexamic acid
3. **Maintenance fluids.** These depend on the source of hypovolaemia. Use the regular fluid prescription (see Chapter 12.3, *Tips for Fluid Prescribing*) for regular maintenance. Estimation of dehydration allows use of a rehydrated weight
   • Patients with burns require higher maintenance due to insensible losses
   • Patients with high NG losses should have these replaced mL/mL with IV fluids
   • Patients with high urinary losses, in diabetes insipidus, should have maintenance fluids plus replacement of high urinary volumes – this can be complicated and a local guideline is essential. These children should be allowed free access to water
4. **Vasopressors and inotropes.** Shock refractory to fluid resuscitation may require vasopressors and inotropes. Discuss with local paediatric intensive care unit (PICU) early
5. **If DKA, insulin.** DKA protocols are very specific. Use a local guideline or the British Society for Paediatric Endocrinology and Diabetes (BSPED) guideline. Insulin infusions, regular rechecking of blood glucose and electrolyte replacement are the key aspects to therapy

Dangerous Diagnosis 2
Diagnosis: Distributive shock

Management Principles
1. **Condition-specific treatment**
   Anaphylaxis:
   - Intramuscular (IM) adrenaline. Patient should be flat with legs raised
   - Steroid (hydrocortisone) and antihistamine (chlorphenamine). See Chapter 13.2 for detailed information on anaphylaxis management.
   Sepsis:
   - Early antibiotics – within an hour, ideally <30 minutes. See Chapter 13.1 for detailed information on sepsis management.
   Neurogenic injury:
   - C-spine stabilisation to prevent further spinal cord injury
   - Urgent neurosurgical review to determine surgical options
   Adrenal crisis:
   - IV hydrocortisone bolus (IM if delay in IV access) and start IV infusion
   - If blood sugar <3 mmol/L, give 2 mL/kg 10% dextrose. Repeat if blood sugar remains low
2. **Fluid resuscitation.** IV fluid boluses as required, followed by maintenance fluids
3. **Vasopressors and inotropes.** If hypotension persists despite euvolemia, discuss with PICU for consideration of vasopressors and inotropes

Dangerous Diagnosis 3
Diagnosis: Cardiogenic shock
All management should be conducted in conjunction with cardiology advice

Management Principles
1. **Treatment of arrhythmia.** Treatment of reversible cardiac rhythm disorder – adenosine, antiarrhythmic agents, cardioversion, pacing
2. **Improve cardiac function.** Medications (guided by paediatric cardiologists and intensivists) aim to reduce systemic vascular resistance, in order to reduce afterload, and increase cardiac contractility. Dobutamine is often used first line. Milrinone is an alternative, particularly if right ventricle function is impaired. Levosimendan (combines inotropic and vasodilating effects) may be used as second line
3. **Diuretics.** Diuretics, such as furosemide, should be given to children with fluid overload and ventricular dysfunction, to return them to euvolaemic state
4. **Reduction of metabolic demands.** Intubation and ventilation, normothermia and sedation can help relieve myocardial stress
5. **IV fluids.** IV fluids may be required in some cases. Aggressive resuscitation should never be used. Fluids should be very cautiously administered (often in restricted volumes) to avoid iatrogenic overload – echocardiography can estimate whether there is preload insufficiency
6. **ECMO.** For patients with cardiogenic shock refractory to conventional therapy, extracorporeal membrane oxygenation (ECMO) can be used for circulatory support

---

Box 2.2.9   Extracorporeal Cardiopulmonary Resuscitation (ECMO)

- ECMO uses a machine similar to a heart–lung bypass machine used in open heart surgery
- Blood from the body is removed, oxygenated and returned
- ECMO is useful in children with severe cardiac or respiratory failure, who have reached the limit of conventional therapies (e.g. ventilation, inotropic support)

- Importantly, ECMO is only appropriate for those who have reversible disease. It is not a treatment on its own, it merely buys time for damaged organs to heal
- The major complication is bleeding, as the circuit is heparinised, which can lead to significant surface/mucosal bleeding and risks intracranial, intrathoracic and intra-abdominal bleeding

Dangerous Diagnosis 4
Diagnosis: Obstructive shock

Management Principles
1. **Condition-specific treatment of reversible causes**
   Tension pneumothorax:
   - **Needle thoracocentesis**: this is immediate, life-saving treatment that should be performed even without radiographical confirmation of pneumothorax. Cannula or needle attached to three-way tap should be inserted in the 2nd intercostal space, mid-clavicular line, above the 3rd rib so as to avoid the neurovascular bundle
   - **Chest drain**: there may have been dramatic relief of symptoms just with thoracocentesis. A chest drain is the definitive treatment, and can now be inserted in more stable conditions
   Cardiac tamponade:
   - **Pericardiocentesis**: should be performed by a competent specialist under ultrasound guidance
   Pulmonary embolism:
   - Urgent senior haematology advice to guide anti-coagulation and consideration of fibrinolytic therapy
2. **Duct-dependent lesions.** If there is suspicion of a duct-dependent obstructive cardiac lesion, a prostaglandin E1 infusion must be immediately started, ideally into a central vein. This might reopen the ductus arteriosus and maintain patency. Transfer to a cardiac surgical centre for definitive corrective surgery

Dangerous Diagnosis 5
Diagnosis: Dissociative shock

Management Principles
1. **Treatment of carbon monoxide poisoning.** 100% oxygen is the mainstay of treatment for carbon monoxide poisoning
2. **If methaemoglobinaemia is suspected: methylene blue**. Methylene blue indirectly reduces methaemoglobin to haemoglobin and can be used in both acute acquired situations and as maintenance therapy in congenital conditions. Ascorbic acid (vitamin C) can be used if methylene blue is contraindicated. Do not use methylene blue in G6PD deficiency or with concurrent serotonergic medications
3. **Treatment of anaemia.** Depending on the cause, anaemia may require packed red blood cell transfusion and iron supplementation

2.3 Syncope

Eleanor Duckworth

University College Hospital, University College London Hospitals NHS Foundation Trust, London, UK

CONTENTS

2.3.1 CHAPTER AT A GLANCE

Box 2.3.1   Chapter at a Glance

- Syncope can be broadly divided into 'cardiac' and 'non-cardiac'
- The history is the most telling part of the assessment and invasive investigations are rarely required
- Some causes of cardiac syncope can increase risk of sudden cardiac death, so detailed assessment is needed

- More commonly, syncope is related to benign conditions, such as vasovagal episodes
- Some conditions, such as seizures and hypoglycaemia, are known as syncope 'mimics'. They may cause loss of consciousness, but since they are not followed by spontaneous recovery, they are not syncope

2.3.2 DEFINITION

- Syncope is a transient loss of consciousness associated with loss of postural tone. It has a rapid onset, short duration and spontaneous recovery
- It is a very common symptom in the paediatric population; 15% will have at least one episode by the end of adolescence

Clinical Guide to Paediatrics, First Edition. Edited by Rachel Varughese and Anna Mathew. Series Editor: Christian Fielder Camm.
© 2022 John Wiley & Sons Ltd. Published 2022 by John Wiley & Sons Ltd.
Companion website: www.wiley.com/go/varughese/paediatrics

2.3.3 DIAGNOSTIC ALGORITHM

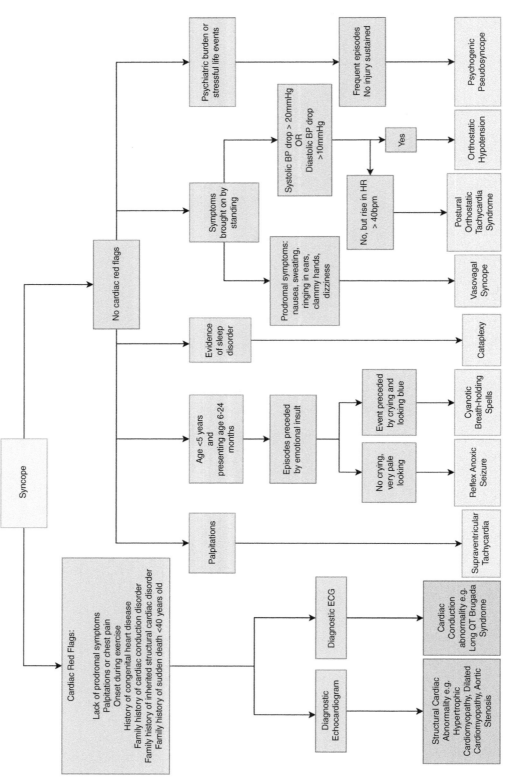

Figure 2.3.1 Diagnostic algorithm for the presentation of syncope.

2.3.4 DIFFERENTIALS LIST

> **Box 2.3.2   Mechanisms of Cardiac Syncope**
>
> Cardiac conditions that lead to abrupt decrease in cardiac output can cause syncope. In general, this happens through one of two mechanisms:
>
> - **Decreased stroke volume:** tends to be related to arrhythmias, usually tachyarrhythmias (bradyarrhythmias very uncommon in children). Conditions resulting in poor contractility, such as myocarditis, also fit into this category
> - **Left ventricular outflow tract obstruction:** compromised systemic blood flow leads to cerebral hypoperfusion

Dangerous Diagnoses

1. Cardiac Conduction Abnormalities
- Inherited conduction abnormalities are caused by genetic mutations in the myocardial ion channels (usually sodium, potassium and calcium channels)
- Genetic mutations are predominantly autosomal dominant, but with variable expression and penetrance
- These predispose the patient to arrhythmias, particularly ventricular tachycardia, which can present as symptoms of syncope, palpitations, chest pain and even sudden cardiac death
- In addition to inherited abnormalities, acquired long QT syndromes may arise from electrolyte disturbances. These are commonly seen in patients with eating disorders. Changes typically resolve as nutrition is restored

> **Box 2.3.3   Inherited Cardiac Conduction Abnormalities That Can Cause Syncope**
>
> Long QT syndrome:
>
> - Prolonged QT interval (over 450 ms in males and 460 ms in females)
> - Causes episodes of ventricular tachycardia (VT), specifically a polymorphic VT called torsades de pointes
> - Usually presents with syncope, or less commonly palpitations or sudden cardiac death
> - Mean age of first presentation is 8 years in boys and 14 years in girls
>
> Brugada syndrome:
>
> - Associated with high risk of ventricular fibrillation (VF) and sudden cardiac death
> - Arrhythmia can be brought out by fever
> - Presents with supraventricular or ventricular tachycardia (SVT or VT), syncope or sudden death
> - There are specific electrocardiogram (ECG) features of ST segment elevation in V1 or V2, but changes can vary from day to day. Repeat recordings with stress testing may be required to confirm the diagnosis
>
> Catecholaminergic polymorphic ventricular tachycardia (CPVT):
>
> - Presents with recurrent abrupt syncope or sudden death
> - CPVT can first present at any age, but most commonly <10 years old
> - Episodes are usually induced by exercise or emotional events
> - ECG is usually normal at rest with occasional sinus bradycardia, so exercise stress testing is very useful in diagnosis
>
> Short QT syndrome:
>
> - Highly lethal and very rare
> - Shortened QT interval caused by early repolarisation predisposes to ventricular arrhythmias
> - 40% of patients will be asymptomatic. Otherwise, presentation may be with dizziness, syncope or sudden cardiac death
> - Neonates specifically present with atrial fibrillation and bradycardia, requiring a pacemaker insertion
> - Arrhythmias are usually triggered by exercise, but can also happen at rest

2. Structural Cardiac Abnormalities
- Any structural abnormality that causes a reduced cardiac output can cause syncope
- Conditions can be inherited or acquired
- The most common mechanism is left ventricular outflow tract obstruction (LVOT)
- Other mechanisms include impaired contractility, myocardial ischaemia or arrhythmia
- Structural heart disease may remain asymptomatic until presentation with syncope or sudden death. The majority of sudden death in athletes is due to underlying structural heart disease

Box 2.3.4   Structural Cardiac Abnormalities That Can Cause Syncope   △△

Hypertrophic cardiomyopathy:

- Hypertrophic cardiomyopathy (HCM) is defined as left ventricular hypertrophy that occurs without ventricular dilatation, in the absence of other explanatory cardiac or systemic disease
- Usually due to an autosomal dominant inherited mutation in a sarcomere gene
- Presents with exertional syncope, chest pain and sudden cardiac death
- Often asymptomatic until adolescence or adulthood
- Most common cause of sudden death in young athletes

Dilated cardiomyopathy:

- Dilated cardiomyopathy (DCM) is the most common form of cardiomyopathy in children
- Characterised by progressive left ventricular dilatation and systolic dysfunction
- Wide range of aetiologies, although two-thirds are idiopathic. Known causes include acute myocarditis, neuromuscular conditions and inborn errors of metabolism
- Presents in the first year of life with congestive heart failure

- Syncope is a less common first presentation
- Poor prognosis: 40% of children require heart transplants or die within 5 years of diagnosis

Coronary artery abnormalities:

- Congenital coronary artery abnormalities include anomalous left coronary artery, where the artery courses between the aorta and pulmonary artery. Compression between these great arteries causes exertional myocardial ischaemia and syncope

Aortic stenosis:

- Severe aortic stenosis causes reduced systemic blood flow, and can cause syncope, particularly during exercise, where demand outweighs supply
- These patients may also have exertional angina, as prolonged systole reduces coronary filling time

Acute myocarditis:

- Myocarditis is an acquired condition, usually due to a viral infection with Coxsackie A/B or adenovirus
- Inflammation of the myocardium impairs contractility and can predispose to arrhythmias

Common Diagnoses

1. Vasovagal Syncope

- Also known as reflex or neurocardiogenic syncope. Accounts for 75% of all paediatric syncope presentations
- Peak incidence is between 15 and 19 years, more common in girls
- Exaggerated alterations in vasomotor tone and heart rate (designed to maintain blood pressure) lead to vasodilation, bradycardia and hypotension, which cause transient cerebral hypoperfusion
- Jerking movements can be unexpectedly marked and mistaken for seizures
- Recovery following syncopal episodes is quick without any confusion (in contrast to postictal phase after epileptic seizures); however, patients can often feel tired afterwards and younger children may go to sleep soon after regaining consciousness

2. Breath-Holding Spells/Reflex Anoxic Seizures

- Believed to be forms of vasovagal syncope seen in young children
- Triggered by an emotional stress – fear, startle or pain, often from a minor injury
- Breath-holding spells are known as 'cyanotic' spells. Reflex anoxic seizures are known as 'pallid' spells. Duration is <1 minute with spontaneous resolution
- Both are benign conditions that do not predispose to epilepsy. Jerking movements may be mistaken for epileptic seizures
- 30% have a family history of similar episodes in childhood
- Age of onset is usually 6–24 months in cyanotic breath-holding and 12–24 months for reflex anoxic seizures. They tend to stop by 5 years of age

3. Orthostatic Hypotension (OH)

- OH is the drop in systolic blood pressure on standing upright
- Usually caused by inadequate increase of total peripheral resistance or heart rate in response to the postural change
- A significant drop in systolic blood pressure (BP) can cause cerebral hypoperfusion and syncope
- Symptoms are often worse after waking up, after meals or after exercise
- It can be exacerbated by hypovolaemia, anaemia, pregnancy and medications

4. Postural Orthostatic Tachycardia Syndrome (POTS)

- POTS is a syndrome in which there are symptoms of orthostatic intolerance or syncope on sitting/standing upright due to autonomic dysfunction. There is an excessive rise in heart rate on standing; however, in contrast to OH, there is no drop in systolic BP
- Exacerbating factors are dehydration, heat, prolonged bed rest, menstruation and alcohol. There is significant diurnal variation, with worse symptoms in the morning
- Associated with other conditions such as chronic fatigue syndrome, irritable bowel syndrome, Ehlers–Danlos syndrome and autoimmune disorders

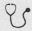

> **Box 2.3.5   Defining Criteria for Orthostatic Hypotension and Postural Orthostatic Tachycardia Syndrome (POTS)**
>
> Orthostatic hypotension:
> - Sustained decrease in systolic blood pressure >20 mmHg or diastolic >10 mmHg within 3 minutes of standing
>
> POTS:
> - *Either* an increase in heart rate (HR) >40 bpm (or absolute HR >120 bpm) within 10 minutes of sitting/standing upright without orthostatic hypotension
>
> - *Or* a history of symptoms of orthostatic intolerance that are relieved by lying down

Diagnoses to Consider

1. Psychogenic Pseudosyncope (PPS)

- PPS is the appearance of transient loss of consciousness in the absence of true loss of consciousness
- Eyes tend to be closed or deviated away from the witness, which is less common with true syncope, and recovery tends to be immediate
- It is considered to be part of a conversion (also known as functional) disorder, rather than intentional malingering

When to consider: in patients with co-existing psychiatric burden or stressful life events, particularly in girls

2. Supraventricular Tachycardia (SVT)

- SVTs are the most common arrhythmias in children, although they rarely present with syncope as their defining feature
- If syncope is present in SVT, it increases the risk of sudden cardiac death
- Presyncope (light-headedness) and syncope are due to reduced cardiac output during a rhythm disturbance
- Most tachyarrhythmia is paroxysmal and so does not lead to heart failure, but it can do if prolonged >48 hours

When to consider: in patients experiencing palpitations with sudden onset and offset of symptoms

3. Cataplexy

- A symptom of narcolepsy where there is sudden, uncontrollable skeletal muscle paralysis or loss of tone
- It is not actually syncope, as although it is brief with full recovery, the patient remains alert and has full memory of the episode
- Muscle weakness in cataplexy is emotionally triggered. Triggering emotions are more commonly positive than negative, such as laughter, excitement or surprise, and patients can often sense an impending episode

When to consider: in those with known narcolepsy or with features of a sleep disorder such as daytime sleepiness, sleep paralysis or vivid hallucinations on falling asleep

2.3.5 KEY HISTORY FEATURES

In addition to the usual paediatric history, all children with syncope should have the following elicited. With the advent of smart phones, many witnesses (parents, carers, schoolteachers) will be able to capture video footage of the episode(s) to help diagnosis.

1. Detailed description of the event from patient and witnesses:

Before	• Environment: was it hot, loud, stressful, emotional? • Actions: were there unusual movements or behaviours? • Posture: how was the patient positioned? • Prodrome: does the patient remember any specific symptoms, or were these voiced to witnesses?
During	• Appearance: colour, eyes open or closed, abnormal movements or postures, incontinence, tongue biting • Duration of loss of consciousness
After	• Duration of recovery • Symptoms: was there confusion, tiredness, chest pain, shortness of breath? • Memory: how much of the episode can be recalled?

2. Previous history of similar episodes:
- How many previous episodes
- Similar or different phenotype
- Frequency of episodes
- Environmental similarities or suspected trigger

3. Family history:
- History of similar episodes in family members (may have to ask grandparents)
- Family history of sudden death

Dangerous Diagnosis 1
Diagnosis: Cardiac conduction abnormalities

Questions
1. **Did the episode start during exercise or emotional stress?** Catecholaminergic polymorphic ventricular tachycardia (CPVT) and short QT are both usually triggered by exercise or emotional stress. It is important to clarify if it occurred *during* exercise, as vasovagal syncope can sometimes occur immediately after exercise
2. **Did the episode occur early in the morning or after a large meal?** In Brugada syndrome, arrhythmias usually occur during sleep or early morning and particularly after a large meal. Fevers can also be a trigger
3. **Was the onset sudden, or was there chest pain or palpitations immediately before the loss of consciousness?** Cardiac syncope is suggested by chest pain or palpitations prior to loss of consciousness, or syncope occurring suddenly without any prodromal symptoms
4. **Is there a family history of arrhythmias, sudden cardiac or unexplained death <40 years old?** Long QT, Brugada, CPVT and short QT are all inherited conditions with predominantly autosomal dominant inheritance, so there is often a family history suggestive of arrhythmias

---

Box 2.3.6   Triggers for Long QT (LQT)

Taking a history for LQT can be challenging, because different types have different triggers:

- LQT1: events are more commonly triggered by exercise (particularly swimming)
- LQT2: events occur in response to emotional stress or during sleep/rest
- LQT3: the majority of arrhythmias occur during sleep/rest

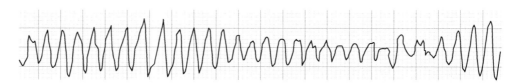

Figure 2.3.2 Torsade de pointes is a polymorphic form of ventricular tachycardia of which patients with long QT syndrome are at risk.

Dangerous Diagnosis 2
Diagnosis: Structural cardiac abnormalities

Questions
1. **Was the episode during exercise?** Syncope from structural cardiac abnormalities are commonly exercise induced, as the heart struggles to meet the increased demands for higher cardiac output.
2. **Were there any symptoms just before the loss of consciousness?** Syncope may be associated with chest pain. If symptoms occurred at rest, it is more likely that there was an arrhythmia, so ask about palpitations
3. **Any previous history of congenital heart disease or cardiac surgery?** Previous congenital heart disease repair can increase the risk of arrhythmias
4. **Any underlying conditions, such as neuromuscular disorders, inborn errors of metabolism or Noonan syndrome, which can be associated with cardiomyopathies?** These conditions may make a diagnosis of cardiomyopathy more likely. The aetiology can also be important in prognostication and treatment, particularly in dilated cardiomyopathy
5. **Is there a family history of structural heart defects (cardiomyopathies or congenital heart disease), sudden cardiac or unexplained death at <40 years old?** Hypertrophic cardiomyopathy and dilated cardiomyopathy can both be inherited (usually autosomal dominant) and so a family history of cardiomyopathy is very important

---

Box 2.3.7   Red Flags for Cardiac Syncope

- Lack of prodromal symptoms
- Palpitations or chest pain during exercise
- History of congenital heart disease
- Family history of arrhythmia, sudden cardiac or unexplained death at <40 years old

Common Diagnosis 1
Diagnosis: Vasovagal syncope

Questions
1. **Have any possible triggers been identified?** Common triggers include prolonged standing, hot environment, fear, pain or blood phobia. There may be 'situational' syncope, which is a reproducible type of vasovagal syncope in response to a predictable precipitant. Triggers include micturition, coughing, sneezing, swallowing and defecation
2. **Were there any prodromal features?** Vasovagal syncope is usually preceded by non-specific prodromal symptoms, including dizziness, nausea, light-headedness, pallor, sweating, palpitations, visual changes and muffled hearing
3. **Were there any abnormal movements?** Contrary to popular belief, vasovagal syncope can be associated with jerking limb movements. These do not have rhythmicity suggestive of a seizure, but can lead to significant anxiety. Videos are very useful
4. **What was the duration?** The duration is short, usually less than a minute, with prompt recovery on assuming the supine position

Common Diagnosis 2
Diagnosis: Breath-holding spells/reflex anoxic seizures

Questions
1. **What is the age of the patient?** Breath-holding spells/reflex anoxic seizures occur in very young children, typically first presenting between 6 to 24 months and usually resolving by 5 years old
2. **Was the episode triggered by an emotional insult?** Breath-holding spells/reflex anoxic seizures are usually triggered by an emotional stress – fear, anger, startle or pain, often from a minor injury
3. **Did the child appear well beforehand?** Patients are usually described as completely well just prior to the event
4. **What behaviour was observed at the start of the event?** Cyanotic breath-holding spells start with crying, whereas reflex anoxic seizures start with a sharp inhalation. Convulsive movements can sometimes be seen
5. **Family history of similar events?** 30% of children diagnosed with reflex anoxic seizures have a family history of similar events in childhood

---

Box 2.3.8   Clinical History of Breath-Holding Spells Compared with Reflex Anoxic Seizures

Cyanotic breath-holding spells	Pallid reflex anoxic seizures
• Initiated by loud crying • Child becomes apnoeic, cyanotic, *then* loses consciousness	• Start silently or with a short gasp • Child becomes pale and loses consciousness, *before* becoming apnoeic and hypotonic

---

Common Diagnosis 3
Diagnosis: Orthostatic hypotension

Questions
1. **Was there a change in position prior to the event?** Syncope from OH occurs just after standing or sitting upright.
2. **Were there prodromal symptoms?** Patients often describe prodromal symptoms similar to those seen in vasovagal syncope, particularly light-headedness and nausea
3. **Any history suggesting an underlying cause for orthostatic hypotension?** There are several predispositions to OH, described in Box 2.3.9

Box 2.3.9   Causes for Orthostatic Hypotension

Mechanism	Examples
Hypovolaemia	Diarrhoea, vomiting, blood loss
Medications altering vasomotor tone/heart rate	Calcium channel blockers, diuretics
Reduced oxygen-carrying capacity of blood	Anaemia
Autonomic nervous system dysfunction	Diabetes, familial dysautonomia
Venous pooling	Pregnancy

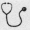

Box 2.3.10   Lifestyle Modifications for Benign Causes of Syncope

- Identify triggers and aim to avoid them
- Cross legs, tense gluteal muscles to increase venous return and improve blood flow to the brain
- Exercise regularly: increases circulatory volume
- Adequate water intake
- Adequate salt intake
- Avoid sudden changes in posture
- Avoid prolonged recumbency
- Avoid exercise in high temperatures
- Avoid large meals
- Avoid skipping meals

Common Diagnosis 4
Diagnosis: Postural orthostatic tachycardia syndrome

Questions
Questions about precipitating events and prodromal symptoms are similar to those for OH. The diagnosis is differentiated by observations: rise in heart rate without BP drop.
1. **Any history of chronic conditions?** POTS has been associated with Ehlers–Danlos syndrome, chronic fatigue syndrome, irritable bowel syndrome and autoimmune disorders

2.3.6 KEY EXAMINATION FEATURES

All patients presenting with syncope should have full cardiovascular and neurological examinations.

Dangerous Diagnosis 1
Diagnosis: Cardiac conduction abnormalities

Examination Findings
1. **Normal examination.** Examination findings are usually normal in conduction abnormalities, unless an arrhythmia occurs at the time of examination
2. **Signs of ongoing arrhythmia.** If there is ongoing haemodynamically significant arrhythmia, syncope, tachycardia, weak pulse and cool peripheries may be observed
3. **Low Body Mass Index (BMI).** Acquired long QT may result from electrolyte abnormalities, commonly seen in patients with eating disorders

Dangerous Diagnosis 2
Diagnosis: Structural cardiac abnormalities

Examination Findings
1. **Systolic murmur.** An ejection systolic murmur indicates left ventricular outflow obstruction – seen in hypertrophic cardiomyopathy (HCM) and aortic stenosis. A pansystolic murmur suggests mitral regurgitation – seen in HCM
2. **Prominent apex beat.** HCM can cause a more prominent, forceful apex beat due to left ventricular hypertrophy
3. **Signs of heart failure.** Pulmonary oedema causes respiratory distress and crackles on auscultation. Hepatic congestion causes hepatomegaly. Chronic respiratory symptoms and high calorie requirements mean many children are small for age

Common Diagnosis 1
Diagnosis: Vasovagal syncope

Examination Findings
1. **Normal examination in a teenager.** Unless examined at the time of syncope, examination will be normal.
2. **Bystanders/paramedic staff observation.** Observers of an episode may note pallor, cold and clammy skin, a slow weak pulse, dilated pupils and occasionally jerking of all limbs

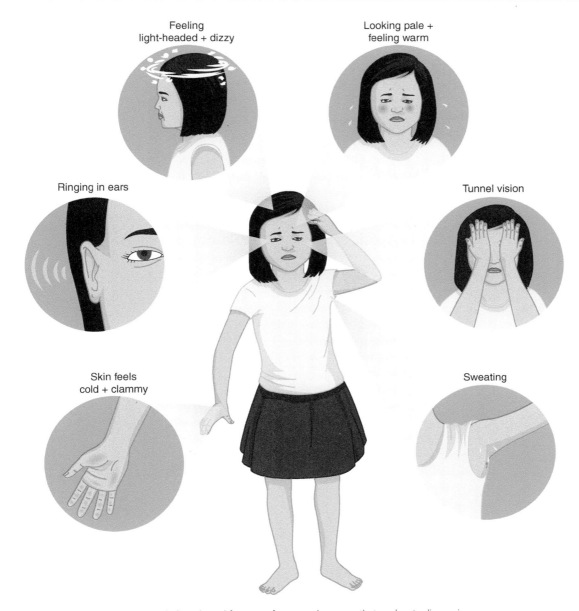

Feeling
light-headed + dizzy

Looking pale +
feeling warm

Ringing in ears

Tunnel vision

Skin feels
cold + clammy

Sweating

Figure 2.3.3 There are several stereotypical prodromal features of vasovagal syncope that are key to diagnosis.

Common Diagnosis 2
Diagnosis: Breath-holding spells/reflex anoxic seizures

Examination Findings
1. Normal examination in a young child. Between episodes, examination will be normal

Common Diagnosis 3
Diagnosis: Orthostatic hypotension

Examination Findings
1. Abnormal lying–standing BP. Diagnostic criteria: sustained decrease in systolic BP >20 mmHg or diastolic >10 mmHg within 3 minutes of standing

Common Diagnosis 4
Diagnosis: Postural orthostatic tachycardia syndrome

Examination Findings
1. **Abnormal lying–standing heart rate.** Diagnostic criteria: there must be a heart rate (HR) rise of >40 bpm (or absolute HR >120 bpm) within 10 minutes of standing upright, but no significant BP drop

2.3.7 KEY INVESTIGATIONS

Most often, if history and examination are reassuring, and the bedside investigations are normal, no further invasive testing is required.

Bedside

Table 2.3.1 Bedside tests of use in patients presenting with syncope

Test	When to perform	Potential result
12-lead ECG	• All children with syncope • To identify conduction abnormalities or LVH	• QT long (>450 ms) or short (<300 ms) • HCM: LVH
Supine and standing blood pressure and heart rate	Suspected: • OH • POTS	• Systolic drop of >20 mmHg or diastolic drop of >10 mmHg indicates OH • Heart rate rise >40 bpm without BP drop indicates POTS
Pregnancy test	• Consider in new syncopal episodes in post-menstrual females	• Urinary HCG positive confirms pregnancy

BP, blood pressure; ECG, electrocardiogram; HCG, human chorionic gonadotropin; HCM, hypertrophic cardiomyopathy; LVH, left ventricular hypertrophy; OH, orthostatic hypotension; POTS, postural orthostatic tachycardia syndrome.

Blood Tests

Table 2.3.2 Blood tests of use in patients presenting with syncope

Test	When to perform	Potential result
FBC	• Suspected anaemia. Anaemia can increase episodes of vasovagal syncope	• Anaemia • ↓ MCV suggests iron deficiency
Iron studies	• Microcytic anaemia – commonest cause of ↓MCV is iron deficiency	• ↓ Serum iron, ↓ferritin, ↑ transferrin/total iron binding capacity confirms iron-deficiency anaemia
TFTs	• Suspected POTS with tachycardia, to rule out hyperthyroidism	• ↓TSH and ↑T4 suggests hyperthyroidism
U&E, LFTs, calcium, phosphate, magnesium	• Suspected cardiac conduction abnormalities, particularly if concurrent eating disorder	• ↓ Na^+, ↓K^+, ↓Ca^{2+}, ↓PO^{3-} and ↓ Mg^{2+} in anorexia • ↑ LFTs seen during refeeding.

Ca, calcium; FBC, full blood count; K, potassium; LFTs, liver function tests; MCV, mean corpuscular volume; Mg, magnesium; Na, sodium; PO, phosphate; POTS, postural orthostatic tachycardia syndrome; TFTs, thyroid function tests; TSH, thyroid-stimulating hormone; U&E, urea and electrolytes

Imaging
Routine imaging is low yield, unless history or physical examination suggests concurrent illness, such as heart failure.

Special

Table 2.3.3 Special tests of use in patients presenting with syncope

Test	When to perform	Potential result
Echocardiogram	• Suspected structural cardiac disease, to look for LV abnormalities, assessment of LVOT obstruction, assessment of heart failure	• Dilated cardiomyopathy ± impaired systolic function • Hypertrophic cardiomyopathy ± impaired diastolic function • Aortic stenosis or LVOT obstruction
Ambulatory ECG	• To pick up paroxysmal arrhythmias. Several types of ambulatory monitors	• May reveal intermittent arrythmias, e.g. SVT. Can correlate events to a symptom diary
Exercise stress testing	• To precipitate and identify conduction abnormalities	• May reveal Brugada syndrome and CPVT, which often have a normal ECG at rest
Head-up tilt testing	• For unexplained clinically significant syncope, to reproduce postural changes in controlled environment. Practice varies significantly across centres	• Vasovagal syncope • Orthostatic hypotension • POTS

CPVT, catecholaminergic polymorphic ventricular tachycardia; ECG, electrocardiogram; LV, left ventricle; LVOT, left ventricular outflow tract; POTS, postural orthostatic tachycardia syndrome; SVT, supraventricular tachycardia

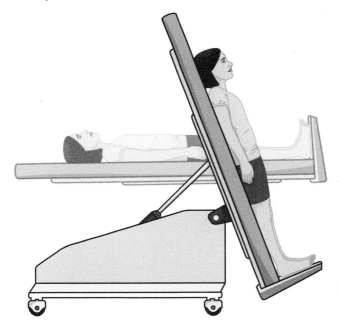

Figure 2.3.4 The tilt-table test. Procedure: the child lies on a bed and is secured to it. The bed is moved slowly from a horizontal to a vertical position, so that the child moves from supine to vertical. Heart rate and blood pressure monitoring is undertaken during this transition to evaluate any drops in systolic and/or diastolic blood pressure, allowing correlation with clinical symptoms of dizziness or syncope. The severity of symptoms, degree in variation of heart rate and blood pressure, and the time taken for onset and offset are analysed together to make a diagnosis.

2.3.8 KEY MANAGEMENT PRINCIPLES

Diagnosis-specific management strategies are outlined here. It is expected that an 'ABCDE' approach to assessment and management is always undertaken (see Chapter 12.1, *The A to E Assessment*).

Dangerous Diagnosis 1
Diagnosis: Cardiac conduction abnormalities

Management Principles
Any patient with red flags for cardiac syncope in history, family history or electrocardiogram (ECG) should be urgently referred to cardiology, who will determine investigations and management. General principles include:

1. Medical management
2. Risk reduction
3. Screening for family members
4. Risk stratification and prevention of sudden cardiac death

Dangerous Diagnosis 2
Diagnosis: Structural cardiac abnormalities

Management Principles
Any patient with red flags for cardiac syncope in history, family history or ECG should be urgently referred to cardiology, who will determine investigations and management. General principles are included here.
1. **HCM: risk reduction.** Treatment in HCM revolves around improving LVOT obstruction. Beta blockers prolong diastole, increase left ventricular filling and hence reduce the obstructive effects. Beta blockers have been shown to reduce risk of sudden cardiac death in HCM. Septal myomectomy may be considered to reduce obstruction if medical management is not effective
2. **DCM: risk reduction.** The majority of patients with DCM have congestive heart failure on presentation and management is centred on this. Medical options include diuretics, beta blockers, angiotensin-converting enzyme (ACE) inhibitors and aldosterone antagonists. In some cases, i.e. inborn errors of metabolism, treatment of the underlying cause can reduce the progression of DCM
3. **Risk stratification and prevention of sudden cardiac death.** Risk stratification guides the decision for implantable cardioverter-defibrillator (ICD) insertion and is condition dependent
4. **Screening for family members.** HCM is most commonly autosomal dominant and so screening is advised for close family members. Only 5% of DCM is due to familial genetic mutations. However, the majority of these mutations have autosomal dominant inheritance and so if there is a known genetic mutation, close family members should be screened
5. **Heart transplant.** Heart transplant is the final management option for progressive heart failure despite treatment

Common Diagnosis 1
Diagnosis: Vasovagal syncope

Management Principles
1. **Reassurance and information.** Vasovagal syncope is benign, but can be troubling for patients and parents. Reassurance is key. It might be helpful to offer a follow-up if anxiety levels are high. The website for STARS (Syncope Trust And Reflex anoxic Seizures; https://www.heartrhythmalliance.org/stars/uk) can be a useful source of information and advice for families
2. **Prevention of future syncopal episodes.** It is important to explain how to identify triggers and avoid further episodes. Patients often achieve symptom control by increasing their fluid and salt intake, particularly in hot weather or when exercising
3. **Iron supplementation.** Anaemia has been implicated in vasovagal syncope, breath-holding spells and reflex anoxic seizures, and so iron supplementation if anaemic may help to reduce episodes

Common Diagnosis 2
Diagnosis: Breath-holding spells/reflex anoxic seizures

Management Principles
1. **Reassurance.** Both cyanotic and pallid episodes can be very frightening to witness. Reassure parents that the spells are not associated with serious outcomes such as sudden infant death, and usually resolve by 4–5 years of age. Suggest the STARS website to those with reflex anoxic seizures
2. **Iron supplementation.** As above, iron supplementation if anaemic may help to reduce syncopal episodes

Common Diagnosis 3
Diagnosis: Orthostatic hypotension

Management Principles
1. **Reassurance.** Reassure parents that there is no serious cardiac or neurological disease
2. **Optimise underlying predispositions.** Avoid dehydration – it can be helpful to give specific fluid targets. Undertake a medication review and, if possible, adjust possible culprits
3. **Lifestyle strategies.** Simple lifestyle measures can be advised, as outlined in Box 2.3.10.

Common Diagnosis 4
Diagnosis: Postural orthostatic tachycardia syndrome

Management Principles
1. **Reassurance.** Reassure parents that there is no serious cardiac or neurological disease
2. **Lifestyle strategies.** Simple lifestyle measures can be advised, as outlined in Box 2.3.10
3. **Compression stockings.** Compression stockings facilitate venous return from the legs, but they are often not well tolerated

2.4 Chest Pain

Emily Operto

Department of Paediatrics, The Royal Brompton Hospital, London, UK

CONTENTS

2.4.1 CHAPTER AT A GLANCE

> **Box 2.4.1 Chapter at a Glance**
>
> - Chest pain is a common presenting complaint in children
> - Although 95–99% of children will have a benign cause for their pain, it is important to identify those with life-threatening conditions that require acute intervention
> - A reassuring history and examination are usually enough to exclude dangerous diagnoses, without the need for invasive investigations
>
> - Chest pain is associated with great societal anxiety, being known as a symptom of serious heart disease in adults
> - Children and their families may also feel significant anxiety, which can impact greatly on quality of life through restriction of activities and school absences. Management of benign conditions requires addressing these concerns

2.4.2 DEFINITION

Chest pain is pain that is felt anywhere in the body cavity between the neck and the diaphragm. This chapter will focus on non-traumatic chest pain only.

2.4.3 DIAGNOSTIC ALGORITHM

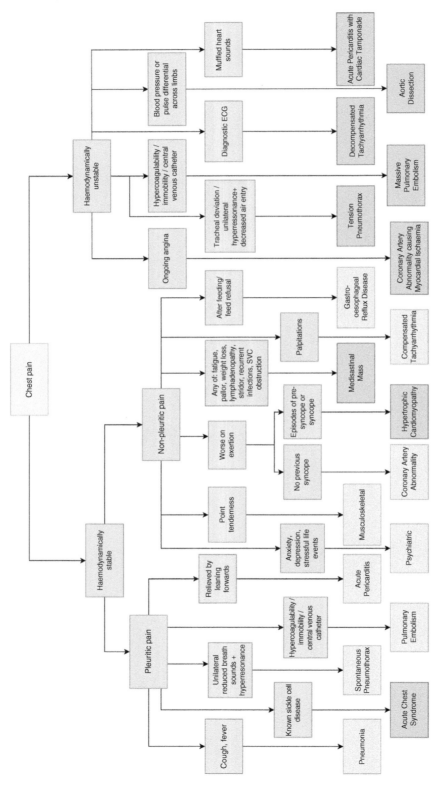

Figure 2.4.1 Diagnostic algorithm for the presentation of chest pain.

2.4.4 DIFFERENTIALS LIST

Dangerous Diagnoses

1. Hypertrophic Cardiomyopathy (HCM)
- HCM is an inherited disease (usually autosomal dominant) characterised by left ventricular hypertrophy, caused by mutations in a variety of sarcomere genes
- Syncope, shortness of breath and exertional chest pain are characteristic
- Chest pain is due to decreased coronary blood flow, causing angina
- Any other heart disease with left ventricular outflow tract obstruction (LVOT), such as aortic stenosis, may cause chest pain in a similar manner
- HCM is the commonest cause of sudden cardiac death in young people and athletes

2. Acute Chest Syndrome (ACS)
- ACS occurs in patients with sickle cell disease (SCD) and can have fatal consequences
- It is caused by sickling of red blood cells in the pulmonary vasculature, vaso-occlusion, ischaemia and endothelial injury
- The highest incidence of ACS is in children <10 years of age
- The trigger is commonly infection in children, but can also be due to pulmonary fat embolism and infarction
- Diagnosis relies on radiographical confirmation of a new pulmonary infiltrate in addition to one symptom from chest pain, fever or respiratory (increased work of breathing, wheeze, cough and hypoxia)

3. Aortic Dissection
- Aortic dissection occurs when tears in the intimal layer of the aorta result in blood entering the intima-media space
- Severe tearing chest pain radiating to the neck or back is characteristic
- Predispositions include Marfan syndrome, homocystinuria, Ehlers–Danlos syndrome and Turner syndrome
- Type A involves the ascending aorta, and is more likely to cause fatal rupture. Type B involves the descending aorta and can lead to downstream organ effects, but is less likely to result in a fatal bleed

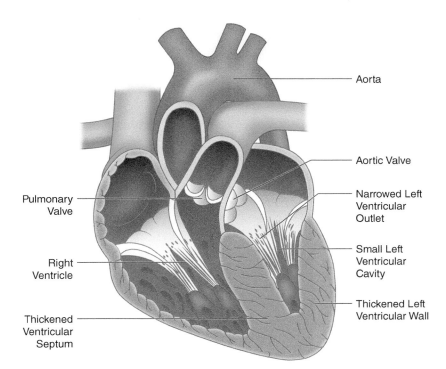

Figure 2.4.2 Hypertrophic cardiomyopathy causes a thickened left ventricular wall and ventricular septum, without dilatation. This effectively narrows the left ventricular outlet.

Common Diagnoses

1. Acute Pericarditis

- Pericarditis is inflammation of the pericardium
- Characteristically results in chest pain that worsens during inspiration or lying flat and improves with leaning forwards
- It is most often caused by viruses (e.g. Coxsackie B, echovirus and adenovirus)
- Additional causative conditions include tuberculosis (TB), human immunodeficiency virus (HIV), recent cardiac surgery, malignancy or trauma
- Acute pericarditis generally has a good prognosis, unless there is cardiac tamponade from pericardial effusion, which is uncommon – 1–2% of cases
- This chapter will not cover purulent pericarditis, a consequence of bacterial pericarditis that rarely causes chest pain and is frequently fatal

Box 2.4.2   Difference between Myocarditis and Pericarditis   △△

	Myocarditis	**Pericarditis**
Disease process	• Inflammation of the myocardium – the heart muscle	• Inflammation of the pericardium – the lining of the heart
Cause	• Usually infection (viral, bacterial or fungal) • Idiopathic	• Infection (usually viral) • Recent cardiac surgery • Non-infectious inflammatory condition, e.g. rheumatological, malignancy • Idiopathic
Chest pain	• Uncommon, unless concomitant pericarditis	• Strongly associated

2. Musculoskeletal Pain

- This accounts for approximately 30% of cases of chest pain in children
- There may be a prior history of trauma, or strenuous chest muscle exercise, but non-traumatic pain is common on its own
- Aetiologies include costochondritis, precordial catch, slipping rib syndrome and fibromyalgia

3. Gastro-oesophageal Reflux Disease (GORD)

- GORD occurs when gastric contents pass into the oesophagus and result in symptoms or complications
- It can cause burning retrosternal chest pain, epigastric pain and difficulty swallowing
- Pain may last minutes to hours and is often associated with meals
- Non-verbal children may present by pounding their chest, self-injurious behaviours (particularly in autism) or as Sandifer syndrome (spasmodic dystonic movements involving arching of the back and posturing of the neck)

4. Psychiatric

- Up to 30% of chest pain is likely to have a psychosomatic cause
- A supportive history underpins this diagnosis

5. Pneumonia

- Chest infection is a common cause of acute paediatric chest pain
- Cough may cause muscle strain, and consolidation itself may cause pleuritic chest pain
- Pneumonia is covered in Chapter 1.3, and will not be discussed further in this chapter

6. Spontaneous Pneumothorax

- Spontaneous pneumothorax is the presence of air in the space between the visceral and the parietal lung pleura
- Results in acute, sharp chest pain and shortness of breath
- Typically occurs in tall, thin male adolescents. Other risk factors include parenchymal lung disease, connective tissue disease (e.g. Marfan or Ehlers–Danlos syndromes), scuba diving, recreational drug use and smoking
- Progression to tension pneumothorax is possible, although not common
- Pneumothorax is covered in Chapter 1.3, and will not be discussed further in this chapter

Box 2.4.3   Musculoskeletal Chest Pain   △△

Differential	Details
Costochondritis	• Point tenderness in the costal cartilages at their joint with the sternum • Can be unilateral or bilateral • No swelling detectable on examination
Precordial catch	• Short, sharp episodes of point tenderness at the cardiac apex or left sternal border • Aetiology is not well understood
Slipping rib syndrome	• Pain caused by impingement on the intercostal nerves by ribs 8–10, when their fibrous connections to each other are weakened
Fibromyalgia	• Common cause of chronic widespread pain • Although it occasionally presents with isolated chest pain, there are usually multiple loci for pain, and associated symptoms of fatigue and cognitive disturbance • Aetiology is not well understood

Diagnoses to Consider
1. Tachyarrhythmias
- Most tachyarrhythmias are initially painless and well tolerated, but if prolonged may cause angina due to reduced coronary filling
- There may be associated palpitations, or children might interpret palpitations as pain
- The most common tachyarrhythmia is supraventricular tachycardia (SVT)

When to consider: in those with palpitations or syncope, associated with sudden onset and offset of symptoms

2. Pulmonary Embolism (PE)
- PEs are rare in children and there is almost always a predisposing risk factor
- The majority of PEs in children do not have haemodynamic effects
- PEs are usually caused by thrombi that originate in the deep veins of the leg
- Characterised by acute-onset pleuritic chest pain, tachycardia and shortness of breath
- A massive PE can cause cardiorespiratory collapse

When to consider: in a patient with acute-onset chest pain and dyspnoea, with predisposing risk factors – see Box 2.4.4.

Box 2.4.4   Risk Factors for Pulmonary Embolism

- Diseases causing a hypercoagulable state, e.g. sickle cell disease, thrombophilias, malignancy
- Recent surgery
- Trauma
- Immobilisation
- Central venous access device
- Dehydration
- Obesity

3. Coronary Artery Abnormalities
- Myocardial infarction is very rare in children, but must be considered if there are underlying coronary artery abnormalities, of which there are several types
- Children can present with typical angina – 'crushing' substernal chest pain, radiation to the left arm, sweating, nausea, vomiting and shortness of breath
- Congenital coronary artery abnormalities include anomalous left coronary artery, where the artery courses between the aorta and pulmonary artery. Compression between these great arteries causes exertional chest pain and even syncope
- Causes include hyperlipidaemia, collagen vascular disease (e.g. systemic lupus erythematosus) and Kawasaki disease, which is associated with coronary artery aneurysm or stenosis
- Coronary vasospasm can be precipitated by use of cocaine, marijuana, amphetamines and synthetic cannabinoids, and is also associated with other vasospastic disorders such as Raynaud's phenomenon or migraine headache

When to consider: if chest pain mainly occurs on exertion, particularly if there is a history of previous Kawasaki or hyperlipidaemia

4. Malignancy
- Chest pain may be caused by mediastinal tumours
- Pain may be due to mass effect on adjacent structures, bleeding within the tumour or rapid growth

- There are usually, but not always, other systemic features of malignancy
- Tumours may be haematological (lymphoma, leukaemia), soft tissue (sarcoma), bony (Ewing's sarcoma) or neuroblastoma. Very occasionally breast masses might affect adolescent females

When to consider: in patients with progressive pain, with systemic features of fevers, weight loss, lymphadenopathy or bone pain

---

Box 2.4.5   Idiopathic Chest Pain

Up to 45% of children with chest pain will be diagnosed with idiopathic chest pain, despite thorough evaluation. Persistence of symptoms is common, and reassurance is important. Symptoms often improve over 3–5 years

---

2.4.5 KEY HISTORY FEATURES

Dangerous Diagnosis 1
Diagnosis: Hypertrophic cardiomyopathy

Questions
1. **Is there a family history of heart disease or sudden death?** There is a family history of cardiomyopathy in approximately 25% of cases. Family history of sudden death under the age of 40 is also suspicious
2. **At what age did the symptoms start?** Clinical symptoms of HCM typically start, or worsen, during puberty
3. **Does chest pain occur with exertion?** Chest pain and disproportionate shortness of breath on exertion make LVOT more likely. There may also be presyncope or syncope during or shortly after exercise
4. **Is there reduced exercise tolerance?** This is normally described as increasing difficulties keeping up in sport, or when playing with friends and siblings, and is suggestive of heart failure

Dangerous Diagnosis 2
Diagnosis: Acute chest syndrome

Questions
1. **Does this patient have suspected or known sickle cell disease?** ACS is a complication of sickle cell disease
2. **Is there a fever?** A temperature >38.5 °C is significant for diagnostic criteria – infection is the most common trigger in children. Patients with sickle cell may well have measured this at home
3. **Are there respiratory symptoms?** Ask about shortness of breath, wheeze or cough
4. **Has there been a recent episode of vaso-occlusive pain?** Vaso-occlusive crisis (VOC) constitutes the main morbidity in patients with sickle cell disease. Almost 50% of ACS occurs within a few days of admission for VOC. Even in those who have not had chest pain at presentation, the immobility, opioid treatment and adjacent pain (e.g. abdominal) lead to hypoventilation and further sickling, precipitating ACS

Dangerous Diagnosis 3
Diagnosis: Aortic dissection

Questions
1. **Was there an abrupt onset to the pain?** Aortic dissection causes sudden-onset pain that is maximal in severity at onset
2. **Is the location of the pain changing?** The evolving dissection may start as anterior chest (ascending aorta) or posterior chest (descending aorta). It can then radiate to the neck, back, flank, abdomen or lower limb due to ischaemia, depending on which arteries become involved
3. **Has there been change in behaviour or cognition?** Aortic dissection can cause neurological deficits in 20% of cases due to involvement of the brachiocephalic, common carotid or intercostal arteries
4. **Is there a known connective tissue disorder?** There is commonly an underlying condition, such as Marfan or Ehlers–Danlos syndrome.
5. **Is there a history of hypertension?** Hypertension is a risk factor for aortic dissection. Primary hypertension is uncommon in children, although it is increasing with childhood obesity. Hypertension is often secondary to renal pathology or endocrine phenomena such as pheochromocytoma

Common Diagnosis 1
Diagnosis: Acute pericarditis

Questions
1. **Is the pain worse on inspiration or lying flat?** Pain is anterior and sharp, worsened by inspiration or lying flat (as both of these actions bring the heart and chest wall into closer contact)
2. **Was there a preceding viral illness or fever?** Pericarditis is most commonly caused by viral infections. There is commonly a low-grade intermittent fever

Common Diagnosis 2
Diagnosis: Musculoskeletal pain

Questions
1. **Can the pain be localised?** Point tenderness is suggestive of musculoskeletal pain. Costo-sternal joint pain is suggestive of costochondritis. Pain at the lower left sternal border or cardiac apex is consistent with precordial catch
2. **Is there pain anywhere else?** Widespread pain suggests fibromyalgia and there may be associated fatigue, sleep disturbance and low mood
3. **Has there been recent muscular strain?** Unaccustomed muscular exertion such as weightlifting may cause chest pain. Muscular strain (e.g. lifting a heavy school bag) also commonly precedes costochondritis
4. **Is the pain constant or intermittent?** Pain of precordial catch tends to be short lasting – seconds to minutes. Costochondritis and slipping rib syndrome may cause intermittent pain

Common Diagnosis 3
Diagnosis: Gastro-oesophageal reflux disease

Questions
1. **How old is the child?** Younger or non-verbal children may be seen to pound their chest. Older children are more likely to describe a burning retrosternal pain that may radiate to the back
2. **Is there food aversion?** Young children may communicate their discomfort by decreased food intake or food aversion
3. **Is there a pattern to the onset of pain?** It usually occurs after meals or awakens the patient from sleep, especially after having eaten a late meal
4. **Does anything relieve the pain?** It may resolve spontaneously or with antacids

Common Diagnosis 4
Diagnosis: Psychiatric

Questions
1. **Have there been recent stressful events?** Ask about illness or death in the family, family separations, exams, school performance, and explore the possibility of bullying
2. **Is there a good quality of sleep?** Sleep disturbance is often an early indicator of psychiatric stress and can cause a vicious cycle of sleep deprivation and stress
3. **Is there a history of non-organic pain?** There may be a history of recurrent non-organic abdominal or limb pain
4. **What does the child think is going on?** Chest pain might represent anxiety or hypochondriasis of a particular disorder. Up to 45% of adolescent patients with chest pain report concern about heart disease or cancer

2.4.6 KEY EXAMINATION FEATURES

Dangerous Diagnosis 1
Diagnosis: Hypertrophic cardiomyopathy

Examination Findings
1. **Systolic murmur.** Patients may develop several types of systolic murmur. The most common are related LVOT (ejection systolic murmur) and mitral regurgitation (apical pan-systolic murmur)
2. **Thrill.** There may be a systolic thrill at the apex or lower left sternal border
3. **Additional heart sounds.** Third or fourth heart sounds are common in young patients
4. **Evidence of heart failure.** Signs include a prominent jugular venous pulse (particularly with a prominent 'a' wave), respiratory distress, crackles on auscultation of the lungs and hepatomegaly

Dangerous Diagnosis 2
Diagnosis: Acute chest syndrome

Examination Findings
1. **Pallor.** Anaemia exacerbates ACS and contributes to hypoxia
2. **Respiratory distress.** Tachypnoea and hypoxia can be marked and there can be rapid progression from mild hypoxia to acute respiratory failure within 24 hours of symptom onset
3. **Change in behaviour or cognition.** Children with SCD are always at risk of neurological complications such as cerebral infarcts and posterior reversible encephalopathy syndrome (PRES). These complications are higher during and after severe ACS. Regular neurological examination should be performed to identify interval change

Dangerous Diagnosis 3
Diagnosis: Aortic dissection

Examination Findings
1. **Hypertension.** Aortic dissection is a cardinal hypertensive emergency, and if haemodynamic stability is preserved, hypertension may still be evident
2. **Pulse or blood pressure differential across limbs.** Subclavian or iliac artery involvement leads to pulse delay (radial–radial/radial–femoral) or blood pressure differential between right arm and other limbs (classic but uncommon finding)
3. **Hypotension.** Late, ominous sign, indicating haemorrhagic shock (from free or contained rupture) or cardiac tamponade (proximal extension)
4. **Muffled heart sounds.** Suggestive of concurrent cardiac tamponade
5. **Neurological deficit – altered mental status.** Cerebral blood flow may be affected, leading to a variety of neurological deficits

Common Diagnosis 1
Diagnosis: Acute pericarditis

Examination Findings
1. **Pericardial rub**. A pericardial rub is highly specific for acute pericarditis. This is a scratching or squeaking sound and is best heard with the diaphragm of a stethoscope over the left sternal border
2. **Patient position.** The patient may naturally be sitting up and leaning forwards to relieve their pain
3. **Muffled heart sounds.** Distant heart sounds suggest secondary pericardial effusion, increasing risk of cardiac tamponade. This is seen in only 1–2% of patients

Common Diagnosis 2
Diagnosis: Musculoskeletal pain

Examination Findings
1. **Reproducible pain.** Pain is replicable with certain movements or application of pressure. In costochondritis, although there is joint pain, there is no joint swelling
2. **Well-localised pain.** Most musculoskeletal pain is well localised, except for fibromyalgia, which may be generalised
3. **Pain on horizontal arm traction.** Pain on horizontal arm traction suggests costochondritis
4. **Pain on chest wall manoeuvres.** This can be done in two ways. Pain on 'passive chest wall stretch' suggests costochondritis. Pain on 'chest wall hooking' suggests slipping rib syndrome
5. **Pain on palpation of a particular muscle.** Indicates chest wall muscle strain

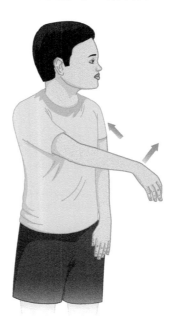

Figure 2.4.3 Horizontal arm traction involves steadily pulling a flexed arm across the patient's chest, while pushing on the opposite shoulder.

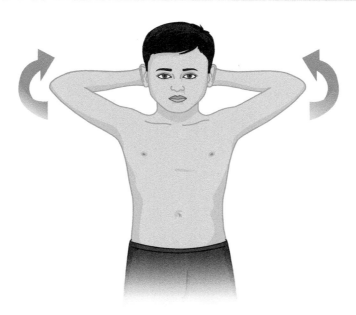

Figure 2.4.4 Passive chest wall stretch, otherwise known as the 'crowing rooster', involves asking the patient to clasp their hands behind their head. The elbows are then passively pulled backwards and upwards.

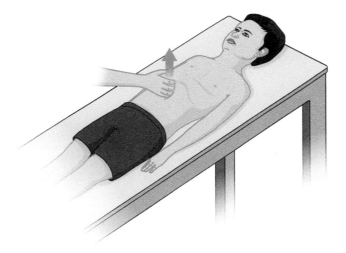

Figure 2.4.5 'Chest wall hooking' involves hooking fingers beneath the costal margin and pulling the ribs forward.

Common Diagnosis 3
Diagnosis: Gastro-oesophageal reflux

Examination Findings
1. **Faltering growth.** Weight and height should be measured and plotted on the appropriate growth chart. Static or slow growth will be reflected as decline from previous centiles
2. **Sandifer syndrome.** This typically occurs in pre-school children and describes specific posturing of back arching with chin lifting. This is only seen during an episode of pain, and parents may have videos
3. **Epigastric pain or diffuse abdominal discomfort.** Children may poorly localise pain from heartburn

Common Diagnosis 4
Diagnosis: Psychiatric

Examination Findings
1. **No signs of organic pathology.** There should be no physical signs indicating other causes of chest pain
2. **Signs of anxiety or depression.** There may be signs alluding to advanced anxiety or depression such as poor eye contact, low mood, limited interactions, hyperactivity or signs of self-harm

2.4.7 KEY INVESTIGATIONS

Not all children will require invasive investigations; often diagnoses are made on clinical evidence from history and examination. Consider carefully which investigations are required for which patient. With a reassuring history, examination and electrocardiogram (ECG), further tests are rarely required.

Bedside

Table 2.4.1 Bedside tests of use in patients presenting with chest pain

Test	When to perform	Potential result
Oxygen saturation	• All children with chest pain • May reveal a need for oxygen supplementation	• Sats <94% indicates hypoxia • Sats 92–94% may be tolerated
ECG	• Essential, non-invasive investigation • Note that the classic 'S1Q3T3' pattern (S wave in V1, Q wave in III and inverted T wave in III) described in PE is actually very rarely seen	• HCM: left ventricular hypertrophy • Aortic dissection: ST depression, less commonly ST elevation • Pericarditis: widespread saddle-shaped ST elevation • Tachyarrhythmia • Coronary vasospasm: ST elevation or depression • PE: Sinus tachycardia
Capillary blood gas (or arterial/venous)	• Only if suspecting dangerous diagnosis • Presence and degree of acidosis guide acute management	• ↑ Lactate if perfusion compromised

ECG, electrocardiogram; HCM, hypertrophic cardiomyopathy; PE, pulmonary embolism

Blood Tests

Table 2.4.2 Blood tests of use in patients presenting with chest pain

Test	When to perform	Potential result
FBC	• Suspected ACS in known SCD	• Hb <90 g/L exacerbates hypoxia and may require transfusion
Hb electrophoresis	• Suspected ACS in known SCD	• HbS >30% may require reduction
U&E + LFTs	Suspected: • HCM • ACS in known SCD • Acute pericarditis • Aortic dissection	• ↑ Urea/creatinine/liver enzymes indicate end-organ impairment • ↑ Urea in renal failure can cause uraemic pericarditis
Blood cultures	Suspected: • ACS in known SCD • Acute pericarditis	• Positive culture confirms bacterial infection • Sensitivities guide antibiotic choice
Crossmatch (extended)	• Suspected ACS in known SCD	• Crossmatched blood • Simple or exchange transfusion may be required
Troponin	• If chest symptoms and ECG are equivocal but angina/myocardial ischaemia suspected • Not be used as a screening tool. If no supporting clinical evidence, raised level is confusing • Reperfusion measures should not be delayed if the clinical diagnosis is clear	• Raised troponin together with clinical evidence of angina indicates myocardial infarction • Raised troponin may indicated myocardial involvement in pericarditis (myopericarditis)
D-dimer	• Very rarely performed in children as not discriminatory	• False positives are high

ACS, acute chest syndrome; ECG, electrocardiogram; FBC, full blood count; Hb, haemoglobin; HCM, hypertrophic cardiomyopathy; LFTs, live function tests; SCD, sickle cell disease; U&E, urea and electrolytes

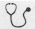

Box 2.4.6 Use of D-Dimer and Wells Score in Children

- A blood test commonly used in adults to aid with diagnosis of pulmonary embolism is the D-dimer. A negative result, together with a low 'Wells Score' (clinical scoring tool for PE) helps to rule out a PE

- However, neither of these performs well in children, with high rates of false negatives and positives. It is therefore recommended that they are not used in the paediatric population

---

Imaging

Table 2.4.3 Imaging modalities of use in patients presenting with chest pain

Test	When to perform	Potential result
Chest x-ray	Suspected: • ACS in known SCD – essential • Complicated pneumonia • Pneumothorax • Malignancy	• ACS: new lung infiltrate is diagnostic • Pneumonia: consolidation • Pneumothorax: absent lung markings/crisp lung edge • Malignancy: mediastinal mass is suggestive
Echocardiogram	• Essential if cardiac or vascular cause is suspected to look for structural and functional abnormalities	• Hypertrophic cardiomyopathy • Other left ventricular outflow tract obstruction • Pericarditis ± pericardial effusion • Tachycardia-induced cardiomyopathy • Coronary artery abnormality
CT/MR angiography	• Investigation of choice in suspected aortic dissection	• Aortic dissection – location and extent
CT pulmonary angiogram	• In a patient with risk factors for venous thromboembolism and suspected PE • Radiation should be carefully considered and only performed if there is genuine suspicion	• PE – size and location

ACS, acute chest syndrome; CT, computed tomography; MR, magnetic resonance; PE, pulmonary embolism; SCD, sickle cell disease

Special

Table 2.4.4 Special tests of use in patients presenting with chest pain

Test	When to perform	Potential result
24-hour Holter ECG monitor	• For paroxysmal arrhythmic events not present during routine ECG	• Intermittent tachyarrhythmias
Exercise tolerance test	• In left ventricular outflow tract obstruction	• Evidence of angina, dyspnoea, palpitations or presyncope on exertion
Cardiac MRI	• Detailed cardiac assessment in known cardiac disease to assess ventricular morphology and inform arrhythmic risk in HCM	• HCM: left ventricular hypertrophy, myocardial fibrosis • Acute pericarditis: bright pericardial thickening ± pericardial effusion
Pericardiocentesis	• In acute pericarditis with effusion • Primarily for therapeutic purposes, with diagnostic potential secondary • Fluid for cytology, tumour markers, Gram stain, cultures	• Positive Gram stain and microbiology indicate causative organism • ↑ Tumour markers/cytology suggest associated malignancy

ECG, electrocardiogram; HCM, hypertrophic cardiomyopathy; MRI, magnetic resonance imaging

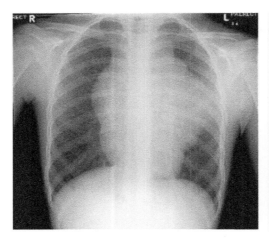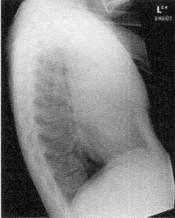

Figure 2.4.6 (A) Anterior and (B) lateral view of an anterior mediastinal mass

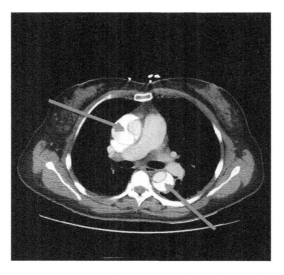

Figure 2.4.7 Axial computed tomography of aortic dissection with involvement of both the ascending and descending aorta. The false lumen (arrows) are opacified by contrast.

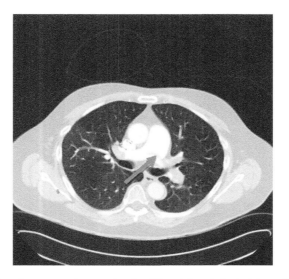

Figure 2.4.8 Computed tomographic pulmonary angiogram showing filling defects in both right and left pulmonary arteries (blue arrow). This is known as a 'saddle embolus' straddling the pulmonary arteries.

2.4.8 KEY MANAGEMENT PRINCIPLES

Diagnosis-specific management strategies are outlined here. It is expected that an 'ABCDE' approach to assessment and management is always undertaken (see Chapter 12.1, *The A to E Assessment*).

Box 2.4.7 World Health Organisation Analgesic Ladder

- **Mild pain** paracetamol ± NSAIDs
- **Moderate pain** weak opioid ± paracetamol ± NSAIDs
- **Severe pain** strong opioid ± paracetamol ± NSAIDs

Dangerous Diagnosis 1
Diagnosis: Hypertrophic cardiomyopathy

Management Principles
1. **Discussion with cardiology + transfer to cardiology centre.** This is a specialist area and cardiologists should guide all management. Will ultimately need transfer to a Paediatric Cardiology centre for assessment, further investigations and management
2. **Medical management.** Medical management of heart failure uses beta blockers or calcium channel blockers (verapamil), but these do not modify the clinical course. Diuretics may be added if heart failure continues to progress

Dangerous Diagnosis 2
Diagnosis: Acute chest syndrome

Management Principles
1. **Adequate oxygenation.** It is extremely important to maintain oxygen saturations ≥95%. Humidified high-flow, non-invasive or mechanical ventilation may be needed in a minority of cases
2. **Fluid resuscitation.** Intravenous (IV) fluids are indicated to correct dehydration or for maintenance fluids. Bolus fluids are only indicated if the patient is shocked; otherwise avoid. Maintenance is usually given at two-thirds to prevent iatrogenic pulmonary oedema
3. **Antibiotics.** All patients require empirical antimicrobials to cover pneumococcal pneumonia (usually third-generation cephalosporin), atypical bacteria (macrolide) and, if severely ill, methicillin-resistant *Staphylococcus aureus* (MRSA; vancomycin)
4. **Analgesia.** Use the World Health Organisation analgesic ladder to provide effective pain relief and prevent splinting. Opioids may be used. Analgesia should be adequate to reduce respiratory splinting and hypoventilation, but should not be so much as to cause respiratory depression
5. **Red blood cell transfusion.** Patients may need a red blood cell transfusion of 10 mL/kg packed red cells if haemoglobin (Hb) is more than 1 g/dL below baseline, or if <9 g/dL. Aim is to target Hb 9–11 g/dL or HbS <30%. Exchange transfusion is usually reserved for those with invasive ventilatory requirements. Crossmatch request should note SCD for extended matching
6. **Prevention of atelectasis.** All patients should perform incentive spirometry by strict routine, for example 2-hourly when awake and 4-hourly at night. Chest physiotherapy is essential. Regular mobilisation helps prevent atelectasis

Dangerous Diagnosis 3
Diagnosis: Aortic dissection

Management Principles
1. **Blood pressure control.** The main goal of initial stabilisation is control of blood pressure, to reduce pulsatile load on the dissection. This reduces risk of extension and rupture
2. **Surgical intervention.** If the dissection is type A, urgent surgery is warranted. Uncomplicated type B dissections may be initially managed conservatively
3. **Analgesia.** Appropriate analgesia helps reduce blood pressure
4. **Endovascular intervention.** In conservatively managed dissections that develop complications, for example end-organ ischaemia or recurrent chest pain, endovascular repair by stent graft may be used
5. **Long-term management.** Long-term management includes serial imaging and blood pressure control

Common Diagnosis 1
Diagnosis: Acute pericarditis

Management Principles
1. **Anti-inflammatory**. Combination therapy of colchicine (3 months) and non-steroidal anti-inflammatory drugs (NSAIDs) are usually recommended. Proton pump inhibitor should be given as cover. NSAIDs are usually tapered 1–2 days after resolution of symptoms
2. **Exercise restriction.** Exercise is restricted until the chest pain resolves and the inflammatory markers are normal. Competitive athletes should not participate for at least 3 months following resolution

3. **Glucocorticoids.** Rarely required, but can be used in patients with contraindications to NSAIDs
4. **Pericardial drain.** If there is a pericardial effusion causing haemodynamic compromise, this should be drained with image guidance

Common Diagnosis 2
Diagnosis: Musculoskeletal pain

Management Principles
1. **Reassurance.** This is the mainstay of management. It is important to convey the benign nature of the diagnosis and likelihood of improvement in time (although this can take months to years)
2. **NSAIDs.** NSAIDs are useful for costochondritis and slipping rib syndrome, but not other causes of musculoskeletal chest pain
3. **Lifestyle change.** Exercise is helpful for all causes. Cognitive behavioural therapy may be useful in fibromyalgia

Common Diagnosis 3
Diagnosis: Gastro-oesophageal reflux disease

Management Principles
1. **Lifestyle change.** There are many simple modifications that can be made to improve gastro-oesophageal reflux. Feed volumes should be reduced if excessive. Thickeners can be used for infants on milk, who can be fed upright. For older patients, avoidance of late evening meals, caffeine, spicy foods and hot drinks can also be useful
2. **Pharmacological therapy.** Pharmacological treatment should start as a 4-week trial to avoid unnecessary medication. Options include Gaviscon, ranitidine or omeprazole
3. **Specialist referral.** If symptoms persist despite pharmacological therapy, referral to gastroenterology should be made to consider endoscopy. Surgical management (fundoplication with or without percutaneous endoscopic gastrostomy (PEG) or percutaneous endoscopic transgastric jejunostomy (PEG-J) insertion) may be necessary in very severe cases or those complicated by underlying conditions

Common Diagnosis 4
Diagnosis: Psychiatric

Management Principles
1. **Reassurance**. Very often, this is all that is required. A clear explanation that there is no evidence for a serious underlying condition is important

2.5 Palpitations

Domenico Sirico

Department of Women's and Children's Health, Paediatric Cardiology Unit, Padua University Hospital, Padua, Italy

CONTENTS

2.5.1 CHAPTER AT A GLANCE

Box 2.5.1   Chapter at a Glance

- Palpitations are a symptom of an abnormality in heart rate or rhythm
- Palpitations can be disturbing to both patients and families and can induce great anxiety about underlying cardiac disease
- Abnormalities in rhythm are known as arrhythmias, and rather than describing each type of arrhythmia, this chapter will focus on the underlying causative conditions
- It is important to differentiate cardiac from non-cardiac causes of palpitations

2.5.2 DEFINITION

Palpitations are an unpleasant subjective feeling or awareness of one's own heartbeats. This usually occurs as a sensation of rapid, irregular or unusually strong heartbeats.

2.5.3 DIAGNOSTIC ALGORITHM

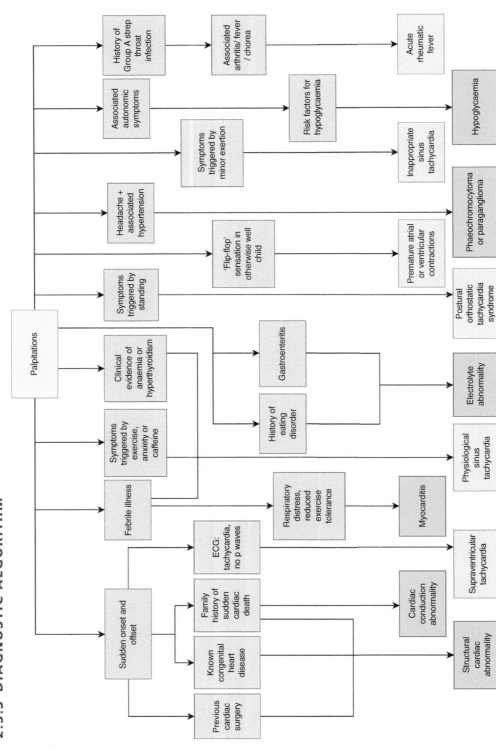

Figure 2.5.1 Diagnostic algorithm for the presentation of palpitations.

2.5.4 DIFFERENTIALS LIST

Box 2.5.2   What Is an Arrhythmia?

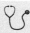

- Arrhythmia is a term describing an irregular heart rhythm or rate
- It is not always pathological – sinus arrhythmia is a normal physiological phenomenon characterised by a raised heart rate during inspiration and decreased heart rate during expiration
- There are many types of pathological arrhythmias. Broadly speaking, arrhythmias can be fast (tachy) or slow (brady)

- The majority of arrhythmias are asymptomatic
- If symptomatic, presentation is usually with palpitations, syncope or sudden death. In this case, tachyarrhythmias are most likely to be the cause
- The specific arrhythmia will be identified on electrocardiogram

Dangerous Diagnoses

1. **Congenital Structural Cardiac Abnormalities**
   - Children with structural cardiac abnormalities are at much higher risk of developing arrhythmias than children with normal hearts
   - Broadly, there are two sub-divisions within this category:
     - Children with surgically corrected structural heart disease
     - Children with inherited structural disease, such as hypertrophic cardiomyopathy (HCM), dilated cardiomyopathy (DCM) or coronary artery abnormalities
   - These structural defects predispose to many types of arrhythmia, including ventricular tachycardia (VT) and torsade de pointes
   - Atrial flutter is particularly associated with surgically repaired or palliated congenital heart disease
   - Accompanying syncope is a significant risk for sudden cardiac death
2. **Cardiac Conduction Abnormalities**
   - Inherited conduction abnormalities, 'channelopathies', are caused by genetic mutations in the myocardial ion channels (usually sodium, potassium and calcium channels)
   - Inheritance is mostly autosomal dominant
   - These predispose the patient to arrhythmias, particularly VT, which can present as symptoms of syncope, palpitations, chest pain and even sudden cardiac death
   - Conditions include long QT syndrome, Brugada syndrome, catecholaminergic polymorphic ventricular tachycardia (CPVT) and short QT syndrome
   - Acquired long QT may result from electrolyte abnormalities, commonly seen in patients with eating disorders
3. **Myocarditis**
   - Myocarditis is an inflammation of the myocardium (heart muscle) usually caused by viral infection with Coxsackie B or, less commonly, other enteroviruses
   - There are three phases in the disease process: the viral infection phase, the inflammatory phase and the dilated cardiomyopathy phase
   - Palpitations are particularly associated with the inflammatory phase, due to impaired ventricular function
   - Palpitations may also be secondary to significant tachycardia

Box 2.5.3   The Three Stages of Viral Myocarditis

1. **Viral infection phase**: prodrome of fever, fatigue and myalgia
2. **Inflammatory phase**: myocyte inflammation and injury leads to impaired ventricular function. This is the primary cause for

arrhythmias and palpitations. This phase is usually self-limiting, with recovery seen over 2–4 weeks
3. **Dilated cardiomyopathy phase**: only occurs in a minority of patients. These patients develop chronic dilation and heart failure

A small subset of patients may develop fulminant myocarditis, where significantly impaired contractility of the inflamed muscle leads to cardiogenic shock

4. **Electrolyte Abnormalities**
   - Hyperkalaemia, hypokalaemia, hypocalcaemia, hypophosphatemia and hypomagnesaemia are all associated with VT and torsade de pointes
   - These are important, reversible causes of arrhythmia

- Magnesium deficiency may cause secondary hypokalaemia and hypocalcaemia
- Mild abnormalities are usually asymptomatic. A derangement significant enough to cause arrhythmia is severe
- Deranged electrolytes may also exacerbate preexisting conditions that predispose to arrhythmias, particularly in those with conduction abnormalities

Common Diagnoses

1. Physiological Sinus Tachycardia
- Any condition that leads to increased metabolic demand may cause tachycardia and hyperdynamic cardiac activity, which may in turn cause palpitations
- Generally, sinus tachycardia is a physiological response to a demand for greater cardiac output and increased sympathetic drive
- Common precipitants are anxiety, physical exercise, caffeine, emotional arousal and fever, but underlying organic conditions such as anaemia and hyperthyroidism should also be considered

2. Paroxysmal Supraventricular Tachycardia (SVT)
- SVT is the most common symptomatic arrhythmia in children, although it is also frequently asymptomatic
- Paroxysmal SVT is most often seen with re-entrant tachycardias involving the AV node, such as AV nodal re-entry tachycardia, and this is how SVT will be used in this chapter
- It is most often caused by an accessory atrioventricular pathway, although it can also be seen in underlying congenital heart disease
- Palpitations are a common complaint in verbal children, who may also complain of chest pain. Syncope is a poor prognostic sign
- SVT is generally well tolerated, although prolonged episodes can cause heart failure

3. Premature Atrial or Ventricular Contractions (PACs or PVCs)
- PACs result from premature depolarisation of an atrial focus. Patients often describe that they feel like their heart 'stops' or 'flip-flops'. They usually appear in healthy children and are the most common sinus arrhythmia of childhood
- PVCs result from premature ventricular depolarisation. Although structural heart disease and ventricular dysfunction should be excluded, PVCs are generally benign and may be detected in up to 50–70% of normal children on 24-hour Holter monitoring

4. Postural Orthostatic Tachycardia Syndrome (POTS)
- POTS is a common disorder among teenage girls that manifests as palpitations, anxiety and dizziness/syncope on sitting/standing up
- POTS is characterised by an excessive increase in heart rate that occurs upon standing without associated hypotension
- The underlying cause is not well described, but is thought to be due to autonomic dysfunction
- POTS is covered in Chapter 2.3, and will not be discussed further in this chapter

---

Box 2.5.4   Anxiety and Panic Attacks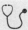

- Anxiety disorders are the most common paediatric psychiatric disorders
- Palpitations are a symptom of tachycardia generated by catecholamine release
- Anxiety is a normal, adaptive part of life. However, it merits specialist assessment when excessive symptoms have a pervasive effect on daily life

- There are several types of anxiety disorder, including panic disorder, which is characterised by recurrent, unexpected panic attacks
- A panic attack is an abrupt, intense surge of discomfort. Typical symptoms include palpitations, sweating, chest pain, nausea and paraesthesias
- Although anxiety is a common cause of palpitations, it is important to exclude underlying conditions that might coexist

---

Box 2.5.5   What Does Supraventricular Tachycardia (SVT) Mean?

- Officially, SVT refers to any tachyarrhythmia arising from above the level of the Bundle of His
- SVTs can be classified either by their site of origin (atria or AV node) or regularity (regular or irregular)
- However, in practice, SVT is almost always used synonymously with re-entry tachycardias

Regular		Irregular
Atrial	**Atrioventricular**	**Atrial**
• Sinus tachycardia	• Atrioventricular re-entry tachycardia (AVRT)	• Atrial fibrillation
• Atrial tachycardia	• AV nodal re-entry tachycardia (AVNRT)	• Atrial flutter
• Atrial flutter		• Multifocal atrial tachycardia
• Inappropriate sinus tachycardia		

Diagnoses to Consider

1. Inappropriate Sinus Tachycardia (IST)
- While normal tachycardia occurs in response to increased metabolic demand, IST causes an elevated heart rate that is disproportionate to demands
- Tachycardia is often noted at rest
- The underlying cause is not fully understood, but sinoatrial node and autonomic nervous system dysfunction are possibilities

When to consider: in children with palpitations at rest, or with very minor exertion, such as moving from lying to sitting

2. Hypoglycaemia
- The autonomic response to hypoglycaemia causes a catecholamine surge that may induce tachycardia with palpitations
- Hypoglycaemia itself is a life-threatening condition
- Palpitations occur as part of an autonomic response to hypoglycaemia, and other features will be present, such as sweating, tremor, hunger and anxiety. Neuroglycopenic symptoms, such as behavioural changes and cognitive impairment, are late signs

When to consider: in children with a known predisposition to hypoglycaemia, such as diabetes or inborn errors of metabolism

---

Box 2.5.6   Phaeochromocytoma and Paraganglioma

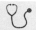

- Phaeochromocytomas and paragangliomas arise from the adrenal medulla and from extra-adrenal origins, respectively
- These are very rare tumours

- The classic triad of symptoms consists of episodic headache, sweating and tachycardia, usually accompanied by hypertension
- Palpitations result from sinus tachycardia, driven by high levels of catecholamines

---

2.5.5 KEY HISTORY FEATURES

Dangerous Diagnosis 1
Diagnosis: Congenital structural cardiac abnormalities

Questions
1. **Is there a history of congenital heart disease?** A history of congenital heart disease, especially with large left-to-right shunts, greatly increases the suspicion of atrial and ventricular tachyarrhythmias
2. **Is there a history of cardiac surgery?** Complex heart surgeries with extensive myocardial scars and suture lines are an independent risk factor for developing arrhythmias
3. **Is there a family history of structural heart defects (cardiomyopathies or congenital heart disease), sudden cardiac or unexplained death at <40 years old?** HCM and DCM can both be inherited (usually autosomal dominant) and so a family history of cardiomyopathy is very important
4. **What are the onset and offset like?** Palpitations caused by serious cardiac arrhythmias usually start and stop abruptly, lasting seconds to minutes. There may be associated chest pain
5. **Do the palpitations occur during exercise?** In significant left ventricular outflow tract (LVOT) obstruction, the heart struggles to meet increased demands for the higher cardiac output required in exercise. Compensatory tachycardia may cause palpitations
6. **Is there associated syncope?** Palpitations associated with syncope may be seen in LVOT obstructions and coronary artery abnormalities

Dangerous Diagnosis 2
Diagnosis: Cardiac conduction abnormalities

Questions
1. **Is there a family history of arrhythmias, sudden cardiac or unexplained death <40 years old?** Long QT, Brugada, CPVT and short QT are all inherited conditions with predominantly autosomal dominant inheritance, so there is often a family history suggestive of arrhythmias
2. **Is there a family history of congenital deafness?** Some inherited channelopathies affecting calcium channels may cause dysfunction of auditory hair cells, as well as sinoatrial node dysfunction
3. **What are the onset and offset like?** Palpitations caused by serious cardiac arrhythmias usually start and stop abruptly, lasting seconds to minutes. There may be associated chest pain
4. **Do palpitations occur early in the morning or after a large meal?** In Brugada syndrome, arrhythmias usually occur during sleep or early morning and particularly after a large meal. Fevers can also be a trigger
5. **Do palpitations start during exercise or emotional stress?** Arrhythmias in CPVT and short QT are both usually triggered by exercise or emotional stress
6. **Do palpitations start with any of the following triggers for long QT?** Different types of long QT syndrome have different environmental triggers. See Chapter 2.3, *Syncope*, Box 2.3.6, *Triggers for Long QT*.
7. **Is there associated syncope?** Syncope may be seen in intermittent ventricular tachyarrhythmias where syncope may be abrupt, with no prodrome.

Dangerous Diagnosis 3
Diagnosis: Myocarditis

Questions
1. **Is there a recent history of viral illness?** Typically, there is a viral prodrome of fever, myalgia, respiratory illness, sore throat and malaise in the weeks prior to presentation
2. **Symptoms of heart failure?** Infants and children often have heart failure at presentation, including symptoms of dyspnoea, exercise intolerance and syncope. Respiratory symptoms may lead to an incorrect presumption of lower respiratory tract infection
3. **Non-specific gastrointestinal symptoms?** Abdominal pain, anorexia and vomiting can predominate at presentation, and often confuse the diagnosis initially

Dangerous Diagnosis 4
Diagnosis: Electrolyte abnormalities

Questions
1. **Is there a history of an eating disorder?** Profound electrolyte abnormalities can occur with nutritional deficits in eating disorders, as well as during the refeeding period
2. **Has there been recent diarrhoea and/or vomiting?** Electrolyte loss in diarrhoea and vomiting can be significant. This is commonly seen in acute gastroenteritis, as well as in patients with chronic malabsorption in cystic fibrosis or ulcerative colitis. Hypovolaemic acute kidney injury can cause hyperkalaemia
3. **Is there diuretic use?** Thiazide diuretics can deplete potassium and magnesium levels. Inappropriate continuation of diuretics during acute hypovolaemia (such as intercurrent gastroenteritis) can precipitate acute kidney injury, leading to hyperkalaemia

Common Diagnosis 1
Diagnosis: Physiological sinus tachycardia

Questions
1. **Are palpitations triggered by physical exercise?** Exercise-induced palpitations may be benign and a consequence of appropriate sinus tachycardia (although exercise may trigger arrhythmia in some underlying cardiac conditions, as above)
2. **What are the onset, duration and offset?** There may be seconds to minutes of increasing awareness, and episodes last minutes to hours, after which heart rate gradually slows down
3. **Have episodes of palpitations been associated with fever?** Fever may produce palpitations as a sensation of increased ventricular stroke volume
4. **Is there a history of drugs that might cause sinus tachycardia?** If age/patient appropriate, ask about stimulants such as caffeine or nicotine, or recreational drugs such as cocaine
5. **Are there known underlying conditions (or symptoms of) that might predispose to a hyperdynamic state?** See Box 2.5.7

Box 2.5.7 Causes of Cardiac Hyperdynamic State		
Condition	**Symptoms**	**Underlying conditions**
Anaemia	Fatigue Breathlessness Pallor	Iron deficiency Sickle cell disease Leukaemia
Hyperthyroidism	Weight loss Hair loss Low tolerance of heat Fatigue Neck swelling (goitre) Prominent eyes (exophthalmos)	Graves' disease
Anxiety	Sweating Chest pain Nausea Paraesthesias	Anxiety disorder Panic disorder Stressful life events (e.g. parental separation, schoolwork, sporting pressure)

Common Diagnosis 2

Diagnosis: Paroxysmal supraventricular tachycardia

Questions
1. **What were the onset and offset?** SVT usually begins and ends suddenly
2. **Do palpitations occur more at rest or with activity?** SVT can occur at any time, mostly at rest, although exercise can be a trigger in some patients
3. **Is there associated presyncope or syncope?** Syncope is not common in SVT, but when present, it is a poor prognostic feature
4. **Are there symptoms of heart failure?** Although generally well tolerated, prolonged SVT can cause heart failure. Symptoms include shortness of breath and reduced exercise tolerance

Common Diagnosis 3

Diagnosis: Premature atrial or ventricular contractions

Questions
1. **Does the patient describe the heartbeat as a 'flip' or a 'jolt' in the chest?** The sensation is often described as a flip-flop, skipped beat or as though the heart has stopped
2. **Are the episodes very short?** Palpitations in PACs and PVCs represent the compensatory heartbeat after the premature depolarisation and then normal rhythm resumes. They are over in a second
3. **Are there any associated symptoms?** There should be no associated symptoms

2.5.6 KEY EXAMINATION FEATURES

Dangerous Diagnosis 1

Diagnosis: Congenital structural cardiac abnormalities

Examination Findings
1. **Surgical scars.** Repair of complex congenital cardiac disease is usually done via sternotomy. Also look for thoracotomy scars (can be quite high in the axilla) and evidence of previous surgical drains. See Chapter 2.1, *Cyanosis*, Figure 2.1.7, *Thoracic Scars*.
2. **Systolic murmur.** An ejection systolic murmur indicates LVOT obstruction – seen in HCM and aortic stenosis. A pansystolic murmur suggests mitral regurgitation – seen in HCM
3. **Prominent apex beat.** HCM can cause a more prominent, forceful apex beat due to left ventricular hypertrophy
4. **Signs of heart failure.** There may be signs of pulmonary oedema (respiratory distress, crackles on auscultation of lungs), hepatic congestion (hepatomegaly) and faltering growth (small for age on height and weight chart)

Dangerous Diagnosis 2

Diagnosis: Cardiac conduction abnormalities

Examination Findings
1. **Surgical scars.** Look for a pacemaker or implantable cardioverter-defibrillator (ICD) scar. See Chapter 2.1, *Cyanosis*, Figure 2.1.7, *Thoracic Scars*.
2. **Normal examination.** Examination findings are usually normal in conduction abnormalities unless an arrhythmia occurs at the time of examination
3. **Low Body Mass Index (BMI).** Eating disorders such as anorexia may lead to acquired long QT

Dangerous Diagnosis 3

Diagnosis: Myocarditis

Examination Findings
1. **Respiratory distress**. Impaired myocardial contractility leads to heart failure. Increased work of breathing are signs of pulmonary congestion
2. **Added heart sounds.** There may be S3 (rapid ventricular filling) and S4 (atrium contracting against stiffened ventricle) heart sounds due to impaired ventricular function
3. **Weak distal pulses.** Poor ventricular contractility leads to weak peripheral pulses
4. **Murmur.** There may be systolic murmurs in keeping with mitral or tricuspid regurgitation, in severe dilatation of the ventricles
5. **Pericardial rub.** Myocarditis alone does not cause a rub, but this might be heard if there is concurrent pericarditis (myopericarditis)
6. **Signs of shock.** Myocarditis can progress to an acute fulminant state, where there are signs of circulatory shock with profound tachycardia, hypotension and altered mental status

Dangerous Diagnosis 4

Diagnosis: Electrolyte abnormalities

There are few useful clinical signs that are specific enough to base a diagnosis upon

Examination Findings

1. **Signs of dehydration.** Clinical signs of dehydration are suggestive of malabsorption or water loss, which is often accompanied by electrolyte loss
2. **Signs of hypocalcaemia.** Hypocalcaemia causes weakness or tetany; there may be a positive Chvostek's sign (twitching of ipsilateral facial muscles when facial nerve tapped in front of tragus) or Trousseau's sign (involuntary carpopedal spasm when upper arm compressed with blood pressure cuff), demonstrating nerve hyperexcitability.

Common Diagnosis 1

Diagnosis: Physiological sinus tachycardia

Examination Findings

1. **Normal examination.** Most often, sinus tachycardia that is brought on by anxiety, exercise, caffeine or emotional arousal will be accompanied by a completely normal examination
2. **Fever.** Sinus tachycardia is generally considered appropriate if there is an increase of approximately 10 bpm for every 1 °C elevation in temperatures above 37 °C. There needs to be careful consideration of whether tachycardia represents sepsis or compensated shock
3. **Signs of anaemia.** Pale palmar creases and conjunctival pallor suggest anaemia
4. **Signs of hyperthyroidism.** Look for a goitre, presence of proptosis and exophthalmos and a fine resting tremor

Common Diagnosis 2

Diagnosis: Paroxysmal supraventricular tachycardia

Examination Findings

1. **Tachycardia.** If examined during an episode, heart rates are between 220 and 280 bpm in infants, and 180 and 240 bpm in older children
2. **Signs of heart failure.** Most tachyarrhythmia is paroxysmal and so does not lead to heart failure, but it can do if prolonged >48 hours. There may be signs of pulmonary oedema (respiratory distress, crackles on auscultation of lungs), hepatic congestion (hepatomegaly) and faltering growth (small for age on height and weight chart)

Common Diagnosis 3

Diagnosis: Premature atrial or ventricular contractions

Examination Findings

1. **Irregular heart rhythm on auscultation.** Patients with frequent PACs and PVCs may have an audibly irregular heart rhythm on auscultation. This should be differentiated from respiratory sinus arrhythmia, which represents the normal increase in heart rate that occurs during inspiration
2. **Normal physical examination.** PACs and PVCs are considered benign in most cases and physical examination is usually normal

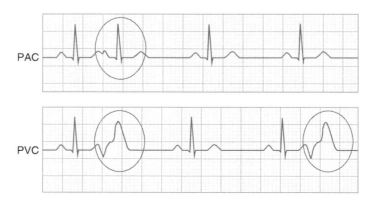

Figure 2.5.2 In premature atrial contractions (PACs), usually the QRS complex occurs prematurely and is preceded by an abnormal P wave morphology. Usually, there is an incomplete compensatory pause. If the abnormal p wave is not followed by a QRS complex, it is considered a non-conducted PAC. Premature ventricular contractions appear as a wide QRS complex earlier than anticipated, with usually full compensatory pause.

2.5.7 KEY INVESTIGATIONS

Not all children will require invasive investigations; often diagnoses are made on clinical evidence from history and examination. Consider carefully which investigations are required for which patient.

Bedside

Table 2.5.1 Bedside tests of use in patients presenting with palpitations

Test	When to perform	Potential result
12-lead ECG	• All patients with palpitations • Defines the rhythm at rest and may be diagnostic if the patient is having symptoms at the time of the ECG recording	• QT interval prolonged (>450 ms) or short (<300 ms) • HCM: LVH • PACs or PVCs • Supraventricular tachycardia • Ventricular tachycardia • Ventricular fibrillation • Torsade de pointes
Blood gas	• Lactate is a marker of peripheral perfusion	• ↑ Lactate indicates poor tissue perfusion
Blood sugar	• Suspected hypoglycaemia	• Level <2.6 mmol/L indicates hypoglycaemia • In diabetic patients, <4 mmol/L is significant
Blood pressure	• All patients with palpitations	• Hypotension indicates decompensated shock
Supine and standing blood pressure and heart rate	• Suspected POTS	• Heart rate rise >40bpm without blood pressure drop indicates POTS

ECG, electrocardiogram; HCM, hypertrophic cardiomyopathy; LVH, left ventricular hypertrophy; PACs, premature atrial contractions; POTS, postural orthostatic tachycardia syndrome; PVCs, premature ventricular contractions

Blood Tests

Table 2.5.2 Blood tests of use in patients presenting with palpitations

Test	When to perform	Potential result
FBC	• Suspected physiological sinus tachycardia due to anaemia	• Anaemia
U&E, phosphate, magnesium	• All patients with palpitations, unless very strong evidence for benign cause • Electrolyte disturbances can affect QT interval and cause VT	• ↑/↓K$^+$, ↓ Ca^{2+}, ↓ phosphate, or ↓ Mg^{2+}
ESR + CRP	• Suspected myocarditis, as markers of inflammation	• ↑ CRP or ESR indicates inflammatory process
BNP + NT-proBNP	• Suspected structural and functional heart disease	↑ BNP and NT-proBNP in: • Myocarditis • Heart failure • Large shunting defects
Troponin (Tn)	• Suspected myocarditis as a marker of myocyte injury	• ↑ Troponin indicates myocardial infarction
TFTs	• Suspected physiological sinus tachycardia due to hyperthyroidism	• ↓ TSH and ↑ T$_4$ indicate hyperthyroidism

BNP, B-type natriuretic peptide; Ca, calcium; CRP, C-reactive protein; FBC, full blood count; ESR, erythrocyte sedimentation rate; K, potassium; Mg, magnesium; NT-proBNP, N-terminal-pro hormone BNP; TFTs, thyroid function tests; TSH, thyroid-stimulating hormone; U&E, urea and electrolytes; VT, ventricular tachycardia

Imaging

Table 2.5.3 Imaging modalities of use in patients presenting with palpitations

Test	When to perform	Potential result
Echocardiogram	• If significant palpitations in history, previous acute tachyarrhythmia • If abnormal ECG or suggestion of structural heart disease • Suspected myocarditis	• Structural cardiac abnormality, e.g. HCM or DCM • Myocarditis

DCM, dilated cardiomyopathy; ECG, electrocardiogram; HCM, hypertrophic cardiomyopathy

Special

Table 2.5.4 Special tests of use in patients presenting with palpitations

Test	When to perform	Potential result
Ambulatory ECG monitoring	• Suspected paroxysmal arrhythmias • Type and duration of ECG monitor (24–72 hr Holter tape, event recorder, implantable loop recorder) should be chosen according to frequency and duration of symptoms	• Confirms intermittent arrhythmias
Exercise tolerance test	• Many tachyarrhythmias only occur with exercise due to increased catecholamine state • If these are suspected, performing an exercise treadmill test may elicit an abnormal tachycardia	• Exercise-induced arrhythmia
Plasma or urine catecholamines and metabolites	• Only if strong suspicions of pheochromocytoma or paraganglioma	• ↑ Level suggestive of neuroendocrine tumour

ECG, electrocardiogram

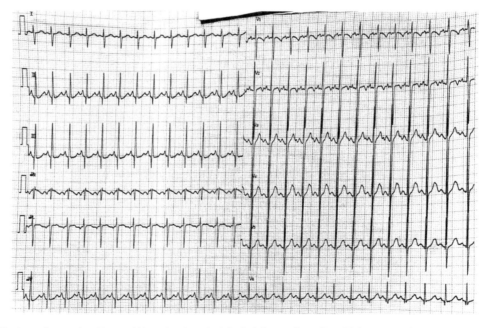

Figure 2.5.3 Electrocardiogram in a 7-year-old boy showing physiological sinus tachycardia, with heart rate of 150 bpm.

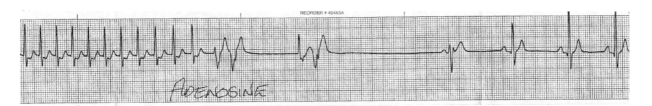

Figure 2.5.4 Supraventricular tachycardia (SVT) is a narrow complex tachycardia, unless there is aberrant conduction, in which case it can appear wide. There are no visible p waves. Here is an electrocardiogram of SVT, which converts to sinus rhythm with the administration of adenosine.

2.5.8 KEY MANAGEMENT PRINCIPLES

Diagnosis-specific management strategies are outlined here. It is expected that an 'ABCDE' approach to assessment and management is always undertaken (see Chapter 12.1, *The A to E Assessment*).
All patients with palpitations must be on continuous cardiac monitoring for the duration of their assessment.

Dangerous Diagnosis 1
Diagnosis: Congenital structural cardiac abnormalities

Management Principles
1. **Urgent referral to cardiology.** Any patient with clinical suspicion of cardiac disease in history, family history or electrocardiogram (ECG) should be referred to cardiology, who will determine investigations and management. General principles are discussed in Chapter 2.3

Dangerous Diagnosis 2
Diagnosis: Cardiac conduction abnormalities

Management Principles
1. **Urgent referral to cardiology.** Any patient with clinical suspicion of cardiac disease in history, family history or ECG should be referred to cardiology, who will determine investigations and management. General principles are discussed in Chapter 2.3

Dangerous Diagnosis 3
Diagnosis: Myocarditis

Management Principles
1. **Paediatric intensive care unit (PICU) involvement.** The high risk of decompensation from arrhythmias or heart failure means early intensive care involvement is essential
2. **Fluid resuscitation.** Most children at presentation will have heart failure. Careful, limited fluid resuscitation must be given
3. **Management of arrhythmias.** Management is highly variable depending on the type of arrhythmia.
   - Any supraventricular/ventricular arrhythmias with haemodynamic instability require DC cardioversion
   - Complete heart block with haemodynamic instability requires pacing
   - Any other arrhythmias require careful discussion, as antiarrhythmic drugs may have negatively inotropic, vasodilatory or proarrhythmic effects that may exacerbate problems
4. **Treatment of heart failure**
   - Mild heart failure: oral diuretics can be used. Angiotensin-converting enzyme inhibitors may be used to reduce afterload
   - Severe heart failure: inotropic support may be required. Cardiac function can be improved by positive pressure ventilation, which reduces afterload and increases systemic oxygen levels
5. **Intravenous immunoglobulin (IVIg).** High-dose IVIg is often used for immunomodulation in severe myocarditis, although evidence is limited as to its benefit

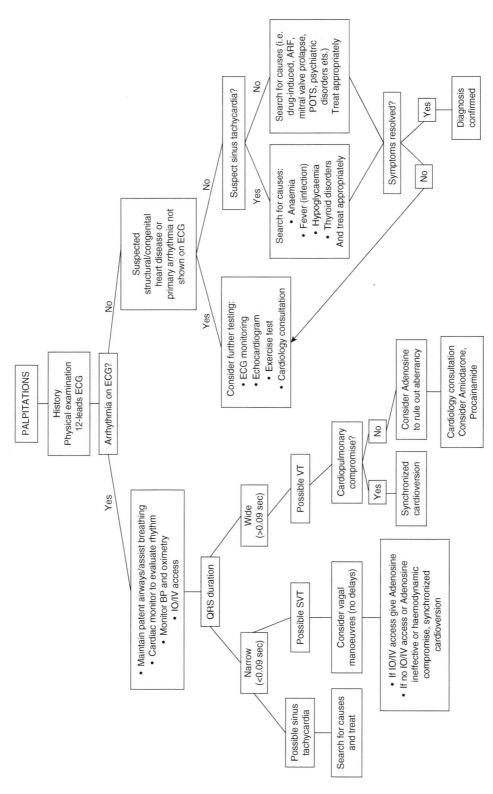

Figure 2.5.5 The electrocardiogram is the definitive tool when assessing and managing children with palpitations. From here, diagnoses can be stratified into life-threatening and non-life-threatening and management chosen accordingly.

6. **Consideration of extracorporeal membrane oxygenation (ECMO).** ECMO should be considered in refractory shock to allow natural healing and recovery of cardiac function

7. **Heart transplant.** Some children with severe heart failure require heart transplantation

Dangerous Diagnosis 4
Diagnosis: Electrolyte abnormalities

Management Principles
1. **Electrolyte replacement.** ECG changes as a result of low levels of electrolytes (potassium, calcium, phosphate or magnesium) require intravenous replacement, in high-dependency or intensive care
2. **Treatment of hyperkalaemia.** Stop all medications containing potassium or potassium-sparing effects. Acute treatment is as below. Severe hyperkalaemia may require dialysis
3. **Maintenance therapy.** Regular monitoring of electrolytes is required after acute treatment. Once electrolytes are in reference range, maintenance may be required if there is ongoing risk of electrolyte loss, e.g. in diarrhoea

---

Box 2.5.8   Intravenous Electrolyte Replacement

Electrolyte to be replaced	Details
Potassium	• Intravenous (IV) potassium chloride 0.2–0.4 mmol/kg/hr • Central access required for concentrations more than 60 mmol/L
Calcium	• IV calcium gluconate 10% 0.5 mL/kg bolus followed by infusion of 0.5–1 mmol/kg/day (max 9 mmol/day) • Central access required for concentrations more than 0.045 mmol/mL
Magnesium	• IV magnesium sulphate 0.2–0.4 mmol/kg over 2 hours • Can cause hypotension so requires blood pressure monitoring
Phosphate	• IV sodium glycerophosphate over 12 hours • Doses vary: 1 mmol/kg (neonate), 0.7 mmol/kg (1 month–2 years), 0.4 mmol/kg (2–8 years), 10 mmol *not per kg* (9–17 years)

Box 2.5.9   Treatment of Hyperkalaemia

- Intravenous calcium gluconate 10% 0.5 mL/kg
- Nebulised salbutamol 2.5 mg (<25 kg) or 5 mg (>25 kg)
- Intravenous insulin bolus 0.1 units/kg **plus**
- Intravenous dextrose bolus 5 mL/kg

- Intravenous insulin infusion 0.1 units/kg/hr **plus**
- Intravenous dextrose 10% + 0.9% sodium chloride at maintenance rate

---

Common Diagnosis 1
Diagnosis: Physiological sinus tachycardia

Management Principles
1. **Treat the underlying disorder.** If due to an underlying condition, such as anaemia or hyperthyroidism, treatment of these will treat the tachycardia. Anxiety may be improved with cognitive behavioural therapy and mental health referral might be required
2. **Lifestyle modifications.** If due to caffeine or other stimulants, avoidance will reduce palpitations

Common Diagnosis 2
Diagnosis: Paroxysmal supraventricular tachycardia

Management Principles
1. **Vagal manoeuvres.** In presence of non-sinus narrow complex (supraventricular) tachycardia and haemodynamic stability, vagal manoeuvres should be attempted first without delay
2. **Adenosine.** Intravenous adenosine is the first-line medical therapy for SVT. It is also useful in haemodynamically stable patients with wide complex tachycardia (this differentiates SVT with aberrant conduction from VT – it will not work in the latter). A 12-lead ECG before, during and after administration is preferable if patient status allows
3. **Synchronised DC cardioversion.** If adenosine is not effective, or in the presence of haemodynamic compromise, patients should receive prompt synchronised DC cardioversion at 0.5–1 J/kg (increased to 2 J/kg if not effective)

Box 2.5.10   Vagal Manoeuvres

- Infants: immerse the head under ice-cold water for 10 seconds
- Young children: place a plastic bag filled with ice over the face for 15–30 seconds

- Older children: encourage bearing down (Valsalva manoeuvre) for 15–20 seconds
- Carotid massage and orbital pressure should not be performed in children

---

Box 2.5.11   Tips for Adenosine Administration

Dosing

Age	Details
<12 years	• Initial dose 0.1 mg/kg rapid bolus (maximum initial dose 6 mg) • If not effective increase dose by 0.1 mg/kg every 1–2 minutes to a maximum single dose of 0.5 mg/kg or 12 mg (whichever is lower), until termination of supraventricular tachycardia
>12 years	• Initially 3 mg • If not effective, increase dose to 6 mg after 1–2 minutes • If not effective, increase dose to 12 mg after a further 1–2 minutes

Tips

- Half-life is very short (seconds). If no central access available, use a proximal large peripheral vein to increase chance of reaching the heart
- If given into a peripheral venous cannula, inject through a three-way tap, followed by a rapid 5–10 mL saline flush
- Monitor (and print) 12-lead electrocardiogram rhythm during adenosine administration

---

Box 2.3.12   Cautions for Adenosine Use
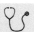

- Do not use adenosine in patients with known second- or third-degree heart block, or sinus node disease
- Be aware that patients with Wolff–Parkinson–White who are treated with adenosine can have atrial fibrillation, which may degenerate into ventricular fibrillation. Keep resuscitation equipment to hand

- Be aware that patients with asthma may experience bronchospasm with adenosine
- Side effects of adenosine include nausea, vomiting, flushing, chest pain and feeling of impending doom

---

Common Diagnosis 3

Diagnosis: Premature atrial or ventricular contractions

Management Principles

1. **Observation and reassurance.** For most PACs, no treatment is indicated as they appear in otherwise healthy children. Occasional PVCs are benign in children, and those with a low burden without underlying heart disease do not require treatment
2. **Lifestyle changes.** For significant PVCs, environmental triggers such as alcohol or caffeine should be identified and avoided
3. **Medical therapy.** First-line treatment for those with symptomatic PVCs is with a beta blocker
4. **Catheter ablation.** If symptoms persist, catheter ablation may be considered, although in complex PVCs further antiarrhythmic drugs may be preferred
5. **Treatment of underlying heart disease.** If there is underlying heart disease, such as HCM, then treatment of the underlying condition may help reduce PVCs

3.1 Fever

Andrew L. Smith

Department of Paediatrics, Children's Services, Homerton University Hospital NHS Foundation Trust, London, UK

CONTENTS

3.1.1 CHAPTER AT A GLANCE

Box 3.1.1 Chapter at a Glance

- Fever is one of the most common paediatric presentations
- There is a wide range of condition severity, from mild self-resolving illness to those with potentially fatal outcomes
- It is important to be able to identify which children have serious underlying causes for their fever, and those who can safely be reassured and discharged, with or without treatment

3.1.2 DEFINITION

- Fever, or pyrexia, is the elevation of body temperature above the normal range (≥37.5 °C)
- The clinical significance of the fever is dependent on the patient's age

Box 3.1.2 Clinical Significance of Fever

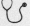

- A temperature of 37.5–37.9 °C is colloquially referred to as a 'low-grade' fever
- A temperature of ≥38.0 °C in a child aged under 3 months is suggestive of a serious bacterial illness (SBI)
- A temperature of ≥39.0 °C in a child aged 3–6 months is suggestive of an SBI
- The peak temperature of a fever in a child aged over 6 months should not be given too much importance in the assessment of the severity of illness, although a temperature of ≥40.0 °C is notable
- A temperature of ≤36.0 °C in a child aged <5 years is suggestive of an SBI

3.1.3 DIAGNOSTIC ALGORITHM

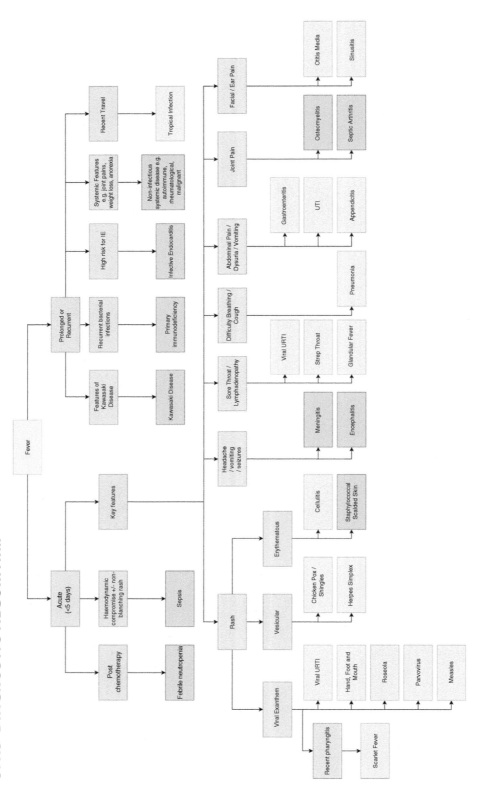

Figure 3.1.1 Diagnostic algorithm for the presentation of fever.

In 2019, a novel coronavirus disease, known as COVID-19 caused a global pandemic, which is still ongoing to publication date in 2022. Cardinal features include cough and loss of smell/taste, but new mutations bring new symptoms and signs, including those more typical of an upper respiratory tract infection (URTI). Since these signs are evolving, COVID-19 is not included separately in this algorithm, but should be considered in all children with fever.

3.1.4 DIFFERENTIALS LIST

Dangerous Diagnoses

1. Sepsis
- The definition of paediatric sepsis is the presence of a systemic inflammatory response syndrome (SIRS) in the presence of, or as a result of, proven or suspected infection
- Can lead to a rapid deterioration and multi-organ failure
- Meningococcal sepsis has reduced in incidence since the implementation of the meningococcal vaccination programme

2. Bacterial Meningitis
- The classic meningism triad of headache, neck stiffness and photophobia will not be described in younger children, so a low index of suspicion is needed in the generally unwell infant
- In the acute setting, it is not possible to differentiate a viral from bacterial cause, so broad-spectrum antibiotics should be given to any patient with suspected meningitis

3. Herpes Encephalitis
- Encephalitis, i.e. inflammation of the brain, is a rare but serious condition
- Viral causes predominate, with herpes simplex being the most common. It can however occur as a consequence of bacterial, fungal and parasitic infections, as well as systemic conditions such as autoimmune diseases
- The clinical presentation can overlap with meningitis, so they are treated similarly in the acute setting

4. Febrile Neutropaenia
- A medical emergency that requires prompt treatment to avoid neutropaenic sepsis and death
- Commonly, the patient is known to be at risk of the condition due to having recently undergone chemotherapy
- Other conditions can lead to neutropaenia though, e.g. bone marrow failure syndromes
- In a patient at high risk of neutropaenia, initial treatment should be given prior to laboratory confirmation of the white cell count

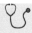

> **Box 3.1.3   Definition of Febrile Neutropaenia**
>
> - A temperature of ≥38.0 °C on at least one occasion and a neutrophil count <0.5 × 10⁹/L; *or*
> - Suspected sepsis in the presence of a temperature <38.0 °C and neutrophils <1.0 × 10⁹/L

5. Septic Arthritis
- Septic arthritis is an orthopaedic emergency and pertains to the infection of a joint leading to inflammation and joint destruction
- Unless prompt treatment is initiated, it is associated with considerable morbidity and mortality
- Orthopaedic involvement should be sought early to assist in definitive diagnosis (joint aspiration) and management (joint wash-out)
- Children with prosthetic joints are at higher risk
- Septic arthritis is associated with osteomyelitis, infection of the bone itself. This can present similarly with pain and erythema

6. Kawasaki Disease
- This systemic medium-vessel vasculitis should always be considered in a child presenting with a fever approaching or exceeding 5 days in duration
- There are clear diagnostic criteria (box 3.1.4). The diagnosis should be considered even if not all criteria are met, as atypical and incomplete forms of Kawasaki disease do exist
- The diagnosis is important to make in order to initiate treatment and implement surveillance for the major complication, coronary artery aneurysms, which can occur in up to 25% of untreated patients
- In the context of COVID-19, it is important to note that many features of Kawasaki Disease overlap with a rare sequelae of COVID-19 known as Paediatric Multisystem Inflammatory Syndrome (PIMS-TS). Details are emerging at time of writing. PIMS-TS seems to affect older children than Kawasaki (average nine years old versus four years old respectively), with abdominal symptoms in addition to the Kawasaki-like features, and a proportion presenting in shock requiring intensive care.

> **Box 3.1.4   Diagnostic Criteria for Kawasaki Disease**
>
> - Fever of at least 5 days' duration, without another explanation
> - Plus four of the following:
>   - Bilateral, non-purulent conjunctivitis
>   - Erythema of lips, oral mucosa, pharynx and tongue (strawberry tongue)
>   - Extremity changes, including erythema and/or oedema of the hands. Desquamation of fingers and toes is a late sign (usually 1–3 weeks after onset of fever)
>   - Polymorphous red rash. Forms include urticaria, maculopapular, target lesions and scarlatiniform (sandpapery)
>   - Cervical lymphadenopathy (usually large and singular)

Common Diagnoses

1. Viral Infections
- Viral infections are incredibly common in children, potentiated by the high infectivity of viruses and the close communion of children in nurseries, schools and at home
- Viruses are common culprits of many of the differentials discussed in this chapter
- Most viral infections are self-limiting and self-resolving
- Viral infections can predispose to secondary bacterial infection, so be wary of prolonged symptoms or patients re-presenting with persistent or progressive symptoms

2. Upper Respiratory Tract Infection (URTI)
- URTI is a broad term, covering a range of diagnoses of the upper airways, including rhinitis, pharyngitis, tonsillitis and sinusitis
- Viral causes are common, but there are notable bacterial infections that are worth considering, e.g. group A *Streptococcus* (GAS) or epiglottitis
- URTIs can, on occasion, progress to have more serious complications, such as a peri-tonsillar abscess (quinsy) or orbital cellulitis

3. Otitis Media
- Acute otitis media is an infection of the middle ear
- It can occur secondary to URTIs and similar pathogens are responsible, i.e. the respiratory viruses along with *Streptococcus pneumonia, Haemophilus influenzae* and *Moraxella catarrhalis*
- It is more common in younger children due to a less acute angle of the Eustachian tube, facilitating transfer of pathogens into the middle ear

4. Urinary Tract Infection (UTI)
- The presentation varies with age, with older children exhibiting the classical symptoms of dysuria, urgency and frequency, and younger children being more generally unwell with abdominal pain, nausea and vomiting
- Left untreated, UTIs in children can progress to cause upper UTIs and irreversible kidney damage
- Remember that Murphy's triad (fever, abdominal pain and vomiting) is suggestive of appendicitis, a diagnosis that may also lead to leucocytes on urine dip. Consider discussion with surgical colleagues if the diagnosis is unclear

5. Scarlet Fever
- Scarlet fever is not as common as it once was, but it has been rising in incidence in recent years for reasons that are not entirely clear, typically affecting children between 2 and 8 years of age
- It is caused by GAS and requires antibiotic treatment to reduce the risk of rheumatic fever
- The classic description is of a florid fine erythematous 'sandpaper' rash, strawberry tongue and fever. The fever may precede the appearance of the skin findings

6. Pneumonia
- Fever may not be the primary presenting symptom in pneumonia, with cough, difficulty in breathing and tachypnoea predominating instead
- Not all patients with suspected pneumonia require a chest x-ray or admission. However, if not adequately treated, a simple pneumonia can progress to more serious complications such as empyema and bronchiectasis
- Pneumonia is covered in Chapter 1.3, and will not be discussed further in this chapter

Diagnoses to Consider

1. Skin Infections
- There are a number of distinct skin infections that can affect children
- These can range from mild infections that can be treated with oral antibiotics to severe infections requiring specialist input
- Skin commensals are most commonly implicated, e.g. *Staphylococcus aureus*, although other organisms can lead to skin infections, especially if secondary to animal bites or in immunocompromised patients
When to consider: in those with skin erythema or induration

2. Infective Endocarditis
- Infection of the lining or valves of the heart, most commonly caused by staphylococcal or streptococcal species, although rarer organisms, including fungi, can be the cause
- The classic examination findings of endocarditis, e.g. Osler's nodes, clubbing etc., are less likely to be present in children
- They may exhibit other examples of immunological and embolic phenomena, e.g. haematuria
When to consider: in patients with known risk factors

Box 3.1.5   Skin Infections in Children   △△

Infection	Features
Impetigo	• Common, localised infection caused by *Staphylococcus* or *Streptococcus* species • Small pustules, which burst creating a yellow crust. Underlying skin may be erythematous and itchy • More serious forms exist, e.g. bullous impetigo
Cellulitis	• Erythematous, warm, swollen area of skin • May have puncture wound/ulcer as a source • Consider an underlying osteomyelitis
Periorbital cellulitis	• Common condition in children • Can mimic an insect bite or allergic reaction • At risk of progressing to an orbital cellulitis
Orbital cellulitis	• Cellulitis posterior to the orbital septum • Causes limitation and pain on eye movement, as well as proptosis • Can be caused by a spreading infection from a sinusitis or peri-orbital cellulitis, directly from the blood or from local trauma • Requires prompt antibiotic treatment and input from ophthalmology and Ear, Nose and Throat • Imaging may be required
Staphylococcal scalded skin syndrome (SSSS)	• Caused by exotoxins released by *Staphylococcus aureus* • Leads to widespread erythema and epidermal breakdown, resulting in a scalded appearance • The vast majority of cases occur in children under 6 years of age • Treatment is with intravenous (IV) antibiotics, monitoring fluid balance, pain and mobility • In severe cases, care should be transferred to a burns unit
Necrotising fasciitis	• A severe subcutaneous infection leading to necrosis of tissue • Surgical debridement is necessary to stop the infection spreading
Eczema herpeticum	• Children with eczema are susceptible to a widespread infection caused by herpes simplex virus • Leads to an acute deterioration of the skin with an erythematous vesicular rash • Treatment with IV aciclovir is necessary, unless it is mild • Predisposes to secondary bacterial cellulitis

Box 3.1.6   Risk Factors for Infective Endocarditis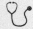

- Known congenital heart disease
- A history of cardiac surgery, in particular those with replacement valves, shunts and patches
- An indwelling central venous catheter
- Immunosuppression
- A previous history of endocarditis
- Illicit intravenous drug use (unlikely in the paediatric population)

3. **Acute Rheumatic Fever (ARF)**
   - ARF is a hypersensitivity reaction due to crossreactivity of antibodies following GAS infection that typically occurs 2–3 weeks after a sore throat
   - Associated fever and pancarditis can cause tachyarrhythmias
   - Other findings include arthralgia, arthritis, erythema marginatum, subcutaneous nodules and chorea
   When to consider: if there is a recent history of tonsillopharyngitis with arthralgia
4. **Tropical Infections**
   - This differential is covered in Chapter 3.2. Nevertheless, it is an important diagnostic consideration in children with risk factors, atypical presentations or prolonged symptoms
   When to consider: in those with a significant travel history

Box 3.1.7   Modified 2015 Jones Criteria for Diagnosis of Acute Rheumatic Fever

Required criteria:
- Evidence of streptococcal infection: positive throat swab for GAS, high ASO and anti-DNAse B titres, scarlet fever

Diagnosis based on:
- Required criteria plus 2 major, *or*
- Required criteria plus 1 major and 2 minor

Major criteria	Minor criteria
• Polyarthritis	• Fever ≥38.5 °C
• Carditis	• Polyarthralgia
• Sydenham chorea	• Prolonged PR interval
• Erythema marginatum	• ESR ≥60 mm/hr or CRP ≥3 mg/L
• Subcutaneous nodules	

Low risk population criteria included only, as incidence in UK is <1/100,000 per year.
ASO, antistreptolysin-O; CRP, C-reactive protein; ESR, erythrocyte sedimentation rate; GAS, group A *Streptococcus*

Box 3.1.8   Non-infectious Causes of Fever   △△

Inflammatory
- Haemophagocytic lymphohistiocytosis (HLH)
- Inflammatory bowel disease
- Juvenile arthritides, e.g. systemic-onset juvenile idiopathic arthritis
- Systemic lupus erythematosus (SLE)
- Vasculitides, e.g. Henoch–Schönlein purpura, Kawasaki disease

Malignancy
- Leukaemia
- Lymphoma

- Neuroblastoma
- Any other malignancy

Medication-related
- Drug-induced fever

Other
- Factitious or induced illness
- Familial periodic fever syndromes
- Sarcoidosis

---

5. **Non-infectious Systemic Disease**
   - Given that fever is a natural response of the body to both infection and inflammation, it can also be a presenting feature of several autoimmune, inflammatory and malignant conditions
   - A thorough systems review is required to assess for any constitutional symptoms, e.g. anorexia, unexplained weight loss, malaise. A clear chronology and description of symptoms is important, e.g. the pattern of joint pains
   - If a patient has one autoimmune condition, they are more susceptible to developing others. If the patient has had previously treated cancer, consider a relapse or secondary complications. Certain syndromes increase the risk of malignancy, e.g. Down syndrome and neurocutaneous syndromes such as neurofibromatosis
   - Examine for pallor, bruising and petechiae – suggestive of underlying pancytopenia, indicating bone marrow suppression. Examine for unexplained masses and focal neurological or ophthalmological signs

   When to consider: if there are systemic, constitutional symptoms, particularly when present over weeks or more
6. **Primary Immunodeficiencies**
   - There are a range of primary immunodeficiency syndromes in which a component of the immune system is missing or dysfunctional. They can range from mild to severe
   - The term does not relate to secondary or acquired immunodeficiencies, i.e. those related to other diseases, splenectomy or immunosuppressive treatments
   - Those with immunodeficiency may exhibit atypical or severe features of common infections. Detail is crucial in the history of a suspected immunodeficiency:
     - A clear chronology of previous infections, i.e. when and how many?

- How they were proven, i.e. culture results, imaging, serology?
- What treatment was required, i.e. did they require admission, oral or intravenous (IV) antibiotics, surgery?

When to consider: in those with recurrent, severe infections, or with a family history of immunodeficiency

---

Box 3.1.9   Features of Immunodeficiency Syndromes

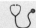

General features	Syndromic features
• Family history of immunodeficiency • Faltering growth • Recurrent proven bacterial infections • Severe infections, i.e. requiring multiple admissions for intravenous antibiotics • Infections caused by atypical or opportunistic pathogens • Deep skin or internal organ abscesses • Extensive candidiasis or warts • Chronic diarrhoea • Non-healing wounds • Persistent leukopaenia	• **Wiskott–Aldrich syndrome:** thrombocytopaenia, eczema • **DiGeorge syndrome:** dysmorphic features, congenital heart disease, hypocalcaemia • **Chédiak–Higashi syndrome:** albinism, neuropathy • **Ataxia-telangiectasia syndrome:** cerebellar ataxia, telangiectasia, growth delay • **Job syndrome:** eczema, skeletal abnormalities, dysmorphic features

---

3.1.5 KEY HISTORY FEATURES

Box 3.1.10   General Approach to History Taking in Children with Fever

Questions

1. **Does the parent/carer feel that the child is behaving like their usual self?** A child who is seriously unwell may have altered behaviour and mood. It is important to take a guardian's report of their child's condition seriously
2. **Has the child completed their immunisation schedule?** In the unimmunised child, thought should be given as to whether they are presenting with one of the conditions protected by vaccinations; see Chapter 12.4, *Childhood Immunisations*.

If the child has recently been vaccinated, i.e. within 24–48 hours prior to presentation, this could be the cause of any fever
3. **Does the child have any past medical history?** Many medical conditions and their treatments can predispose to infection, e.g. congenital or acquired immunodeficiency syndromes, post-splenectomy, immunosuppressant drugs, chemotherapy

---

Dangerous Diagnosis 1
Diagnosis: Sepsis

Questions
1. **What is the timeframe of the child's illness?** Sepsis can progress rapidly, so the rate of progression is important. A child may go from having a few petechiae in the morning to a fulminant rash by the afternoon
2. **Has there been a preceding illness to this presentation?** Sepsis is usually the progression of a previously localised infection
3. **In a newborn infant presenting in the first few days of life, were there any perinatal risk factors for sepsis?** Early-onset neonatal sepsis is a diagnosis in its own right, caused by specific pathogens, e.g. group B *Streptococcus*, *Escherichia coli*. There are well-established risk factors that should have been highlighted at the time of birth, which should be reviewed if the baby presents within the first 3 days of life
4. **How is the child behaving?** Parents may report a difference in behaviour from baseline. Cognitive or behavioural change are very concerning for end-organ hypoperfusion, due to sepsis
5. **What has their urine output been?** Children with sepsis can develop hypovolaemic and distributive shock and may have profound fluid replacement requirements. Ask about reduced urine output, estimated by the number of wet nappies or toilet visits

> **Box 3.1.11   Risk Factors for Early-Onset Neonatal Sepsis**
>
> - Maternal group B *Streptococcus* colonisation
> - Previous invasive group B *Streptococcus* infection in sibling
> - Preterm infant (<37 weeks' gestation)
> - Prolonged rupture of membranes (>18 hours)
> - Suspected or confirmed infection in a sibling in a multiple pregnancy
>
> - Maternal antibiotics given for suspected sepsis within 24 hours of delivery
> - Intrapartum maternal pyrexia (>38.0 °C) or suspected/confirmed chorioamnionitis

Dangerous Diagnosis 2
Diagnosis: Bacterial meningitis

Questions
1. **Is there any headache, neck stiffness or photophobia?** This is the classic symptom triad of meningism, i.e. meningeal irritation. Younger children will not complain of these symptoms, so a high index of suspicion is required in this age group
2. **Have there been any seizures?** 'Febrile seizures' are common in young children and it can be difficult to differentiate these from seizures due to underlying meningitis. Have a low threshold for suspecting meningitis, especially if the seizure is focal or prolonged
3. **Does the patient have an intra-cerebral shunt in situ or have they recently undergone neurosurgery?** Some children will have an indwelling shunt to alleviate hydrocephalus. Shunts, along with a history of recent neurosurgery, increase the risk of meningitis
4. **Is there vomiting/nausea?** Vomiting is a common non-specific symptom of bacterial meningitis and may indicate raised intracranial pressure

Dangerous Diagnosis 3
Diagnosis: Herpes encephalitis

Questions
1. **Was there any preceding illness?** Encephalitis often occurs a couple of days after symptoms of a non-specific viral infection
2. **Is there any history of herpetic lesions or suspected contact with herpes simplex?** Ask about vesicular lesions in the recent history or exposure to herpetic lesions elsewhere, e.g. from kissing a parent affected with a cold sore
3. **Is there an altered mental state (e.g. confusion), headache or seizures?** These symptoms are associated with encephalitis. Discuss baseline cognitive function with parents and whether they have noticed any deviation

Dangerous Diagnosis 4
Diagnosis: Febrile neutropaenia

Questions
1. **Is the patient known to be at risk of neutropaenia?** Most commonly, patients presenting with febrile neutropaenia will be known to have risk factors (e.g. chemotherapy). However, it is possible that this is the presenting event of a cyclical neutropaenia or bone marrow failure syndrome
2. **If an oncology patient, when was the last course of chemotherapy?** Patients are most vulnerable to develop febrile neutropaenia in the nadir, which typically occurs around 7–14 days following chemotherapy
3. **Does the patient have central line access, e.g. a Hickmann line, port or peripherally inserted central catheter (PICC) line?** If so, has it been accessed recently? Many children with oncology and other chronic illnesses have central venous access to facilitate regular phlebotomy and medication administration. Always consider a line infection, especially if fevers/rigors occur during or shortly after the line is accessed
4. **Is the patient known to be colonised with any resistant organisms?** The family might be aware of this or it might be documented in previous records. If resistant organisms are present, microbiology advice should be sought urgently regarding appropriate antibiotics
5. **Are any medications contraindicated during their treatment?** Given their toxicity, certain antibiotics are contraindicated in certain chemotherapy regimens or patients, e.g. piperacillin-tazobactam (if receiving high-dose methotrexate) or aminoglycosides (renal malignancies or impairment)

Dangerous Diagnosis 5
Diagnosis: Septic arthritis

Questions
1. **Is there any reported joint or bone pain or a limp?** A child with fever and joint pain should be considered to have septic arthritis until proven otherwise. Pain may be referred to a nearby joint
2. **Is there any history of injury or surgery to the joint?** In younger children, it is more common for infection to spread directly from an osteomyelitis or via the blood (haematogenous spread). However, in older children, infection secondary to trauma or surgical intervention can occur

Dangerous Diagnosis 6
Diagnosis: Kawasaki disease

Questions
1. **Has there been a fever for 5 days?** Kawasaki's disease is a clinical diagnosis that relies on a fever of at least 5 days. Many of the other features can be picked up in the examination; however, they are not always present at the same time, and it is useful to ask whether any have come and gone
2. **Has the child had a recent sore throat?** The symptoms of Kawasaki disease can mimic streptococcal tonsillitis. This diagnosis should be considered as an alternative differential
3. **What ethnicity is the child?** Kawasaki disease is more common in those of East Asian descent
4. **Have any other family members had Kawasaki disease before?** Although not fully understood, there is a familial tendency to Kawasaki disease, particularly in those with previously affected siblings

Common Diagnosis 1
Diagnosis: Viral infection

Questions
1. **What is the exact progression of the symptoms?** Many infections follow a well-described progression from a prodrome illness to development of rash and recovery
2. **Has the child been in contact with anyone with similar symptoms?** Viruses are highly contagious, so it is common for them to spread around nurseries, schools and siblings. The incubation period of different viruses is variable, but symptoms usually occur within 1–7 days of exposure. Varicella, measles, mumps and rubella generally have a longer incubation period, i.e. 2–3 weeks
3. **How long have symptoms been present?** Viral infections can follow on one after the other and they can also predispose to secondary bacterial infection. It is imperative to get a clear chronology of symptoms, including any days where the patient was fever/symptom free

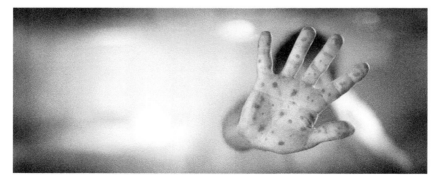

Figure 3.1.2 Vesicles on the palm in hand, food and mouth disease, usually caused by an enterovirus infection, most commonly Coxsackie A16. Source: Reproduced with permission of Getty Images.

Table 3.1.1 Viral causes of fever in children

Diagnosis	Causative virus(es)	Key features
'The flu'	Influenza type A, B or C	• Fever, coryza, cough, myalgia and fatigue
Upper respiratory tract infections (URTIs)	Rhinovirus, adenovirus, coronavirus (e.g. COVID-19), metapneumovirus, parainfluenza, respiratory syncytial virus (RSV)	• Coryza, sneezing, mild conjunctivitis, sore throat, cough and malaise • May lead to sinusitis and otitis media • Parainfluenza typically causes croup (laryngotracheobronchitis) • May lead to bronchiolitis in children under 18 months • COVID-19, caused by coronavirus SARS-CoV-2, is associated with cough and anosmia
Infectious mononucleosis (glandular fever)	Epstein–Barr virus (EBV)	• May be asymptomatic or cause a mild URTI-type illness • In adolescents causes fever, sore throat, lymphadenopathy and fatigue • Malaise may persist for several weeks
Roseola infantum (sixth disease)	Human herpesvirus 6 or 7	• 2–3 days of high fever, followed by non-pruritic maculopapular rash once the fever subsides • Most common in children under 2 years of age
Slapped cheek (erythema infectiosum/fifth disease)	Parvovirus B19	• URTI symptoms followed by pruritic maculopapular rash, classically on cheeks but can be over whole body • Adolescents can have reactive arthritis • Can precipitate aplastic crises in those with haematological disorders
Hand, foot and mouth disease	Coxsackie A	• URTI symptoms followed by flat red spots in the mouth, palms, soles, buttocks and groin, which may blister
Chicken pox, shingles	Varicella zoster virus (VZV)	• Rash progresses through different phases, papular, vesicular and pustular, with crops at different stages • Highly contagious from before rash until all lesions are crusted over • Serious complications: bacterial superinfection/toxic shock, encephalitis, cerebellitis, pneumonia and disseminated infection in the immunocompromised host • Reactivation leads to shingles
Herpetic whitlow, cold sores, gingivostomatitis	Herpes simplex virus (HSV)	• HSV causes a range of conditions, from a localised rash on the fingers (herpetic whitlow) to generalised infection (e.g. eczema herpeticum) • Infection of the oral mucosa leads to gingivostomatitis
Measles	Measles	• Prodrome of fever, cough, coryza, conjunctivitis and diarrhoea • Pathognomonic 'Koplik spots': small red spots with a bluish-white centre on buccal mucosa • Maculopapular rash develops on the face, spreading to trunk and extremities, fading in the order of appearance, and may coalesce and desquamate • Complications can occur, including neurological, respiratory and gastrointestinal
Mumps	Mumps	• Causes fever, malaise and parotitis (usually bilateral) • Complications: encephalitis, orchitis and pancreatitis
German measles	Rubella	• Mild disease with prodrome of fever, headache and coryza, followed by rash • Rash is initially discrete non-pruritic macules starting on the face, which may coalesce and extend to the trunk and extremities • Risk of congenital rubella syndrome in the foetus of a non-immune pregnant mother

Common Diagnosis 2
Diagnosis: Upper respiratory tract infection

Questions
1. **Has the child been in contact with anyone with similar symptoms?** Given that the vast majority of URTIs are caused by viral infections, there is often a history of exposure within the previous week
2. **How long have symptoms been present?** Normal children may have eight or more viral URTIs a year and they can seemingly follow on, one after the other. Symptoms from one infection can also last up to 2 weeks. Ask about symptom-free days
3. **Is there any facial pain?** Pain behind the eyes is suggestive of a possible sinusitis. Pain on eye movement should raise the suspicion of an orbital cellulitis, which can be a complication of sinusitis

Common Diagnosis 3
Diagnosis: Otitis media

Questions
1. **Is there any reported ear pain or is the child pulling at their ear?** Pain is common in otitis media
2. **Is there any history of otitis media?** Some children are vulnerable to developing recurrent acute otitis media or more chronic forms
3. **Any discharge from the ear?** Occasionally, the tympanic membrane can perforate, which can lead to a discharge (otorrhoea)
4. **Any recent illness?** Otitis media is caused by pathogens associated with URTIs

Common Diagnosis 4
Diagnosis: Urinary tract infection

Questions
1. **Is there a history of dysuria, urgency or frequency?** These classic symptoms of a UTI may be present in older children and teenagers. Young children may be more non-specifically unwell, with abdominal pain and vomiting. The urine may be foul-smelling
2. **If the patient has previously been toilet trained, have they started wetting themselves again?** Secondary enuresis usually has a precipitating factor. This can be a UTI. Importantly, enuresis can also be associated with stressful events, e.g. problems at school, home or sexual abuse.
3. **Is this their first episode of a UTI?** Recurrent UTIs raise the suspicion of a structural issue of the urinary tract or potential renal damage
4. **Is there any blood in the urine?** Blood in the urine is generally pathological and warrants further investigation. Consider, however, whether the patient is menstruating if of an appropriate age

Common Diagnosis 5
Diagnosis: Scarlet fever

Questions
1. **What is the progression of symptoms?** There may be a prodrome of fever, sore throat, headache, vomiting and myalgia. After 1–2 days, a florid rash develops. The rash starts on the neck and trunk, extending to extremities
2. **Has the child been in contact with anyone with similar symptoms?** The incubation period is relatively short at 2–4 days, so there may be a recent contact that can be remembered

3.1.6 KEY EXAMINATION FEATURES

> **Box 3.1.12   General Approach to Examination in Children with Fever**
>
> Patients with sepsis can deteriorate quickly and become very unwell. A thorough 'A to E' assessment should be performed (see Chapter 12.1, *The A to E Assessment*)
> In particular look out for:
>
> - A: signs of airway obstruction
> - B: tachypnoea, difficulty breathing, wheeze and hypoxia
> - C: tachycardia, hypotension, prolonged capillary refill time and changes in colour
> - D: reduced consciousness/tone, seizures, altered behaviour or signs of raised intracranial pressure
> - E: temperature abnormalities, glucose and electrolyte abnormalities, rashes

Dangerous Diagnosis 1
Diagnosis: Sepsis

Examination Findings
1. **Altered mental status.** Children may be drowsy, lethargic, confused or irritable. In addition, lack of response to social cues and a weak, high-pitched or continuous cry are all concerning
2. **Non-blanching rash (petechiae/purpura).** Many conditions can cause petechiae, e.g. cough or vomit-induced petechiae in the distribution of the superior vena cava. However, in the presence of fever, consideration must be given to sepsis. If there is a non-blanching purpuric rash or petechial rash, strongly consider sepsis
3. **Signs of poor perfusion.** Systemic cytokine release causes vasodilation and fluid leak from capillaries, resulting in poor perfusion. Signs include increased capillary refill time, lactic acidosis, oliguria and altered mental status
4. **Signs of shock.** Capillary leak can cause distributive shock. Hypotension and poor perfusion refractory to volume resuscitation suggest septic (distributive) shock and need urgent escalation of care
5. **Bleeding.** Excessive bleeding may be due to thrombocytopenia as a result of disseminated intravascular coagulation

Dangerous Diagnosis 2
Diagnosis: Bacterial meningitis

Examination Findings
1. **Bulging fontanelle**. In children whose cranial sutures are yet to fuse, i.e. those under 12 months of age, there may be a bulging fontanelle
2. **Meningism.** Meningism causes restriction of neck flexion: a child who can put their chin on their chest is not meningitic. Reduction in neck movement is not a reliable sign in babies: look for irritability (a high-pitched or moaning, inconsolable cry) instead. See Chapter 8.1, *Headache*, Figure 8.1.4. *Detecting meningism on clinical examination*
3. **Photophobia.** If the child is truly photophobic, they will probably either keep their eyes closed or ask for the lights to be turned off
4. **Altered mental status.** This includes confusion, delirium, drowsiness and impaired consciousness
5. **Appears systemically unwell.** Children with infective meningitis nearly always appear systemically unwell and may have signs consistent with sepsis. The exception is tuberculous meningitis, which can be more insidious
6. **Non-blanching purpuric rash.** Meningococcal septicaemia may lead to disseminated intravascular coagulation (DIC), causing a purpuric rash (normally in the setting of circulatory collapse). Absence of a rash does not rule out meningitis.

Dangerous Diagnosis 3
Diagnosis: Herpes encephalitis

Examination Findings
1. **Focal neurology.** Examine limbs and cranial nerves carefully for focal neurological deficit. There may also be seizures
2. **Altered mental state.** Look for confusion, delirium, drowsiness and impaired consciousness
3. **Herpetic skin lesions.** Assess for any herpetic lesions – groups of vesicular lesions on an erythematous base
4. **Evidence of other viral infections.** Other causes of encephalitis should also be considered, including searching for insect bites, chickenpox or features of systemic disease

Dangerous Diagnosis 4
Diagnosis: Febrile neutropaenia

Examination Findings
1. **Erythema tracking along central line.** This is a concerning feature suggestive of central line infection. Also look for pain, swelling and discharge
2. **Mucositis.** Following chemotherapy, patients are vulnerable to having mucositis. This can be exquisitely tender and predisposes to infection due to mucous membrane breakdown
3. **Perianal infection.** Patients are vulnerable to perianal lesions and infection. An examination of the groin and perianal region is therefore mandatory, maintaining patient dignity as much as possible
4. **The absence of infective signs is not reassuring.** In the absence of a functioning immune system, signs of infection may not be present. It may not be possible to localise the cause of the fever, but the patient may still be at risk of overwhelming neutropaenic sepsis

Dangerous Diagnosis 5
Diagnosis: Septic arthritis

Examination Findings
1. **Swelling or erythema of the joint.** These common findings of inflammation are usually detectable in superficial joints, although they may be harder to identify in joints covered by more subcutaneous tissue, e.g. the hip. A joint effusion may be detectable
2. **Reduced range of movement.** Pain-limiting range of movement can present as a limp if affecting a lower-limb joint in a mobile child. Younger children with a hip arthritis may hold their hip flexed, abducted and externally rotated
3. **Signs of osteomyelitis.** Localised bone pain near the joint with overlying erythema is suggestive of an associated osteomyelitis. Occasionally, a sinus tract may be visible, connecting the bone infection to the skin

Dangerous Diagnosis 6
Diagnosis: Kawasaki disease

Examination Findings
The diagnosis of Kawasaki disease is clinical and requires satisfaction of certain key features (see Box 3.1.4).
1. **Persistent fever.** Fever is often minimally responsive to antipyretics
2. **Irritability.** Children with Kawasaki disease tend to be very miserable, out of proportion to their clinical findings
3. **Cervical lymphadenopathy.** Lymphadenopathy tends to be limited to the cervical area, mostly the anterior cervical nodes
4. **Conjunctivitis.** Conjunctivitis is bilateral and non-exudative, with marked erythema, and is present in more than 90% of patients. Children may also be photophobic
5. **Mucositis.** This manifests as cracked, red lips and a 'strawberry tongue'
6. **Rash.** There are many types of rash associated with Kawasaki disease. A widespread maculopapular rash over the trunk and limbs is common. The characteristic desquamation of palms and soles is a late sign
7. **Reactivation at BCG site.** In children who have received a BCG vaccination, there may be a reactivation of the scar, with erythema or crust formation
8. **Are there tonsillar exudates?** Bacterial tonsillitis is an important differential of Kawasaki disease. The presence of pharyngitis with tonsillar exudates points away from Kawasaki disease

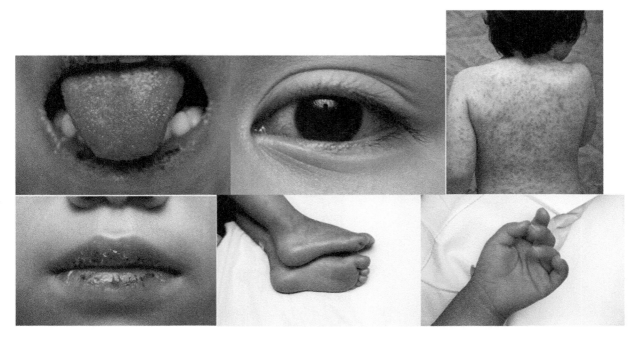

Figure 3.1.3 Findings in Kawasaki disease. (A) Strawberry tongue; (B) non-purulent conjunctivitis; (C) maculopapular red rash; (D) erythematous peeling lips; (E) erythema of feet; (F) erythema of hands. Courtesy of Kawasaki Disease Foundation.

Common Diagnosis 1
Diagnosis: Viral infection

Examination Findings
1. **Features of specific conditions.** Certain viral infections are associated with typical rashes or examination findings, beyond the scope of this chapter

Common Diagnosis 2
Diagnosis: Upper respiratory tract infection

Examination Findings
1. **Rhinitis/conjunctivitis.** The typical child with a simple URTI is coryzal. They may have a cough and can appear miserable, especially when febrile
2. **Tonsillar enlargement/erythema/exudate.** It is common for children to have enlarged tonsils, which may be erythematous and have white/yellow exudate on them
3. **Lymphadenopathy.** Lymphadenopathy is common in URTIs, typically in the anterior cervical chain. If tender and unilateral, it is more suggestive of a GAS throat infection
4. **Facial tenderness.** Tenderness on pressing superficially over the sinuses is suggestive of an underlying sinusitis

---

Box 3.1.13   Features Suggestive of More Than an Upper Respiratory Tract Infection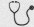

- An asymmetrical swelling in the throat, deviating the uvula, is suggestive of a peritonsillar abscess (quinsy)
- A pseudomembrane over the tonsils is suggestive of diphtheria, although this is now rare due to successful vaccination programmes

---

Common Diagnosis 3
Diagnosis: Otitis media

Examination Findings
1. **Pulling ear.** Younger children may visibly pull on the ear on the side of the infection as an indication of discomfort
2. **Characteristic otoscopy findings.** See Box 3.1.14

Box 3.1.14   Findings on Otoscopy in Otitis Media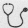

- A red/cloudy tympanic membrane
- Air-fluid level in the middle ear
- Bulging tympanic membrane
- A perforated tympanic membrane may be present. If there is discharge, it might not be possible to visualise this

---

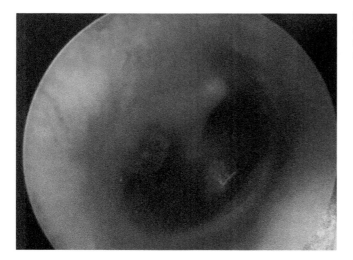

Figure 3.1.4 Dull and retracted tympanic membrane as seen in otitis media on otoscopy. Source: Reproduced with permission from Newell, S.J., and Darling, J.C. (2014). *Paediatrics lecture notes*. Chichester: Wiley Blackwell.

Common Diagnosis 4
Diagnosis: Urinary tract infection

Examination Findings
1. **Suprapubic or renal angle tenderness.** Lower UTIs can be associated with suprapubic tenderness on palpation, whereas pyelonephritis may cause flank pain
2. **Abdominal masses.** UTIs are associated with structural abnormalities of the kidneys and urinary tract, as well as children with constipation
3. **Spinal anomalies.** Those with spinal problems, such as spina bifida, may have a neurogenic bladder, where poor emptying increases risk of UTI
4. **Genital discharge or balanitis/vulvovaginitis.** These signs are suggestive of an alternative diagnosis. Consider sexually transmitted diseases in sexually active adolescents or if there is a concern about sexual abuse

---

Box 3.1.15 Categorising Urinary Tract Infections (UTIs)

Term	Definition
Upper UTI (pyelonephritis)	• Children with bacteriuria and fever >38.0 °C; *or* • Children with a fever <38.0 °C with loin pain/tenderness
Lower UTI (cystitis)	• Children with bacteriuria but no features of an upper UTI
Recurrent UTI	• ≥2 episodes of upper UTI • 1 episode of upper UTI plus ≥1 episode of lower UTI • ≥3 episodes of lower UTI
Atypical UTI	• Infection with non-*Escherichia coli* organism • Seriously unwell/septic • Poor urine flow • Abdominal or bladder mass • Raised creatinine • Failure to respond to appropriate antibiotic within 48 hours

---

Common Diagnosis 5
Diagnosis: Scarlet fever

Examination Findings
1. **Scarlatiniform rash.** Classic features of this rash are described in Box 3.1.16
2. **Flushed cheeks/circumoral pallor.** The face is usually spared from the scarlatiniform rash, but the cheeks may be red, with sparing in the perioral region
3. **Strawberry tongue.** Initially, the tongue has red papillae seen through a white coating. This later desquamates, leaving a red tongue with prominent papillae
4. **Throat.** The tonsils may appear red and swollen with exudate

---

Box 3.1.16 Description of Rash in Scarlet Fever

- A coarse texture, described as sandpaper rash, with fine papules on an erythematous base
- May be more prominent in skin creases
- Pastia's lines: confluent petechiae forming red lines in skin creases
- May desquamate

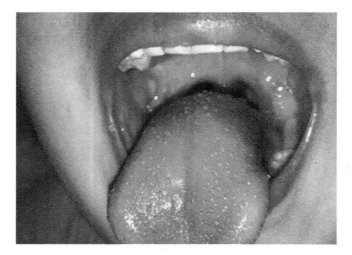

Figure 3.1.5 Strawberry tongue in scarlet fever. Source: Reproduced with permission of Shutterstock.

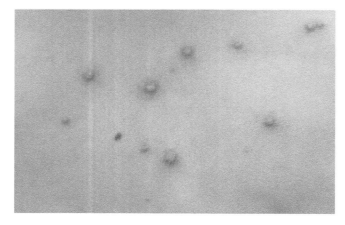

Figure 3.1.6 The classic rash of chickenpox involves pruritic, fluid-filled vesicles on an erythematous base. Source: Reproduced with permission of Shutterstock.

3.1.7 KEY INVESTIGATIONS

In children with a clinical focus of viral or uncomplicated bacterial infection and no evidence of sepsis, blood tests may not be necessary.

Bedside

Table 3.1.2 Bedside tests of use in patients presenting with fever

Test	When to perform	Potential result
Throat swab	Suspected: • Scarlet fever • Rheumatic fever	• Pure growth of an organism supports infection • Sensitivities guide antibiotic choice
Urine dipstick	• Suspected UTI	• See Box 3.1.17 for a guide to interpretation • Remember, leucocyte esterase can be present in the urine due to infections other than UTIs

Table 3.1.2 (Continued)

Test	When to perform	Potential result
Urine MC&S *must be clean catch	• If positive urine dipstick • If strong clinical suspicion of UTI despite negative urine dipstick • In infants <6 months as urine dipstick not sensitive • If patient unwell, consider catheter sample	• Pure growth of an organism supports infection • Sensitivities guide antibiotic choice
Blood gas	• If systemically unwell	• ↓ pH and ↑CO_2 indicates respiratory acidosis • ↓ pH, ↓ HCO_3, ↑lactate indicate metabolic acidosis, suggestive of poor perfusion • ↑/↓ Glucose may occur in sepsis
NPA	• With suspected respiratory viral infection, *if knowing result is felt to be useful*	• Respiratory virus, e.g. respiratory syncytial virus (RSV) • Knowing result is not always necessary, but children with the same viruses can be 'cohorted' together

CO_2, carbon dioxide; HCO_3, bicarbonate; MC&S, microscopy, culture and sensitivity; NPA, nasopharyngeal aspirate; UTI, urinary tract infection

Blood Tests

Table 3.1.3 Blood tests of use in patients presenting with fever

Test	When to perform	Potential result
Blood culture (ideally take prior to commencing antibiotics)	• All children <3 months of age Suspected: • Sepsis • Meningitis • Infective endocarditis – take three separate sets	• Pure growth of an organism supports infection • Sensitivities guide antibiotic choice
FBC	• All systemically unwell children • White cell counts useful in assessing for infection and haematological malignancy • Neutrophils crucial in assessment of febrile neutropaenia • Platelets count useful if petechiae	• Normocytic anaemia in chronic disease • ↓/↑ WCC in infection (usually neutrophilia if bacterial, lymphocytosis in viral) • ↓ Platelets in DIC • ↑ Platelets in chronic inflammation • Pancytopenia: malignancy, bone marrow failure syndrome
Blood film	• Suspected malignancy	• Peripheral blast cells are indicative of malignancy • 'Left shift' suggests a population of young neutrophils being produced in response to infection • Platelet clumping may explain underestimated counts in FBC
U&E	• If systemically unwell • Severe dehydration	• ↑ Urea and creatinine indicates acute kidney injury, which can result from poor perfusion in sepsis or severe dehydration
CRP	• If systemically unwell • To guide suspicions of invasive infections, such as septic arthritis • Lacks specificity, so interpret with history and examination	• Significant ↑ in bacterial infections • Less marked ↑ in viral infections • Rise can be delayed, so serious illness should not be discounted in the presence of a low CRP if there is clinical concern
Calcium and magnesium	Suspected: • Sepsis • Meningitis	• ↓ Ca^{2+} and ↓ Mg^{2+} in sepsis, particularly meningococcal septicaemia
ESR	• Consider as an adjunct in monitoring inflammation	• ↑ In infection and inflammation
Clotting screen	• Only in systemically unwell patients with clinical evidence of sepsis	• ↑ INR/APTT and ↓ fibrinogen levels occur in DIC • Fibrinogen is an acute-phase reactant, so may be raised in infection

APTT, activated partial thromboplastin time; Ca, calcium; CRP, C-reactive protein; DIC, disseminated intravascular coagulation; ESR, erythrocyte sedimentation rate; FBC, full blood count; INR, international normalised ratio; Mg, magnesium; U&E, urea and electrolytes; WCC, white cell count

Imaging

Table 3.1.4 Imaging modalities of use in patients presenting with fever

Test	When to perform	Potential result
Chest x-ray	• Suspected complicated pneumonia	• Pneumonia: consolidation • Complications of pneumonia: abscess, empyema • Mediastinal lymphadenopathy: wide mediastinum
Limb x-ray	• Suspected septic arthritis	• See Chapter 10.1, *Limp*, Box 10.1.10 *Radiological Findings in Septic Arthritis*
Joint ultrasound	• Suspected septic arthritis, for diagnosis and to help guide aspiration	
Urinary tract ultrasound	• In atypical or complicated UTIs – see Box 3.1.20	• Structural urinary tract lesions • Dilatation or hydronephrosis
Magnetic resonance imaging (MRI) brain	• If presenting with focal neurology or significantly altered mental status • To rule out space-occupying lesion prior to lumbar puncture	• Brain abscess • In encephalitis there may be evidence of high signal intensity in the temporal lobes, but a normal scan does not rule it out
MRI bone	• Suspected osteomyelitis and septic arthritis – more sensitive and specific for early damage	• Subchondral bone changes, perisynovial oedema, synovial enhancement with contrast

Special

Table 3.1.5 Special tests of use in patients presenting with fever

Test	When to perform	Potential result
CSF, MC&S and PCR (should not delay administration of antibiotics)	• Suspected meningitis or encephalitis • Do not perform LP if systemically unstable, raised intracranial pressure, coagulation abnormalities or cellulitis over the spine • If suspected viral meningitis or encephalitis, specifically request *viral PCR*	• See Box 3.1.18 for a guide to interpretation • PCR can give rapid results for bacterial and viral infections • Confirmed organism determines duration of antibiotic treatment and whether steroids are indicated
Anti-streptolysin O titre (ASOT)	• Suspected GAS throat infection or ARF	• ↑ Titres suggest recent GAS infection • There can be a delay in rise initially, so a low titre with a strong suspicion of GAS infection does not exclude it
Echocardiogram	Suspected: • Kawasaki disease • Infective endocarditis	• Kawasaki disease: coronary artery aneurysms • Infective endocarditis: endocardial vegetations
Heterophile antibody test	• Rapid test for suspected EBV infection	• Positive test suggestive of acute EBV • False positives in other viral and autoimmune conditions
Immunodeficiency tests	• Suspected immunodeficiency • A number of possible tests are available • They should generally be ordered on the advice of an immunologist • Genetic studies are available for certain disorders	Tests vary: • Quantitative assays: mannose-binding lectin, leucocyte subsets, general and specific Ig levels • Functional tests: T-cell proliferation studies, complement function and the nitroblue tetrazolium test
Serology	• Although it will not be justified in all cases, immunological testing for serology can aid in the diagnosis of specific infections	• IgM positive: suggestive of an acute infection • IgG positive and IgM negative: suggestive of past infection
Whole-blood PCR for bacterial and viral DNA/RNA	• Suspected bacterial meningitis to detect *Neisseria meningitidis* • PCR can also be used to quantify viral loads in presumed systemic viral infections in vulnerable groups	• Detection of a DNA/RNA of a specific virus or bacterium is supportive of that pathogen causing infection • Trends in viral load are useful to monitor treatment

ARF, acute rheumatic fever; CSF, cerebrospinal fluid; EBV, Epstein–Barr virus; GAS, group A *Streptococcus*; Ig, immunoglobulin; LP, lumbar puncture; MC&S, microscopy, culture and sensitivity; PCR, polymerase chain reaction

Box 3.1.17   Interpretation of Urine Dipstick

Leucocyte esterase	Nitrites	Interpretation
Positive	Positive	• Treat as UTI
Negative	Positive	• Start antibiotics • Formal diagnosis depends on culture
Positive	Negative	• Only start antibiotics if clinical evidence of UTI • Formal diagnosis depends on urine culture
Negative	Negative	• UTI unlikely • Repeat or send urine for culture if clinically suggestive of UTI

UTI, urinary tract infection

Box 3.1.18   Interpretation of Cerebrospinal Fluid (CSF)

Diagnosis	Appearance	White cells	Protein	Glucose
Bacterial meningitis	Cloudy	High (typically neutrophils)	High	Low
Viral meningitis	Clear	High (typically lymphocytes)	Normal or high	Normal or low
Tuberculous meningitis	Clear or cloudy	High (typically lymphocytes)	High	Very low
Encephalitis	Clear	Normal or raised lymphocytes	Normal or high	Normal or low

Note: further tests will be performed on CSF samples, including Gram stain and bacterial culture.
If requested, polymerase chain reaction (PCR) tests can be performed to look for viruses or bacteria

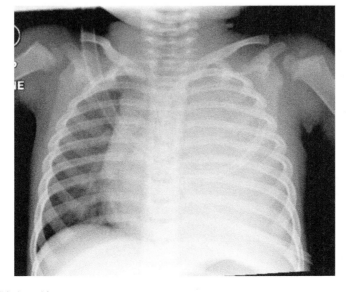

Figure 3.1.7 Left-sided consolidation with empyema.

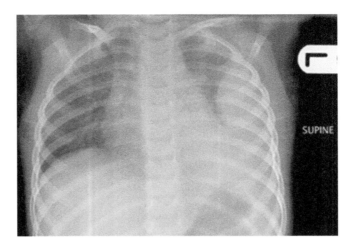

Figure 3.1.8 Left-sided empyema with a clear convexity due to the pleural collection.

3.1.8 KEY MANAGEMENT PRINCIPLES

Diagnosis-specific management strategies are outlined here. It is expected that an 'ABCDE' approach to assessment and management is considered standard practice (see Chapter 12.1, *The A to E Assessment*). If the diagnosis is unclear and sepsis is possible, it is essential to commence treatment for sepsis while diagnostic evaluation continues.

Dangerous Diagnosis 1
Diagnosis: Sepsis

Management Principles
1. **Urgent broad-spectrum antibiotics.** This is the most important aspect to the management of sepsis. Antibiotics should be given within 60 minutes of sepsis being suspected, ideally within 30 minutes. IV antibiotics are preferred; if no IV access, IO should be obtained, and if in the community, IM can be given. For detailed discussion of the management of sepsis, see Chapter 13.1, *Sepsis Management*

Dangerous Diagnosis 2
Diagnosis: Bacterial meningitis

Management Principles
1. **Urgent broad-spectrum antibiotics.** In the community setting, intramuscular benzylpenicillin should be given. In hospital a third-generation cephalosporin is used, usually high-dose IV ceftriaxone. Cefotaxime is often used in children <6 weeks old due to the risk of jaundice with ceftriaxone
2. **Consider adjuvant antimicrobials.** Amoxicillin: to cover for *Listeria monocytogenes* in children <3 months of age. Anti-staphylococcal antibiotics: if intra-cerebral shunts are in situ. Aciclovir: if a herpes simplex meningoencephalitis is suspected. Vancomycin: in those who have recently travelled outside the UK or with prolonged, multiple exposure to antibiotics
3. **Dexamethasone.** In children over 3 months of age, dexamethasone is recommended if any of the following cerebrospinal fluid (CSF) findings are present:
   - Frankly purulent CSF
   - CSF white cell count (WCC) >1000/μL
   - Protein concentration >1 g/L in the context of raised CSF WCC
   - Bacteria present on Gram stain

   Dexamethasone should be given at the time of, or as soon as possible after, the first dose of antibiotics. This can reduce the risk of hearing impairment and other long-term neurological damage
4. **Monitor for deterioration.** Very close monitoring for signs of deterioration is required, with respiration, pulse, blood pressure, oxygen saturations and Glasgow Coma Scale score. Rapid deterioration is possible, regardless of initial severity
5. **Audiology follow-up.** All patients with confirmed bacterial meningitis should undergo audiology follow-up due to the risk of associated sensorineural deafness

6. **Alert public health authorities.** Confirmed bacterial meningitis is a public health concern and the appropriate authorities should be informed. Contact tracing might be required, with prophylactic antibiotics provided to high-risk contacts

Dangerous Diagnosis 3
Diagnosis: Herpes encephalitis

Management Principles
1. **Aciclovir.** IV aciclovir is indicated if encephalitis is suspected, as herpes is the most common cause. Antibiotics are usually started as well, since it is difficult to differentiate between meningitis and encephalitis in the acute setting and they can occur together
2. **Alert public health authorities.** Viral encephalitis is a notifiable disease
3. **Treatment of complications.** Treatment of seizures should be managed with anticonvulsant medication. For management of raised intracranial pressure (ICP), see Chapter 13.5, *Raised Intracranial Pressure Management*

Dangerous Diagnosis 4
Diagnosis: Febrile neutropaenia

Management Principles
1. **Urgent extended-spectrum antibiotics.** Antibiotics should be given as per local guidelines – often piperacillin-tazobactam. When making antibiotic choice, consider known resistant organisms, contraindications and extra cover for line/endo-prosthetic infections
2. **Consider central line sustainability.** Antibiotics should ideally be given through the central line, even if a line infection is suspected. It may be possible to 'salvage' the line and the decision to remove it should be made in discussion with the tertiary treatment centre
3. **Length of treatment.** If the patient remains clinically well with negative blood cultures, consideration can be given to converting to oral antibiotics after 48 hours. In some high-risk patients, this may not be possible
4. **Supportive therapy.** Febrile neutropaenia typically occurs at predictable points post chemotherapy, which also coincides with the height of other symptoms, e.g. mucositis. Other symptom-control medications may include analgesia, mouthwashes and antiemetics

Dangerous Diagnosis 5
Diagnosis: Septic arthritis

Management Principles
1. **Joint aspiration.** Aspiration of the joint is useful in both confirming the diagnosis and culturing the causative organism
2. **Joint lavage.** A joint lavage is required to reduce complications and may be arthroscopic or open
3. **Antibiotics.** Commencement of appropriate IV antibiotics is crucial – use local guidelines. Typically, anti-staphylococcal antibiotics are used, given this is the most common causative organism
4. **Follow-up.** Children with a diagnosis of septic arthritis should have ongoing orthopaedic follow-up to monitor for complications and ensure growth of the joint has not been impaired

Dangerous Diagnosis 6
Diagnosis: Kawasaki disease

Management Principles
1. **Intravenous immunoglobulin (IVIg).** Standard treatment consists of high-dose IVIg. High-dose IVIg administered within 10 days of the beginning of the disease decreases the risk of coronary aneurysm by more than 5 times. Re-treatment with IVIg can be considered if there is persistence or recurrence of fever within 2 weeks of the first treatment
2. **Aspirin.** Dose is controversial, but generally high-dose aspirin is prescribed initially, with variable evidence for when to reduce to low-dose. Continuation is dependent on the presence of coronary artery abnormalities
3. **Cardiac follow-up.** Cardiology review is essential to monitor for development of coronary artery abnormalities, diagnosed with echocardiography
4. **Glucocorticoids.** Glucocorticoid treatment with prednisolone should be considered for those at high risk for IVIg resistance, or in those who do not respond. Various scores, such as the Kobayashi score, determine risk of IVIg resistance; however, these are not commonly used in the UK

Box 3.1.19   Intravenous Immunoglobulin (IVIg)

- IVIg is a blood product, requiring caution when administering, due to possible allergic reactions
- The recommended dose for Kawasaki disease is 2 g/kg, to be given as an infusion over 8–12 hours
- The mechanism of action in Kawasaki disease is not fully understood, but it has anti-inflammatory effects

Common Diagnosis 1
Diagnosis: Viral infection

Management Principles
1. **Reassurance, safety-netting and monitoring for resolution.** The majority of viral infections resolve without issue. Appropriate safety-netting advice should be given to the parents to monitor for complications such as secondary bacterial infection
2. **Notify public health authorities.** Certain viral infections are notifiable diseases, including measles, mumps and rubella
3. **Antivirals if appropriate.** There are only a limited number of antiviral medications in common use. Complicated or prolonged infections with viruses in the herpes family may warrant use of aciclovir

Common Diagnosis 2
Diagnosis: Upper respiratory tract infection

Management Principles
1. **Reassurance, safety-netting and monitoring for resolution.** The majority of URTIs are caused by viruses and will resolve spontaneously. Appropriate safety-netting advice should be given
2. **Supportive therapies.** Saline drops for nasal congestion can be useful in younger children who are nasal breathers. Paracetamol and ibuprofen can help control associated pain
3. **Antibiotics if bacterial infection suspected.** If the patient is systemically well, it is reasonable to provide a delayed prescription, for use if symptoms do not improve. Antibiotics should be given if the patient is systemically unwell, has a significant comorbidity or has signs of a complication, e.g. abscess/cellulitis
4. **Consider Ear, Nose and Throat (ENT) referral.** Routine referrals can be sent for chronic sinusitis or if children have recurrent tonsillitis (≥5 times a year, with disruption of daily activities) or evidence of sleep apnoea

Common Diagnosis 3
Diagnosis: Otitis media

Management Principles
1. **Reassurance, safety-netting and monitoring for resolution.** The vast majority of acute otitis media cases will resolve spontaneously within a few days, but it can last for a week. Appropriate safety-netting advice should be given
2. **Consideration of antibiotics.** Immediate antibiotics should be given in the following groups:
   - Systemically very unwell, i.e. signs of sepsis
   - High risk of or suspected complications, e.g. craniofacial abnormalities, immunodeficiency
   In other groups, consider a delayed antibiotic prescription for use if symptoms do not improve. Those most likely to benefit from antibiotics are those with discharge following a perforated tympanic membrane, or children under 2 years of age, with bilateral otitis media
3. **Supportive therapies.** Paracetamol and ibuprofen can be used to control associated pain. Evidence does not support the use of decongestants or antihistamines
4. **Specialist referral.** Children with recurrent otitis media, or signs of chronic forms, warrant ENT referral. Audiology referral may be justified if there are concerns of hearing loss in chronic otitis media

Common Diagnosis 4
Diagnosis: Urinary tract infection

Management Principles
1. **Antibiotics.** Consult local guidelines – first-line antibiotics vary widely. For simple lower UTIs, a short course of oral antibiotics can be given. Admit for IV antibiotics if concerns of an upper UTI or in high-risk patients

2. **Follow-up investigations.** If certain criteria are met, the child may require follow-up investigations. This is to assess for structural abnormalities, reflux and renal scarring

3. **Preventative measures.** There are several simple supportive therapies to help treat and prevent UTIs, including:
   - High fluid intake
   - Regular voiding and 'double micturition', i.e. encouraging the child to sit on the toilet twice in quick succession
   - Avoiding constipation
   - Good hygiene
   - Low-dose prophylactic antibiotics in high-risk groups

Box 3.1.20   Investigations Following Urinary Tract Infection (UTI)

***Escherichia Coli* UTI responding well to treatment within 48 hours**

<6 months	USS within 6 weeks
>6 months	No further imaging needed

Non-*E. Coli* UTI responding well to treatment within 48 hours
If no other features of atypical infection:

<6 months	USS within 6 weeks, MCUG, DMSA 4–6 months
6 months–3 years	USS within 6 weeks, DMSA 4–6 months
>3 years	USS within 6 weeks

If other features of atypical infection:

<6 months	Urgent USS, MCUG, DMSA 4–6 months
6 months–3 years	Urgent USS, MCUG, DMSA 4–6 months
>3 years	Urgent USS

Recurrent UTI

<6 months	Urgent USS, MCUG, DMSA 4–6 months
6 months–3 years	USS within 6 weeks, DMSA 4–6 months
>3 years	USS within 6 weeks, DMSA 4–6 months

Note: MCUG should always be considered if there is dilatation on ultrasound scan, poor urine flow or there is a family history of vesico-ureteric reflux.
DMSA, dimercaptosuccinic acid; MCUG, micturating cystourethrogram; USS, ultrasound scan
Source: Adapted from National Institute for Health and Care Excellence (2018). Urinary tract infection in under 16s: diagnosis and management. Clinical guideline CG54. London: NICE.

Common Diagnosis 5
Diagnosis: Scarlet fever

Management Principles
1. **Antibiotics.** Consult local guidelines. Typical choice is a 10-day course of phenoxymethylpenicillin (penicillin V) or a shorter course of a macrolide
2. **Alert public health authorities.** Scarlet fever is a notifiable disease

3.2 Fever in the Returning Traveller

Andrew L. Smith

Department of Paediatrics, Children's Services, Homerton University Hospital NHS Foundation Trust, London, UK

CONTENTS

3.2.1 CHAPTER AT A GLANCE

Box 3.2.1   Chapter at a Glance

- International travel is increasingly common. Around 10% of travellers seek medical attention either while abroad, or after returning home
- Fever is common among travellers, often caused by a self-limiting illness
- Incubation periods for infective illnesses vary, meaning that timescale for suspicion depends on type of infection. Travel history should cover the last 12 months

- There are many pathogens that can cause disease in travellers, ranging over viral, bacterial, fungal and parasitic infections
- This chapter provides a snapshot of some of these infections; however, a fully comprehensive review is not possible given the scale of this subject

3.2.2 DEFINITION

- Fever, or pyrexia, is the elevation of body temperature above the normal range (≥37.5 °C)
- The definition of 'returning traveller' depends on the suspected illness, due to varying incubation periods, but should include any person with travel to high-risk areas in the past 12 months

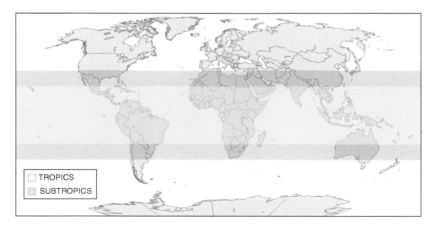

Figure 3.2.1 The Tropics and the Subtropics.

Clinical Guide to Paediatrics, First Edition. Edited by Rachel Varughese and Anna Mathew. Series Editor: Christian Fielder Camm.
© 2022 John Wiley & Sons Ltd. Published 2022 by John Wiley & Sons Ltd.
Companion website: www.wiley.com/go/varughese/paediatrics

3.2.3 DIAGNOSTIC ALGORITHM

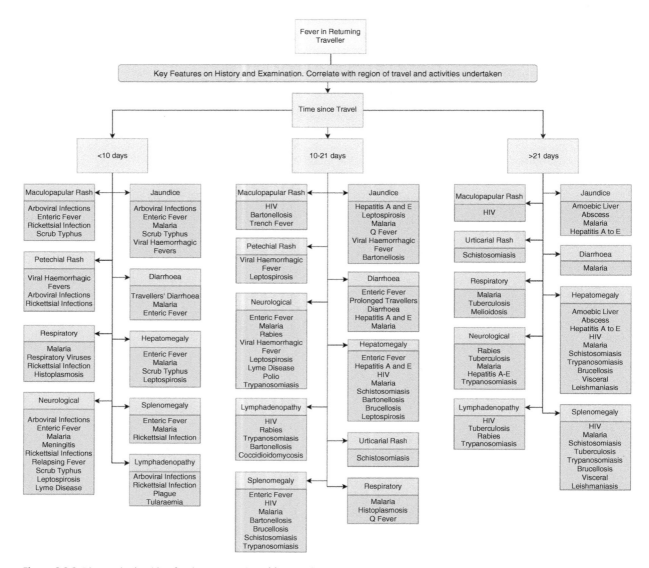

Figure 3.2.2 Diagnostic algorithm for the presentation of fever in the returning traveller.

3.2.4 DIFFERENTIALS LIST

Dangerous Diagnoses

1. Malaria

- Incubation period typically 7–30 days, but can be delayed for many months
- Malaria must be considered in all febrile patients returning from a malaria zone, even if prophylactic medications and precautions were taken
- *Plasmodium falciparum* is the most common cause and the most likely to lead to serious complications; symptoms typically present within 2 months of exposure
- *P. vivax, P. ovale* and *P. malariae* are the other major human pathogens. They generally produce a milder illness, but may present later
- Cerebral malaria is the most serious complication

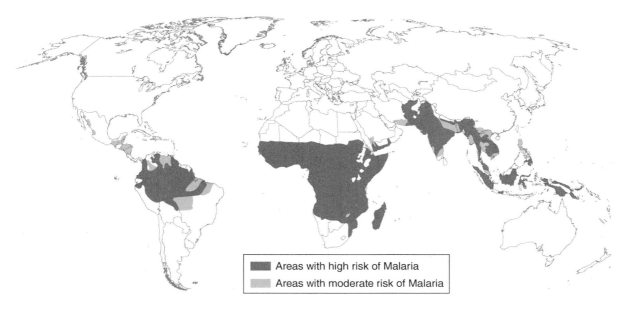

Figure 3.2.3 Areas with endemic malaria, requiring travel precautions.

2. Enteric Fever (Typhoid and Paratyphoid)
- Incubation period typically up to 21 days
- Caused by *Salmonella enterica* serotype Typhi or Paratyphi A, B or C. These are referred to respectively as typhoid and paratyphoid fever, and collectively as enteric fever
- Transmission can be direct faecal-oral, or through consumption of water or food contaminated by faeces
- Major risk factors are countries with endemic disease, with poor access to food, water and sanitation
- Chronic, asymptomatic carriage may occur, typically in the biliary tract

3. Rickettsial Infection (Typhus, Spotted Fever)
- Incubation period typically <10 days
- Mostly transmitted by bites from ectoparasites such as fleas, lice, mites and ticks
- Fever is usually of an abrupt onset and non-specific symptoms predominate, e.g. headache, myalgia and nausea/vomiting
- Rashes are common, along with an eschar (dark crusty ulcer) at the bite site. If severe, multi-organ failure is possible
- Common organisms are broadly divided into the spotted fever group and the typhus group and include *Rickettsia rickettsii* (Rocky Mountain spotted fever), *R. prowazekii* (epidemic typhus), *R. typhi* (endemic typhus) and *Orientia tsutsugamushi* (scrub typhus)

4. Tuberculosis (TB)
- Incubation period may vary from 2 weeks to over a year
- *Mycobacterium tuberculosis* infection is often considered with tropical diseases. However, TB prevalence rates in the UK are high in large urban areas, especially in London and Birmingham
- TB can cause a wide variety of diseases, from the classic pulmonary disease to lymphadenitis, meningitis, genitourinary, cutaneous and bone infections
- Generally insidious in onset, usually with systemic symptoms (e.g. weight loss, night sweats and malaise)
- Children are more likely to progress to active disease due to relatively immature immune systems

5. Human Immunodeficiency Virus (HIV)
- Most people infected with HIV experience a short flu-like illness, due to seroconversion (production of antibodies) within 2–6 weeks of infection. They may not have symptoms after this for several years
- Most children infected with HIV acquire it via vertical transmission, the prevention, investigation and management of which are not covered in this text
- Should always be considered in children from high-risk groups, e.g. known family contacts with HIV, refugee families, sexual abuse victims, or adolescents involved in high-risk activities, e.g. unprotected sexual intercourse
- While not curative, treatments are very successful. Left untreated, HIV infection leads to acquired immunodeficiency syndrome (AIDS) and death
- There should be a low threshold for testing if children are presenting with other infections that are associated with HIV

6. Rabies
- Incubation period is typically 20–60 days
- A severe disease caused by viruses of the *Lyssavirus* genus
- Worldwide, it is primarily transmitted from the bites or scratches of dogs or bats
- Once infected, the virus travels along the peripheral nerves to the central nervous system (CNS). The incubation period therefore depends on the site of the bite
- Symptoms are heralded by pain, pruritus or paraesthesia at the site of inoculation. This is followed by fever and psychological disturbances, including hydrophobia, confusion, hypersalivation and agitation
- Once symptoms appear, the disease is almost universally fatal, even with specialist intensive care. Management is targeted at disease control, exposure prevention and post-exposure prophylaxis with immunoglobulin and vaccines

7. Viral Haemorrhagic Fever (VHF)
- Incubation period is between 2 days and 3 weeks
- The VHFs are a spectrum of serious conditions caused by a variety of viruses from different families
- VHFs, as the name suggests, are typified by fever and haemorrhage. However, during the initial stages of disease, only non-specific symptoms predominate
- Disease severity ranges from mild to life-threatening
- Most of these viruses have zoonotic reservoirs. In those with mammal hosts, human acquisition is through ingestion of contaminated food, direct contact through broken skin or occasionally aerosol transmission. In those with arthropod hosts (mosquitoes, ticks, sand-flies), transmission is via a bite
- Once there is human infection, human-to-human transmission occurs via blood, bodily fluids or aerosol
- Some of the causative agents are incredibly infectious and dangerous (e.g. Ebola virus up to 90% mortality). As such, intensive quarantine of infected patients is required

Common Diagnoses
1. Traveller's Diarrhoea
- Incubation period typically 6–48 hours
- Diarrhoea is one of the most commonly encountered symptoms during travel. Younger children are more likely to develop diarrhoea and are more likely to suffer severe forms
- Dysentery is typified by blood in the stool, fever and abdominal cramps
- Pathogens are mostly acquired via contaminated food and water
- A range of causative pathogens exists
- Onset is usually rapid, but if symptoms are prolonged, then consideration should be given to a protozoal or helminth cause

---

Box 3.2.2   Common Causes of Travellers' Diarrhoea

Viral
- Norovirus
- Rotavirus

Bacterial
- *Campylobacter jejuni*
- Enterotoxigenic or enteroaggregative *Escherichia coli*
- *Salmonella* spp.
- *Shigella* spp.
- *Vibrio cholerae**

Other†
- *Cryptosporidium parvum*
- *Entamoeba histolytica*
- *Giardia lamblia*
- *Schistosoma* spp.
- *Strongyloides stercoralis*

* Rare in travellers; † Rare; more likely to cause prolonged symptoms

---

2. Self-Limiting Arbovirus Infection
- Incubation periods vary depending on the virus, but are typically between 2 and 15 days
- Arbovirus describes a variety of viruses from different families, transmitted by arthropods (**ar**thropod-**bo**rne **virus**)
- Arboviruses occur worldwide, with different viruses predominating in different regions

- Many will remain asymptomatic, but if clinical features are present, they will generally fall into one of three clinical syndromes:
  - a self-limiting disease typified by fever, arthralgia, myalgia, headache, vomiting and rash
  - a viral haemorrhagic fever (discussed in Dangerous Diagnoses)
  - CNS infection (meningoencephalitis, not discussed in detail in this chapter)
- Dengue has the highest global prevalence and usually causes a mild illness with a fever-rash syndrome. Repeated infection increases the risk of developing haemorrhagic fever
- Other common arboviruses include yellow fever, chikungunya, West Nile virus, Colorado tick fever, Japanese encephalitis, Rift Valley fever virus and Zika virus

3. Viral Hepatitis
- There are five viral hepatitis viruses: A, B, C, D and E. They come from different virus families
- Hepatitis A and E are transmitted through the faecal-oral route, usually via contaminated water and food. They have no chronic state, but can cause fulminant liver failure in some. They are the most common viral hepatitides in children. Incubation period is up to 2 months
- Hepatitis B and C are transmitted sexually, parenterally or vertically. Infection with these viruses may lead to chronic carriage and long-term sequalae. Incubation period is up to 6 months
- Hepatitis D only affects those with Hepatitis B, as it is an incomplete virus that requires the helper function of hepatitis B in order to replicate
- Vaccinations for hepatitis A and B are widely available, with a hepatitis E vaccine in use in China

4. Respiratory Infections
- Upper/lower respiratory tract infections are common in the returned traveller
- Awareness of epidemics, e.g. of influenza or coronavirus infections (MERS-CoV, COVID-19), is useful to risk-stratify patients and implement appropriate treatments
- The vast majority are caused by common viral and bacterial causes seen worldwide; these are discussed in Chapter 3.1 and are not considered further in this chapter

Diagnoses to Consider
These diagnoses are not covered further in this chapter as many are rare, requiring specialist investigation. They are provided here to give the reader an idea of the wide spectrum of possible diseases.

1. Bacterial Infections
- Bartonellosis – *Bartonella* spp.
- Brucellosis – *Brucella* spp.
- Leptospirosis (Weil's disease) – *Leptospira* spp.
- Lyme disease – *Borrelia burgdorferi*
- Melioidosis – *Burkholderia pseudomallei*
- Plague – *Yersinia pestis*
- Q fever – *Coxiella burnetti*
- Relapsing fever – *Borrelia* spp.
- Tularaemia – *Francisella tularensis*

2. Fungal Infections
- Coccidioidomycosis – *Coccidioides* spp.
- Histoplasmosis – *Histoplasma capsulatum*

3. Protozoal Infections
- African trypanosomiasis (sleeping sickness) – *Trypanosoma brucei*
- American trypanosomiasis (Chagas' Disease) – *Trypanosoma cruzi*
- Amoebiasis – *Entamoeba histolytica*
- Visceral leishmaniasis (kala-azar/'black fever') – *Leishmania* spp.

4. Helminth Infections
- Acute schistosomiasis – *Schistosoma* spp.
- Lymphatic filariasis (elephantiasis) – *Wichereria bancrofti Brugia* spp.

Box 3.2.3   Always Remember Sepsis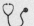

- Any infection can cause sepsis and it should always be considered and treated aggressively. Although many of the conditions in this chapter can cause serious illness, those that are common are common
- Sepsis is covered in detail in Chapters 3.1 and 13.1 and will not be covered further here

3.2.5 KEY HISTORY FEATURES

General Approach to History Taking for Fever in the Returning Traveller

Questions
1. **Where did the patient travel to and how long for, including transit points/stopovers?**
   - This is a crucial question to categorise which infections the patient is at risk from
   - A general overview of region-specific infections is provided in Figure 3.2.7 later in the chapter. It is also worth considering the season at the time of travel
   - A travel history of at least 12 months should be sought
   - There are several websites that provide up-to-date information on disease risk for different countries and regions, such as that of the World Health Organisation
2. **When did they travel and when did the symptoms start?** This question, combined with a knowledge of the incubation times of various pathogens, can help narrow down the differential diagnosis
3. **What activities were undertaken when abroad?** It is important to pick up specific risk factors, e.g.:
   - Exposure to animals, local or in game parks/farms, including exposure to slaughtered animals during hunting
   - Swimming in unclean water and/or caving
   - If deemed relevant, i.e. in adolescents, enquiry about high-risk activities such as sexual activity, tattoos and body piercings

   Although the significance of exposures may not be known to the generalist, having the information will prove critical when discussing with infection specialists
4. **What were their diet and water supply?** Exposure to unclean water as well as undercooked or contaminated foodstuffs will increase the risk of several conditions
5. **Are they aware of any contact with possible infection, e.g. unwell contacts, bites or knowledge of any disease outbreaks?**
   - Children who are visiting families abroad are more likely to be integrated into the local communities, increasing the risk of exposure to unwell contacts, even attendance at funerals
   - They may recall specifically being bitten by an animal, mosquito, mite or tick, increasing the risk of a vector-borne disease
   - Exposure to disease outbreaks can also occur on cruise ships, e.g. infective diarrhoea, or within hotels, e.g. Legionnaires' disease
6. **Did they undertake pre-travel health planning, including appropriate vaccinations and prophylaxis?**
   - No vaccination or disease prophylaxis treatment is 100% effective; nevertheless, their use is worth enquiring about
   - Children visiting families abroad are less likely to adhere to such preventative measures, sometimes potentiated by a parental belief that they are immune to diseases if they grew up in the region
7. **Did they receive treatment for any disease while abroad?**
   - Infective symptoms can sometimes appear while the traveller is still abroad. In these cases, they may have sought local medical advice and potentially received treatment
   - Partial treatment may cloud the diagnostic picture and if symptoms persist despite treatment, it may suggest an underlying antimicrobial resistance
   - If the patient has been admitted to hospital abroad, this increases the risk of a multi-drug resistant pathogen
8. **Are they known to have any preexisting medical conditions, in particular those predisposing to immunosuppression, or are they taking regular medications?**
   - Children with immunosuppression, both primary and secondary, will be more susceptible to the effects of tropical infections; a lower threshold for observation and treatment should be employed
   - Some medications indicated in the treatment of tropical infections are contraindicated in those with glucose-6-phosphate dehydrogenase (G6PD) deficiency

   In additional to the general history questions, use diagnosis-specific questions to hone the differential.

Dangerous Diagnosis 1
Diagnosis: Malaria

Questions
1. **Any sore throat, myalgia, diarrhoea or vomiting?** These are common symptoms of malaria in children, often leading to a misdiagnosis of a simple viral infection, and may impair the absorption of oral treatments
2. **Have there been any neurological complications, e.g. seizures, loss of consciousness?** While cerebral malaria is the most important complication to detect, indirect neurological phenomena are common in malaria, e.g. from hypoglycaemia or hyponatraemia

3. **Is there dark urine?** Haemoglobinuria is a well-known complication of malaria, due to haemolysis, mostly seen in falciparum infection
4. **Was the child affected by mosquito bites while abroad?** Although covered in the general approach, mosquito bites are a central part of the diagnosis and should not be missed

Dangerous Diagnosis 2
Diagnosis: Enteric fever

Questions
1. **Any gastrointestinal symptoms?** There can be either constipation or diarrhoea, with diarrhoea more common after the first week. In severe cases, peritonitis and intestinal perforation can occur
2. **Any neurological or psychiatric symptoms?** These can range from headache and disordered sleep to psychosis and encephalopathy
3. **Any nosebleeds?** Minor bleeding can be seen in the early stages of the disease. Massive haemorrhage can occur if left untreated

---

Box 3.2.4   Classic Description of Enteric Fever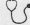

- First week: rising fever
- Second week: persistent fever, abdominal pain, rose spots

- Third week: worsening of symptoms, with risk of complications including bleeding, peritonitis, encephalitis and septic shock

---

Dangerous Diagnosis 3
Diagnosis: Rickettsial infection

Questions
1. **Has there been a headache?** The headache is typically frontal and may be unremitting
2. **Any psychiatric symptoms?** An acute confusional state is relatively common in epidemic typhus and scrub typhus
3. **Have there been any recent bites?** Although covered in the general approach, flea/lice/mite/tick bites are a central part of the diagnosis and should not be missed

Dangerous Diagnosis 4
Diagnosis: Tuberculosis

Questions
1. **Any known contact with someone with unexplained respiratory symptoms**? It is especially important to explore exposure risk when considering TB, including uninvestigated symptomatic close contacts. Investigation of the contact may yield positive results that will guide management.
2. **Any constitutional symptoms?** The features of TB are non-specific, but have typically been present for longer than other respiratory infections. Prolonged fever with the presence of night sweats and weight loss/faltering growth should raise the suspicion of TB, but their absence does not exclude it
3. **Any localising symptoms?** The precise symptomatology will vary depending on the site of infection

---

Box 3.2.5   Risk Factors for Tuberculosis (TB)

- Recent close contact to person with known active TB
- Recent immigrants (<5 years) from high-prevalence countries
- Residents of high-risk congregate settings
- Recent travel to country with endemic TB and having had extended contact with residents

- Children exposed to adults at high risk (intravenous drug users, employees in high-risk areas)
- Known human immunodeficiency virus infection or immunosuppression

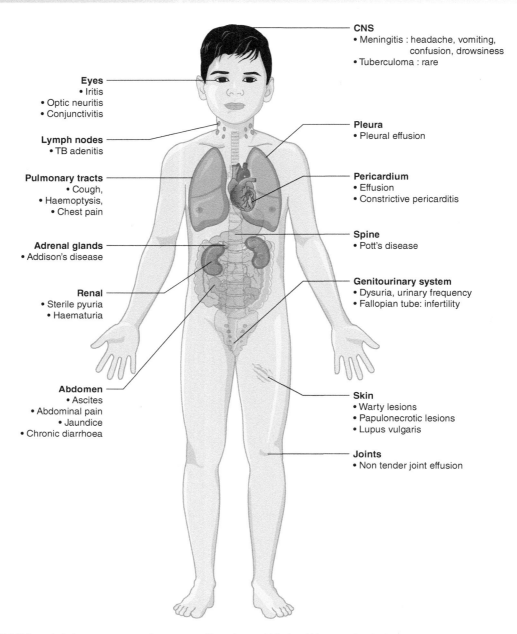

CNS
- Meningitis : headache, vomiting, confusion, drowsiness
- Tuberculoma : rare

Eyes
- Iritis
- Optic neuritis
- Conjunctivitis

Lymph nodes
- TB adenitis

Pulmonary tracts
- Cough,
- Haemoptysis,
- Chest pain

Adrenal glands
- Addison's disease

Renal
- Sterile pyuria
- Haematuria

Abdomen
- Ascites
- Abdominal pain
- Jaundice
- Chronic diarrhoea

Pleura
- Pleural effusion

Pericardium
- Effusion
- Constrictive pericarditis

Spine
- Pott's disease

Genitourinary system
- Dysuria, urinary frequency
- Fallopian tube: infertility

Skin
- Warty lesions
- Papulonecrotic lesions
- Lupus vulgaris

Joints
- Non tender joint effusion

Figure 3.2.4 Tuberculosis has many extra-pulmonary manifestations, which should be considered when conducting a clinical examination. In the context of exposure, any of these signs should prompt investigation.

Dangerous Diagnosis 5
Diagnosis: Human immunodeficiency virus

Questions
1. **Any specific risk of exposure?** This may include possible exposure from a positive family member or unprotected sexual intercourse
2. **Any symptoms typical of seroconversion illness?** Symptoms may resemble flu, with fever, fatigue, sore throat, maculo-papular rash, headache, myalgia and lymphadenopathy. Duration is usually 1–2 weeks
3. **Is there a history of recurrent infections?** Common presenting features include a history of recurrent upper respiratory tract infections, pneumonia, otitis media or other atypical bacterial/fungal/viral infections

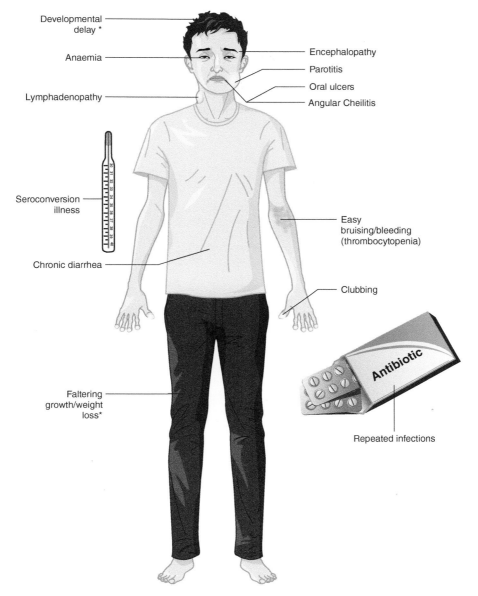

Developmental delay *

Anaemia

Lymphadenopathy

Encephalopathy

Parotitis

Oral ulcers

Angular Cheilitis

Seroconversion illness

Chronic diarrhea

Easy bruising/bleeding (thrombocytopenia)

Clubbing

Faltering growth/weight loss*

Repeated infections

Figure 3.2.5 Signs and symptoms associated with human immunodeficiency virus (HIV) infection. *Mostly seen in those who have acquired HIV by vertical transmission.

Box 3.2.6   Conditions Associated with Human Immunodeficiency Virus (HIV) Infection

Bacterial	Viral	Fungal	Others
• Recurrent bacterial infections • *Pneumocystis jiroveci* pneumonia • Mycobacterial infections • Necrotising gingivitis	• CMV disease • Herpes zoster • Widespread *Molluscum contagiosum* • Chronic HSV • Oral hairy leucoplakia (EBV) • Kaposi sarcoma (HHV-8)	• Oesophageal candidiasis • Invasive fungal disease	• Seborrheic dermatitis • Non-Hodgkin lymphoma • CNS toxoplasmosis • HIV nephropathy • HIV cardiomyopathy • Lymphoid interstitial pneumonitis

CMV, cytomegalovirus; CNS, central nervous system; EBV, Epstein–Barr virus; HHV, human herpesvirus; HSV, herpes simplex virus

Dangerous Diagnosis 6
Diagnosis: Rabies

Questions
1. **Is there a known exposure to a possibly infected animal?** Bites from any dog or bat while abroad should be considered as a possible source of rabies.
2. **Is the animal still alive?** The animal will typically die within 2 weeks of being infected
3. **Has the patient previously received a rabies vaccination, and if so, when?** This impacts management and decisions about whether immunoglobulin treatment is required, as discussed in the management section

Dangerous Diagnosis 7
Diagnosis: Viral haemorrhagic fever

Questions
1. **Any exposure to a known case or source?** This is important to stratify risk of disease. Exposure to unwell patients with fever and bleeding is notable, as well as exposure to animals and their excrement, in particular rodents and bats. Most VHFs are acquired in rural areas and if the exposure was more than 3 weeks prior to symptom onset, a VHF can be ruled out
2. **Fever, diarrhoea, arthralgia, rash or headache?** These non-specific symptoms may form an initial prodrome in VHF
3. **Any history suggestive of easy bleeding?** Ask about mucosal bleeding, oozing from grazes or venepuncture sites, haematemesis, haematuria or blood in the stool
4. **Any abdominal pain?** In VHF, particularly in severe dengue fever, abdominal pain can be marked

Common Diagnosis 1
Diagnosis: Travellers' diarrhoea

Questions
1. **Change in stool frequency or consistency?** There is a wide variety of normal stool habits in children, but a primary infective diarrhoea is likely if there has been a change from normal for that patient
2. **Any associated symptoms?** Travellers' diarrhoea is often associated with fever, abdominal pain, urgency, vomiting and bloody stools

Common Diagnosis 2
Diagnosis: Self-limiting arbovirus infection

Questions
1. **Fever, arthralgia, rash or headache?** The presence of these non-specific symptoms constitutes a common syndrome of arboviral infection. Many of these infections may be mistaken for flu, and are not formally diagnosed
2. **Have there been any recent bites?** Arthropod bites are a central part of the diagnosis and should not be missed
3. **Are there any features of severe disease?** Severe disease may manifest as haemorrhage (discussed above) or meningoencephalitis. Description of bleeding or neurological symptoms should prompt urgent reconsideration of a more serious clinical course

Common Diagnosis 3
Diagnosis: Viral hepatitis

Questions
1. **Fever, headache, nausea and vomiting, diarrhoea?** These are common symptoms of a prodromal phase of acute hepatitis infection. Diarrhoea is common in young children, whereas constipation is more common in adults
2. **Is the urine dark or faeces pale?** Although they are typically a feature of biliary obstruction, dark urine and pale stools can occur due to transient conjugated hyperbilirubinaemia in many acute hepatic illnesses
3. **Any abdominal pain?** There may be abdominal pain, particularly in the right upper quadrant, and diarrhoea
4. **Any previous history of viral hepatitis?** Previous infection with hepatitis A or E provides immunity
5. **Any contact with infected individuals?** Consider household contacts with hepatitis A or E, or needle sharing in adolescents engaging in substance misuse (risk of hepatitis B and C)

3.2.6 KEY EXAMINATION FEATURES

Many of the conditions discussed will only have non-specific findings on examination. A very thorough clinical examination is required, assessing carefully for any rashes, bite marks and other subtle clinical signs.

Dangerous Diagnosis 1
Diagnosis: Malaria

Examination Findings
1. **Signs of haemolytic anaemia.** Haemolysis of infected red cells causes pallor and jaundice
2. **Hepatosplenomegaly.** Hepatosplenomegaly is immune-mediated, with deposition of immune complexes in Kupffer cells in the liver and spleen, and reticuloendothelial cell hyperplasia
3. **Any features of severe malaria?** See Box 3.2.7

Box 3.2.7   Features of Severe Malaria

Clinical features	Lab features
• Reduced urine output	• Acidosis (base deficit >8 mEq/L, bicarbonate <15 mmol/L or lactate >5 mmol/L)
• Impaired consciousness	• Hyperparasitaemia (>10%)
• Multiple seizures	• Hypoglycaemia (<2.2 mmol/L)
• Extreme weakness	• Jaundice (serum bilirubin >50 μmol/L)
• Significant bleeding	• Severe anaemia (<5.0 g/L in children <12 years, <7.0 g/L in children ≥ 12 years)
• Pulmonary oedema	• Acute kidney injury (raised urea and creatinine)
• Shock	

Dangerous Diagnosis 2
Diagnosis: Enteric fever

Examination Findings
1. **Rose spots.** These are faint pink macules present on the trunk and abdomen that appear after the onset of fever. They are not easily visible on those with dark skin
2. **Relative bradycardia.** An absence of rise in heart rate with fever may be seen
3. **Evidence of peritonitis or intestinal perforation.** Diffuse abdominal rigidity, guarding, severe pain or evidence of ileus (vomiting, distension, absent flatus/stool). If present, urgent surgical review is imperative
4. **Encephalopathy.** In severe disease, there may be enteric encephalopathy, with altered or decreased mental state

Dangerous Diagnosis 3
Diagnosis: Rickettsial infection

Examination Findings
1. **Features of rash.** The rashes of rickettsial infections are typically maculopapular, but may become petechial or even purpuric as they progress
2. **Lymphadenopathy.** Either local or generalised lymphadenopathy can occur; this is more prominent in the typhus group
3. **Evidence of complications, e.g. cardiovascular, neurological.** There are several possible complications, more so in the spotted fever group
4. **Relative bradycardia.** An absence of rise in heart rate with fever may be seen

---

Box 3.2.8   Rashes of Rickettsial Infections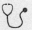

- **Spotted fever.** Rash is typically centripetal, starting on the extremities and spreading to the trunk. It typically spares the face, but involvement of the scrotum or vulva can be seen

- **Typhus.** Rash typically starts centrally and spreads to the extremities, sparing the face, palms and soles

---

Box 3.2.9   Complications of Rickettsial Infections

- **Cardiac**: myocarditis, arrhythmias, hypotension, heart failure
- **Neurological**: meningoencephalitis, seizures, focal neurology
- **Respiratory**: pneumonitis, pulmonary oedema
- **Ophthalmological**: conjunctivitis, retinal disease

Dangerous Diagnosis 4
Diagnosis: Tuberculosis

Examination Findings
1. **Pulmonary signs.** Signs of respiratory involvement with tachypnoea, crepitations and pleural effusions may indicate active pulmonary TB
2. **Lymphadenopathy.** Lymphadenitis is one of the commonest extra-pulmonary manifestations of TB. In the cervical region, it is known as scrofula
3. **Neurological features.** Features of TB meningitis can be insidious. Nuchal rigidity, altered reflexes and cranial nerve palsies may be seen, especially the sixth cranial nerve. Abnormal movements and posturing, seizures and coma can occur in the late stages

---

Box 3.2.10   Tuberculosis (TB) Is Predominantly a Clinical Diagnosis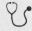

Confirmatory laboratory testing in TB is achieved in less than 50% of cases. Diagnosis relies on:

- History of close contact with TB
- Positive tuberculin skin test or interferon-gamma release assay
- Suggestive clinical features ± chest x-ray changes

Dangerous Diagnosis 5
Diagnosis: Human immunodeficiency virus

Examination Findings
1. **Lymphadenopathy.** Lymphadenopathy is a common sign during seroconversion and is frequently associated with hepatosplenomegaly
2. **Oral candidiasis.** Opportunistic oral infections are a common source of morbidity in children with HIV. These are usually seen later in infection, but may also be seen during seroconversion
   Note that signs are often non-specific and there may be no immediate clinical features

Dangerous Diagnosis 6
Diagnosis: Rabies

Examination Findings
1. **Hydrophobia and aerophobia.** Most patients with rabies will exhibit hydrophobia, a fear of drinking. This is related to painful spasms on attempts to drink. Aerophobia is typified by painful spasms caused by air being blown on the face
2. **Hypersalivation.** Infected animals and individuals will hypersalivate. This is caused by the virus replicating in the salivary glands
3. **Mental state.** Patients may become restless, hyperactive and confused. They can become aggressive, attempting to bite others. These furious episodes may be interspersed with periods of calm
4. **Neurological signs.** A wide variety of signs may be encountered, ranging from muscle fasciculations or seizures to coma. Autonomic dysfunction can occur, with fever, tachycardia and hypertension. A minority of patients will exhibit a paralytic rabies, which may be mistaken for Guillain–Barré syndrome

Dangerous Diagnosis 7
Diagnosis: Viral haemorrhagic fever

Examination Findings
1. **Evidence of bleeding.** Bleeding is the cardinal sign of VHF. Look for petechial or purpuric rash, mucosal bleeding and venepuncture oozing. In advanced stages there can be bleeding from eyes and ears
2. **Shock.** Hypovolaemic shock may manifest as tachycardia, hypotension, prolonged capillary refill time or altered mental state

Box 3.2.11   Clinical Features of Viral Haemorrhagic Fevers

Early features	Late features
• Abdominal pain	• Acidosis
• Chest pain	• Ascites
• Conjunctivitis	• Disseminated intravascular coagulation
• Mucosal bleeding	• Encephalopathy
• Oedema	• Haematemesis
• Petechiae	• Liver failure
• Pharyngitis	• Pleural effusions
• Rash	• Renal failure
• Venepuncture oozing	• Shock

Common Diagnosis 1
Diagnosis: Travellers' diarrhoea

Examination Findings
1. **Dehydration.** Assessment of hydration status is important to decide whether admission is required for intravenous fluid replacement
2. **Are there features of other disease?** Rule out more serious diagnoses. Consider other tropical infections – many of the conditions described in this chapter may cause diarrhoea, e.g. malaria and enteric fever. Alternatively, this may be a presentation of underlying pathology, e.g. coeliac disease or inflammatory bowel disease

Common Diagnosis 2
Diagnosis: Self-limiting arbovirus infection

Examination Findings
1. **Rash.** The rash can be variable, from a maculopapular rash to confluent erythema to petechiae
2. **Absence of features of severe disease.** Arbovirus infections can cause a number of complications. In the simple, self-limiting syndrome, there should be no features of viral haemorrhagic fever, liver failure or meningoencephalitis

Box 3.2.12   Tourniquet Test

The tourniquet test is part of the World Health Organisation case definition for dengue:

- A blood pressure cuff is inflated to halfway between systolic and diastolic pressure and left for 5 minutes
- A positive test is the presence of >20 petechiae in a 2.5 cm² area below the level of the blood pressure cuff
- A positive result indicates capillary fragility, which can be found in patients with both dengue fever and dengue haemorrhagic fever

Common Diagnosis 3
Diagnosis: Viral hepatitis

Examination Findings
1. **Jaundice.** Usually occurs 1 week after onset of symptoms of mild fever
2. **Hepatomegaly.** Hepatomegaly, which may be tender, often presents at the same time as jaundice
3. **Rash.** A maculopapular rash is a common extrahepatic manifestation of hepatitis A and E. In children with acute hepatitis B infection, there may be a papular acrodermatitis of the face, extremities and trunk (which, in addition to lymphadenopathy, is known as Gianotti–Crosti syndrome)
4. **Signs of cirrhosis or fulminant liver failure.** Although most infections are self-limiting, some will progress to chronic liver failure or fulminant liver failure, so encephalopathy, evidence of coagulopathy, malaise, ascites and malnutrition may be evident. Those with chronic disease may develop finger clubbing

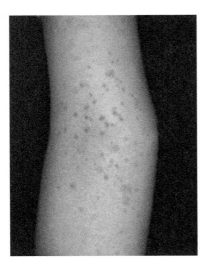

Figure 3.2.6 Petechiae in the antecubital fossa following the tourniquet test for dengue. Source: Reproduced with permission from Shutterstock.

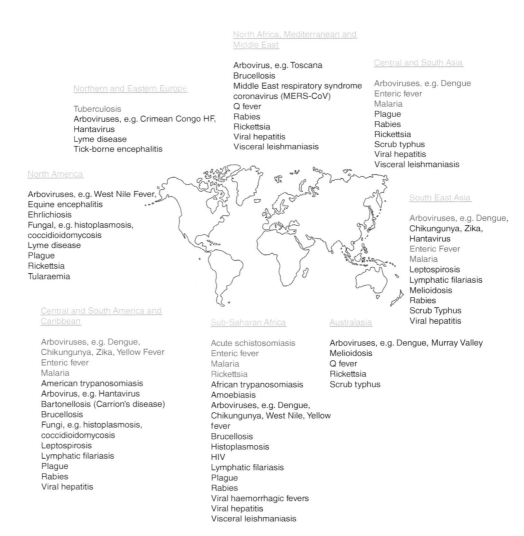

North Africa, Mediterranean and Middle East

Arbovirus, e.g. Toscana
Brucellosis
Middle East respiratory syndrome coronavirus (MERS-CoV)
Q fever
Rabies
Rickettsia
Viral hepatitis
Visceral leishmaniasis

Central and South Asia

Arboviruses, e.g. Dengue
Enteric fever
Malaria
Plague
Rabies
Rickettsia
Scrub typhus
Viral hepatitis
Visceral leishmaniasis

Northern and Eastern Europe

Tuberculosis
Arboviruses, e.g. Crimean Congo HF, Hantavirus
Lyme disease
Tick-borne encephalitis

North America

Arboviruses, e.g. West Nile Fever, Equine encephalitis
Ehrlichiosis
Fungal, e.g. histoplasmosis, coccidioidomycosis
Lyme disease
Plague
Rickettsia
Tularaemia

South East Asia

Arboviruses, e.g. Dengue, Chikungunya, Zika, Hantavirus
Enteric Fever
Malaria
Leptospirosis
Lymphatic filariasis
Melioidosis
Rabies
Scrub Typhus
Viral hepatitis

Central and South America and Caribbean

Arboviruses, e.g. Dengue, Chikungunya, Zika, Yellow Fever
Enteric fever
Malaria
American trypanosomiasis
Arbovirus, e.g. Hantavirus
Bartonellosis (Carrion's disease)
Brucellosis
Fungi, e.g. histoplasmosis, coccidioidomycosis
Leptospirosis
Lymphatic filariasis
Plague
Rabies
Viral hepatitis

Sub-Saharan Africa

Acute schistosomiasis
Enteric fever
Malaria
Rickettsia
African trypanosomiasis
Amoebiasis
Arboviruses, e.g. Dengue, Chikungunya, West Nile, Yellow fever
Brucellosis
Histoplasmosis
HIV
Lymphatic filariasis
Plague
Rabies
Viral haemorrhagic fevers
Viral hepatitis
Visceral leishmaniasis

Australasia

Arboviruses, e.g. Dengue, Murray Valley
Melioidosis
Q fever
Rickettsia
Scrub typhus

Figure 3.2.7 The differential diagnosis for tropical infections is wide. This world map demonstrating region-specific infections can help to narrow down possible differential diagnoses, but remember that some of these are rare, and those that are common are common. Diagnoses in red should be particularly considered.

3.2.7 KEY INVESTIGATIONS

Note that if sending potentially highly contagious samples to the laboratory, these should be transported appropriately, and laboratory staff informed so appropriate precautions can be taken. Not all children will require invasive investigations, particularly if a clear and benign diagnosis is suspected from history and examination.

Bedside

Table 3.2.1 Bedside tests of use in returning travellers presenting with fever

Test	When to perform	Potential result
Samples for microscopy, culture and/or polymerase chain reaction (PCR) testing	• Depending on suspected infection, these may include throat swab, nasopharyngeal aspirates, wound swabs, urine samples, stool cultures • Isolating a causative organism helps guide management	• A pure growth of an organism is supportive of infection • Some tropical pathogens are difficult to culture
Urinalysis	Suspected: • Leptospirosis • Malaria • Schistosomiasis	• Proteinuria and haematuria indicate renal involvement, seen in any of these infections

Blood Tests

Table 3.2.2 Blood tests of use in returning travellers presenting with fever

Test	When to perform	Potential result
Blood gas	• If systemically unwell	• ↓ pH and ↑ CO_2 indicate respiratory acidosis • ↓ pH, ↓ HCO_3, ↑lactate indicate metabolic acidosis, suggestive of poor perfusion • ↑/↓ Glucose may occur in sepsis • ↓ pH, ↑ lactate and ↓ glucose are features of severe malaria
Blood culture (ideally take prior to commencing antibiotics)	• All children with fever as returning travellers, unless strong clinical evidence for benign cause	• Pure growth of an organism supports infection • Sensitivities guide antibiotic choice • Many of the pathogens discussed in this chapter take a long time to culture or may not be detected on blood culture at all
FBC	• All patients systemically unwell or with uncertain diagnosis • Anaemia is a feature of several infectious diseases • White cell counts useful in differentiating infections • Platelets count useful if petechiae or bleeding • Underlying red cell disorders, e.g. G6PD, thalassaemia, can predispose to complications	• Hb <7.0 g/L is a feature of severe malaria • Microcytic anaemia in helminth infection • Pancytopaenia in visceral leishmaniasis and brucellosis • ↓/↑ WCC may be present in several infections • ↑ Neutrophils in bacterial infection • ↑ Eosinophils in parasitic or fungal infections • ↓ Platelets in malaria, enteric fever, viral infections (dengue, HIV) and severe sepsis
U&E	Suspected • Severe infection • Severe dehydration	• ↑Urea and creatinine indicate acute kidney injury • Acute kidney injury is a feature of severe malaria
LFTs	• Suspected tropical infection – many affect the liver • Certain antimicrobials cause derangements in liver function, so having a baseline is useful	• ↑ Bilirubin ± ↑ALT/AST (transaminitis) in malaria, viral hepatitis, enteric fever, leptospirosis, arboviruses • ↑ ALP in those with an amoebic liver abscess
CRP	• If systemically unwell	• Significant ↑ in bacterial infections • Less marked ↑ in viral infections

Table 3.2.2 (Continued)

Test	When to perform	Potential result
ESR	• Consider as an adjunct in monitoring inflammation	• ESR ↑ in infection and inflammation
Clotting	• If systemically unwell, septic or signs of bleeding	• ↑ INR/APTT and ↓ fibrinogen levels occur in DIC, seen in VHF and sepsis
Serology	• Serological testing is the mainstay of diagnosis for many conditions discussed (often requiring specialist labs)	• IgM positive: suggestive of an acute infection • IgG positive and IgM negative: suggestive of past infection
Malarial blood film	• A thick and thin blood film is mandatory in all febrile patients returning from a malaria region • If negative, it should be repeated up to three times over 48–72 hours	• Confirms malaria • Provides quantification and speciation of the parasitaemia • False negatives can occur if interpreted by inexperienced staff
Malaria rapid antigen test	• A useful adjunct in the diagnosis of malaria	• Confirms malaria, but cannot infer the level of parasitaemia or speciation • False positives and negatives can occur
HIV test	• In patients with risk of exposure or who have associated illnesses • Several rapid diagnostic tests are also available	• Confirms HIV • Serological testing cannot be used in children <12 months due to the possibility of maternal antibodies being present
Interferon-gamma release assay	• An adjunctive test in the diagnosis of *Mycobacterium tuberculosis*	• Positive result provides support for TB, but does not differentiate between active and latent
Sample save	Given the broad range of differentials, the exact tests required may not have been decided at the time of initial blood sampling. Extra samples to save in the lab allow future testing	

ALP, alkaline phosphatase; ALT, alanine aminotransferase; APTT, activated partial thromboplastin time; AST, aspartate aminotransferase; CO_2, carbon dioxide; CRP, C-reactive protein; DIC, disseminated intravascular coagulation; ESR, erythrocyte sedimentation rate; FBC, full blood count; G6PD, glucose-6-phosphate dehydrogenase; Hb, haemoglobin; HCO_3, bicarbonate; HIV, human immunodeficiency virus; Ig, immunoglobulin; INR, international normalised ratio; LFTs, liver function tests; TB, tuberculosis; U&E, urea and electrolytes; VHF, viral haemorrhagic fever; WCC, white cell count

Imaging

Table 3.2.3 Imaging modalities of use in returning travellers presenting with fever

Test	When to perform	Potential result
Chest x-ray	Suspected: • TB • Respiratory infection	• TB: hilar lymphadenopathy/consolidation with possible cavitation/miliary TB (widespread opacities)/pleural involvement • Pneumonia: consolidation
Targeted ultrasound scan	Suspected: • Hepatosplenomegaly • Lymphadenopathy • Abscesses in pyrexia of unknown origin	• Characterises hepatosplenomegaly • Characterises lymphadenopathy or lymphadenitis • Confirms abscess
CT/MRI brain	• If neurological features suggesting a cerebral infective source or involvement	• Features are often non-specific and require correlation with history • There may be abscess, haemorrhage, cerebral oedema, ischaemia or evidence of meningoencephalitis

CT, computed tomography; MRI, magnetic resonance imaging; TB, tuberculosis

Special

Table 3.2.4 Special tests of use in returning travellers presenting with fever

Test	When to perform	Potential result
Tuberculin skin testing	• Measures level of induration present following the administration of a purified protein derivative of *Mycobacterium tuberculosis*	• Positive result has varying thresholds, depending on the pre-test probability from risk factors
Mycobacterial culture + acid-fast bacilli smear	• Specimens should be collected from any site where infection is suspected • In those suspected of having pulmonary tuberculosis (TB), use gastric lavage or induced sputum	• Confirms TB • Diagnostic yield generally poor (approximately one-third of specimens)
Lumbar puncture (LP)	• If suspected meningitis or encephalitis • If suspected TB in <12 months, perform LP regardless of neurological signs • If unusual infection suspected, discuss with lab first to ensure correct testing is performed	• See Chapter 3.1, *Fever*, Box 3.1.18, *Interpretation of Cerebrospinal Fluid (CSF)*

3.2.8 KEY MANAGEMENT PRINCIPLES

Diagnosis-specific management strategies are outlined here. It is expected that an 'ABCDE' approach to assessment and management is always undertaken (see Chapter 12.1, *The A to E Assessment*).

Box 3.2.13   General Management Principles

Infection control precautions

- The human-to-human infectivity of the pathogens discussed in this chapter varies
- Appropriate barrier nursing should be employed if patients are presenting with respiratory symptoms, diarrhoea, vomiting, rashes or bleeding. This may include the need for face masks to limit airborne spread

- High-level quarantine will be required if certain pathogens are suspected, e.g. viral haemorrhagic fevers
- Patients who have been admitted to hospitals abroad should be considered for isolation as a matter of routine, pending culture results, due to the risk of multi-drug-resistant organisms

Notifying public health authorities

- Many of the conditions discussed in this chapter are notifiable diseases
- The exact list of notifiable diseases and pathogens varies between countries, but those notifiable in the UK are listed at https://www.gov.uk/guidance/notifiable-diseases-and-causative-organisms-how-to-report#list-of-notifiable-diseases

- Public health authorities need to be informed to facilitate disease monitoring, assist with contact tracing and implement measures to avoid disease outbreaks

Determine which patients to admit

- Admit all patients who are systemically unwell
- Deciding which stable patients to admit can be difficult and will depend on local resources and policies. Discuss with a consultant and an infectious disease specialist

- All patients with suspected contagious infections will require isolation

---

Dangerous Diagnosis 1
Diagnosis: Malaria

Management Principles

1. **Anti-malarial treatments.** In general, first-line therapy in severe falciparum malaria is intravenous (IV) artesunate or, if unavailable, IV quinine. First-line oral therapy is artemether-lumefantrine, with alternatives being atovaquone-proguanil, or quinine with doxycycline or clindamycin. Doxycycline should be avoided in children under 12 years of age due to the risk of dental staining and hypoplasia. In *P. vivax* or *P. ovale* infection, primaquine is required to eradicate dormant parasites. This should be used with caution in patients with G6PD deficiency
2. **Broad-spectrum antibiotics.** Children with severe malaria should also receive standard broad-spectrum antibiotics until bacterial infection can be ruled out

3. **Admission.** A low threshold for admission at the commencement of treatment is advised. Children with malaria can deteriorate rapidly and close observation is warranted

4. **Preventative advice.** Despite the widely held belief, infection does not confer protection to re-infection. Advice should be given about preventative and prophylactic measures for future travel

Dangerous Diagnosis 2
Diagnosis: Enteric fever

Management Principles
1. **Antibiotics.** Multi-drug resistance is a growing concern in the treatment of enteric fever, with the most appropriate drug treatment varying dependent on the area of travel. Generally, ceftriaxone is indicated in the systemically unwell patient. A carbapenem may be indicated if the pathogen is likely to be an extended-spectrum beta-lactamase–producing organism. Treatment should be guided by local policy, susceptibility of cultured organisms and response of the patient to therapy

2. **Dexamethasone.** In patients with severe disease, i.e. encephalopathy or shock, adjuvant IV dexamethasone has been shown to reduce mortality

3. **Treatment of complications.** This may include surgical review if peritonitis or a typhoid abscess is suspected

Dangerous Diagnosis 3
Diagnosis: Rickettsial infection

Management Principles
1. **Doxycyline.** Decision to treat is based upon clinical suspicion, as organisms are difficult to culture, and serological testing can be slow and treatment should not be delayed. Doxycycline is the treatment of choice for all ages, for 7–14 days. Although usually contraindicated in children (dental staining, enamel hypoplasia), it is felt that the benefit outweighs the risks, especially given the generally short treatment course

2. **Cephalosporin.** Since symptoms and signs may overlap with meningococcal infection (headache, cognitive disturbance, rash), consider adding a third-generation cephalosporin if diagnosis is uncertain

3. **Monitoring.** If suspicion does not meet the threshold for antibiotic treatment, consider outpatient monitoring for 24–48 hours before discharge

Dangerous Diagnosis 4
Diagnosis: Tuberculosis

Management Principles
1. **Antibiotics.** The management of TB requires a prolonged course of treatment, minimum 6 months, with multiple antibiotic medications. Encouragement must be given to support the child and family in completing the full course. For some, directly observed therapy (DOT) is required. Treatment should be overseen by a specialist. There are many possible interactions with other medications

   A typical starting regime would be 6 months of isoniazid and rifampicin, with ethambutamol and pyrazinamide added as well for the first 2 months. Pyridoxine is also administered when Isoniazid is prescribed. The regimen will be tailored if the risk of multi-drug-resistant TB is high or confirmed, or if there is central nervous system involvement.

2. **Contact tracing.** Contact tracing and screening should be performed, using a tuberculin skin test. If present, treatment of latent disease is usually with a 3-month course of isoniazid and rifampicin

Dangerous Diagnosis 5
Diagnosis: Human immunodeficiency virus

Management Principles
Patients with a positive HIV result should be referred to a specialist service, as treatment is complex. Treatment principles include:
- Antiretroviral agents
- Prophylactic medications to reduce opportunistic infections
- Psychosocial support
- Prevention of transmission

Dangerous Diagnosis 6
Diagnosis: Rabies

Management Principles
1. **Wound care.** If presenting immediately after any animal bite, the wound should be cleaned thoroughly, ensuring no debris remains. Use of antiseptic solutions, such iodine, is required. If possible, the wound should not be sutured but left to heal by secondary intention
2. **Vaccination.** Administer a rabies vaccine on day 0. This is repeated on day 3. If there was no pre-exposure prophylaxis, repeat dose on days 7 and 14. If immunosuppressed, a fifth dose on day 28 is given
3. **Immunoglobulin.** If no previous rabies vaccination, rabies immunoglobulin (RIg) should be given (20 IU/kg). The wound site should be inoculated directly with as much as possible, with any excess being given as an intramuscular (IM) injection into a deltoid muscle different from the one used for vaccination. In those with pre-exposure vaccine prophylaxis, RIG is not indicated
4. **Treating possible co-infection.** Anti-tetanus measures should be taken as required, along with the commencement of antibiotics to minimise the risk of a wound infection
5. **Palliation.** In those unlikely to survive or at risk of a poor neurological outcome, a palliative approach may be adopted

Dangerous Diagnosis 7
Diagnosis: Viral haemorrhagic fever

Management Principles
1. **Appropriate isolation and safety.** Many VHFs are highly infectious and can spread directly between humans. Strict high-level quarantine is required and ideally the patient should be cared for in an infectious disease centre with negative pressure room capabilities
2. **Ribavirin.** Treatment with ribavirin is indicated for many causes of VHF, although it is ineffective for Ebola, Marburg, dengue and yellow fever
3. **Supportive treatments.** Patients can become critically unwell, requiring fluid and blood product support and analgesia. A Critical Care setting may be required

Common Diagnosis 1
Diagnosis: Travellers' diarrhoea

Management Principles
1. **Rehydration.** Maintaining hydration is key. This may be helped with the use of an oral rehydration solution, a widely available or easily made mixture of water, salt and sugar. Nasogastric or IV fluids may be required based on dehydration status
2. **Antimicrobials.** Many cases will resolve spontaneously. However, in dysentery, antibiotics, e.g. ciprofloxacin or ceftriaxone, may be indicated. If a protozoal cause is suspected or confirmed, metronidazole is indicated. Mebendazole is used in helminth infections
3. **Loperamide.** Use of loperamide is common in adults, but opinion is divided on its use in children. Consider in mild to moderate diarrhoea in older children to reduce the frequency of stool and length of illness. Avoid in children less than 3 years of age and those with dysentery, as there is an increased risk of adverse events, e.g. toxic megacolon
4. **Prevention.** Advice to limit infection in future travels includes scrupulous hygiene practices, use of bottled water and avoidance of high-risk foods, e.g. uncooked food washed in water
5. **Monitoring for post-infective phenomena.** Diarrhoea may persist despite treatment due to transient lactose intolerance following Giardia, or a post-infectious enteropathy. There are reports of the onset of irritable bowel syndrome following gastroenteritis

Common Diagnosis 2
Diagnosis: Self-limiting arbovirus infection

Management Principles
1. **Supportive therapy.** Most cases are self-limiting and supportive therapy with oral rehydration and paracetamol is appropriate
2. **Prevention.** Advice on appropriate prevention for future travel is useful, e.g. avoidance of bites using barrier methods and insect repellents. Vaccinations for yellow fever (required for travel to certain regions) and Japanese encephalitis exist for travel to high-risk areas

Common Diagnosis 3
Diagnosis: Viral hepatitis

Management Principles
1. **Symptomatic treatment.** Managing nausea, ensuring adequate hydration and nutrition, and rest are the mainstays of treatment. Avoidance of hepatotoxic drugs is essential. Older children must be advised to avoid alcohol
2. **Antiviral treatment.** No routine antivirals are indicated in viral hepatitis. The primary aim in chronic infection is to prevent progression to cirrhosis or liver failure. Chronic hepatitis B may be treated with pegylated interferon alfa and nucleoside or nucleotide analogues. Chronic hepatitis C may be treated with interferon alfa and ribavirin
3. **Liver transplant.** Liver transplant may be required in severe cases of liver failure

3.3 Lymphadenopathy

Tim Sell and Rachel Varughese

Department of Paediatrics, Oxford University Hospitals NHS Foundation Trust, Oxford, UK

CONTENTS

3.3.1 CHAPTER AT A GLANCE

Box 3.3.1 Chapter at a Glance

- Lymphadenopathy is a physiological part of childhood, the vast majority of which is benign
- Enlarged lymph nodes in the neck, termed cervical lymphadenopathy, form the most common presentation in paediatrics, due to the common nature of upper respiratory tract infections
- Other palpable lymph nodes may be found in the supraclavicular, axillary and inguinal anatomical areas

- It is important not to over-investigate simple cases, but to recognise those representative of serious underlying illness
- A child with persistent or generalised lymphadenopathy, or lymph node >2 cm, always warrants investigation

3.3.2 DEFINITION

- Lymphadenopathy refers to enlargement of lymph nodes
- Size threshold is dependent on region and age, but <1 cm is likely to be normal
- Localised lymphadenopathy describes enlarged lymph nodes in only one region
- Generalised lymphadenopathy describes enlarged lymph nodes in more than one anatomical area
- 'Lymphadenitis' means inflammation of the lymph nodes, often due to infection of the node itself

Clinical Guide to Paediatrics, First Edition. Edited by Rachel Varughese and Anna Mathew. Series Editor: Christian Fielder Camm.
© 2022 John Wiley & Sons Ltd. Published 2022 by John Wiley & Sons Ltd.
Companion website: www.wiley.com/go/varughese/paediatrics

3.3.3 DIAGNOSTIC ALGORITHM

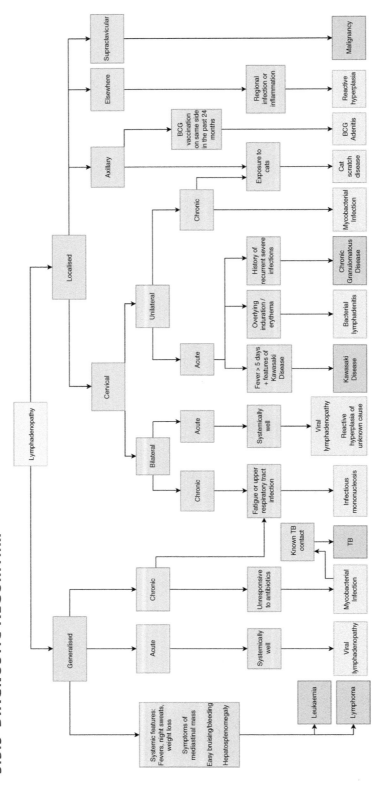

Figure 3.3.1 Diagnostic algorithm for the presentation of lymphadenopathy.

3.3.4 DIFFERENTIALS LIST

Dangerous Diagnoses

1. Acute Lymphoblastic Leukaemia (ALL)
- Malignant proliferation of white cell precursors (blasts) in the bone marrow
- Most common form of childhood cancer (about one-third of all paediatric cancers)
- Occurs at all ages, peak is between 2 and 4 years old
- There is a spectrum of presentations
- Classified according to:
  - Speed of progression (acute much more common than chronic)
  - Morphology (acute lymphoblastic leukaemia and acute myeloid leukaemia)
  - Cytochemistry, immunophenotype and cytogenetics

2. Lymphoma
- Malignant proliferation of lymphoid cells
- There are two main types: Hodgkin and non-Hodgkin
- Generally presents more insidiously than leukaemia, as unilateral lymphadenopathy
- Frequency increases with age, most common in teenagers
- Staged I–IV depending on spread of malignancy

3. Kawasaki Disease
- Systemic, inflammatory illness, causing medium-vessel vasculitis
- It is the second most common vasculitis in childhood, after Henoch–Schönlein purpura
- Nodes are typically >1.5 cm and painful
- Typically affects children 6 months – 5 years old
- Children with affected first-degree relatives are more at risk, suggesting genetic predisposition
- Most common in children of East Asian descent, and boys are more susceptible than girls
- Diagnosis is clinical, with evidence of systemic inflammation (fever for at least 5 days) accompanied by other signs of mucocutaneous inflammation
- Usually self-limiting; however, there is potential for serious complications, such as coronary artery aneurysms and heart failure
- It is the most common cause of acquired heart disease in children in developed countries
- Kawasaki disease is covered in detail in Chapter 3.1, and will not be discussed further in this chapter

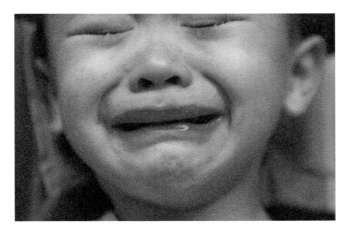

Figure 3.3.2 Children with Kawasaki disease are often very miserable, out of proportion to clinical findings. This boy also has typical dry, red, cracked lips. Courtesy of the Kawasaki Disease Foundation.

Box 3.3.2   Lymphadenopathy Associated with Solid Tumours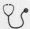

Lymphadenopathy may also result from metastases from solid tumours, such as:

- Rhabdomyosarcoma
- Neuroblastoma

Common Diagnoses
1. Viral Lymphadenopathy
- Most common form of reactive hyperplasia
- Usually represents transient response to simple infection
- Nodes are usually rubbery and non-tender, and should not be significantly enlarged >1 cm
- Most commonly affects cervical lymph nodes, due to the predisposition for infections in the oral cavity and pharynx
- Lymphadenopathy may persist for weeks to months, far outlasting the clinical infection
- Recurrent mild upper respiratory tract infections may lead parents to worry that lymphadenopathy is persistent

---

Box 3.3.3   Reactive Hyperplasia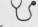

- Reactive lymphoid hyperplasia is a reversible enlargement of lymphoid tissue in response to an antigenic stimulus
- It is a normal physiological reaction to infection and inflammation

- Lymph nodes are small, rubbery, mobile, minimally tender and discrete, otherwise known as 'shotty'
- There should be no overlying skin changes

---

2. Bacterial Lymphadenitis
- Bacterial infection of the lymph node, commonly unilateral
- Most common in toddlers and early school-age children
- Nodes may be tender and fluctuant, most commonly occurring in the anterior cervical region
- The majority are caused by local bacterial infection, e.g. throat infections, scalp or dental infections. Most common organisms are *Staphylococcus aureus* and group A *Streptococci*

3. Infectious Mononucleosis
- Otherwise known as glandular fever, this is usually caused by Epstein–Barr virus (EBV), a common herpes virus, for which humans are the main reservoir. Cytomegalovirus (CMV) is also a cause
- Lymphadenopathy is classically symmetrical, involving posterior more than anterior cervical nodes, and may also affect axillary and inguinal nodes
- Characterised by a triad of fever, tonsillar pharyngitis and lymphadenopathy
- Infection is subclinical in up to 90% of children. Symptomatic infection is more common in adolescence, leading to EBV being termed the 'kissing disease', due to spread by intimate contact, as virus is shed in salivary secretions
- Chronic fatigue is a recognised complication

4. Cat-Scratch Disease
- Cat-scratch disease is one of many clinical syndromes that can be caused by *Bartonella henselae* bacteria
- It is caused by a bite or scratch from a cat, particularly a kitten
- Typically, symptoms are of a low-grade fever, and localised tender lymphadenopathy that develops 3 days – 3 weeks after exposure

Diagnoses to Consider
1. Mycobacterial Infection
- Either atypical mycobacteria or tuberculosis (TB)
- Non-tuberculous mycobacteria usually occurs in children under 5 years old. *Mycobacterium avium* and *M. scrofulaceum* account for most cases in children
- TB is less common, but should be considered if there is a positive history of visiting an endemic area or meeting a known TB contact
- Usually presents with long-term lymphadenopathy and symptoms not responding to antibiotics (weeks to months)

When to consider: in those with chronic lymphadenopathy not responding to routine antibiotics

2. Chronic Granulomatous Disease (CGD)
- Rare inherited (autosomal recessive or X-linked recessive) condition resulting in phagocyte defects, causing immunodeficiency with particular vulnerability to fungal and bacterial infections
- Presents in the neonatal or infant period with generalised lymphadenopathy, recurrent abscesses and recurrent pneumonia
- The child may present with faltering growth and recurrent infections
- Children are prone to granuloma formation, particularly affecting the gastrointestinal and genitourinary tracts

When to consider: in those with a history of recurrent, severe infections

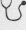

Box 3.3.4 Organisms Affecting Children with Chronic Granulomatous Disease (CGD)

Children with CGD are affected by recurrent severe fungal and bacterial infections:

- Fungal organisms: *Candida albicans, Aspergillus fumigatus*
- Bacterial organisms: *Staphylococcus aureus, Pseudomonas aeruginosa, Nocardia asteroides, Salmonella typhi*

3. BCG Lymphadenitis
- BCG lymphadenitis is the most common complication of the BCG vaccine
- Enlarged ipsilateral lymph nodes after BCG vaccination are common. These usually regress over a period of a few weeks
- Occasionally, lymph nodes may become fluctuant, with inflammation of overlying skin, indicative of suppurative lymphadenitis
- Suppurative lymphadenitis can also have an unprovoked onset at any time within 24 months of vaccination, although most cases are within 6 months
- Newborns are at higher risk of lymphadenitis
- In serious immunodeficiency states, systemic disseminated BCG infection is possible after vaccination
- Non-suppurative adenitis is usually self-resolving. Management is with conservative methods and reassurance. Suppurative adenitis requires needle aspiration. If this fails, surgical excision is indicated

When to consider: in those with lymphadenopathy on the same side as a recent BCG vaccination

4. Human Immunodeficiency Virus (HIV)
- HIV is a retrovirus affecting the T-lymphocytes of the immune system
- Rare as primary presentation in children (even sexually active teenagers) in the UK, especially since improved antenatal testing has dramatically reduced vertical transmission
- Lymphadenopathy is a common symptom of primary HIV infection during 'seroconversion illness', where antibodies are produced
- Travel and contact history is important
- Vulnerability to opportunistic infections increases as the disease progresses and, if left untreated, acquired immunodeficiency syndrome (AIDS) will develop
- HIV is covered in Chapter 3.2

When to consider: in those with known contact history

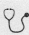

Box 3.3.5 Non-infective Causes of Lymphadenopathy

Dermatological conditions

- Eczema
- Psoriasis
- Insect bites

Iatrogenic

- Vaccine induced
- Drug hypersensitivity (e.g. phenytoin, carbamazepine, penicillins, cephalosporins)

Autoimmune

- Arthritis
- Systemic lupus erythematosus
- Dermatomyositis

Infiltrative diseases

- Sarcoidosis
- Amyloidosis

Metabolic

- Gaucher
- Niemann–Pick

Lymphoproliferative disorders

- Rosai-Dorfman disease
- Castleman disease
- Langerhans cell histiocytosis

Box 3.3.6　Mimics of Lymphadenopathy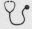

Salivary gland abnormalities

- Infection
- Stones

Congenital anomalies

- Branchial cleft cyst
- Cystic hygroma
- Thyroglossal cyst

- Salivary cyst
- Sternocleidomastoid pseudo-tumour

Soft tissue abnormalities

- Lipoma
- Swelling from trauma or insect bite
- Dermoid cyst

Thyroid nodule

3.3.5 KEY HISTORY FEATURES

Box 3.3.7　Key Aspects of History in Children with Lymphadenopathy

- Duration of enlargement
- Progression of symptoms
- Site and laterality of affected lymph nodes
- Associated constitutional symptoms
- Immunisation status

- Exposures:
  - Unwell contacts
  - Animals
  - Insect bites
  - Medications
  - Travel

Dangerous Diagnosis 1
Diagnosis: Acute lymphoblastic leukaemia

Questions
1. **Has there been weight loss?** Weight loss should raise worry for malignancy. This may be associated with anorexia
2. **Have there been fevers at home?** A history of fever is present in over 50% of children at the time of presentation and may be secondary to the leukaemia, or due to infection
3. **Has the child been complaining of abdominal pain?** At time of presentation, hepatomegaly and/or splenomegaly are common findings. These may manifest as abdominal distension or pain
4. **Any history of limp or 'growing pains'?** Occasionally, bone pain and joint pain may have been explained away as 'growing pains' until specifically asked about. There may be a limp or refusal to bear weight
5. **Has there been reduced exercise tolerance?** Bone marrow failure causes a pancytopenia (anaemia, leukopenia and thrombocytopenia). There may be shortness of breath, fatigue or reduced exercise tolerance resulting from anaemia
6. **Is there a history of recurrent infections, or easy bleeding/bruising?** Bone marrow suppression can result in neutropaenia (leading to increased susceptibility to infections) and thrombocytopaenia (may result in bleeding)
7. **Are there concurrent syndromes associated with an increased risk for leukaemia?** Some genetic syndromes, e.g. Down syndrome, ataxia-telangiectasia and neurofibromatosis type 1, are associated with increased risk
8. **Neurological symptoms.** Symptoms relating to raised intracranial pressure, including early-morning headache and vomiting, suggest central nervous system involvement

Dangerous Diagnosis 2
Diagnosis: Lymphoma
Clinical symptoms depend on location of the lymphoma, which often presents with symptoms from local compression of structures.

Questions
1. **What age is the child?** Lymphoma can present at any age, but is significantly more common with advancing age (mainly from adolescence onwards)
2. **Are there any systemic ('B') symptoms?** B symptoms include weight loss, night sweats and fever and have important implications for staging and prognosis

3. **Has there been shortness of breath or difficulty in swallowing?** Symptoms of lymphoma are a result of compression of surrounding structures. Mediastinal masses may cause shortness of breath, particularly on lying flat, and dysphagia
4. **Has the child been complaining of abdominal pain?** In advanced-stage lymphoma, there may be hepatomegaly and/or splenomegaly

Common Diagnosis 1
Diagnosis: Viral lymphadenopathy

Questions
1. **Are there, or have there recently been, coryzal symptoms?** Viral lymphadenopathy is precipitated by upper respiratory tract infections and there will usually be intercurrent or recent symptoms of runny nose, cough or fevers
2. **Is the child otherwise well?** The lymphadenopathy will usually have been discovered by chance by the parents, with no other associated symptoms

Common Diagnosis 2
Diagnosis: Bacterial lymphadenitis

Questions
1. **Is the child complaining of pain?** Acute bacterial adenitis tends to cause larger lymph nodes. The rapid expansion of the swelling stretches the capsule and can be painful
2. **Is there a source of infection in the area drained by the lymph node?** Lymphatic drainage roughly follows the veins in the body, meaning that lymph nodes drain downstream from an infection. Dental abscesses, tonsillitis or scalp folliculitis will lead to cervical lymph node involvement. Axillary lymph node involvement may follow cellulitis in an arm

Common Diagnosis 3
Diagnosis: Infectious mononucleosis

Questions
1. **Has there been a fever or sore throat?** Along with lymphadenopathy, fever and pharyngitis make up the classic triad of infectious mononucleosis
2. **Is the child lethargic?** Glandular fever classically causes lethargy. Parents may report that the child is waking later in the mornings and struggling with energy levels. Fatigue may be persistent and have a significant impact on school work
3. **Has the child had antibiotics for tonsillitis?** Infectious mononucleosis causes exudative tonsils, which may have prompted antibiotic administration. These would have had no effect on the pharyngitis, but may have provoked a widespread maculopapular rash

Common Diagnosis 4
Diagnosis: Cat-scratch disease

Questions
1. **Has the child been exposed to cats?** The classic history is of a child who has been playing with kittens
2. **When was the exposure?** The onset is usually between 3 days and 3 weeks after the exposure
3. **Are there any flu-like symptoms?** Systemic symptoms mimic flu, with fever, malaise, fatigue and headache

---

Box 3.3.8 Clinical Features Concerning for Malignancy or Granulomatous Disease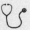

- Systemic symptoms: fever >7 days, night sweats, weight loss
- Supraclavicular nodes
- Generalised lymphadenopathy
- Painless nodes
- Firm/hard consistency
- Fixed or matted nodes
- Progressive course
- Nodes >1 cm (neonates) or >2 cm in children
- Absence of local infective/inflammatory causes

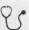

Box 3.3.9   Supraclavicular Lymphadenopathy

- Approximately 75% of supraclavicular lymphadenopathy in children is associated with malignancy
- Right-sided adenopathy is suggestive of mediastinal lymphadenopathy

- Left-sided adenopathy is suggestive of intra-abdominal malignancy. This is sometimes called 'Virchow's node'

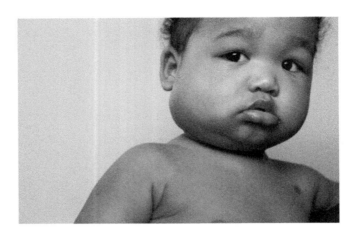

Figure 3.3.3 Child with cervical lymphadenopathy. Courtesy of the Kawasaki Disease Foundation.

3.3.6 KEY EXAMINATION FEATURES

Box 3.3.10   Stratification of Cervical Lymphadenopathy by Laterality

	Acute <2 weeks	Subacute/chronic >2 weeks
Unilateral	1. **Bacterial lymphadenitis** 2. **Group A *Streptococcus* throat infection** 3. **Kawasaki Disease** 4. Chronic granulomatous disease 5. Malignancy	1. **Non-tuberculous mycobacteria** 2. **Cat-scratch disease** 3. Tuberculosis 4. Toxoplasmosis 5. BCG adenitis 6. Malignancy
Bilateral	1. **Viral lymphadenopathy** 2. Infectious mononucleosis 3. Group A *Streptococcus* throat infection 4. Non-tuberculous mycobacteria 5. Malignancy	1. **Infectious mononucleosis** 2. Human immunodeficiency virus (HIV) 3. Tuberculosis 4. Toxoplasmosis 5. Malignancy

Note: Commonest causes in each category are in bold

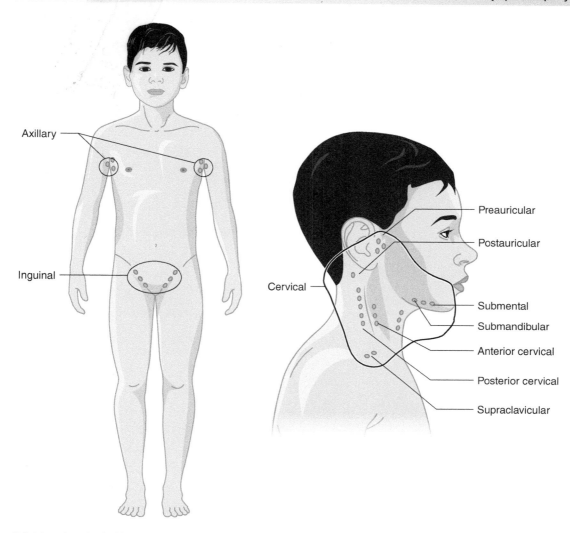

Figure 3.3.4 Location of palpable peripheral lymph nodes.

Dangerous Diagnosis 1
Diagnosis: Acute lymphoblastic leukaemia

Examination Findings
1. **Painless lymphadenopathy.** Typical lymphadenopathy of ALL is non-tender and firm. Enlarged, matted nodes are particularly concerning
2. **Pallor.** Bone marrow failure causes anaemia. Pallor can be seen in the conjunctivae or palmar creases
3. **Bruising.** A tendency to easy bruising (or petechiae) may present as multiple bruises or bruising on uncommon areas. In leukaemia, this is due to thrombocytopenia from bone marrow failure
4. **Hepatosplenomegaly.** Hepatomegaly and splenomegaly are present in up to 90% of children presenting with leukaemia. The abdomen may be distended
5. **Limp.** Bone pain is a common presentation. In young children this may manifest as a limp or refusal to bear weight

Dangerous Diagnosis 2
Diagnosis: Lymphoma

Examination Findings
1. **Painless lymphadenopathy.** Lymphadenopathy is non-tender, firm and may be widespread, particularly in the cervical, supraclavicular and axillary regions. Aggregates of lymph nodes >6 cm in diameter are known as 'bulky lymphadenopathy' and are relevant to prognostication
2. **Increased work of breathing when lying flat.** Lymphoma commonly presents as symptoms due to compression of surrounding structures. Respiratory distress worsened on lying flat is particularly concerning for a mediastinal mass. Up to 75% of children with Hodgkin lymphoma have a mediastinal mass on x-ray at presentation
3. **Signs of superior vena cava (SVC) syndrome.** SVC syndrome, from compression of the SVC, is an emergency. There may be neck and facial swelling, arm swelling and distended veins over the anterior chest wall
4. **Cachexia.** The child may have lost weight and thus look cachectic
5. **Scratch marks.** Children with Hodgkin lymphoma in particular may suffer from pruritus, known as paraneoplastic pruritis. This can precede other clinical signs by weeks or even months
6. **Hepatosplenomegaly.** Hepatomegaly and splenomegaly may be present in advanced lymphoma

Common Diagnosis 1
Diagnosis: Viral lymphadenitis

Examination Findings
1. **Small lymph nodes.** There will be multiple small lymph nodes scattered throughout the cervical chains bilaterally, which are painless on palpation
2. **Systemically well child.** The child may have a viral upper respiratory tract infection, with evidence of coryza, pharyngitis or cough, but will be generally healthy

Common Diagnosis 2
Diagnosis: Bacterial lymphadenitis

Examination Findings
1. **Unilateral large lymphadenitis.** Bacterial adenitis is most likely to be unilateral, although there may be bilateral lymphadenopathy with other smaller, non-inflamed lymph nodes. The affected lymph node is markedly enlarged, often >3 cm
2. **Signs of local bacterial infection.** Depending on the location of the lymph node swelling, look for signs of bacterial infection in the local area, including dental abscess, tonsillitis or cellulitis
3. **Inflammation of overlying skin.** Overlying skin may be erythematous, warm and indurated. Occasionally there may be purulent exudate if a sinus is formed
4. **Fluctuance on palpation.** Enlarged lymph nodes can rupture, leading to an abscess. This may need surgical drainage
5. **Is the child systemically well?** A bacterial lymphadenitis can develop into sepsis, so the child should be assessed and managed for sepsis if they are systemically unwell

Common Diagnosis 3
Diagnosis: Infectious mononucleosis

Examination Findings
1. **Symmetrical posterior triangle cervical lymphadenopathy.** Lymphadenopathy is classically symmetrical. It is often prominent in posterior triangles of the neck, in contrast to tonsillitis, which tends mainly to affect the anterior cervical chain. Nodes may be tender
2. **Generalised lymphadenopathy.** As opposed to other upper respiratory tract infections, there may be axillary and inguinal lymphadenopathy

3. **Splenomegaly.** Splenomegaly is seen in over 50% of patients. If splenic enlargement is present, this may cause abdominal pain. It usually recedes by the third week
4. **Maculopapular rash.** Although this is classically associated with amoxicillin, a generalised rash can occur, even without provocation by antibiotics
5. **'Whitewash' tonsils.** The tonsils can have the appearance of having pus present – on closer inspection this will be more confluent than the classical exudative spots of tonsillitis. There may also be palatal petechiae

Common Diagnosis 4
Diagnosis: Cat-scratch disease

Examination Findings
1. **Swelling at site of bite/scratch.** There may be swelling or a blister at the site of bacterial entry. If it is several weeks after inoculation, this may simply be a small papule. These usually heal without a scar
2. **Axillary lymphadenopathy.** Affected lymph nodes are usually axillary, as inoculation sites tend to be on the arms. About 25% of children also have isolated cervical lymph nodes
3. **Tender, fluctuant lymph nodes.** Lymph nodes are tender, and about 30% of children develop suppurative disease
4. **Hepatosplenomegaly.** Although uncommon, it is important to be aware that visceral organ involvement can result in hepatomegaly and/or splenomegaly

---

Box 3.3.11   Complications of Cat-Scratch Disease

- Hepatosplenic disease
- Neuroretinitis
- Endocarditis

- Parinaud's oculoglandular syndrome: unilateral granulomatous follicular conjunctivitis + ipsilateral regional lymphadenopathy
- Encephalopathy

3.3.7 KEY INVESTIGATIONS

Systemically well children with cervical lymphadenopathy and clinical evidence of reactive hyperplasia are unlikely to require any further investigations. If necessary, monitor children with serial examinations every few weeks until regression.

Bedside

Table 3.3.1 Bedside tests of use in patients presenting with lymphadenopathy

Test	When to perform	Potential result
Throat swab MC&S ± viral PCR	Those presenting with pharyngitis or exudates on the tonsils	• Pure growth of an organism supports infection • Sensitivities guide antibiotic choice

MC&S, microscopy, culture and sensitivity; PCR, polymerase chain reaction

Blood Tests

Table 3.3.2 Blood tests of use in patients presenting with lymphadenopathy

Test	When to perform	Potential result
FBC	• All patients systemically unwell • White cell counts useful in assessing for infection and haematological malignancy • Neutrophils crucial in assessment of febrile neutropaenia	• ↓/↑ WCC in infection (usually neutrophilia if bacterial, lymphocytosis in viral) • ↑ Platelets in Kawasaki disease • Pancytopenia: malignancy, bone marrow failure syndrome • ↑ Monocytes seen in CGD and lymphoma
Blood film	• Suspected malignancy • Other infections, such as infectious mononucleosis, may have an abnormal blood film	• Peripheral blast cells indicate malignancy • 'Left shift' of neutrophils suggests infection • Abnormal lymphocytes with nucleoli within nuclei are present in mononucleosis
CRP	• Suspected serious underlying infection or inflammatory process	• Significant ↑ in bacterial infections • Less marked ↑ in viral infections
LDH	• Suspected malignancy	• ↑ LDH signifies increased cell turnover
EBV serology	• Suspected infectious mononucleosis • Serology ideal, as monospot may be falsely negative in children	• Confirms EBV infection
HIV antibodies and antigen	• Suspected HIV infection	• Negative result rules out HIV • If positive, need to do HIV RNA level
ASOT	• Suspected bacterial lymphadenitis secondary to GAS throat infection	• Indicates GAS infection • Note that positive result may indicate colonisation
Bartonella henselae serology	• Suspected cat-scratch disease	• Positive serology confirms diagnosis
Blood culture	• If systemically unwell	• Positive culture confirms bacterial infection • Sensitivities guide antibiotic choice

ASOT, anti-streptolysin O titre; CGD, chronic granulomatous disease; CRP, C-reactive protein; EBV, Epstein–Barr virus; FBC, full blood count; GAS, group A *Streptococcus*; HIV, human immunodeficiency virus; LDH, lactate dehydrogenase; WCC, white cell count

Imaging

Table 3.3.3 Imaging tests of use in patients presenting with lymphadenopathy

Test	When to perform	Potential result
Chest x-ray	Suspected: • Mycobacterial infection • CGD • HIV • Malignancy	• Pulmonary TB: Infiltrates, consolidation, ± effusion, ± hilar lymphadenopathy • Pneumonia in CGD/HIV: consolidation • Malignancy: mediastinal lymphadenopathy
Lymph node ultrasound	• If fluctuant swelling, to detect presence and extent of abscess	• Characterisation of abscess • Alternative diagnosis of congenital cystic abnormality

CGD, chronic granulomatous disease; HIV, human immunodeficiency virus; TB, tuberculosis

Special

Table 3.3.4 Special tests of use in patients presenting with lymphadenopathy

Test	When to perform	Potential result
Biopsy (usually excisional) – histopathology and microbiology	• If failure to respond to empirical therapy or chronic lymphadenopathy of uncertain cause • If malignancy strongly suspected	• Microbial isolation of causative agent • Cytological diagnosis of lymphoma
Neutrophil function tests	• If suspecting CGD – measures neutrophil superoxide production	• Confirmation of qualitative neutrophil defect
Tuberculin skin testing	• If suspicious of tuberculous mycobacterial infection • Only confirms exposure, with no distinction between acute or past infection	• Induration is measured. Positive result depends on pre-test probability • Non-tuberculous mycobacterial infection yields false positive • Test is positive after BCG vaccination
Mycobacterial culture + acid-fast bacilli smear	• Specimens should be collected from any site where infection is suspected • In those suspected of having pulmonary TB, use gastric lavage or induced sputum	• Confirms TB • Diagnostic yield generally poor (approximately one-third of specimens)

CGD, chronic granulomatous disease; TB, tuberculosis

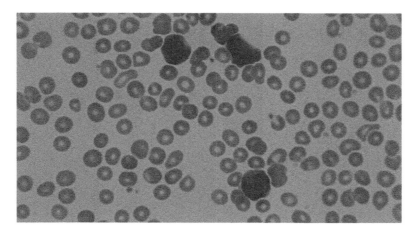

Figure 3.3.5 Blood film showing three large blasts in a patient with precursor B-ALL (acute lymphoblastic leukaemia).

3.3.8 KEY MANAGEMENT PRINCIPLES

Diagnosis-specific management strategies are outlined here. It is expected that an 'ABCDE' approach to assessment and management is always undertaken (see Chapter 12.1, *The A to E Assessment*).

Dangerous Diagnosis 1
Diagnosis: Acute lymphoblastic leukaemia

Management Principles
1. **Refer to tertiary paediatric oncology unit and ALL work-up.** Once the initial diagnosis is made, refer to the tertiary paediatric oncology centre. There is extensive work-up that guides management, including blood tests (baseline organ function, viral screen, cytogenetics, infection markers, blood group), lumbar puncture, baseline imaging and bone marrow aspiration
2. **Immunocompromise precautions.** Most newly diagnosed patients are immunocompromised. Standard procedure involves strict infection control with side room isolation. Patients with neutropenic pyrexia or sepsis should have immediate broad-spectrum antibiotics and management as per local protocol

3. **Supportive treatment if risk of leukostasis.** Patients with high white blood cell counts are at risk of tumour lysis syndrome. Interim treatment, until definitive cytoreductive chemotherapy is started, includes steroids, hyperhydration with 0.9% saline, allopurinol or rasburicase. The appropriate treatment will be determined by local protocol and advice from a local tertiary paediatric oncology service
4. **Trials.** Most patients will be enrolled into current national clinical trials for treatment. Treatment is generally split into stage 1 (induction), stage 2 (consolidation) and stage 3 (maintenance)

Dangerous Diagnosis 2
Diagnosis: Lymphoma

Management Principles
1. **Involvement of tertiary oncology service.** Early referral to a tertiary paediatric oncology service is advised for definitive management
2. **Immunocompromise precautions.** Most newly diagnosed patients are immunocompromised. Standard procedure involves strict infection control with side room isolation. Patients with neutropenic pyrexia or sepsis should have immediate broad-spectrum antibiotics and management as per local protocol
3. **Avoid giving steroids until lymphoma has been ruled out.** Administration of steroids can precipitate tumour lysis syndrome and make the diagnosis more difficult

Common Diagnosis 1
Diagnosis: Viral lymphadenopathy

Management Principles
1. **Reassurance and safety netting.** Very often, viral lymphadenopathy is noticed once the initial infection is already resolving. Reassurance of normal history and examination is important. Safety net advice about any emerging systemic features should be given

Common Diagnosis 2
Diagnosis: Bacterial lymphadenitis

Management Principles
1. **Antibiotics.** The most common organisms causing bacterial lymphadenopathy are streptococci and staphylococci. Co-amoxiclav is therefore a good empirical treatment and oral may be appropriate if the patient is systemically well. If discharged, a review after 2 weeks of treatment is useful to make sure that the lymph node has responded to treatment
2. **Surgical drainage.** If the swelling is fluctuant, then an Ear, Nose and Throat (ENT; if cervical) or surgical (if elsewhere in the body) opinion should be sought

Common Diagnosis 3
Diagnosis: Infectious mononucleosis

Management Principles
1. **Symptomatic treatment.** Fluid replacement may be needed if severe pharyngitis precludes adequate oral intake. Analgesia and antipyretics are useful
2. **Avoid contact sports.** The child needs to be advised to avoid contact sports for 6 months as there is a risk of splenic rupture
3. **Be aware of potential neurological complications.** Rarely, Guillain–Barré syndrome, meningoencephalitis and cranial nerve palsies can follow infectious mononucleosis

Common Diagnosis 4
Diagnosis: Cat-scratch disease

Management Principles
1. **Antibiotics.** Even in those with presumed cat-scratch disease, without laboratory confirmation, treatment is indicated. Generally, a 5-day course of azithromycin is recommended. Alternative options are 7 days of clarithromycin, rifampicin or co-trimoxazole
2. **Review after 3 weeks.** If lymphadenitis has not resolved after 3–4 weeks, re-treatment with azithromycin and additional rifampicin is indicated
3. **Needle aspiration.** In suppurative lymphadenopathy, needle aspiration may speed up resolution and provide symptomatic relief

4.1 Bruising

Rachel Varughese

Department of Paediatrics, Oxford University Hospitals NHS Foundation Trust, Oxford, UK

CONTENTS

4.1.1 CHAPTER AT A GLANCE

> **Box 4.1.1   Chapter at a Glance**
>
> - Bruising is a common occurrence in the life of a mobile child and is often due to accidental injury sustained during routine play
> - There are four key questions to answer:
>   - Is this bruising normal?
>   - Is this bruising due to inflicted injury?
>   - Is this bruising due to a bleeding disorder?
> - Is this bruising due to another medical condition?
> - 'Easy' bruising is suggestive of an underlying medical condition. This is defined as bruising without a history of significant injury, or bruising that is out of proportion to a minor trauma
> - There may be overlap between bruising conditions and inflicted injury

4.1.2 DEFINITION

A bruise is a collection of blood beneath the skin, resulting from bleeding into subcutaneous tissues from nearby vessels.

Clinical Guide to Paediatrics, First Edition. Edited by Rachel Varughese and Anna Mathew. Series Editor: Christian Fielder Camm.
© 2022 John Wiley & Sons Ltd. Published 2022 by John Wiley & Sons Ltd.
Companion website: www.wiley.com/go/varughese/paediatrics

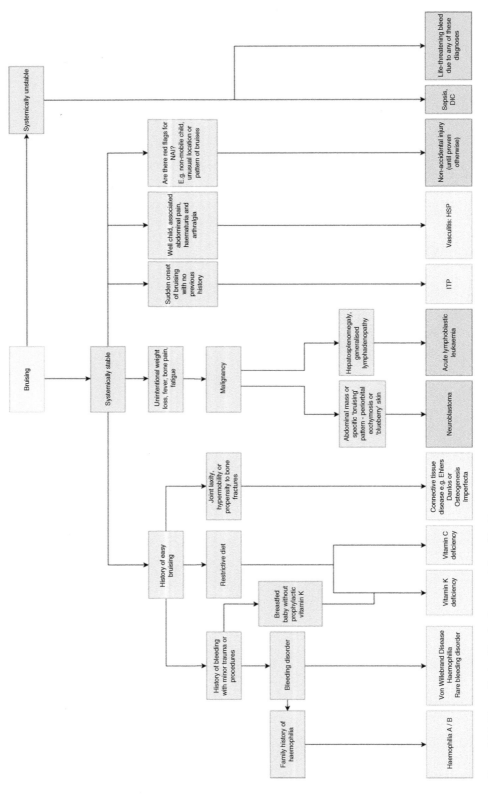

Figure 4.1.1 Diagnostic algorithm for the presentation of bruising.

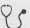

Box 4.1.2   Features of a Normal Bruise

- Mobile child
- Small in size
- Non-distinct borders
- Rounded shape

- Front of body
- Near bony prominences
- No recognisable shape or pattern
- No clustering

4.1.4 DIFFERENTIALS LIST

Dangerous Diagnoses

1. Non-accidental Injury (NAI)
- Bruising is a key external sign seen in NAI, which is covered in more detail in the safeguarding section (see Chapter 12.5, *Safeguarding*)
- In a non-mobile child, bruising is a serious concern for NAI and should be considered as a safeguarding priority
- Careful history will be key in establishing the consistency and plausibility of an alternative mechanism

Box 4.1.3   Red Flags for Non-accidental Injury in a Child with Bruising

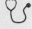

- **Mobility**: non-mobile children
- **Location**: ears, neck, feet, buttocks, torso, back of body, not overlying bony prominence
- **Pattern**: reminiscent of distinctive shape, e.g. handprint, shoe, cord, belt, bite or ligature marks

- **Distribution**: cluster of bruises
- **History**: appearance of bruise inconsistent with mechanism described

2. Acute Lymphoblastic Leukaemia (ALL)
- ALL is the commonest childhood cancer, with most cases affecting children aged 0–5 years
- It involves bone marrow production of excess numbers of immature white blood cells, known as blasts
- The production of blasts in ALL disrupts the bone marrow production of red blood cells and platelets
- Reduction in platelet number may cause easy bruising, as well as unusual bleeding of gums and nasal mucosa, or purpuric rashes
- ALL is covered in Chapter 3.3 and will not be discussed further in this chapter

3. Neuroblastoma
- A neuroblastoma is a solid tumour of neuroblasts, immature cells destined to become sympathetic nerve cells or cells of the adrenal medulla
- It is the most frequent extra-cranial solid tumour in children and commonly arises from the adrenal glands, but can occur anywhere along the sympathetic chain
- Most children affected are <5 years old
- Neuroblastoma can cause bruising through bone marrow infiltration or metastases to skin of orbits
- Neuroblastoma typically presents as an abdominal mass. As such, detailed discussion is included in Chapter 5.2, and it will not be addressed further in this chapter

Box 4.1.4   Mechanisms of Bruising in Neuroblastoma

Neuroblastoma has three ways of causing or mimicking bruising:

- Infiltration of bone marrow leads to a reduction in platelet numbers
- Metastases to the skin can cause bruise-like lesions that are nodular and blue or purple in colour. These are sometimes referred to as having a 'blueberry' appearance

- Neuroblastoma frequently metastasises to the orbit. The presentation of this is periorbital ecchymosis, sometimes referred to as 'racoon' eyes. Deposition of blood in the eyelids can be mistaken for bruising

Common Diagnoses

1. Immune Thrombocytopenia (ITP)
- Previously described as idiopathic thrombocytopenic purpura, immune thrombocytopenia is the most common acquired disorder of coagulation
- Autoantibodies directed against platelet membrane antigens cause accelerated clearance as well as inhibited production, leading to a profound decrease in platelet number

- ITP can be primary or secondary (see Box 4.1.5)
- Children can present at any age, with a peak between 2–5 years and again during adolescence

---

Box 4.1.5   Primary and Secondary Immune Thrombocytopenia (ITP)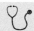

- The cause of primary ITP is unknown, but viral and environmental triggers are often suspected

- In secondary ITP, the precipitant is known, such as medication, immune deficiency or systemic illness, and management includes the need to treat the underlying condition

---

2. Von Willebrand Disease (VWD)

- VWD is the most common inherited coagulation disorder, with an incidence of up to 1% in the general population
- VWD is due to a quantitative or functional reduction in von Willebrand factor (VWF), which under normal conditions acts as a bridging molecule at sites of vascular injury and promotes platelet aggregation

---

Box 4.1.6   Three Subtypes of Von Willebrand Disease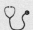

Types are characterised by the deficiency of von Willebrand factor (VWF):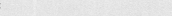

- Type 1: reduced-level VWF
- Type 2: dysfunctional VWF

- Type 3: absent/undetectable VWF

---

3. Haemophilia

- The next most common coagulation disorders are factor VIII deficiency (haemophilia A) and factor IX deficiency (haemophilia B)
- These are X-linked recessive conditions. As such, most patients are male (females are affected in very rare circumstances or in a mild form as symptomatic carriers)
- Haemophilia is classed as mild, moderate or severe, depending on the residual baseline clotting factor level
- Bleeding sites vary depending on age and disease severity. Newborns may present with intracranial bleeds, cephalohaematoma and excess bleeding at sites of medical intervention such as venepuncture or circumcision
- Children commonly present with bruising, joint/musculoskeletal bleeding or gastrointestinal bleeding

4. Ehlers–Danlos Syndrome (EDS)

- Many connective tissue diseases, in particular EDS, are associated with bruising
- There are several subtypes, many of which share the same risk factors for bruising
- Affected children with joint laxity tend to fall more easily due to reduced joint and muscle control
- Furthermore, fragility of dermal capillaries and poor structural integrity to the skin contribute to easy bruising

---

Box 4.1.7   Osteogenesis Imperfecta (OI)

- OI is another connective tissue disease that may cause bruising
- OI is a rare condition, with several subtypes, characterised by fragile bones that fracture easily

- Severity is variable across the four subtypes and also within affected families
- Easy bruising, although the mechanism is not fully understood, is thought to be due to vascular and skin fragility

---

Diagnoses to Consider

1. Nutritional Deficiencies

- Vitamin deficiencies can be associated with bruising, seen in particular with vitamin K and C deficiency
- Vitamin C is a requirement in the diet, because humans cannot synthesise endogenous vitamin C. Scurvy is uncommon in the developed world, but can occur in restrictive diets
- Vitamin K is essential in the activation of clotting factor 2 (prothrombin), as well as 7, 9 and 10. Humans do not store much vitamin K and rely on nutritional intake

When to consider: in children with large unexplained bruises and a history of a restricted diet

Box 4.1.8   Vitamin C Deficiency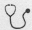

- Initially, symptoms are non-specific, including anorexia, lethargy, weakness and depression

- Untreated, severe vitamin C deficiency results in defective collagen synthesis and fragility of capillary connective tissue, leading to bruising and increased bleeding tendency

Box 4.1.9   Vitamin K Deficiency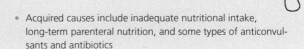

- Deficiency is universal in newborn babies due to the lack of placental transfer in utero
- Hereditary vitamin K deficiency is possible, but extremely rare

- Acquired causes include inadequate nutritional intake, long-term parenteral nutrition, and some types of anticonvulsants and antibiotics

Box 4.1.10   Dietary Sources of Vitamins C and K

Vitamin C–rich foods	Vitamin K–rich foods
Oranges, red and green peppers, strawberries, blackcurrants, broccoli, Brussels sprouts, potatoes	Broccoli, spinach, kale, lettuce, chard, cabbage, cauliflower, vegetable oils, cereals

2. Vasculitis

- Vasculitides, such as immunoglobulin A (IgA) vasculitis, also known as Henoch–Schönlein purpura (HSP), can cause palpable purpura. These are often painful or tender
- HSP is characterised by the tetrad of palpable purpura, arthritis/arthralgia, abdominal pain and renal disease. It is covered in more detail in Chapter 9.2

When to consider: in those with tender purpura on lower-limb extensor surfaces and buttocks

3. Sepsis

- Always remember that extensive bruising may be seen in systemic infections such as meningococcal septicaemia, causing disseminated intravascular coagulation (DIC)
- It is included here, rather than in the 'dangerous diagnoses' section, since bruising will not be the primary presenting complaint of sepsis
- Sepsis is covered in detail elsewhere, in Chapter 3.1

When to consider: in those with evidence of infection and systemic compromise

Box 4.1.11   Rare Bleeding Disorders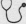

There are many other types of rare inherited and acquired bleeding disorders, which fall into three broad categories: coagulation disorders, fibrinogen disorders and platelet disorders:

Coagulation disorders

- Inherited deficiencies of a variety of factors may be associated with clinical bleeding

- Mostly autosomal recessive and include factor 2, 5, 7, 10, 11, 13 and combined deficiencies

Fibrinogen disorders

- Fibrinogen is essential for normal haemostasis as a precursor of fibrin, which is vital in coagulation by binding and supporting platelets and thrombin

Acquired platelet disorders

- Can occur in association with several conditions, including liver disease, renal disease, malignancy or due to autoimmune causes

- There are a large number of rare inherited causes, mostly affecting platelet function, such as Glanzmann thrombasthenia and Wiskott–Aldrich syndrome

Box 4.1.12   Alternative Diagnoses Masquerading as Bruises   △△

Diagnosis	Detail
Slate grey naevus	• Previously known as Mongolian blue spot • Extremely common congenital skin lesion in non-Caucasian infants • Results from arrested melanocyte progression in the lower part of the dermis, during migration from the neural crest to the epidermis • Lesion is macular and blue-grey in colour, most often affecting the buttocks and back
Haemangioma	• Haemangiomas are collections of blood vessels beneath the skin • Superficial haemangiomas are usually raised and red, not representing bruises at all, but deep haemangiomas can be blue in colour and less prominent • May develop over first weeks of life and grow rapidly for 3 months, after which they tend to plateau and shrink
Dermal melanocytosis	• Melanocytic naevi deep within the dermis appear as blue-grey-purple lesions • They can occur anywhere on the body, but three types are commonly described: naevus of Ota: forehead/periocular; naevus of Hori: cheeks; and naevus of Ito: shoulder girdle • Can be congenital or acquired and may darken through childhood
Erythema multiforme	• Hypersensitivity reaction, usually to viruses, e.g. herpes simplex, less commonly to drugs • Starts in lower limbs and spreads to trunk and face • Lesions are dusky red and may be referred to as 'target' lesions as they have a dark centre, surrounded by a pale area, circumscribed by a red ring
Erythema nodosum	• These are purple-red bumps that are initially painful, but gradually fade to look like bruises • Related to inflammatory bowel disease, systemic lupus erythematosus, tuberculosis and drug reactions. May also be idiopathic
Incontinentia pigmenti	• X-linked dominant condition with characteristic skin lesions • Initially (stage 1 and 2), lesions are blisters followed by wart-like crusting, but stage 3 can mimic bruises as flat hyperpigmented patches develop
Skin staining from ink	• Stains from ink or dyes can be so convincing of bruising that child protection examinations might even be arranged
Phytophotodermatitis	• Photosensitive reaction following exposure to certain plants, initially starting as blistering, but followed by post-inflammatory hyperpigmentation that may persist for months

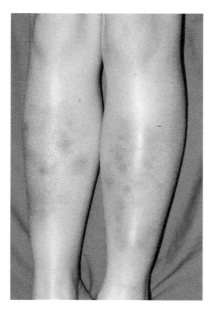

Figure 4.1.2 Erythema nodosum. Source: Reproduced with permission from Newell, S.J., and Darling, J.C. (2014). *Paediatrics lecture notes*. Chichester: Wiley Blackwell.

4.1.5 KEY HISTORY FEATURES

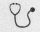

> **Box 4.1.13   Assessment Is Targeted at Answering These Four Questions**
>
> - Is this normal?
> - Is this due to inflicted injury?
>
> - Is there an underlying bleeding disorder?
> - Is there an underlying alternative medical condition?

Dangerous Diagnosis 1
Diagnosis: Non-accidental injury

Questions
1. **How did the bruise happen?** Careful, open-ended history taking is essential. Do not suggest mechanisms of injury. Often, due to the nature of clerking, the history might be taken several times by people of increasing seniority. This can be frustrating for parents, but is essential in establishing consistency. If age appropriate, the child can be questioned separately, in a sensitive manner
2. **Who does the child spend time with?** It is important to establish a clear picture of who looks after the child. Multiple people might have shared responsibility, including parents, family members, childminders and school
3. **Is the family known to social services?** It is important to establish whether there is a background of other child protection issues. Any child can be a victim of NAI, whether the family is known to social services or not. However, this information is useful in determining risk and potential further involvement of social care
4. **Are there any other known injuries?** Other injuries may be revealed on examination, but it is essential to ask about other known injuries first. This encourages disclosure and allows a detailed history to be taken about circumstances
5. **Have there been previous presentations with injuries?** It is possible that previous injuries may not have appeared suspicious, but a pattern of presentation with bruises, fractures or other injuries is very important to reveal

Common Diagnosis 1
Diagnosis: Immune thrombocytopenia

Questions
1. **What was the onset of the bruising?** ITP tends to cause the sudden appearance of bruising or mucocutaneous bleeding
2. **Are there any other symptoms?** The child is often otherwise well – the absence of systemic symptoms is consistent with ITP
3. **Has there been a recent viral infection?** Approximately 60% of children with ITP will have had a viral infection in the past 4 weeks

Common Diagnosis 2
Diagnosis: Von Willebrand disease

Questions
1. **Do bruises occur without trauma, or with unusually minor trauma?** The key here is to ascertain whether there is easy bruising, which is either unprovoked or related to a very mild injury
2. **Has the child been exposed to a 'bleeding challenge' before and how was this tolerated?** Exposures that count as a bleeding challenge include invasive dental procedures, surgery, menstruation or childbirth (of course, this is unusual in the paediatric population). Did they bleed excessively or require unexpected blood products?
3. **Have there been frequent or prolonged episodes of mucocutaneous bleeding?** Epistaxis is the typical example of mucocutaneous bleeding. Episodes longer than 10 minutes are significant

Common Diagnosis 3
Diagnosis: Haemophilia

Questions
1. **Do bruises occur without trauma, or with unusually minor trauma?** The key here is to ascertain whether there is easy bruising, which is either unprovoked or related to a very mild injury
2. **Have they undergone any minor procedures and how was this tolerated?** Patients with mild haemophilia may have delayed bleeding after minor surgery such as tooth extraction

3. **Has there been bleeding in response to minor injury?** This is slightly different to asking about easy bruising. Bleeds might include subgaleal bleeds and cephalohaematomas in infancy, frenulum and oral injuries (particularly in toddlers), joint bleeds and large forehead 'egg' haematomas

Common Diagnosis 4
Diagnosis: Ehlers–Danlos syndrome

Questions
1. **Have there been previous joint dislocations?** Children with common forms of EDS have mutations in genes encoding collagen, making them likely to have joint instability
2. **Is there joint or musculoskeletal pain?** Joint and muscular laxity leads to chronic pain in many affected individuals
3. **Is there family history of EDS?** Depending on the subtype, EDS may be sporadic or inherited in an autosomal recessive or autosomal dominant manner

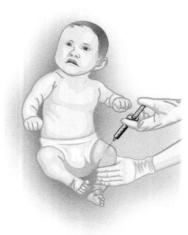

Figure 4.1.3 Newborn babies require vitamin K at birth. This is commonly given as a single intramuscular injection, but can be given in serial oral doses if parents prefer. Vitamin K prevents 'vitamin K deficiency bleeding', also known as 'haemorrhagic disease of the newborn'.

4.1.6 KEY EXAMINATION FEATURES

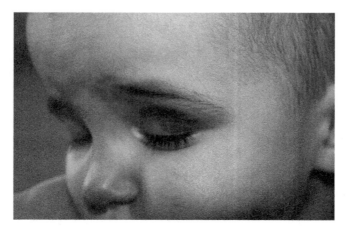

Figure 4.1.4 Always consider non-accidental injury in any bruising in a child. Source: Reproduced with permission from Shutterstock.

Dangerous Diagnosis 1

Diagnosis: Non-accidental injury

Examination Findings

1. **Suspicious pattern of bruises.** Suspicious bruises include those in unusual clusters or patterned like an instrument of assault. See Box 4.1.3 for red-flag features
2. **Unkempt appearance.** Children suffering from NAI do not have a stereotyped appearance. However, it is important to look carefully for signs of neglect, e.g. unclean clothes, dirty nails, dental caries
3. **Other injuries.** Unfortunately, there are many signs that might represent NAI – see box 4.1.14

Box 4.1.14   Concerning Features of Non-accidental Injury

Signs of inflicted injury include, but are not limited to:

- Lacerations
- Thermal injuries:
  - Implement
  - Immersion
- Cold injury
- Fracture

- Spinal injury
- Oral injury, e.g. frenulum tear
- Signs of sexual abuse:
  - Trauma
  - Pregnancy
  - Sexually transmitted infections

See also Chapter 12.5, *Safeguarding, Figures 12.5.2 and 12.5.3, Suspicious areas for bruising from the front and back.*

Common Diagnosis 1

Diagnosis: Immune thrombocytopenia

Examination Findings

1. **Macular petechial or purpuric lesions.** Isolated purpura or petechiae may be the only examination finding. Children are generally well. Serious bleeding is uncommon (1–3%)

Common Diagnosis 2

Diagnosis: Von Willebrand disease

Examination Findings

1. **Bleeding.** Besides easy bruising and mucocutaneous bleeding, there may be no other specific signs

Common Diagnosis 3

Diagnosis: Haemophilia

Examination Findings

1. **Bleeding.** Easy bruising and excessive bleeding are the key signs
2. **Haemophilic arthropathy.** In severe haemophilia, multiple episodes of haemarthrosis in a target joint lead to persistent joint disease

Common Diagnosis 4

Diagnosis: Ehlers–Danlos syndrome

Examination Findings

1. **Joint hypermobility.** This is the hallmark of most subsets of EDS. On diagnosis, many children may have noticed their hypermobility and will be more than happy to demonstrate. Objective assessment is by the Beighton score
2. **Hyperextendable skin.** Hyperelasticity is demonstrated by stretching the skin at least 4 cm, e.g. on the ventral aspect of the forearm

Box 4.1.15   Beighton Score for Hypermobility Assessment: Score >4 suggestive of hypermobility

Criteria	Left	Right
Passive dorsiflexion of the fifth finger >90 degrees with forearm flat	/1	/1
Passive apposition of the thumb to the flexor aspect of the forearm	/1	/1
Hyperextension of elbow >10 degrees	/1	/1
Hyperextension of the knee >10 degrees	/1	/1
Flexion of waist with palms on the floor (and with the knees fully extended)	/1	
		Total /9

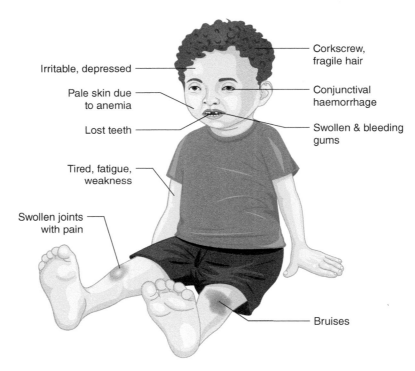

Irritable, depressed

Pale skin due to anemia

Lost teeth

Tired, fatigue, weakness

Swollen joints with pain

Corkscrew, fragile hair

Conjunctival haemorrhage

Swollen & bleeding gums

Bruises

Figure 4.1.5 Vitamin C deficiency was classically associated with sailors due to their severely restricted diet. 'Scurvy' is rare these days, as dietary intake is usually enough to prevent severe vitamin C deficiency.

Box 4.1.16   Can Bruises Be Dated from Their Appearance?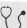

- It is often expected that the age of bruises can be estimated by their colour
- This has largely been disregarded, as it is now felt that the progression in colour of bruises differs significantly between patients

- However, the presence of multiple injuries sustained at different timepoints (as is sometimes seen with old rib fractures) is highly suggestive of non-accidental injury

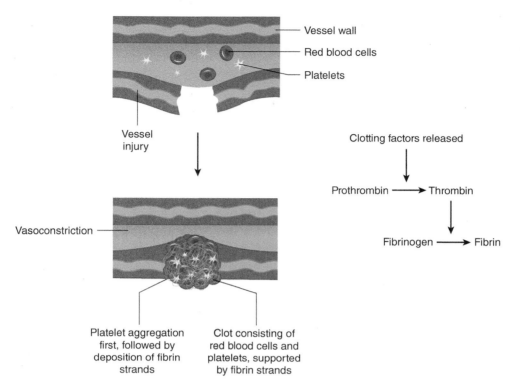

Figure 4.1.6 Damage to a blood vessel triggers a cascade of reactions. Endothelial damage induces vasoconstriction at the site of injury. Platelets are activated and start to aggregate with assistance of von Willebrand factor, creating a plug, with red blood cells. Once fibrinogen (soluble) has been converted to fibrin (insoluble) by the coagulation cascade, fibrin strands deposit at the plug to stabilise the clot. Defects to any part of this process lead to excessive bruising and bleeding.

4.1.7 KEY INVESTIGATIONS

In those with clear clinical evidence of 'normal', non-suspicious bruising, further investigations may not be warranted. All other patients presenting with bruising will require further tests.

Bedside Tests

Table 4.1.1 Bedside tests of use in patients presenting with bruising

Test	When to perform	Potential result
Blood gas	Suspected: • Sepsis • Severe bleeding	• ↓ pH, ↓ HCO$_3$, ↑ lactate indicate metabolic acidosis, suggestive of sepsis or severe bleeding • ↑/↓ Glucose may occur in sepsis • Hb level can often be estimated
Urine dipstick	• Suspected HSP	• Proteinuria and haematuria indicative of renal involvement in HSP

Hb, haemoglobin; HCO$_3$, bicarbonate; HSP, Henoch–Schönlein purpura

Blood Tests

Table 4.1.2 Blood tests of use in patients presenting with bruising

Test	When to perform	Potential result
FBC	• All patients with bruising	• Pancytopenia: bone marrow failure, suggestive of malignancy • Isolated ↓ platelets: ITP or if unwell, consumption in DIC • ↓ Hb in suspected bleeding disorder
Blood film	• All patients with bruising	• Peripheral blasts: leukaemia • Platelet count might be falsely low on FBC due to platelet aggregation, but clumps are obvious on examination of film • Platelet size helps diagnose rare platelet disorders that cause thrombocytopenia
LDH	• If malignancy suspected	• ↑ LDH: increased cell turnover
PT/INR	• All patients with bruising • To look for extrinsic clotting pathway dysfunction (vitamin K–dependent factors)	• ↑ PT/INR: vitamin K deficiency, DIC
APTT	• All patients with bruising • To assess intrinsic and common clotting pathways	• Prolonged in VWD and haemophilia • Might accompany PT prolongation in severe rare factor deficiencies and DIC

APTT, activated partial thromboplastin time; DIC, disseminated intravascular coagulation; FBC, full blood count; Hb, haemoglobin; INR, international normalised ratio; ITP, immune thrombocytopenia; LDH, lactate dehydrogenase; PT, prothrombin time; VWD, von Willebrand disease

Imaging

Table 4.1.3 Imaging modalities of use in patients presenting with bruising

Test	When to perform	Potential result
Skeletal survey	• Suspected NAI • To assess for old or intercurrent fractures	• Fractures of skull, chest, spine, pelvis, upper limbs, lower limbs
CT head	Suspected: • NAI • Bleeding disorder with neurological symptoms	• NAI: variety of findings possible, subdural haemorrhage, subarachnoid bleed, ischaemic injury, skull fractures • Bleeding disorder: any intracranial bleeding
MRI head	Suspected: • NAI • Bleeding disorder with neurological symptoms • Intracranial malignancy	• MRI might better identify parenchymal injury, bleeds of varying age, malignancy
Abdominal ultrasound	• Suspected intra-abdominal malignancy	• Neuroblastoma: heterogeneous mass with internal vascularity
CT/MRI abdomen	• If USS demonstrative of mass suspicious for neuroblastoma	• Heterogenous mass, possibly with calcifications

CT, computed tomography; MRI, magnetic resonance imaging; NAI, non-accidental injury; USS, ultrasound scan

Special

Table 4.1.4 Special tests of use in patients presenting with bruising

Test	When to perform	Potential result
Fibrinogen	• Suspected impaired clot formation • To guide cryoprecipitate use in active bleeding	• ↓ Fibrinogen: consumption (e.g. in DIC), or fibrinogen disorder
Thrombin time	• Evaluation of patient with prolonged PT and APTT	• Suggestion of fibrinogen disorder or sample heparin contamination

Table 4.1.4 (Continued)

Test	When to perform	Potential result
Mixing study	• If PT/APTT prolonged, mixing distinguishes between factor deficiency or factor inhibitor (inhibitor can develop in children given exogenous factor as treatment)	• Factor deficiency correctable by addition of normal plasma (mixing) • Factor inhibitor suspected if mixing does not correct abnormal PT/APTT
Factor activity levels	• Suspected bleeding disorder and prolonged APTT that corrects on mixing	• ↓ Level of factor, e.g. factor VIII
VWD screening	• Suspected bleeding disorder • Involves measure of VWF antigen (quantitative) and VWF activity (functional)	• Antigen level or factor activity <30% suggestive of VWD (note that Factor VIII activity might be reduced as this factor relies on VWF for stability)
Ophthalmic review	• If suspecting NAI	• Retinal haemorrhages may suggest shaking
Urine catecholamine studies	• VMA and HVA are products of catecholamine breakdown by neuroblastoma cells • Highly sensitive and specific for neuroblastoma	• Raised VMA or HVA in neuroblastoma

APTT, activated partial thromboplastin time; DIC, disseminated intravascular coagulation; HVA, homovanillic acid; NAI, non-accidental injury; PT, prothrombin time; VMA, vanillylmandelic acid; VWD, von Willebrand disease; VWF, von Willebrand factor

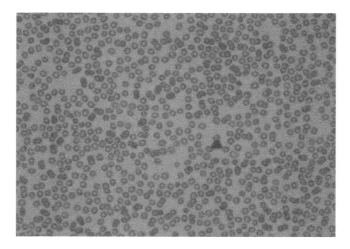

Figure 4.1.7 Thrombocytopenia and one reactive lymphocyte in a child with immune thrombocytopenia.

4.1.8 KEY MANAGEMENT PRINCIPLES

Diagnosis-specific management strategies are outlined here. It is expected that an 'ABCDE' approach to assessment and management is always undertaken (see Chapter 12.1).

Dangerous Diagnosis 1

See Chapter 12.5, *Safeguarding* for principles on escalating safeguarding concerns.

Diagnosis: Non-accidental injury
Management Principles
1. **Escalate to senior.** In any suspicion of NAI, concerns must be shared with the whole team and escalated to the consultant, or most senior clinician available
2. **Safeguarding team.** Safeguarding team structure differs among hospitals, but there will always be a protocol for who to contact and how to share information between agencies, e.g. social services and police
3. **Communication with family.** Open communication is very important. Safeguarding investigations follow a national set of guidelines and this can be helpful to mention when explaining the next steps. It is important to emphasise that all measures are to provide the best possible care for the child in question

Common Diagnosis 1
Diagnosis: Immune thrombocytopenia

Management Principles
1. **Activity restriction and education.** Children with ITP should be advised to restrict activities that carry a risk of bleeding from traumatic injury, e.g. contact sports. These decisions are collaborative with the family and there is no strict guidance. Protective helmets should be used when cycling. Education of risks and safety net advice for excessive bleeding should be discussed
2. **Avoidance of antiplatelet medications.** Non-steroidal anti-inflammatory drugs (NSAIDs) including ibuprofen should be avoided, although clinically significant bleeding with these drugs is unlikely
3. **Menstrual control.** Females who menstruate can consider hormonal therapy to inhibit menses and prevent severe menorrhagia
4. **Watchful waiting.** Most children will remain clinically stable, without dangerous bleeding. In the absence of significant bleeding, there is no strict numerical threshold for platelet count, and even <10,000/μL can be tolerated
5. **Tranexamic acid.** Although this has no effect on platelets, it is helpful in promoting clots with mucosal bleeding (e.g. gum or nose) or heavy periods
6. **Intravenous immunoglobulin (IVIg).** IVIG infusion is effective in 75% of patients, by halting the immune destruction of platelets. It is indicated in significant bleeding. Effects last up to 6 weeks
7. **Platelet transfusion.** The effect of a platelet transfusion is very short-lived, lasting only 24 hours. It is only indicated as an emergency treatment in severe or life-threatening bleeding
8. **Steroids.** Occasionally, steroids can be used to increase platelet count, but this decreases as soon as steroids are stopped. Side effects are common
9. **Splenectomy.** In ITP, most platelets are destroyed in the spleen. However, splenectomy is a major operation, leaving children vulnerable to lifelong risk of infection by encapsulated organisms. It may be considered in chronic ITP, with recurrent severe bleeding
10. **Monitor platelet count.** Monitoring of platelet counts should be regular. This varies between units, but might initially be weekly, with spacing when improvement is seen. The majority of children recover spontaneously within 3–6 months

Common Diagnosis 2
Diagnosis: Von Willebrand disease

Management Principles
1. **Refer to haematology tertiary centre.** Patients with VWD should be referred to a haematology specialist service, which can perform further assessment to determine the bleeding phenotype of the child
2. **Education.** There is no definitive treatment for VWD. Education on avoiding and managing minor bleeds is important, including when to seek help for prolonged bleeding
3. **Treatment for bleeding.** Specific treatment options include desmopressin, which promotes the release of endogenous VWF from endothelial storage sites. VWF concentrates can also be used
4. **Menstrual control.** Females who menstruate can consider hormonal therapy to inhibit menses and prevent severe menorrhagia

Common Diagnosis 3
Diagnosis: Haemophilia

Management Principles
1. **Haemophilia specialist service.** Most regions will have a haemophilia specialist service and patients should be referred there for tertiary oversight. This is essential in coordinating a multidisciplinary team approach to counselling, education, chronic care and managing complications
2. **Factor replacement therapy.** Decisions regarding treatment are individualised, and involve weighing up long-term prophylaxis, short-term prophylaxis and on-demand treatment. Factor replacement also carries the risk of inhibitor development, where neutralising antibodies are formed to exogenous factor, which is recognised as foreign. There are a variety of factors available for haemophilia A and B
3. **Evolving treatment options.** Advanced treatment options include monoclonal antibody therapy, gene therapy and cellular therapy

Common Diagnosis 4
Diagnosis: Ehlers–Danlos syndrome

Management Principles
1. **Multidisciplinary team (MDT) approach.** Specific treatment depends on the type of disorder, but all patients will require several members of the MDT. These may include physiotherapy, occupational therapy, psychology and school
2. **Analgesia.** Simple analgesia should be introduced and paracetamol can be effective. In general, NSAIDs should be avoided as a long-term solution, due to the risk of thrombocytopenia that might exacerbate easy bruising
3. **Avoidance of contact sports.** Due to increased risk of injury through bruising, skin fragility or bone fragility (depending on the type), risks of heavy exercise and contact sports should be considered

4.2 Pallor

Rachel Varughese

Department of Paediatrics, Oxford University Hospitals NHS Foundation Trust, Oxford, UK

CONTENTS

4.2.1 CHAPTER AT A GLANCE

Box 4.2.1 Chapter at a Glance

- Pallor can be acute or chronic
- Pallor is often representative of anaemia, but can be present in conditions affecting perfusion, where blood is redistributed away from surface capillaries

- When acute, it is more likely to represent a serious underlying condition
- Chronic pallor may have an insidious onset that is not immediately noticeable to caretakers in regular contact with the child

4.2.2 DEFINITION

Pallor is a description of unusually pale skin compared to the normal complexion.
Anaemia is a condition where there is either a reduced number of red blood cells, or reduced haemoglobin concentration within them.

Clinical Guide to Paediatrics, First Edition. Edited by Rachel Varughese and Anna Mathew. Series Editor: Christian Fielder Camm.
© 2022 John Wiley & Sons Ltd. Published 2022 by John Wiley & Sons Ltd.
Companion website: www.wiley.com/go/varughese/paediatrics

4.2.3 DIAGNOSTIC ALGORITHM

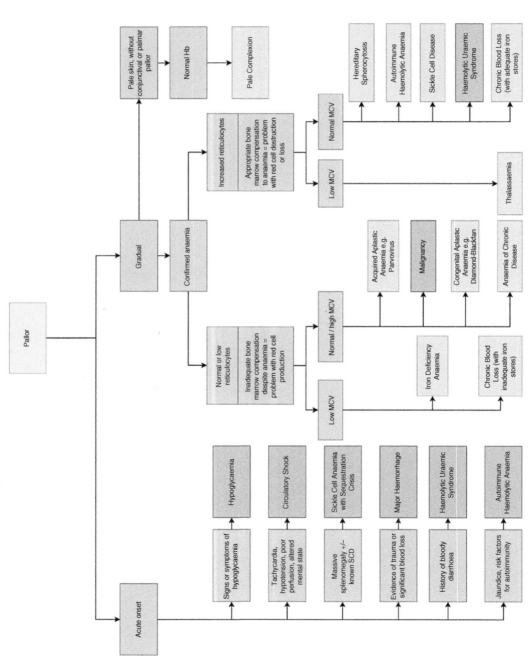

Figure 4.2.1 Diagnostic algorithm for the presentation of pallor.

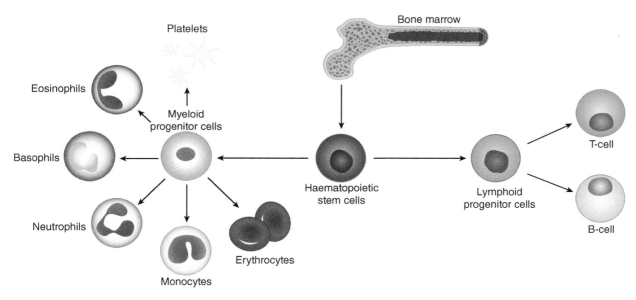

Figure 4.2.2 Haematopoietic stem cells are pluripotent and reside in the bone marrow. These have the potential to become myeloid or lymphoid progenitor cells, which can then follow differentiation pathways to become a specific type of blood cell. All blood cells can be divided into three main cell lines: red blood cells (erythrocytes), white blood cells (lymphocytes, monocytes, neutrophils, basophils and eosinophils) and platelets.

Box 4.2.2   Three Key Questions to Ask about Anaemia   ΔΔ

- Is this due to blood loss?
- Is this due to increased red blood cell destruction?
- Is this due to decreased red blood cell production?

4.2.4 DIFFERENTIALS LIST

Dangerous Diagnoses

1. Major Haemorrhage
- Major haemorrhage is a life-threatening cause of pallor
- Pallor, primarily due to anaemia, may be exacerbated by reduced perfusion in hypovolaemic shock
- The initial haemoglobin concentration (Hb) may be misleadingly normal in acute blood loss due to delayed equilibrium
- In children, major haemorrhage is most often due to major trauma
- Other important causes include post-operative bleeding, gastrointestinal bleeding, pulmonary haemorrhage and inflicted injury

2. Autoimmune Haemolytic Anaemia (AIHA)
- AIHA is a group of conditions where autoantibody binding to red blood cells causes premature erythrocyte destruction
- Anaemia results from haemolysis
- AIHA can be subdivided into warm and cold (based on the thermal reactivity of the autoantibodies) and primary and secondary (based on the absence or presence of a precipitating condition)

3. Haemolytic Uraemic Syndrome (HUS)
- Triad of microangiopathic haemolytic anaemia (MAHA), thrombocytopenia and acute kidney injury (AKI)
- Anaemia results from haemolysis: platelet microthrombi in glomeruli cause mechanical shearing of red blood cells
- Renal impairment can be severe, requiring dialysis
- There are several causes, of which Shiga toxin-producing *Escherichia coli* (typically *E. coli* 0157) is the best known

- Other causes include complement gene mutations, *Streptococcus pneumoniae*, human immunodeficiency virus (HIV), complement autoantibodies
- *E. coli* HUS is preceded by a diarrhoeal illness, usually involving bloody diarrhoea and abdominal pain

---

Box 4.2.3   Warm vs Cold Autoimmune Haemolytic Anaemia (AIHA)   △△

The categorisation of AIHA into warm and cold describes the temperature at which autoantibodies preferentially bind to the red cells

Warm-reactive AIHA

- The most common primary AIHA in children (up to 90%)
- Immunoglobin (Ig) G binds to red cells at normal body temperature, 37 °C
- Haemolysis takes place mostly in the spleen

Cold-reactive AIHA

- Less common in children (approx. 10%)
- Often precipitated by infection, e.g. *Mycoplasma pneumoniae* or Epstein–Barr virus
- IgM binds red cells when exposed to cold temperatures, at an optimum temperature of 3–5 °C
- Cold-induced symptoms affect the extremities, or on swallowing cold liquids

---

Box 4.2.4   Primary vs Secondary Autoimmune Haemolytic Anaemia (AIHA)   △△

Primary AIHA

- Approximately 45% of cases
- No evidence of underlying illness

Secondary AIHA

- Approximately 55% of cases
- Precipitated by another systemic illness:
  - Autoimmune diseases: systemic lupus erythematosus, Sjögren syndrome, juvenile idiopathic arthritis, dermatomyositis, type 1 diabetes mellitus

- Immunodeficiency: common variable immunodeficiency, Wiskott–Aldrich syndrome
- Malignancy: Hodgkin lymphoma, acute lymphoblastic leukaemia
- Infection: *Mycoplasma pneumoniae*, Epstein–Barr virus, measles, varicella
- Post transplant
- Medications: penicillins, cephalosporins, macrolides

Box 4.2.5   Evans Syndrome   △△

- Triad of autoimmune haemolytic anaemia (AIHA), immune thrombocytopaenia (ITP) and autoimmune neutropaenia
- AIHA often presents first, followed by ITP ± neutropaenia, which may develop months or years later

- Chronic and recurrent disease more common than in AIHA alone
- Underlying autoimmune lymphoproliferative syndrome is common

---

Box 4.2.6   Thrombotic Thrombocytopaenic Purpura (TTP)   △△

- TTP is a thrombotic microangiopathy with several similarities to haemolytic uraemic syndrome
- It is rare in children, typically affecting young adults
- Small-vessel platelet microthrombi cause thrombocytopaenia and microangiopathic haemolytic anaemia

- Caused by reduced activity of ADAMTS13 – a von Willebrand factor – cleaving protease

---

4. Malignancy

- Anaemia is a common feature of many malignancies
- The commonest mechanism is bone marrow infiltration, where normal haematopoiesis is disrupted
- Leukaemias and lymphomas as well as solid tumours, such as neuroblastoma, can involve bone marrow
- There is usually associated thrombocytopenia and leukopaenia
- Malignancy can also precipitate secondary AIHA

Box 4.2.7   Non-haematological Causes of Pallor   △△

Conditions where perfusion is poor deviate blood flow away from the skin, causing pallor. This is often the result of adrenergic cutaneous vasoconstriction. Causes are frequently potentially life-threatening and include the following:

- Circulatory shock
  - Distributive, e.g. sepsis, anaphylaxis
  - Hypovolaemia, e.g. dehydration, haemorrhage
  - Neurological, e.g. traumatic brain injury, spinal cord injury
- Cardiogenic, e.g. cardiac failure, arrhythmia
- Obstructive, e.g. tension pneumothorax, cardiac tamponade
- Dissociative, e.g. methemoglobinemia, cyanide poisoning
- Hypoglycaemia

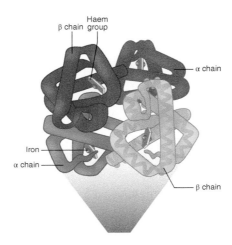

Figure 4.2.3 The haemoglobin molecule is made up of two alpha globin chains and two beta globin chains. Each globin chain is associated with a haem group, containing iron. This is known as a tetrahedral structure.

Common Diagnoses
1. Iron-Deficiency Anaemia (IDA)
- Commonest cause of anaemia in childhood
- Iron is essential for haem synthesis, required for haemoglobin formation
- In IDA there is insufficient total body iron to support haem synthesis, leading to decreased erythrocyte production
- IDA is commonly due to a nutritional deficit, although it can also be a result of chronic blood loss or malabsorption (e.g. in short bowel syndrome)
- IDA is usually seen in toddlers, where dietary iron may be insufficient to support rapid growth
- Fussy eaters, or those who drink a lot of cow's milk, are particularly at risk
- Iron deficiency may also exacerbate several other types of anaemia

2. Sickle Cell Anaemia
- Sickle cell disease (SCD) is an autosomal recessive condition caused by a mutation in the beta globin chain of the haemoglobin molecule
- This results in abnormal haemoglobin, which polymerises in deoxygenated conditions, causing red cells to deform
- These stiff, deformed, 'sickled' cells can lead to vascular occlusion, causing a myriad of complications, including haemolytic anaemia
- Presentation is usually in early childhood, with pallor and periodic episodes of pain. However, SCD can also present with life-threatening anaemia if exacerbated by splenic sequestration or aplastic crises
- With a few rare exceptions, those with sickle cell trait are completely normal and may not be aware they are carriers
- There are a number of variations where those heterozygous for the sickle mutation co-inherit another beta globin mutation such as thalassaemia or haemoglobin C

Box 4.2.8   Acute Pallor in Sickle Cell Disease (SCD): Could It Be a Splenic Sequestration Crisis?   △△

- An important cause of life-threatening anaemia in SCD is splenic sequestration
- Red blood cells rapidly pool within the spleen, causing sudden anaemia and hypovolaemic shock
- In those with known SCD, diagnosis of sequestration crisis will be more straightforward; however, it could be the first presenting symptom in up to 20% of patients
- Acute pallor accompanied by rapid splenic enlargement, with markedly decreased haemoglobin, should prompt urgent consideration of this diagnosis

- Splenic sequestration can occur in any SCD patient who has not undergone splenic auto-infarction. Children with homozygous SCD may be rendered functionally asplenic by 4 years of age
- Management involves aggressive fluid replacement, which should be crystalloid until emergency red blood cell transfusion is available
- Splenectomy is recommended in children who have had two or more episodes of splenic sequestration

Box 4.2.9   Anaemia of Chronic Disease

- Many chronic diseases are associated with a normocytic anaemia
- Although classically associated with inflammatory conditions (infection, rheumatological, malignancy), almost any chronic disease can be associated with anaemia, including obesity
- Anaemia results from dysregulation of iron homeostasis resulting in decreased erythropoiesis
- A key factor in the pathophysiology of anaemia of chronic disease is hepcidin, produced in response to inflammation

- Hepcidin is a negative regulator of iron, decreasing gastrointestinal absorption and decreasing iron release from macrophages. (Normally, macrophages ingest old red blood cells and release the iron, which can then be used for haem synthesis)
- In those with renal insufficiency, additional factors exacerbate anaemia. There is reduced urinary excretion of hepcidin. There is also decreased production of renal erythropoietin, essential in stimulating stem cell differentiation into erythrocytes

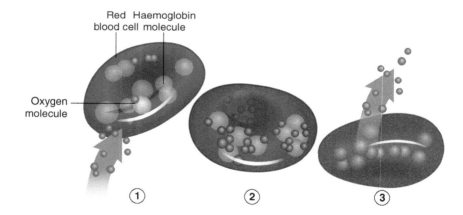

Figure 4.2.4 Under normal circumstances, oxygen is collected from the lungs (1), bonds to haemoglobin (2) and is released in the peripheral tissues (3). Haemoglobin molecules remain as isolated units in the red cell, whether they are oxygen bound or not, and red cells remain disc shaped.

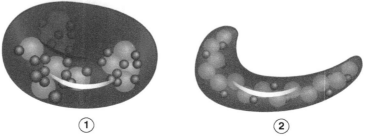

Figure 4.2.5 In sickle cell disease, haemoglobin only exists as isolated units while oxygen is bound (1). When oxygen is released to the tissues (2), the haemoglobin molecules polymerise and stick together. These polymers are rigid, distorting the cell into a sickle shape. When haemoglobin binds again to oxygen, the molecules revert to being isolated, and the usual disc shape of the cell is resumed.

Diagnoses to Consider

1. Thalassaemia

- The thalassaemias are a collection of disorders affecting the globin chains in haemoglobin. Either the alpha or beta chain can be affected, resulting in an uneven ratio of chains
- Inheritance is autosomal recessive
- Prevalence is most common among those of Mediterranean, Asian or North African descent
- Anaemia results from impaired erythropoiesis and haemolysis, caused by precipitation of 'spare' unpaired globin chains
- Thalassaemias can be categorised as 'alpha' and 'beta' and 'major' and 'minor'
- Anaemia is microcytic of variable severity, depending on the type and number of chains affected
- Clinical findings include bone deformities (seen in severe forms due to bone marrow proliferation – see Box 4.2.21 later in the chapter), hepatosplenomegaly (as a result of chronic haemolysis) and faltering growth

When to consider: in those with a known family history of thalassaemia, foetal death or from high-risk areas of the world

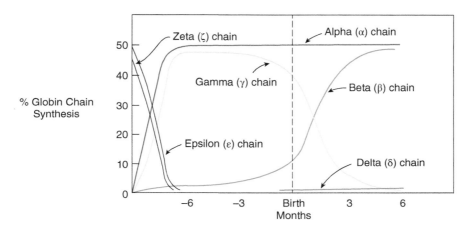

Figure 4.2.6 There are several types of globin chains involved in haemoglobin. At birth, Hb is primarily HbF ($2\alpha + 2\gamma$). Over a period of months, this ratio evolves into the final adult ratio. Adult haemoglobin is made up of 97% HbA ($2\alpha + 2\beta$), and 3% HbF and HbA 2 ($2\alpha + 2\delta$). Because γ is used instead of β in early infancy, β-thalassaemia is usually asymptomatic until 3–4 months of age, when HbF declines and HbA2 increases.

2. Hereditary Spherocytosis (HS)

- HS is the result of one of several genetic mutations coding for red blood cell membrane proteins
- These defects lead to a spherical, rather than biconcave, red blood cell shape
- The spherocytes are abnormally fragile, and are destroyed during passage through the spleen, resulting in a haemolytic anaemia
- HS is most common in patients of northern European ancestry
- Most inheritance is autosomal dominant, although there are recessive forms
- There is a huge spectrum of disease severity (from asymptomatic to severe haemolysis) and age of presentation (from foetal to advanced adult)

When to consider: in those with a family history of HS

Box 4.2.10   Types of Alpha Thalassaemia

There are four alpha globin genes, as a pair on each chromosome. Mutations tend to be deletions, resulting in total loss of one or more chains

Condition	Alpha chains affected	Clinical outcome
Alpha thalassaemia minima	Loss of one chain	Silent carrier state
Alpha thalassaemia minor	Loss of two chains	Mild microcytic anaemia
Haemoglobin H disease	Loss of three chains	Variable severity from mild anaemia to hydrops fetalis
Alpha thalassaemia major	Loss of four chains	Incompatible with live birth, causing hydrops fetalis

Box 4.2.11   Types of Beta Thalassaemia

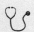

There are two beta globin genes, one on each chromosome. Mutations can result in absent ($\beta°$) or decreased ($\beta\downarrow$) beta globin production. Normal beta globin gene is denoted by β.

Condition	Beta globin production	Clinical outcome
Beta thalassaemia minor	β $\beta\downarrow$ or β $\beta°$	Mild microcytic anaemia
Beta thalassaemia intermedia	$\beta\downarrow$ $\beta\downarrow$	Moderate microcytic anaemia
Beta thalassaemia major	$\beta°$ $\beta°$ or $\beta°$ $\beta\downarrow$	Severe microcytic anaemia with transfusion dependency

3. Parvovirus-Induced Aplastic Anaemia

- One of the best-described viral causes of aplastic anaemia is parvovirus B19
- The resulting aplasia often only affects red cell production, although occasionally platelets and white cells are also affected
- Aplasia is usually transient but can be severe
- In a non-immune pregnant woman, profound foetal anaemia and death can occur
- Parvovirus B19 typically affects those with underlying haemolytic anaemias, such as chronic haemolysis (SCD, HS, thalassaemia), who usually rely on accelerated erythrocyte production
- Those with immunocompromise are also at increased risk, due to inability to clear the viraemia quickly
- However, parvovirus B19–induced aplastic anaemia has also been described in previously healthy children

When to consider: in those with contact history with parvovirus B19

Box 4.2.12   Aplastic Anaemia

- Aplastic anaemia results from failure of bone marrow haematopoiesis
- In most cases, there is loss or damage to pluripotent haematopoietic stem cells, meaning all three cell lines are affected – red cells, white cells and platelets
- Although parvovirus is the most commonly described cause of aplastic crises, there are many other causes of aplastic anaemia:

- Idiopathic (up to 80%)
- Radiation exposure
- Medications, e.g. chemotherapy (expected), systemic chloramphenicol, sulphonamides, carbamazepine
- Toxic chemicals, e.g. benzene
- Infections: Epstein–Barr virus, human immunodeficiency virus
- Hepatitis
- Pregnancy

Box 4.2.13   Chronic Blood Loss

- Repeated loss of small amounts of blood may cause anaemia
- If there are inadequate iron stores, this may lead to an iron-deficiency anaemia (IDA)
- In adequate iron stores, blood loss causes a normocytic anaemia
- Consider in children who have an IDA without a dietary history consistent with nutritional deficit

- Heavy menstrual bleeding is a common cause among teenage females
- Other causes include Meckel diverticulum, inflammatory bowel disease, repeated nose bleeds, lung pathology or renal pathology
- Family history of intestinal polyps, malignancy and bleeding tendency is important

4.2.5 KEY HISTORY FEATURES

Before a thorough history is taken, an assessment should be conducted to determine whether the patient is seriously systemically unwell. If they are, consider whether shock, hypoglycaemia or massive haemorrhage is the underlying cause, and instigate supportive measures.

Box 4.2.14   Symptoms of Anaemia

- Lethargy
- Shortness of breath
- Reduced exercise tolerance
- Palpitations

Note that children with chronic anaemia may compensate very well, and may not necessarily have symptoms of anaemia

---

Dangerous Diagnosis 1
Diagnosis: Major haemorrhage

Questions
1. **Is pallor acute?** Major haemorrhage will cause an acute, rapid drop in haemoglobin with rapid onset of pallor
2. **Is there a history of trauma?** Internal major haemorrhage sites include chest, pelvis, abdomen and long bones. A history of trauma to any of these sites should prompt urgent investigation. There may also be obvious external bleeding. Always consider non-accidental injury
3. **Is there a history of severe blood loss?** Non-traumatic blood loss, for example with a miscarriage, should also be considered
4. **Does the child take anticoagulant or antiplatelet medications?** Medications that disrupt physiological clotting may exacerbate haemorrhage

Dangerous Diagnosis 2
Diagnosis: Autoimmune haemolytic anaemia

Questions
1. **Is pallor acute?** AIHA may cause acute, rapidly progressive haemolysis. This is important to recognise as the result can be a life-threatening anaemia. In most cases, however, AIHA is of gradual onset
2. **Has there been a fever?** Warm AIHA is associated with fever in approximately 50% of presentations
3. **Have symptoms been brought on by cold exposure?** Those with cold-reactive AIHA may have cold-induced symptoms of acrocyanosis (purple discoloration due to venous congestion) on the extremities – fingers, toes, nose and ears
4. **Has there been a change in urine colour?** In cold-reactive AIHA, there may be haemoglobinuria due to intravascular haemolysis, which causes dark urine
5. **Are there any concurrent conditions or medications that may have triggered secondary AIHA?** Several underlying illnesses and medications can trigger secondary AIHA (see Box 4.2.4). Be sure to ask about symptoms of recent infectious illnesses, which may have been considered insignificant
6. **Is there a family history of autoimmunity?** 10–15% of patients may have a family history of autoimmunity

Dangerous Diagnosis 3
Diagnosis: Haemolytic uraemic syndrome

Questions
1. **Has there been abdominal pain or diarrhoea?** There is often a prodromal illness, with abdominal pain, vomiting and diarrhoea, 5–10 days prior to development of HUS. Ongoing abdominal pain should be noted, as severe HUS can cause serious gastrointestinal manifestations such as bowel necrosis, perforation and intussusception
2. **Is there a history of bloody diarrhoea?** Children with HUS typically have a history of bloody diarrhoea following infection with *E. coli* 0157, the most common bacterial agent
3. **Has there been any contact with farm animals or ingestion of contaminated or unpasteurised foods?** *E. coli* are found normally in the intestines of animals, particularly cattle, and can be picked up from contaminated or uncooked meats and vegetables, or water contaminated with faeces containing *E. coli*.
4. **What is the urine output like?** In severe AKI, urine output may be significantly reduced or absent. Although haematuria is a feature of the disease, this is commonly microscopic and may not be reported
5. **Is pallor acute?** The haemolysis, which is due to mechanical shearing of red cells, can be severe and rapid, causing acute pallor

Dangerous Diagnosis 4
Diagnosis: Malignancy

Questions
1. **Any concerning systemic symptoms?** Fever, weight loss, fatigue and night sweats are very concerning for malignancy
2. **Has there been easy bruising or recurrent infections?** Easy bruising/bleeding (thrombocytopaenia) and recurrent infections (leukopaenia) are seen in many malignancies due to bone marrow infiltration
3. **Any limb pains?** Bone pain is a concerning feature of malignancy. In young children this may manifest as a limp or refusal to bear weight
4. **Any abdominal pain?** Abdominal pain can be a direct result of a tumour (e.g. neuroblastoma), lymphadenopathy or organomegaly

Common Diagnosis 1
Diagnosis: Iron-deficiency anaemia

Questions
1. **Over what timeframe did pallor develop?** IDA develops over months. Pallor may first be recognised by somebody who does not have regular contact with the child
2. **What is the child's diet like?** The most common scenario for IDA is a child who is fussy with solid foods, or who drinks excessive cow's milk. Iron-rich foods are important from 6 months of age. Cow's (and other animal's) milk does not contain enough iron and reduces the appetite
3. **Are there symptoms concerning for coeliac disease?** Malabsorption in coeliac disease can cause IDA. Ask about chronic diarrhoea (although a small minority may have constipation), anorexia, abdominal distension and abdominal pain. Stools may be bulky, foul-smelling and may float
4. **Are there any perinatal risk factors for iron deficiency?** Newborns rely on maternal–foetal iron transfer, the majority of which occurs during the third trimester of pregnancy. Children within the first 6 months of life may have increased risk for IDA based on a variety of perinatal risk factors
5. **Craving for non-food items?** This is known as pica, and is an uncommon phenomenon seen in IDA. Children with developmental delay are much more likely to be affected

---

Box 4.2.15 Perinatal Risk Factors for Iron-Deficiency Anaemia

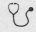

- Prematurity
- Maternal iron deficiency
- Perinatal haemorrhage
- Twin-to-twin transfusion syndrome

Common Diagnosis 2
Diagnosis: Sickle cell anaemia

Questions
1. **Is there a family history of sickle cell anaemia or known sickle cell trait?** Sickle cell anaemia is an autosomal recessive condition. A child born to two carriers of SCD will have a 25% chance of inheriting SCD and a 50% chance of being a carrier. All children born in the UK will be tested for SCD as part of the newborn screening programme
2. **What age is the patient?** Due to the presence of HbF, SCD is not clinically apparent at birth. During the first few months of life, the concentration of HbS rises as HbF declines. Children commonly present at a few months old
3. **What ethnicity is the family?** SCD is most common in those with African ancestry. Variants, such as sickle-beta thalassaemia, are more likely in Mediterranean populations
4. **Over what timeframe did pallor develop?** In sickle cell anaemia, pallor usually becomes evident over weeks to months. Very acute pallor, over hours to days, should prompt consideration of a sequestration crisis.
5. **Have there been episodes of unexplained pain?** Painful crises, particularly in cold environments, are a result of vaso-occlusion of sickle cells
6. **Have there been recurrent infections?** Increased risk of infections results from functional hyposplenism, which may start in the first few months of life. This particularly risks infection from encapsulated organisms, although risks of all infection, including viral, are increased

	Hb^A	Hb^S
Hb^A	Hb^A Hb^A	Hb^A Hb^S
Hb^S	Hb^S Hb^A	Hb^S Hb^S

Figure 4.2.7 Sickle cell disease is autosomal recessive. Offspring born to parents who are both carriers have a 50% chance of being carriers (yellow) and a 25% chance of being affected (orange).

Box 4.2.16   Symptoms of Erythema Infectiosum: Parvovirus B19

Timescale	Symptoms
Initially	• Fever, coryza, headache, myalgia, nausea, diarrhoea, pruritus
1 week later	• Erythematous malar rash, circumoral pallor • Onset of rash usually heralds termination of systemic symptoms
2 weeks later	• Reticular rash on trunk and extremities

Box 4.2.17   Other Causes of Anaemia

Condition	Characteristics
Vitamin B$_{12}$ deficiency	• May be due to dietary insufficiency, a strict vegan diet or underlying malabsorption, e.g. coeliac disease
Folate deficiency	• May be due to underlying malabsorption, e.g. coeliac disease
Transient erythroblastopaenia of childhood	• Transient reduction in erythrocyte precursors related to recent viral illness, followed by spontaneous recovery
Diamond–Blackfan syndrome	• Congenital hypoplastic anaemia affecting red blood cell line only, due to reduction in erythrocyte precursors
Fanconi anaemia	• Congenital hypoplastic anaemia affecting all three bone marrow cell lines, resulting in pancytopaenia • Multiple associated abnormalities, including abnormalities of the thumbs and radii
Sideroblastic anaemia	• Despite normal amounts of iron, there is a functional defect with its use in haem synthesis, causing iron accumulation within red blood cells
Red cell membrane defects	• Aside from hereditary spherocytosis, other defects exist such as elliptocytosis, predisposing to haemolysis
Red cell enzyme defects	• Pyruvate kinase deficiency and some types of glucose-6-phosphate dehydrogenase (G6PD) deficiency predispose to haemolysis

Box 4.2.18   General Examination Features Seen in Anaemia

- **Pallor:** in darker skin pallor is not immediately obvious, so carefully examine mucous membranes, nailbeds, conjunctivae and palmar creases
- **Flow murmur:** systolic murmur due to hyperdynamic state

- **Reduced exercise tolerance:** breathlessness, lethargy and fatigue are all common signs of anaemia. This is difficult to appreciate in younger children

4.2.6 KEY EXAMINATION FEATURES

Dangerous Diagnosis 1

Diagnosis: Major haemorrhage

Examination Findings
1. **Evidence of shock.** Tachycardia, hypotension and prolonged capillary refill time are signs of hypovolaemic shock
2. **Narrow pulse pressure.** Narrow pulse pressure (<30 mmHg) is caused by compensatory increased systemic vascular resistance in hypovolaemia
3. **Evidence of internal bleeding.** Classic internal bleeding sites with potential for major blood loss are the thorax, abdomen, pelvis and long bones
4. **Old bruises or abrasions.** Children with evidence of suspiciously distributed bruises or abrasions are concerning for non-accidental injury

Box 4.2.19   Locations at Risk of Major Haemorrhage

- **Haemothorax:** respiratory distress, ipsilateral reduced air entry and dullness to percussion
- **Abdominal bleed:** abdominal pain, haematemesis, melaena, abdominal wall bruising, guarding, distension and peritonism

- **Pelvic bleed:** abdominal pain, flank pain, back pain, flank bruising
- **Long bone bleed:** deformity from fracture, soft tissue swelling, bruising. Evidence of distal vascular or neurological compromise indicates compartment syndrome

Dangerous Diagnosis 2

Diagnosis: Autoimmune haemolytic anaemia

Examination Findings
1. **Jaundice.** Due to haemolysis, patients are often jaundiced. In darker skin tones dermal jaundice may not be immediately obvious, so sclera should always be examined
2. **Minimal organomegaly.** Although liver and spleen are often palpable, they should not be significantly enlarged. The presence of massive organomegaly should prompt consideration of an alternative diagnosis

Dangerous Diagnosis 3

Diagnosis: Haemolytic uraemic syndrome

Examination Findings
1. **Fluid overload, hypertension.** Acute renal failure causes impaired filtration, leading to oliguria or anuria and fluid overload, with oedema. Hypertension is caused by fluid overload as well as renal impairment
2. **Jaundice.** Due to haemolysis, patients are often jaundiced. In darker skin tones dermal jaundice may not be immediately obvious, so sclera should always be examined. Hepatomegaly is a frequent finding
3. **Abnormal neurology.** Lethargy worsens over time as the combination of haemolysis, dehydration and uraemia progresses. Focal neurological deficits, or even seizures, can occur due to cerebral microvascular damage, though this is fortunately rare

Dangerous Diagnosis 4

Diagnosis: Malignancy

Examination Findings
1. **Bruising or petechiae.** These are suggestive of thrombocytopaenia
2. **Lymphadenopathy.** There may be generalised lymphadenopathy, typically non-tender and firm. Enlarged, matted nodes are particularly concerning

3. **Hepatosplenomegaly.** Palpable organomegaly is common at diagnosis of haematological malignancies
4. **Abdominal mass.** A palpable abdominal mass may indicate a tumour. Neuroblastoma most commonly affects the adrenal glands, but can occur anywhere along the sympathetic tract

Common Diagnosis 1

Diagnosis: Iron-deficiency anaemia

Examination Findings

1. **Pallor in the setting of an otherwise well child.** IDA usually causes a mild disease, where anaemia is suspected due to pallor or is an incidental finding
2. **Nail changes.** Iron deficiency causes koilonychia, which is concave or 'spoon-shaped' nails
3. **Angular stomatitis.** Also known as cheilitis, this is inflammation at the corners of the mouth. Vitamin B_{12} deficiency is also a cause, so should be considered as a differential diagnosis
4. **Faltering growth.** Height and weight should be measured and plotted on an appropriate growth chart. Poor growth can result directly from IDA, or may be a feature of underlying malabsorption, e.g. in coeliac disease

Common Diagnosis 2

Diagnosis: Sickle cell anaemia

Examination Findings

1. **Jaundice.** Jaundice results from haemolysis. This can be subtle in dark-skinned children, but should be seen easily in the sclera. It is unconjugated, so stool colour should be normal
2. **Splenomegaly.** There is commonly splenomegaly during the first decade of life; however, due to auto-infarction, the spleen often undergoes progressive atrophy. Rapidly enlarging splenomegaly is indicative of a sequestration crisis. Persistence of splenomegaly may indicate hypersplenism, where the enlarged spleen is associated with significant anaemia, thrombocytopenia and neutropenia

---

Box 4.2.20   Acute Complications of Sickle Cell Disease

- Infections
- Severe anaemia: exacerbating factors include splenic sequestration or aplastic crisis
- Sequelae of vaso-occlusion:
  - Vaso-occlusive pain
  - Dactylitis
  - Acute chest syndrome

- Stroke
- Renal infarction
- Bone infarction
- Myocardial infarction
- Priapism
- Venous thromboembolism
- Avascular necrosis of the femoral head

Box 4.2.21   Bony Changes in Thalassaemia

Bone change	Mechanism
Frontal bossing	Expansion of bone marrow
Maxillary bone overgrowth	
Malar eminence overgrowth	
Shortening of limbs	Premature fusion of epiphyses
Osteopaenia	Thinning of cortex as a result of widened marrow
Osteoporosis	
Bone masses	Invasion of bone marrow into cortex

4.2.7 KEY INVESTIGATIONS

Not all children will require invasive investigations; often diagnoses are made on clinical evidence from history and examination. Consider carefully which investigations are required for which patient.

Bedside

Table 4.2.1 Bedside tests of use in patients presenting with pallor

Test	When to perform	Potential result
Blood gas	• Systemically unwell children	• Rapid estimation of Hb • ↓ pH, ↓ HCO_3, ↑ lactate: metabolic acidosis in sepsis, severe dehydration
Urine dip	• Suspected HUS	• + Blood, + protein: renal involvement in HUS
Blood sugar	• If history or signs of hypoglycaemia	• <2.6 mmol/L: Hypoglycaemia as the cause for pallor

Hb, haemoglobin; HCO_3, bicarbonate; HUS, haemolytic uraemic syndrome

Blood Tests

Table 4.2.2 Blood tests of use in patients presenting with pallor

Test	When to Perform	Potential Result
FBC	• All children with pallor	• See Boxes 4.2.22–4.2.24 for guides to interpretation
Reticulocyte count	• All children with pallor • Differentiates between decreased red cell production and increased red cell destruction	• ↑/↔: haemolysis, blood loss • ↓: bone marrow failure, aplastic crisis • See Box 4.2.25
Blood film	• All children with pallor	• See Box 4.2.26
DAT	• All children with pallor, to assess for autoimmune haemolysis	• +ve DAT: autoimmune haemolysis • −ve DAT: not autoimmune
Iron	• All children with pallor	• ↓ in IDA • ↑/↔ in thalassaemia • ↓ in anaemia of chronic disease
Transferrin saturation	• All children with pallor	• ↓ in IDA • ↔ in thalassaemia • ↓ in anaemia of chronic disease • ↑ in iron overload
Ferritin	• All children with pallor • Is an acute-phase reactant and will be elevated in inflammation	• ↓ in IDA • ↑/↔ in thalassaemia • ↑ in anaemia of chronic disease
TIBC	• All children with pallor	• ↑ in IDA • ↔ in thalassaemia • ↓ in anaemia of chronic disease
U&E	• Suspected HUS	• ↑ Urea, ↑creatinine in HUS with acute renal impairment
Group and save + crossmatch	• If transfusion expected	• Allows provision of crossmatched packed red cells

DAT, direct antiglobulin test; FBC, full blood count; HUS, haemolytic uraemic syndrome; IDA, iron-deficiency anaemia; TIBC, total iron-binding capacity; U&E, urea and electrolytes

Imaging

Table 4.2.3 Imaging modalities of use in patients presenting with pallor
A variety of imaging techniques may be required to investigate acute and chronic blood loss, depending on the suspected diagnosis

Test	When to perform	Potential result
Abdominal ultrasound scan	Suspected: • Abdominal trauma • Abdominal malignancy	• Major abdominal haemorrhage (can be performed in A&E) • May demonstrate malignancy or intrabdominal lymphadenopathy
Chest x-ray	Suspected: • Malignancy • Chest trauma	• Malignancy: mediastinal lymphadenopathy • Chest trauma: haemothorax

Special

Table 4.2.4 Special tests of use in patients presenting with pallor

Test	When to perform	Potential result
Haemoglobin electrophoresis	Suspected: • Sickle cell disease • Thalassaemias	• Reveals abnormal haemoglobin(s)

Box 4.2.22   Haemoglobin Normal Reference Ranges

Age	Haemoglobin g/L
Newborns	170–220
1 week	150–200
1 month	110–150
6 months–2 years	110–130
2–6 years	115–135
6–12 years	125–145
12–18 years	140

Box 4.2.23   Interpreting the Full Blood Count

The full blood count provides a wealth of information in a child with pallor

Item	Details
Haemoglobin (Hb)	• Hb is a measure of the concentration of haemoglobin in whole blood, expressed in g/L. Normal values vary with age • Decreased Hb confirms anaemia as the cause for pallor
Haematocrit (HCT)	• HCT is the percentage of whole blood occupied by red blood cells (RBCs)
Mean corpuscular volume (MCV)	• MCV measures the volume of individual RBCs • Low MCV: 'microcytic' anaemia • Normal MCV: 'normocytic' anaemia • High MCV: 'macrocytic' anaemia

(Continued)

Box 4.2.23   (Continued)

Item	Details
Mean corpuscular haemoglobin concentration (MCHC)	• MCHC measures the concentration of Hb within RBCs • Low MCHC: 'hypochromic anaemia' • Normal MCHC: 'normochromic anaemia' • High MCHC: 'hyperchromic anaemia'
White cell count (WCC)	• Low WCC: abnormal bone marrow function or infection • High WCC: infection or acute leukaemia
Platelets	• Low platelets: abnormal bone marrow function, peripheral consumption (e.g. in haemolytic uraemic syndrome, thrombocytic thrombocytopaenic purpura, Evans syndrome) • High platelets: infection, iron deficiency

The combination of anaemia, leukopaenia and thrombocytopaenia is highly suggestive of abnormal bone marrow function, either due to infiltration (e.g. malignancy) or functional aplasia

Box 4.2.24   Using the Mean Corpuscular Volume (MCV) to Narrow Differential Diagnoses in Anaemia

Microcytic anaemia	Normocytic anaemia	Macrocytic anaemia
• Iron-deficiency anaemia • Thalassaemia	• Anaemia of chronic disease • Blood loss • Haemolytic anaemias: autoimmune haemolytic anaemia, sickle cell disease, haemolytic uraemic syndrome, thrombotic thrombocytopaenic purpura, hereditary spherocytosis	• Vitamin B12 deficiency • Folate deficiency • Diamond–Blackfan anaemia • Aplastic anaemia

*Anaemia of chronic disease can also be microcytic

Box 4.2.25   Interpretation of Reticulocyte Count

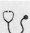

• Reticulocytes are immature red blood cells
• Maturation takes place after 24–48 days into mature erythrocytes
• The reticulocyte count is expressed as a percentage of total red cells. It must therefore be corrected for the degree of anaemia
• Corrected reticulocyte count = reticulocyte count × Hb/Hb^N (where Hb^N is the normal age-appropriate haemoglobin level)
• In the presence of anaemia, interpretation is generally divided into an elevated or a normal/low count

Elevated count	• Demonstrates appropriate bone marrow response to anaemia • Suggestive of increased red blood cell loss • Consider haemolysis or bleeding*
Normal/low count	• Indicates lack of compensatory erythropoiesis • Suggestive of inadequate bone marrow production • Consider causes of aplastic/hypoplastic anaemia, or bone marrow infiltration

*Note that if there are inadequate iron stores, erythropoiesis will be affected, and reticulocytes will not be raised

Box 4.2.26   Blood Film Findings in Children with Anaemia

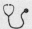

The blood film is an essential part of evaluating anaemia:

• Red blood cell (RBC) size confirms microcytosis, normocytosis or macrocytosis
• RBC appearance may be suggestive of particular condition
• Leukocyte appearance:
  • Increased neutrophils or toxic granulation: seen in infection

Box 4.2.26   (Continued)

- Hypersegmented neutrophils: vitamin B$_{12}$ or folate deficiency
- Blasts: seen in leukaemia and lymphoma
- Platelet appearance:
  - Thrombocytopenia may be reported on automatic counters when there is platelet clumping. Blood film can confirm true thrombocytopenia

RBC appearance	Clinical scenario
Biconcave disc with one-third of the diameter occupied by central pallor	Normal
Numerous nucleated RBCs	Haemolysis – suggestive of rapid turnover
Increased central pallor – 'hypochromic'	Iron-deficiency anaemia and thalassaemia
Schistocytes – fragmented cells	Microangiopathic haemolytic anaemias
Sickle cells	Diagnostic of sickle cell disease (SCD)
Poikilocytes – pencil-shaped cells	Iron deficiency or thalassaemia
Target cells	Thalassaemia
Howell–Jolly bodies	Splenic hypofunction (e.g. SCD, hereditary spherocytosis)
Heinz bodies	Glucose-6-phosphate dehydrogenase (G6PD) deficiency
Elliptocytes	Hereditary elliptocytosis
Basophilic stippling	Lead poisoning, thalassaemia, SCD

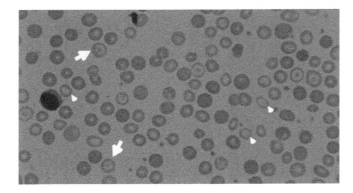

Figure 4.2.8 Microcytic hypochromic red cells (arrowhead) and target cells (large arrows) in a patient with iron-deficiency anaemia.

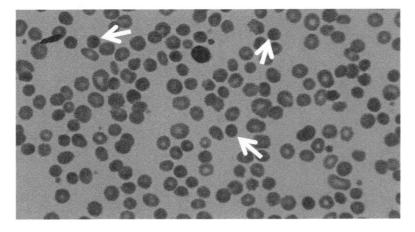

Figure 4.2.9 Spherocytes (some of which are indicated by arrows) in a patient with hereditary spherocytosis.

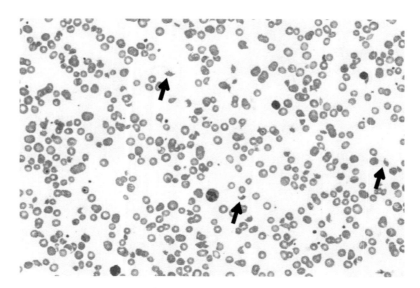

Figure 4.2.10 Red cell fragments (some of which are indicated by arrows) in a patient with atypical haemolytic uraemic syndrome.

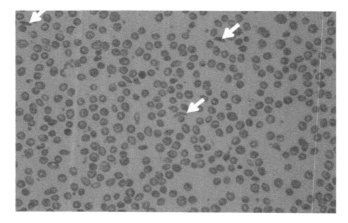

Figure 4.2.11 Three sickle-shaped red cells (arrows) in a patient with sickle cell anaemia. Polychromasia and target cells are present too. Patient also has alpha plus thalassaemia.

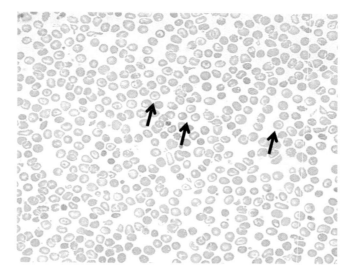

Figure 4.2.12 Blood film showing multiple target cells and microcytic red cells in a newborn with haemoglobin H disease.

4.2.8 KEY MANAGEMENT PRINCIPLES

Management of these haematological disorders can be complicated. Many will require specialist haematology input and detailed description is beyond the scope of this chapter, which covers general principles only.

Diagnosis-specific management strategies are outlined here. It is expected that an 'ABCDE' approach to assessment and management is always undertaken (see Chapter 12.1, *The A to E Assessment*).

Dangerous Diagnosis 1
Diagnosis: Major haemorrhage

Management Principles
1. **Simple measures to control bleeding.** Depending on the nature of bleeding, simple measures such as pressure/elevation may be useful
2. **Major haemorrhage protocol.** Every hospital should have a major haemorrhage protocol, which can be activated by calling the switchboard (similar to a crash call). This allocates an emergency porter to facilitate rapid supply of blood components and rapid transport of blood samples
3. **Reversal of anticoagulation.** Children on anticoagulation may require reversal. Urgently consult a haematologist for advice
4. **Red blood cell transfusion.** Packed red blood cell transfusion will be necessary and should be given as O negative emergency blood until crossmatched blood is available. While waiting for blood, crystalloid or colloid fluids can be given for resuscitation.
5. **Prevent coagulopathy.** Platelets and fresh frozen plasma (FFP) will be required. Cryoprecipitate may also be useful if fibrinogen is depleted
6. **Tranexamic acid.** Intravenous (IV) tranexamic acid can be used as a haemostatic agent in those with active bleeding
7. **Surgical management.** Surgical management may be the definitive treatment, and early involvement of surgical colleagues is imperative. Consider interventional radiology

Dangerous Diagnosis 2
Diagnosis: Autoimmune haemolytic anaemia

Management Principles
1. **Urgent transfusion in those presenting with life-threatening anaemia.** Children who present as unstable, with severe anaemia, require urgent red blood cell transfusion. Discussion with haematology and transfusion specialists should take place urgently, to discuss identification of compatible red blood cells
2. **Further investigation for secondary causes.** In all new cases, further evaluation for secondary causes will be required, at the advice of a haematologist
3. **Warm AIHA: medical treatment.** Warm-reactive AIHA usually requires pharmacological treatment. Glucocorticoids are first line, and the dose is dependent on the severity of the anaemia
4. **Cold AIHA: conservative.** Most cold-reactive AIHA is self-limiting and does not require treatment. Management is directed towards cold avoidance. All IV fluids should be warmed before giving. For those with significant chronic anaemia, rituximab can be used (off-label) to reduce antibody production
5. **Monitoring.** Regular monitoring of Hb and reticulocyte count is required and will be guided by a haematologist

Dangerous Diagnosis 3
Diagnosis: Haemolytic uraemic syndrome

Management Principles
1. **Careful fluid replacement.** In children deemed to be clinically dehydrated (due to vomiting, diarrhoea or decreased intake), careful fluid replacement is required to restore euvolaemia
2. **Strict fluid balance.** Fluid overload is a huge problem with HUS, due to oliguria/anuria, resulting in heart failure, pulmonary oedema and exacerbation of hypertension. Weight should be monitored twice a day. In those with normal/increased intravascular volume and decreased urine output, fluid intake should be restricted to insensible losses plus urinary output
3. **Transfusion.** Packed red cell transfusion should be considered for Hb <60 g/L or if the patient is significantly symptomatic. The goal is to restore Hb to 80–90 g/L, and not to normal, to avoid complications of fluid overload. Platelet transfusion is not commonly required, but may be required in active bleeding
4. **Antibiotics.** If HUS is thought to be secondary to an infectious cause, antibiotics are vital. Use local policy to determine antibiotic choice. Ensure that nephrotoxic medications are avoided

5. **Antihypertensives.** Fluid overload can be associated with hypertension. Renal impairment may aggravate renin-driven hypertension and require antihypertensive therapy. Advice varies over whether calcium channel blockers or angiotensin-converting enzyme (ACE) inhibitors are used as first line

6. **Dialysis.** Peritoneal or haemodialysis is indicated in significant electrolyte abnormalities, uraemia and severe fluid overload

Dangerous Diagnosis 4
Diagnosis: Malignancy

Management Principles
1. **Refer to tertiary oncology centre.** Management is highly variable depending on type of malignancy identified. Discussion of possible options is outside the scope of this chapter, but is discussed elsewhere in Chapters 3.3 and 4.1. All new diagnoses of malignancy must be discussed with the local tertiary oncology centre

Common Diagnosis 1
Diagnosis: Iron-deficiency anaemia

Management Principles
1. **Iron supplementation.** Oral elemental iron can be given by tablets or liquid. The dose is 3–6 mg/kg (max 200 mg) daily given in 2–3 divided doses. Note that different preparations contain different amounts of ferrous iron (e.g. ferrous fumarate 200 mg contains 65 mg ferrous iron). Warn parents about black stools as a common side effect, and avoidance of constipation
2. **Monitor Hb.** It is sensible to recheck Hb after 2–4 weeks of iron supplementation. Continue treatment for 3 months to replenish iron stores. For those at high risk of recurrent IDA (e.g. coeliac disease, menorrhagia), consider an ongoing prophylactic dose
3. **Dietary modifications.** Dietician referral may be useful. Dietary iron should be increased. Vitamin C helps in absorption of iron. Avoid tea, which reduces gastrointestinal absorption of iron
4. **Avoid excessive cow's milk.** Cow's milk should not be offered to children under 12 months, who should receive infant formula or breast milk as their primary milk drink. Even in those over 1 year, cow's milk should be limited to 500 mL per day

---

Box 4.2.27   Foods Rich in Iron

- Fortified formula
- Fortified cereals
- Meat
- Beans
- Lentils
- Eggs

- Fish
- Raisins
- Prunes
- Leafy green vegetables
- Oatmeal
- Tuna

Common Diagnosis 2
Diagnosis: Sickle cell anaemia
Management is extremely complicated given the heterogeneity of presentation and complications. Treatment is based on prevention, as well as treatment of complications.

Management Principles
1. **Early recognition of infection.** Infection makes up a large part of the morbidity in children with SCD. Parents should be educated about recognising infection. A written plan should be given about seeking medical review in the event of a fever
2. **Antibiotic prophylaxis.** Prophylactic penicillin should start by 3 months of age. Lifelong prophylaxis is required, but full adherence is particularly important up to 5 years old
3. **Immunisations.** All immunisations on the childhood immunisation programme should be given. Several additional vaccines are also indicated (see Box 4.2.28)
4. **Red blood cell transfusions.** In SCD, symptomatic anaemia is superimposed upon chronic anaemia. Knowledge of baseline Hb level is essential in interpreting the extent of acute anaemia and guiding whether a transfusion is required. Transfusion is usually indicated for symptomatic anaemia with Hb >20 g/L below baseline
5. **Hydroxyurea.** Hydroxyurea (hydroxycarbamide) is used to prevent acute chest syndrome and painful crises. As there is a risk of myelosuppression, it is only indicated in those with recurrent episodes

6. **Treatment of complications.** Delineating treatment of complications is beyond the scope of this chapter, but many require emergency treatment, such as sequestration, painful crises, acute chest syndrome, sepsis and stroke

7. **Education.** Parents should be advised on the importance of keeping children warm, avoiding sudden drops in temperature and ensuring good hydration

8. **Psychological support.** Children may need psychological support, particularly if they have frequent painful crises

9. **Haematopoietic stem cell transplantation from matched sibling donor.** This is the only definitive cure for SCD and is only indicated in children younger than 17 years old. It can be considered in those with severe SCD-related complications that have not responded to hydroxyurea

---

Box 4.2.28   Recommended Additional Immunisations in Children with Sickle Cell Disease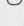

- Pneumococcal polysaccharide vaccine at 2 years, and then every 5 years
- Influenza vaccine annually from 6 months old
- Hepatitis B vaccine at 12, 13 and 18 months
- Meningitis ACWY vaccination for travel to high-risk areas

Box 4.2.29   Iron Overload

- Iron overload is a common side effect in those with any chronic anaemias (e.g. sickle cell, thalassaemia, Diamond–Blackfan anaemia) requiring repeated transfusions
- Iron overload is particularly common in thalassaemia major and intermedia, due to the ineffective erythropoiesis that promotes increased intestinal iron uptake
- Affected organs:
- Liver: cirrhosis
- Heart: cardiac haemosiderosis
- Pituitary: hypogonadism, hypothyroidism, growth impairment
- Thyroid: hypothyroidism
- Pancreas: insulin resistance
- Iron chelation, such as with desferrioxamine, is an essential part of treatment, in order to prevent excess iron deposition in organs

5.1 Abdominal Pain

Gillian Rivlin and Rachel Varughese

Department of Paediatrics, Oxford University Hospitals NHS Foundation Trust, Oxford, UK

CONTENTS

5.1.1 CHAPTER AT A GLANCE

> **Box 5.1.1   Chapter at a Glance**
>
> - Abdominal pain in children can signify underlying conditions of varying severity, from benign to life-threatening
> - Unlike in adults, children may not experience localised pain, and so other associated features help identify differential diagnoses
>
> - Concealed trauma from inflicted injury or an ectopic pregnancy should always be considered if the history is inconsistent

5.1.2 DEFINITION

Pain or discomfort originating from the abdominal cavity. Abdominal pain can be acute or chronic and either localised or diffuse.

Clinical Guide to Paediatrics, First Edition. Edited by Rachel Varughese and Anna Mathew. Series Editor: Christian Fielder Camm.
© 2022 John Wiley & Sons Ltd. Published 2022 by John Wiley & Sons Ltd.
Companion website: www.wiley.com/go/varughese/paediatrics

5.1.3 DIAGNOSTIC ALGORITHM

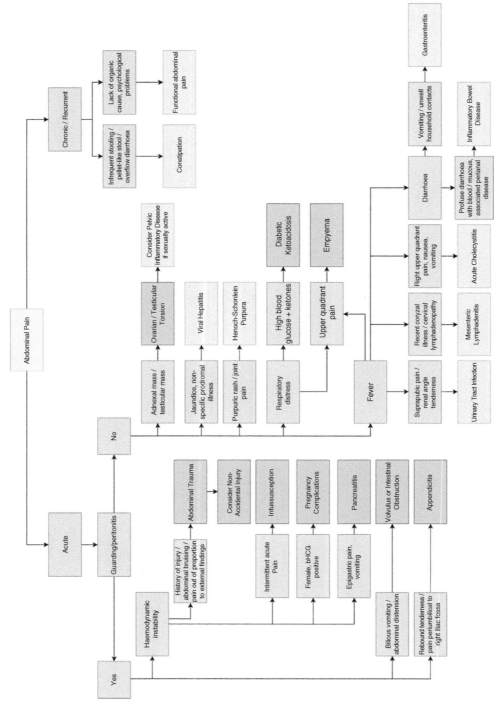

Figure 5.1.1 Diagnostic algorithm for the presentation of abdominal pain.

5.1.4 DIFFERENTIALS LIST

Dangerous Diagnoses

1. Acute Appendicitis
- Appendicitis is inflammation of the appendix, which is a small pouch connected to the colon at the level of the caecum
- If the lumen becomes blocked (often with normal or hardened stool: a 'faecolith'), it fills with mucus and bacteria multiply within it
- As the pressure rises within the lumen, it eventually infarcts and leads to perforation
- Causes acute-onset abdominal pain, classically originating in the periumbilical region and then localising to the right iliac fossa

2. Acute Pancreatitis
- Inflammation of the pancreas requiring prompt treatment, as some cases can be life-threatening
- Causes acute-onset abdominal pain, which is often epigastric, and at times radiating to the back
- Common causes of pancreatitis in children include infections, gallstones, abdominal trauma, high triglycerides and some medicines

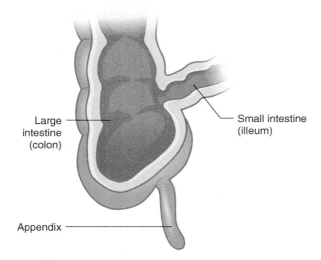

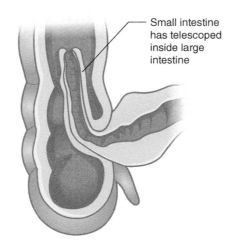

Figure 5.1.2 Intussusception: an intussusception can involve the telescoping of any part of the gut into another. Most commonly, however, it is ileo-colic, where the ileum goes within the colon.

3. Abdominal Trauma
- Blunt or penetrating abdominal injury
- Internal abdominal damage may not be outwardly obvious. Consider if known history of trauma, or abdominal pain out of proportion to examination findings
- Consider possibility of concealed trauma in non-accidental injury

4. Intussusception
- More common in children <2 years old (3–12 months)
- Intermittent colicky abdominal pain with increasing bouts of fever, lethargy, vomiting, drawing up of knees and redcurrant jelly stools
- Inconsolable crying is characteristic
- Occasionally seen in older children with Henoch–Schönlein Purpura (HSP)

5. Intestinal Obstruction
- Partial or complete blockage of bowel, preventing normal bowel movement
- Always consider whether the obstruction may be compressing the bowel from outside, lies within the bowel wall or within the lumen of the bowel

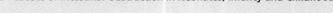

Box 5.1.2   Causes of Intestinal Obstruction in Neonates, Infancy and Childhood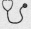

- Meconium plug
- Imperforate anus
- Congenital hypertrophic pyloric stenosis
- Hirschsprung disease
- Malrotation leading to volvulus
- Atresia/stenosis: duodenum, jejunum, ileum
- Annular pancreas
- Strangulated inguinal hernia
- Ileocaecal intussusception
- Meckel's diverticulum
- Post-operative adhesions

6. Volvulus
- Volvulus in children often results from intestinal malrotation, where a loop of intestine twists around its mesenteric attachment, often because the mesentery on which the gut hangs is unusually narrow at its base
- Without the normal wide-based mesentery, it is easier for the gut to swing and twist on a narrow base
- Mostly affects those under 1 year of age
- The small bowel twists around the superior mesenteric artery, compromising the vascular supply to the midgut

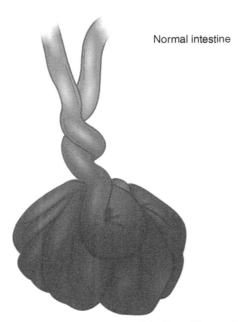

Normal intestine

Intestine with vascular compromise

Figure 5.1.3 Volvulus: twisting of the gut, usually on a base of narrow mesentery, causes compromised blood supply.

7. Testicular or Ovarian Torsion
- **Testicular torsion:** most common urological emergency caused by the twisting of the testis on the spermatic cord, leading to vascular ischaemia and necrosis
- **Ovarian torsion:** ovary twists on its attachment to other structures, leading to ischaemia and necrosis

Box 5.1.3   Testicular and Ovarian Torsion

Diagnosis	Presentation	Outcome
Testicular torsion	<li> Acute abdominal and groin pain, scrotal oedema, erythema <li> Acutely tender testicle lies higher and transverse in comparison to unaffected testicle. No relief on lifting affected testicle <li> Differentials include torsion of appendix testis, epididymitis	<li> Testicular damage is determined by length of time taken from onset of symptoms to surgery and untwisting, as well as the degree of cord twist
Ovarian torsion	<li> Sudden, acute one-sided lower abdominal or pelvic pain, with nausea and vomiting <li> Risk factors include ovarian cysts, tumours and pregnancy	<li> Diagnosis is often delayed and compounded by waiting for radiological diagnosis <li> Preservation of ovarian function directly correlates to time from onset of symptoms to surgery and untwisting the torsion

8. Pregnancy Complications
- Beware of undiagnosed pregnancies in females of childbearing age
- Miscarriage, ectopic pregnancy or preterm labour can present as acute abdominal pain

Box 5.1.4   Diabetic Ketoacidosis (DKA)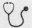

- DKA is a life-threatening cause of abdominal pain in new or known diagnoses of type 1 diabetes mellitus
- Abdominal pain is a cardinal sign of DKA. Mechanism is poorly understood, however considered to be due to gastritis, gastric distension, ileus, mesenteric ischaemia and rapid expansion of the hepatic capsule

- It rarely presents with abdominal pain alone and may be accompanied by respiratory distress (Kussmaul breathing), dehydration and altered mental status

Common Diagnoses
1. Functional Abdominal Pain
- Abdominal pain without an organic cause
- Acute or chronic pain, which is often vague and described as persistent and central
- Diagnosis should only be made after exclusion of other possible organic causes. There may be a family history of functional disorders such as irritable bowel syndrome (IBS) or migraine
2. Urinary Tract Infection (UTI)
- Caused by microorganisms in the urinary tract
- Boys tend to present within the first year of life, after which the prevalence is higher in girls
- Presentation varies according to age, with those under 1 year often presenting with fever, vomiting, lethargy, irritability and poor feeding. Older children may present with dysuria, increased urinary frequency and urgency, back pain and fever
- Urinary tract infections are covered in detail in Chapter 3.1, and will not be discussed further here
3. Viral Hepatitis
- Caused by infection with hepatotrophic viruses (e.g. hepatitis A, B and C) and non-hepatotrophic viruses, including herpes simplex virus (HSV), Epstein–Barr virus (EBV), cytomegalovirus (CMV) and enteroviruses
- Typical prodrome includes progressive jaundice, lethargy, anorexia, nausea, abdominal pain, myalgia and sometimes fever
- Although most infections are self-limiting, fulminant liver failure can develop and carries a mortality of 70% without appropriate treatment
- Viral hepatitis is covered in detail in Chapters 3.2 and 5.5, and will not be discussed further in this chapter

4. Gastroenteritis
- Infectious diarrhoea usually associated with abdominal pain, nausea and vomiting
- Can be associated with low-grade fever, fatigue, headache and muscle pain
- Gastroenteritis is covered in detail in Chapter 5.3, and will not be discussed further in this chapter

5. Constipation
- Common paediatric problem with a prevalence of 3% worldwide during childhood
- Defined as infrequent bowel movements or difficult passage of stools, typically fewer than 3 times per week
- Constipation is covered in detail in Chapter 5.2, and will not be discussed further in this chapter

Diagnoses to Consider

1. Mesenteric Lymphadenitis
- Self-limiting inflammation of mesenteric lymph nodes
- Often intercurrent or recent upper respiratory tract infection (URTI) associated with diffuse abdominal pain

When to consider: in otherwise unexplained abdominal pain, particularly if evidence of extra-abdominal lymphadenopathy

2. Acute Cholecystitis
- Inflammation of the gall bladder, often associated with cholelithiasis
- Abdominal pain (right upper quadrant), fever, rigors, nausea and vomiting are frequent presenting symptoms
- Children with haemolytic diseases, such as sickle cell disease, hereditary spherocytosis, glucose-6-phosphate dehydrogenase (G6PD) deficiency and thalassaemia are at risk of pigment gallstones, as a result of red blood cell destruction
- Many other comorbidities increase the risk of gallstones, including Wilson's disease, obesity, cystic fibrosis, Crohn's disease and previous gut resection

When to consider: in children with previous symptoms or risk factors for gallstones

3. Inflammatory Bowel Disease (IBD)
- Chronic inflammatory bowel change. IBD is an umbrella term encompassing Crohn's disease and ulcerative colitis
- Those with a genetic predisposition develop IBD, which is a dysregulated mucosal immune response to intestinal microflora
- IBD is covered in detail in Chapter 5.4

When to consider: in those with weeks or more of a history of diarrhoea and weight loss

4. Henoch–Schönlein Purpura (HSP)
- Systemic immunoglobulin (Ig) A vasculitis affecting the joints, skin, mucosal membranes and kidneys
- HSP can present with an acute abdomen and acute intussusception should be considered
- Typical presentation is with a purpuric rash on the lower half of the body and arthralgias/arthritis affecting knees, ankles and wrists
- Painful scrotal oedema is noted occasionally in affected boys
- HSP is covered in detail in Chapters 9.2 and 10.2

When to consider: in children with palpable purpura on lower-limb extensor surfaces and buttocks

---

Box 5.1.5   Clinical Presentation of Henoch–Schönlein Purpura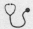

Finding	Detail
Rash	• Description: evolves usually from hives to palpable purpuric rash. Purpuric rash ranges from small dots to bigger bruises and ecchymosis • Distribution: backs of the legs, buttocks, arms initially. Can spread to involve other parts of the body, front of legs, back and chest
Abdominal pain	• Intensity varies from mild to severe • May be associated with vomiting. In such cases, acute intussusception should be ruled out
Arthritis	• Inflammation and pain in the joints of the ankles and knees are more common than in the wrist and elbows
Renal involvement	• Haematuria and proteinuria are often seen • Progressive glomerulonephritis with high blood pressure is a complication

---

Box 5.1.6   Pneumonia and Complications

Pneumonias can be complicated by pleural effusions and empyemas, all of which can cause referred pain to the abdomen. These typically present with upper quadrant pain on the affected side

5.1.5 KEY HISTORY FEATURES

Box 5.1.7   Red Flag Symptoms Seen in Abdominal Pain

Finding	Detail
Unexplained fever	
Involuntary weight loss	
Back pain	
Upper gastrointestinal symptoms	• Difficulty swallowing (dysphagia) • Painful swallowing (odynophagia) • Significant vomiting (bilious, protracted, projectile or otherwise worrisome)
Change in bowel habit	• Chronic severe diarrhoea (≥3 loose or watery stools per day for more than 2 weeks) • Nocturnal diarrhoea • Bloody diarrhoea • Melaena (black, tarry stools)
Urinary symptoms	• Change in bladder function • Dysuria • Haematuria • Flank pain
Skin changes	• Urticarial rash • Angioedema
Family history	• Inflammatory bowel disease • Coeliac disease • Peptic ulcer disease

Dangerous Diagnosis 1
Diagnosis: Acute appendicitis

Questions
1. **Has the intensity and location of the pain changed?** Appendicitis typically presents with peri-umbilical pain, which localises to the right iliac fossa 6–48 hours later. Younger children may have difficulty localising the pain. Children may be reluctant to move because of the severity of the pain
2. **Has there been any anorexia or nausea?** Important associated symptoms of appendicitis are explored by using the Paediatric Appendicitis Score (PAS)

Box 5.1.8   Paediatric Appendicitis Score

The Paediatric Appendicitis Score (PAS) is applicable to patients between 3 and 18 years of age with abdominal pain of ≤4 days, to predict the likelihood of appendicitis. Not suitable for use in patients with known gastrointestinal disease, pregnancy or previous abdominal surgery.

Sign/symptom	Scoring
Fever (temp in axilla >38 °C)	1
Anorexia	1
Nausea or vomiting	1
Pain on cough/percussion or hopping	2
Right iliac fossa (RIF) tenderness	2
Migration of pain (from central to RIF)	1
White cell count (WCC) >10 × 10^9/L	1
Neutrophils >7.5 × 10^9/L	1

Low risk (≤4), equivocal (4–6) and high risk (>6)

Dangerous Diagnosis 2
Diagnosis: Acute pancreatitis

Questions
1. **How quickly have symptoms progressed?** Acute pancreatitis often presents with a progressively unwell child over hours, with severe abdominal pain, persistent vomiting and fever
2. **Is there a history supporting a concomitant viral or bacterial infection?** Mumps, measles, influenza, EBV, mycoplasma and some Gram-negative bacterial infections may cause pancreatitis
3. **Any blunt abdominal trauma?** Blunt trauma to the abdomen could be a precipitating cause, and non-accidental injury should be part of the consideration
4. **Is the child on any long-term medication?** Medication such as sodium valproate, azathioprine, steroids, anticoagulants, mercaptopurine and mesalazine can precipitate pancreatitis

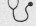

> **Box 5.1.9   Risk Factors for Pancreatitis**
>
> - Juvenile idiopathic arthritis
> - Systemic lupus erythematosus
> - Haemolytic uraemic syndrome
> - Henoch–Schönlein purpura
> - Kawasaki disease
> - Inflammatory bowel disease
> - Cystic fibrosis
> - Anorexia nervosa

Dangerous Diagnosis 3
Diagnosis: Abdominal trauma

Questions
1. **Is there a history of trauma and, if so, what was the mechanism?** In a patient known to have a traumatic injury, understanding the mechanism of injury is vital in deciding on abdominal imaging. Blunt abdominal trauma is common with road traffic accidents, falls and assaults. The liver and spleen are the most commonly injured organs in blunt abdominal trauma
2. **Is the history consistent with symptoms?** If the history from parents is inconsistent with symptoms, or continuously changing, there should be a high level of suspicion of non-accidental injury

Dangerous Diagnosis 4
Diagnosis: Intussusception

Questions
1. **What is the age of the patient?** Intussusception is most common in children under 2 years of age. Older children are unlikely candidates, unless they have HSP
2. **What is the nature of the pain?** There may be intermittent crying with drawing up of the knees, followed by pain-free periods. (This is due to intermittent invagination of the intestinal tract, leading to oedema of the intestinal wall, until spontaneous reduction is no longer possible, ultimately resulting in bowel wall ischaemia)
3. **Has the child opened their bowels recently?** Diarrhoea is not uncommon initially. Rectal bleeding with the classic 'redcurrant jelly' stool is a late sign suggestive of bowel ischaemia and infarction

Dangerous Diagnosis 5
Diagnosis: Intestinal obstruction

Questions
1. **Is there a history of previous abdominal surgery?** Patients who have previously undergone abdominal surgery are more likely to form adhesions. Adhesions allow the bowel to kink or twist, causing a total or partial obstruction of the intestine
2. **Have they been vomiting?** Green bilious vomit suggests mechanical obstruction, at or distal to the duodenum. A proximal gastrointestinal obstruction above the level of the ampulla of Vater (where bile drains into the duodenum) will be non-bilious
3. **When did the child last open their bowels and are they passing flatus?** Children with intestinal obstruction will be unable to open bowels or pass flatus

Dangerous Diagnosis 6
Diagnosis: Volvulus

Questions
1. **How old is the child?** In the paediatric population, volvulus is most common in infants, 3–12 months. In this population, patients often present with inconsolable crying
2. **Is there bilious vomiting?** An acute presentation with bilious vomiting and abdominal distension is common in volvulus and helps differentiate from intussusception

Dangerous Diagnosis 7
Diagnosis: Testicular or ovarian torsion

Questions
1. **Is the patient sexually active?** Young people who have no history of sexual activity are unlikely to have pelvic inflammatory disease or epididymitis, therefore making torsion the most likely cause
2. **Does the testicle lie in an abnormal position?** Testicular torsion is described as a high-lying testicle in a transverse position. Pain is not relieved with lifting of the testicle and pain can be referred to the lower abdomen
3. **Is there a history of ovarian cysts?** Ovarian cysts are more likely to lead to ovarian torsion; however, in premenarchal girls around 50% have been found to have normal ovaries

Dangerous Diagnosis 8
Diagnosis: Pregnancy complications

Questions
1. **Is there a known pregnancy?** It is not uncommon for a young female person to be unaware of her pregnancy or have avoided seeking medical assistance for pregnancy. Always consider the possibility of an ectopic pregnancy
2. **Is there vaginal bleeding?** Vaginal bleeding may represent a ruptured ectopic, impending miscarriage or early premature delivery

Common Diagnosis 1
Diagnosis: Functional abdominal pain

Questions
1. **What are the duration and frequency of symptoms?** This diagnosis should be considered in children and adolescents who experience recurrent (>3 episodes) and prolonged abdominal pain (>3 months) with no associated red flag symptoms
2. **Have there been any stressful life events?** Stressful stimuli include parental separation, bullying, exams, changing schools and competitive hobbies. These may all contribute to functional abdominal pain
3. **Is the patient male or female?** Girls are more likely to be affected with functional abdominal pain

5.1.6 KEY EXAMINATION FEATURES

All children should be examined for features of peritonitis, which may indicate serious infection or rupture of an abdominal organ. Peritonitis should be considered if there is significant diffuse abdominal tenderness, rebound tenderness or guarding.

Dangerous Diagnosis 1
Diagnosis: Acute appendicitis

Examination Findings
1. **Tenderness in the right iliac fossa.** Positive McBurney's sign, demonstrated by pressing over the right iliac fossa: eliciting acute pain demonstrates irritation of the overlying peritoneum
2. **Position of patient.** Patients prefer to lie still with hips flexed in order not to stretch the irritated peritoneum
3. **Pain elicited with specific manoeuvres.** In some patients applying pressure over the left iliac fossa elicits Rovsing's sign. Abdominal pain can also be elicited by asking a patient to jump or cough

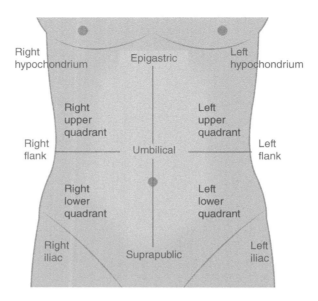

Figure 5.1.4 Abdominal regions can either be divided into nine areas (red) or quadrants (blue). Use these when describing localised abdominal pain.

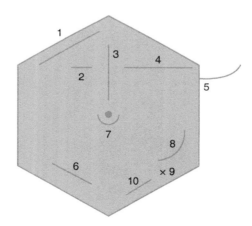

Figure 5.1.5 Abdominal scars. **1. Kocher's incision:** hepatic surgery, biliary atresia, cholecystectomy. **2. Ramstedt's procedure:** pyloromyotomy. **3. Midline laparotomy:** Nissen's fundoplication, major abdominal surgery. **4. Transverse upper abdominal incision:** splenectomy, repair of congenital diaphragmatic hernia. **5. Lateral thoracolumbar incision:** renal surgery (nephrectomy). **6. Grid-iron incision:** appendicectomy. **7. Sub-umbilical incision:** exomphalos repair, gastroschisis repair. **8. Hockey-stick incision:** renal transplant. **9. Point incision:** drains, laparoscopic ports. **10. Inguinal incision:** inguinal hernia repair.

Box 5.1.10	Clinical Signs Supporting Diagnosis of Acute Appendicitis
Sign	**Details**
McBurney's	Palpation over the right iliac fossa elicits pain over that area
Rovsing's	Palpation over the left lower quadrant elicits pain in the right lower quadrant

Dangerous Diagnosis 2
Diagnosis: Acute pancreatitis

Examination Findings
1. **Unwell-looking patient.** The child will often look very ill, taking up an antalgic position, with hips and knees bent and lying on one side. They may have signs of shock with poor peripheral perfusion, tachycardia and hypotension
2. **Abdominal distension.** The abdomen may be tender on palpation, and a mass may be palpable
3. **Cullen or Grey Turner sign.** A bluish discoloration seen around the umbilicus (Cullen sign) or over the flanks (Grey Turner sign) are signs of haemorrhagic pancreatitis, the most severe form of acute pancreatitis, associated with a high mortality

Dangerous Diagnosis 3
Diagnosis: Abdominal trauma

Examination Findings
1. **Bruising/ecchymosis.** When present over the anterior and posterior abdomen, bruising/ecchymosis increases the likelihood of serious intra-abdominal injury from blunt trauma
2. **Guarding.** Signs of peritonism, such as guarding, also increase the likelihood of intra-abdominal injury
3. **Abdominal distension and rigidity.** These also increase the likelihood of intra-abdominal injury

Dangerous Diagnosis 4
Diagnosis: Intussusception

Examination Findings
1. **Focal abdominal tenderness.** Focal tenderness in the right upper quadrant or upper abdomen may be present, but the absence of pain on palpation should not exclude a diagnosis of intussusception
2. **Palpable 'sausage-shaped' mass.** 50–70% of patients present with a sausage-shaped mass in the right abdomen that may cross the midline in the epigastrium, which can be accompanied by a feeling of emptiness on palpation of the right lower quadrant (Dance's sign)
3. **Bloody stool.** 50% of patients have bloody stools and a further 25% will have occult blood. Redcurrant jelly stool is late sign of intussusception

Dangerous Diagnosis 5
Diagnosis: Intestinal obstruction

Examination Findings
1. **Abdominal distension.** Obstructed passage of food or liquid will lead to abdominal distension
2. **Hyperactive bowel sounds initially, loss of bowel sounds later.** Bowel sounds are initially hyperactive, as an obstruction progresses due to accumulation of fluid and gas build-up in the intestinal tract with increased peristaltic movement. Later, bowel sounds become tinkling or absent. Important to listen for at least 2 minutes before concluding that bowel sounds are absent

Dangerous Diagnosis 6
Diagnosis: Volvulus

Examination Findings
1. **Abdominal distension.** Abdominal distension, particularly when accompanied by bilious vomiting, suggests midgut obstruction
2. **Poor peripheral perfusion, tachycardia, hypotension.** Shock is late sign of bowel ischaemia. The child may look 'toxic' and extremely unwell

Dangerous Diagnosis 7
Diagnosis: Testicular or ovarian torsion

Examination Findings
1. **Localised pain.** Localised testicular tenderness is suggestive of torsion until proven otherwise. Ovarian torsion is associated with unilateral abdominal pain, usually localised to the iliac fossa
2. **Hard testis with absent cremasteric reflex.** A hard testis along with swelling, nausea/vomiting, high-lying position and absent cremasteric reflex are strong predictors of testicular torsion
3. **Adnexal mass.** A mass in a girl with unilateral abdominal pain and associated nausea and vomiting should raise clinical suspicion of ovarian torsion

Dangerous Diagnosis 8
Diagnosis: Pregnancy complications

Examination Findings
1. **Lower abdominal tenderness.** The onset of pain in ectopic pregnancies can vary widely and symptoms can be extremely vague. In females of childbearing age with lower abdominal pain and vaginal bleeding, ectopic pregnancy should be considered
2. **Unwell-looking patient.** Ruptured ectopic pregnancies can lead to haemodynamic instability. Patients experiencing a miscarriage are susceptible to extensive rapid bleeding and can quickly become haemodynamically unstable

Common Diagnosis 1
Diagnosis: Functional abdominal pain

Examination Findings
1. **Normal examination.** Patients with longstanding abdominal pain and a normal examination are unlikely to have a serious underlying pathology

5.1.7 KEY INVESTIGATIONS

Not all children will require invasive investigations; often diagnoses are made on clinical evidence from history and examination. Consider carefully which investigations are required for which patient.

Bedside

Table 5.1.1 Bedside tests of use in patients presenting with abdominal pain

Test	When to perform	Potential result
Blood sugar	• Normal result rules out DKA • Hypoglycaemia can result from reduced oral intake	• >10 mmol/L: significant stress • >11 mmol/L: consider DKA • <2.6 mmol/L: consider ketotic hypoglycaemia secondary to gastroenteritis
Blood gas (capillary or venous)	• All systemically unwell children • Quick results to determine metabolic or respiratory derangement	• ↓ pH, ↓ HCO_3, ↑ lactate suggests sepsis • ↓ pH, ↑ PCO_2: respiratory pathology, e.g. empyema
Stool MC&S	• Profuse or bloody diarrhoea	• Identification of infective pathogen
Urine dipstick	Suspected: • UTI • HSP	• Nitrites, leucocytes suggest a UTI • Haematuria, proteinuria suggest renal involvement in HSP
Urine culture	• If positive urine dipstick	• Positive culture confirms bacterial infection • Sensitivities guide antibiotic choice
Urine βHCG	• All pubertal or post-pubertal girls	• Positive result will confirm pregnancy
Blood pressure	• Suspected HSP	• Hypertension indicates renal involvement in HSP

DKA, diabetic ketoacidosis; HCO_3, bicarbonate; HSP, Henoch–Schönlein purpura; MC&S, microscopy, culture and sensitivity; PCO_2, partial pressure of carbon dioxide; UTI, urinary tract infection

Blood Tests

Table 5.1.2 Blood tests of use in patients presenting with abdominal pain

Test	When to perform	Potential result
FBC	• Consider in all patients with abdominal pain unless clear evidence of benign cause	• ↑ WCC suggests infection • Beware falsely reassuring Hb in acute haemorrhage
CRP	• Consider in all patients with abdominal pain unless clear evidence of benign cause	• Significant ↑ in bacterial infections • Less marked ↑ in viral infections • Rise can be delayed, so serious illness should not be discounted in the presence of a low CRP if there is clinical concern
Blood culture	• All systemically unwell children	• Positive culture confirms bacterial infection • Sensitivities guide antibiotic choice
U&E	• All systemically unwell children • To assess electrolytes • To look for AKI	• ↑ Urea/creatinine indicates AKI, seen in hypovolaemic states, HSP, DKA • Abnormal electrolytes in gastroenteritis, IBD, depending on predominant upper/lower gastrointestinal losses
Complement and autoimmune profile	• Suspected HSP with renal involvement	• Positive ANA, dsDNA, ANCA, low C3/C4 support diagnosis of HSP
LFTs	Suspected: • Hepatitis • Cholecystitis • Pancreatitis • Abdominal trauma	• ↑ Bilirubin in hepatitis, cholecystitis, pancreatitis • ↑ AST/ALT indicates hepatocellular injury • ↑ ALP suggests cholestasis, although this is not specific to liver disease • ↑ γ-GT in pancreatitis
Amylase, lipase	• Suspected pancreatitis	• ↑ Amylase and lipase in pancreatitis
Hepatitis serology	• Suspected viral hepatitis	• Positive hepatitis A/B/C (± D and E) serology
Crossmatch	• If surgery imminent or expected	• Prepares crossmatched blood products

AKI, acute kidney injury; ALP, alkaline phosphatase; ALT, alanine aminotransferase; ANA, antinuclear antibody; ANCA, antineutrophil cytoplasmic antibody; AST, aspartate aminotransferase; CRP, C-reactive protein; DKA, diabetic ketoacidosis; dsDNA, double-stranded DNA; FBC, full blood count; γ-GT, gamma-glutamyltransferase; Hb, haemoglobin; HSP, Henoch–Schönlein purpura; IBD, inflammatory bowel disease; LFTs, liver function tests; U&E, urea and electrolytes; WCC, white cell count

Imaging

Table 5.1.3 Imaging modalities of use in patients presenting with abdominal pain

Test	When to perform	Potential result
Ultrasound	• Consider in all acute abdominal pain	• Can diagnose appendicitis, pancreatitis, abdominal trauma (splenic/hepatic/renal), intussusception, volvulus, ectopic pregnancy, ovarian and testicular torsion, empyema, pyelonephritis, mesenteric lymphadenitis, and cholecystitis/cholelithiasis
Abdominal x-ray	Suspected: • Intestinal obstruction • Perforation • Constipation with diagnostic uncertainty	• Distended loops of bowel and fluid levels may suggest intestinal obstruction • Air under the diaphragm will suggest intestinal perforation • Faecal loading in constipation • Toxic megacolon may be seen in inflammatory bowel disease • Radio-opaque gallstones
Chest x-ray	• Suspected chest infection	• Identification of pneumonia or empyema
CT abdomen or MRI abdomen	• If concerns about serious intra-abdominal pathology unable to be determined by ultrasound	• Will diagnose most conditions in this chapter

CT, computed tomography; MRI, magnetic resonance imaging

Special

Table 5.1.4 Special tests of use in patients presenting with abdominal pain

Test	When to perform	Potential result
Lower gastrointestinal endoscopy/biopsy	• Suspected IBD • Assessment of extent of bowel involvement, mucosal changes, strictures, and to obtain biopsies	• Evidence of mucosal changes supporting inflammation, polyps, strictures • Biopsies may show typical histological changes of IBD
ERCP	• To investigate recurrent pancreatitis	• Will determine abnormalities in the pancreatic and biliary ductal systems
MRCP	• Obstructive jaundice • Particularly useful for assessing the biliary system	• May identify gallstones or other biliary tract abnormalities
Urine protein/creatinine ratio	• To quantify proteinuria in HSP	• Level of proteinuria will indicate a nephritic/nephrotic picture in HSP and guide management

ERCP, endoscopic retrograde cholangiopancreatography; HSP, Henoch–Schönlein purpura; IBD, inflammatory bowel disease; MRCP, magnetic resonance cholangio pancreatogram

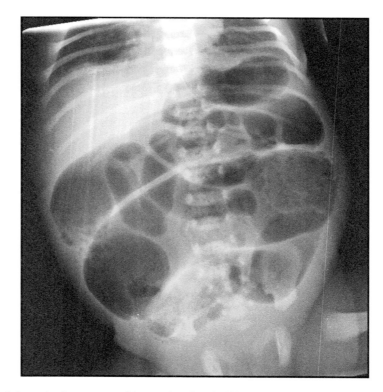

Figure 5.1.6 Low intestinal obstruction in a neonate with meconium ileus (bubbly appearance of meconium visible in flanks).

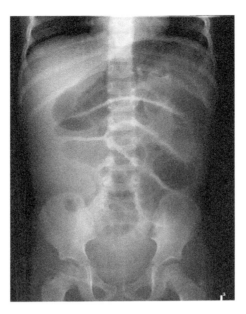

Figure 5.1.7 Abdominal x-ray in a 2-year-old with intussusception, shown by the crescent of gas in the right lower quadrant. Under normal circumstances, ultrasound is the preferred imaging modality.

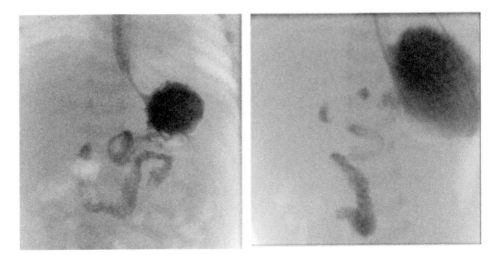

Figure 5.1.8 Contrast study demonstrating a normal duodenojejunal (DJ) flexure on the left (shown left of the vertebral column and at the level of the pylorus). On the right, the duodenum is spiralling, with an incorrectly positioned DJ flexure, demonstrating a malrotation with midgut volvulus.

5.1.8 KEY MANAGEMENT PRINCIPLES

Diagnosis-specific management strategies are outlined here. It is expected that an 'ABCDE' approach to assessment and management is always undertaken (see Chapter 12.1, *The A to E Assessment*).

Dangerous Diagnosis 1
Diagnosis: Appendicitis

Management Principles
1. **Nil by mouth.** Patients suspected of having appendicitis should be kept nil by mouth, to prepare for surgery
2. **Appendicectomy.** Once appendicitis is diagnosed, refer to the surgical team for consideration of surgical intervention to minimise complications
3. **Antimicrobials.** Local protocols vary regarding use of antibiotics and should be followed where suggested

Dangerous Diagnosis 2
Diagnosis: Acute pancreatitis

Management Principles
1. **Pain relief.** Adequate and appropriate pain relief is an important first step, if necessary with morphine
2. **Nutritional support.** Make patient nil by mouth, and provide fluid and electrolyte supplementation with intravenous (IV) fluids initially. Lipase and amylase levels and control of pain will determine when gradual introduction of enteral fluids and food can be initiated. An nasojejunal (NJ) tube may be needed initially to reduce stimulation of the pancreas to produce pancreatic enzymes. A low-fat diet is started initially
3. **Treatment of infection.** In mild cases of pancreatitis, prophylactic antibiotics are probably not necessary, but in moderate to severe cases they should be considered. Advice from the gastroenterology team should be sought
4. **Enzyme inhibition therapy.** Treatment with pancreatic protease inhibitors will need specialist advice

Dangerous Diagnosis 3
Diagnosis: Abdominal trauma

Management Principles
1. **Prompt surgical and trauma evaluation.** Paediatric surgeons should be involved as soon as possible. Advanced Paediatric Life Support (APLS) trauma protocols should be followed and any life-threatening injuries treated. Emergency laparotomy may be required for diagnostic purposes, or for treatment
2. **Imaging.** Haemodynamically stable patients with signs of intra-abdominal injury should undergo emergency computed tomography (CT)

Dangerous Diagnosis 4
Diagnosis: Intussusception

Management Principles
1. **Non-operative management.** Haemodynamically stable patients are able to undergo pneumatic or hydrostatic reduction, where air or water is instilled under pressure through the rectum to 'push' out the intussusceptum

---

Box 5.1.11　Non-operative Reduction of Intussusception

Pneumatic vs hydrostatic

- Largely dependent on user preference. Conflicting evidence about which is superior
- Pneumatic technique involves instillation of air via a Foley catheter or equivalent

- Hydrostatic technique involves instillation of normal saline or contrast, with hydrostatic pressure induced by placing the reservoir 1 m above the patient

Image-guided technique

- Fluoroscopy is required for pneumatic reduction, as air obscures ultrasound

- Ultrasound can be used for hydrostatic reduction, in which case saline can be used. This limits the exposure to ionising radiation

Risks

- Bowel perforation is a risk, seen in <1% of patients. Patients with signs of peritonism should not have non-operative reduction attempted

2. **Operative management.** Indications for surgery are haemodynamic instability, evidence of peritonism or perforation, or failure of non-operative methods. Intra-operative attempts can be made to reduce the intussusceptum, but often this requires resection and primary end-to-end anastomosis

3. **Antimicrobials.** Antibiotics are not indicated in stable patients who have undergone non-operative management. In patients who show progressive symptoms or signs of sepsis or perforation, antibiotics should be given according to local protocols

Dangerous Diagnosis 5
Diagnosis: Intestinal obstruction

Management Principles
1. **Nil by mouth and gastric decompression.** All patients should be kept nil by mouth and a nasogastric (NG) tube should be inserted to decompress the stomach and placed on free drainage. Output should be closely monitored, as NG losses may require replacement

2. **Fluid management and antibiotics.** IV fluids for maintenance will be required as a minimum, with further fluids indicated as determined by clinical assessment of peripheral perfusion status and levels of hydration. The surgical team and local protocols will determine antibiotic administration

3. **Surgical intervention.** Referral should be made to the surgical team. Unstable patients may require emergency laparotomy

Dangerous Diagnosis 6
Diagnosis: Volvulus

Management Principles
Follow the management principles for intestinal obstruction.

Dangerous Diagnosis 7
Diagnosis: Testicular or ovarian torsion

Management Principles
1. **Pain relief.** Ensure that patients are kept comfortable using simple analgesia and escalating treatment as necessary
2. **Surgical intervention**
3. **Testicular torsion:** ideally an ultrasound scan can be quickly performed first; however, this should not delay definitive treatment and referral to a urologist should be done urgently
4. **Ovarian torsion:** urgent assessment by a paediatric surgeon (or gynaecologist with paediatric expertise in older children) is needed and urgent exploration of the pelvis considered

Dangerous Diagnosis 8
Diagnosis: Pregnancy complications

Management Principles
1. **Management of blood loss.** Patients with evidence of a ruptured ectopic pregnancy or significant blood loss through miscarriage should be actively managed and shock treated appropriately
2. **Obstetric and gynaecological review.** Urgent gynaecological assessment should be organised for examination with or without surgical intervention for any child with abdominal pain and a positive pregnancy test. In the event of threatened preterm labour, urgent review by a midwife and obstetrician is required

---

Box 5.1.12   Cervical Shock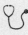

In addition to haemorrhagic shock that might be seen in miscarriage, always consider cervical shock. Cervical shock results from vagal stimulation triggered by dilatation of the cervical canal, causing hypotension and bradycardia, which do not resolve with fluid resuscitation. Evacuation of the retained products of conception can facilitate immediate relief

---

Common Diagnosis 1
Diagnosis: Functional abdominal pain

Management Principles
1. **Parental reassurance.** Reassuring parents that there is no underlying significant pathology (by reiterating negative findings) is crucial to the ongoing management of patients with chronic abdominal pain
2. **Psychological input.** Patients may need referral to the paediatric psychology service to help them to manage their pain

5.2 Abdominal Mass

Catarina Pinto Carr

Department of Paediatrics, East Surrey Hospital, Surrey and Sussex Healthcare NHS Trust, UK

CONTENTS

5.2.1 CHAPTER AT A GLANCE

Box 5.2.1   Chapter at a Glance

- There are a wide range of differentials to be considered for a child presenting with an abdominal mass. These range from benign to serious
- In babies, most masses are caused by hydronephrosis, the majority of which resolve with time
- In older children, constipation is the most common cause for an abdominal mass
- If you are satisfied there is no constipation and the diagnosis remains unclear, the most useful initial investigation is often an ultrasound

5.2.2 DEFINITION

A localised enlargement or swelling within the abdominal cavity, which may be palpated or cause visible swelling.

Clinical Guide to Paediatrics, First Edition. Edited by Rachel Varughese and Anna Mathew. Series Editor: Christian Fielder Camm.
© 2022 John Wiley & Sons Ltd. Published 2022 by John Wiley & Sons Ltd.
Companion website: www.wiley.com/go/varughese/paediatrics

5.2.3 DIAGNOSTIC ALGORITHM

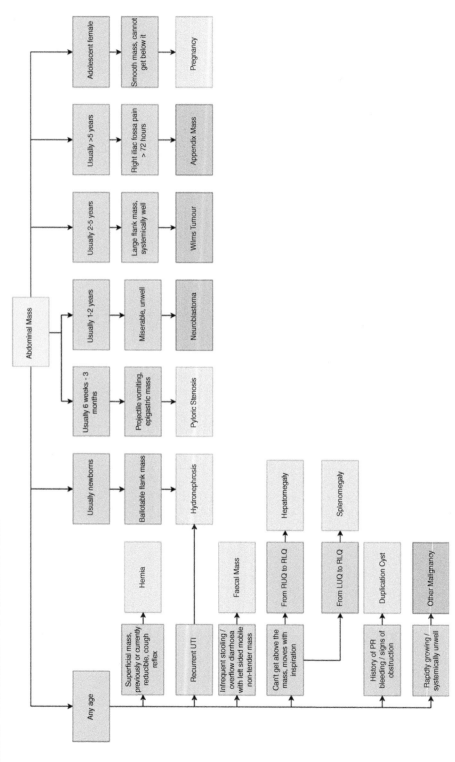

Figure 5.2.1 Diagnostic algorithm for the presentation of abdominal mass.

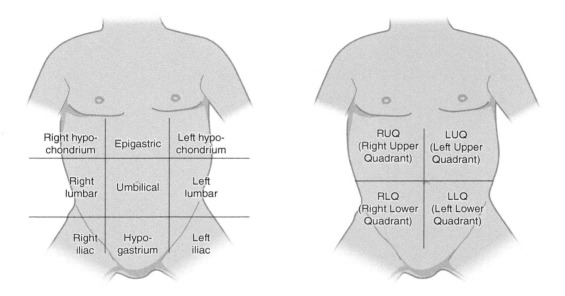

Figure 5.2.2 The anatomical areas of the abdomen or the simplified four quadrants. Consider the organs and possible pathologies found in each area as you work through the chapter.

5.2.4 DIFFERENTIALS LIST

Dangerous Diagnoses

1. Neuroblastoma
- Neural crest cell tumour arising anywhere along the sympathetic chain or in the adrenal gland
- Two-thirds of neuroblastomas are intra-abdominal masses – often adrenal
- Neuroblastoma is the most common cancer seen in babies and comprises 15–20% of cancers in the 0–4 years age range
- It is the most common extra-cranial solid tumour seen in childhood

2. Wilms' Tumour
- Also called nephroblastoma, Wilms' tumour is an embryonal renal neoplasm
- Most cases are sporadic, but children with certain syndromes such as Beckwith–Weidemann syndrome are at increased risk
- Wilms' tumour typically presents between the ages of 2 and 5 years and accounts for 5% of all childhood cancers
- Can present with an abdominal mass or as an incidental finding following a scan for haematuria
- Wilms' is rare over 10 years, when a renal malignancy is more likely to be a renal cell carcinoma

3. Other Malignancy
- Other tumours can arise from the tissue of abdominal organs (e.g. hepatoblastoma from the liver), their embryonic precursors (e.g. germ cell tumours) or from the connective tissue in the abdomen (e.g. sarcoma)
- Leukaemia and lymphoma can also infiltrate the liver, spleen or intra-abdominal lymph nodes and result in a mass
- Malignancy should be considered in any child presenting with an unexplained mass, especially if they are losing weight or complaining of diffuse symptoms

---

Box 5.2.2   Pyloric Stenosis   △△

- Pyloric stenosis results from hypertrophy of the pyloric sphincter
- It classically presents from 2–6 weeks of age with projectile vomiting, and on feeding an 'olive'-shaped mass may be palpated in the epigastric region
- This mass is the hypertrophied muscular pylorus
- Pyloric stenosis is discussed in more detail in Chapter 5.3

Box 5.2.3   Intussusception   △△

- More common in children under 2 years of age (3–12 months)
- Classically presents with intermittent colicky abdominal pain and possibly redcurrant jelly stools
- Occasionally seen in older children with Henoch–Schönlein Purpura

- Present with a sausage-shaped mass in the right abdomen, which can be accompanied by a feeling of emptiness on palpation of the right lower quadrant (Dance's sign)
- Intussusception is discussed in more detail in Chapters 5.1 and 5.4

Box 5.2.4   The Most Common Childhood Cancers   △△

Type of cancer	Percentage of all childhood cancers
Leukaemia	32%
Central nervous system tumours	18%
Lymphoma	11%
Neuroblastoma	6%
Soft tissue sarcomas	6%
Wilms' tumours	5%
Germ cell tumours	5%
Bone tumours	4%
Other tumours	8%

Common Diagnoses
1. Hydronephrosis
- The majority of abdominal masses in infants arise from the kidneys
- Most kidney masses are as a result of hydronephrosis, though rarer causes should always be considered
- Hydronephrosis is the abnormal dilatation of the renal pelvis and calyces, and in paediatrics it is usually congenital
- Hydronephrosis can also develop later in life, due to infection, obstructing renal calculi and masses

Box 5.2.5   Causes of Congenital Hydronephrosis   △△

Underlying pathology	Anatomical location
Obstruction	Pelvi-ureteric junction (PUJ) Vesico-ureteric junction (VUJ) Posterior urethral valves (PUV)
Reflux	Vesico-ureteric reflux (VUR)
Multicystic dysplastic kidney	Cysts replace renal tissue → non-functioning kidney

Box 5.2.6   Rarer Causes of Renal Mass   △△

- **Other renal malignancies:** aside from Wilms', these include mesoblastic nephroma (usually newborns) and renal cell carcinoma (usually adolescents)
- **Renal vein thrombosis:** can present with a flank mass, frank haematuria and thrombocytopaenia. Usually seen in infants of diabetic mothers or in babies as a result of intrauterine foetal distress or underlying hypercoagulability

- **Polycystic kidney disease:** can also cause bilateral renal masses. In the more common autosomal dominant form, enlarged cystic kidneys may be palpated from late childhood onwards, but kidney function is usually maintained until adulthood. However, the rarer autosomal recessive form can present with bilateral renal masses and end-stage renal failure in infancy

2. Constipation
- Constipation affects up to 30% of children at some point during childhood
- In the context of severe constipation, stool can sometimes be felt as a discrete mass
- In school-age children, this is the most likely cause of an abdominal mass and can also cause faltering growth
- It is important to exclude serious underlying causes, including spinal abnormalities, neuromuscular problems, Hirschsprung disease, bowel obstruction and pelvic malignancy

3. Splenomegaly
- The spleen is not usually palpable in well children, though the spleen tip can occasionally be felt in healthy neonates or slim healthy children
- There are several causes of splenomegaly in children, as a result of underlying pathology

Box 5.2.7   Causes of Splenomegaly: use the mnemonic 'IIITCH'   ΔΔ

Cause	Examples
Infectious	Epstein–Barr virus, cytomegalovirus
Inflammatory	Systemic lupus erythematosus, juvenile idiopathic arthritis
Infiltrative	Leukaemia, lymphoma, rarer storage disorders
Traumatic	Traumatic splenic rupture, e.g. bicycle or road trauma
Congestive	Right-sided cardiac failure (usually along with hepatomegaly)
Haematological	Sickle cell disease, thalassaemia, hereditary spherocytosis

4. Hepatomegaly
- The liver can be palpated in some healthy infants and children; however, this is usually less than 2 cm below the costal margin
- Percussing for the lower and upper borders of the liver can help determine if it is truly enlarged or just displaced downwards, for example by hyperinflation of the lungs
- There are several causes of hepatomegaly in children, as a result of underlying pathology

Box 5.2.8   Causes of Hepatomegaly   ΔΔ

Cause	Examples
Infectious	Congenital, e.g. cytomegalovirus, rubella Postnatally acquired, e.g. hepatitis A/B/C, Epstein–Barr virus
Inflammatory	Autoimmune hepatitis, drug-induced hepatitis
Infiltrative	Leukaemia, lymphoma, fatty liver disease, enzyme disorders, e.g. alpha 1-antitrypsin deficiency, Wilson's disease and lysosomal storage diseases
Primary liver malignancy	Hepatoblastoma (usually <5 years), hepatocellular carcinoma (usually >5 years)
Congestive	Right-sided cardiac failure, Budd–Chiari syndrome (hepatic venous outflow obstruction)
Biliary obstruction	Choledochal cyst, cholestasis, e.g. in cystic fibrosis

5. Abdominal Wall Hernia
- A hernia is a protrusion of an organ through the body wall that usually contains it
- Abdominal hernias commonly contain bowel, or less commonly an ovary, and these tissues can become incarcerated (stuck) or strangulated (incarcerated hernia with vascular compromise)
- The most commonly encountered abdominal wall hernias in children are inguinal and umbilical
- However, hernias through surgical scars (incisional hernias), around stomas (parastomal hernias) or through other weak spots in the abdominal wall (e.g. epigastric hernias through the linea alba) can occur. See Chapter 5.1, *Abdominal Pain*, Figure 5.1.5, *Abdominal scars*

Diagnoses to Consider

1. Appendix Masses
- An appendix mass is a walled-off collection resulting from an already perforated appendix
- Roughly 1 in 10 children with appendicitis presents with a mass

When to consider: in any child with a tender right iliac fossa mass. Parents may describe swinging fevers

2. Pregnancy
- Must be considered in any pubertal female
- If considering pregnancy and encountering a tender abdominal mass, remember that ectopic pregnancy is an emergency
- It is important to ask about sexual activity in an open manner, ideally without the parents present. If the patient is sexually active, it is important to establish whether they are practising safe sex and to signpost them to resources and services if not. It is also very important to make sure there are no safeguarding concerns, e.g. if there are signs of sexual exploitation or grooming

When to consider: in any pubertal female with an abdominal mass

---

Box 5.2.9 Gastrointestinal Duplication Cysts

- Duplication cysts are congenital cysts, which may form anywhere along the gastrointestinal (GI) tract, usually not connected with the bowel lumen
- Can present with an otherwise asymptomatic mass at any age, or cause GI obstruction, volvulus, intussusception or rectal bleeding

---

Box 5.2.10 Bezoars

- A rare but fascinating cause of abdominal mass and gastrointestinal obstruction
- Accumulation of undigested material, such as milk and mucous (lactobezoar) in infants, or hair (trichobezoar) in older children with compulsive hair eating
- Usually in the stomach, becoming palpable as epigastric masses
- Management is usually surgical

5.2.5 KEY HISTORY FEATURES

Dangerous Diagnosis 1
Diagnosis: Neuroblastoma

Questions

1. **Is there any general malaise or faltering growth?** Children with neuroblastoma often have an insidious history of general deterioration with fatigue, diffuse bony pain, weakness and loss of appetite
2. **Are there any associated symptoms affecting the skin, eyes or coordination?** Neuroblastoma has a broad spectrum of clinical presentations, depending on the location of the primary tumour, its metastases and potential paraneoplastic effects

---

Box 5.2.11 Varied Presentations of Neuroblastoma

Pathophysiology	Examples	Description	Explanation
Primary tumour local effect	Horner's syndrome: 'ipsilateral meiosis, partial ptosis, enophthalmia and anhydrosis'	Unilateral constricted pupil, drooping eyelid, sunken eye and reduced sweating over the face	Occurs on same side of a tumour disrupting the sympathetic chain, either in the neck (cervical chain) or abdomen (paravertebral chain)
Metastasis local effect	Proptosis and periorbital ecchymoses	Protruding eyes, best noted observing from above, and 'racoon' eyes with bruising around the eye	Metastases to the orbit
	Subcutaneous nodules	Firm, bluish, non-tender nodules	Metastases to skin, commonly in infantile neuroblastoma
Paraneoplastic syndrome	Opsoclonus-myoclonus syndrome	'Dancing eyes' syndrome: multidirectional nystagmus, involuntary muscle twitches and cerebellar ataxia	Autoantibodies directed against central nervous system
	Secretory diarrhoea	Intractable diarrhoea and associated hypokalaemia, which persists with fasting	Tumour secretion of vasoactive intestinal polypeptide

Dangerous Diagnosis 2
Diagnosis: Wilms' Tumour

Questions
1. **Despite a mass, is the child otherwise well?** Children with Wilms' are often surprisingly well at presentation, especially when considering the large mass that may be evident. They are usually asymptomatic
2. **Has there been any blood in the urine?** Other than discomfort and occasional constipation due to mass effect, the most common symptom at the time of diagnosis is haematuria
3. **Does the child have any predisposing risk factors for developing a Wilms' tumour?** The cause of Wilms' tumour is unknown; however, children with certain underlying conditions are more at risk

---

Box 5.2.12   Risk Factors for Wilms' Tumour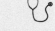

- Wilms' tumour gene disorders: WT1, CTNNB1 or AMER1
- Family history of Wilms' tumour
- Beckwith–Wiedemann syndrome

- Denys Drash syndrome
- WAGR (Wilms' tumour, Aniridia, Genitourinary anomalies, 'Retardation') syndrome

---

Dangerous Diagnosis 3
Diagnosis: Other Malignancy

Questions
1. **Has the mass changed in size since it was first noticed?** Masses related to leukaemia and lymphoma grow rapidly. In contrast, some tumours, such as teratomas, grow very slowly
2. **Does the child look pale, has there been any bruising?** Suspect leukaemia in a child with pallor and easy bruising
3. **Are there systemic symptoms?** Fever, weight loss and night sweats are important indicators of a poorer prognosis in lymphoma
4. **Is there any evidence of mass effect?** Abdominal lymphomas often present with gastrointestinal obstruction. Many abdominal tumours may cause constipation or urinary symptoms

Common Diagnosis 1
Diagnosis: Hydronephrosis

Questions
1. **Is there a history of a urinary tract infection (UTI)?** Abnormalities of the genitourinary (GU) tract can result in varying degrees of obstruction and stagnant urine. This will dramatically increase the risk of infection
2. **Is there evidence of faltering growth?** In infants, an acute UTI will most likely present with unexplained fever and often vomiting. However, some babies have chronically infected urine, and this should be considered when assessing a child with faltering growth
3. **Is the urinary stream normal?** Particularly important for baby boys, where a weak or dribbling urinary stream may suggest posterior urethral valves
4. **Were the antenatal scans normal?** Check if the mother received routine antenatal care with the usual scans, as hydronephrosis and other GU tract abnormalities are often detected antenatally

Common Diagnosis 2
Diagnosis: Constipation

Questions
1. **How often does the child open their bowels and is it associated with pain or distress?** Constipation is more likely if children do not pass stools at least 3 times a week. Constipation can be painful, with both griping abdominal pain and anal fissures
2. **How much water does the child drink in a 24-hour period?** Many children do not drink enough fluids in a day, compounding the constipation. See Box 5.2.14
3. **What is the stool like?** A paediatric Bristol Stool Chart will be helpful to get the child involved in describing their stool. Classically constipation occurs with the passage of firm dry stool
4. **Do they have accidents?** As a child's colon is highly distensible, hard stool can accumulate, stretching the rectum, which reduces the defecation reflex. Overflow diarrhoea, with liquid stool bypassing the impacted stool, may result in a history of

frequent liquid stool, often with soiling. It can be a significant cause of distress and bullying in children. Children may complain of smears (skid marks) in their underwear.

5. **Are there any other medical conditions?** Constipation is very common in children without any significant medical history. However, children with cerebral palsy, spina bifida, developmental delay or psychological difficulties are more prone to constipation

6. **Are there any red flags for constipation?** Red flags suggest a serious underlying cause or condition, such as Hirschsprung disease (congenital aganglionic megacolon), neurological causes or anal anomalies, and warrant urgent specialist advice and management

Bristol Stool Chart		
Appearance	**Type**	**Description**
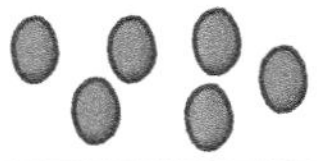	1	Hard lumps
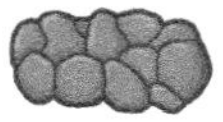	2	Sausage-shaped but lumpy
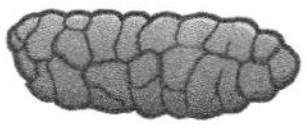	3	Sausage shaped, cracks on surface
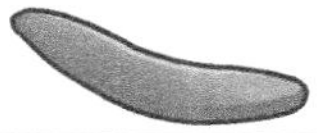	4	Sausage-shaped, smooth surface
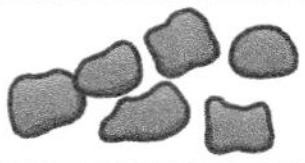	5	Soft blobs
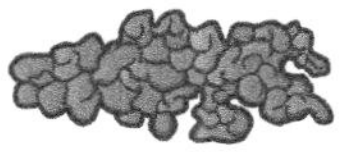	6	Fluffy pieces, mushy appearance
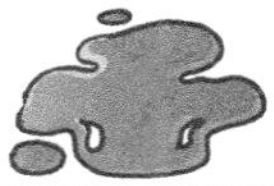	7	Watery, entirely liquid

Figure 5.2.3 A Bristol Stool Chart is an extremely useful tool in determining stool consistency in children. Interpretation: types 1–2 suggest constipation, types 3–4 normal stool, types 5–7 may indicate diarrhoea and urgency.

Box 5.2.13　Red and Amber Flags for Constipation

Red flags	Amber flags
Constipation from birth	Faltering growth
Delay in passing meconium for more than 48 hours in a term baby	Developmental delay
Abdominal distension, vomiting	Triggered by introduction of cow's milk
Family history of Hirschsprung disease	Safeguarding concerns
Ribbon stools	
Leg weakness/motor delay	
Abnormality of anus: anteriorly placed, fissures, tight or patulous	
Abnormality of lumbosacral, gluteal region: sacral agenesis, sacral pit, hairy patch, naevi	

Source: Adapted from National Institute for Health and Care Excellence (2017). Constipation in children and young people: diagnosis and management. Clinical guideline [CG99]. London: NICE.

Box 5.2.14   Suggested Daily Fluid Intake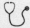

	Total intake per day, including water contained by food	Water obtained by drinks per day
0–6 months	700 mL, assumed to be from breast milk	
7–12 months	800 mL from milk and complementary foods and beverages	600 mL
1–3 years	1300 mL	900 mL
4–8 years	1700 mL	1200 mL
Boys 9–13 years	2400 mL	1800 mL
Girls 9–13 years	2100 mL	1600 mL
Boys 13–18 years	3300 mL	2600 mL
Girls 13–18 years	2300 mL	1800 mL

Source: Adapted from National Institute for Health and Care Excellence (2017). Constipation in children. https://cks.nice.org.uk/topics/constipation-in-children/management/management. London: NICE.

Common Diagnosis 3
Diagnosis: Splenomegaly

Questions
1. **Has there been a fever?** This suggests an infectious pathology, especially if associated with general viral signs such as a sore throat in Epstein–Barr virus (EBV)
2. **Is there a history of bruising, pallor, weight loss or lymphadenopathy?** This is concerning for an underlying malignancy
3. **Is there a history of occasional jaundice and/or anaemia?** If there is jaundice (with or without anaemia), consider haemolytic problems such as spherocytosis and glucose 6 phosphate dehydrogenase (G6PD) deficiency. In chronic anaemia, consider thalassaemia. Have a higher index of suspicion in children from Mediterranean backgrounds
4. **Is there a history of joint pain, eye problems or unusual rashes?** This suggests an inflammatory or rheumatological problem, e.g. systemic lupus erythematosus (SLE), juvenile idiopathic arthritis (JIA)

Common Diagnosis 4
Diagnosis: Hepatomegaly

Questions
1. **Does the child have nausea and/or loss of appetite?** Hepatomegaly does not necessarily mean that the function of the liver will be impaired; however, if it is, these are the most common initial symptoms. Later symptoms include jaundice, tendency to bruise and bleed easily, ascites and progressive confusion
2. **Has there been recent fever, travel or new medication?** Fever might suggest acute infection causing liver swelling. Especially consider EBV if there is a sore throat, or hepatitis A if there is a history of travel. Though rare, some medications are hepatotoxic, e.g. aspirin causing Reye's syndrome
3. **Is there a risk of prenatal congenital infection?** Consider this if there was incomplete antenatal care or concern about symmetrical intrauterine growth restriction (IUGR)
4. **Is development progressing normally?** The lysosomal storage diseases that also cause hepatomegaly, e.g. Hunter syndrome or Tay–Sachs disease, are associated with marked neurodevelopmental delay
5. **Is there a family history of any inherited conditions?** Many inherited conditions can cause hepatomegaly. Cystic fibrosis is the most common genetic disease in the UK, and alongside the respiratory problems, many older children also develop hepatomegaly as a result of biliary obstruction and steatosis

Common Diagnosis 5
Diagnosis: Abdominal wall hernia

Questions
1. **Is there a history of a lump that 'comes and goes', especially noticeable when the child is crying, straining or coughing?** An abdominal wall hernia will protrude further when intra-abdominal pressure is raised

2. Has the lump ever become stuck? Has there been associated pain or vomiting? Any hernia has the potential to become irreducible, though inguinal hernias are generally the highest risk. Consider an incarcerated hernia in any child with gastrointestinal obstruction, especially if there is a prior history of a lump

5.2.6 KEY EXAMINATION FEATURES

Box 5.2.15   Key Points to Consider When Examining a Mass

- Where is the mass?
- Is it tender?
- What size is it (in finger breadths or cm)?
- Are the contours smooth or irregular?
- Is it hard, soft or fluctuant?

- Does it move, for example with inspiration?
- Is it ballotable?
- Is it dull or resonant to percussion?
- Can you get above it and/or below it?
- Are any local lymph nodes (i.e. inguinal) enlarged?

Box 5.2.16   Examination Tips to Ensure a Soft and Relaxed Tummy

- Ideally the child should be laid flat and kept distracted and relaxed
- For babies, sucking on a dummy/gloved finger or distracting with jingling keys may help. It may be beneficial to examine a baby's abdomen while they are feeding

- Young children may prefer to lie in their parents' arms and elicit a parent's help for distraction with songs/toys or sticker rewards
- Older children and teens will often relax while chatting about their interests during the examination

Dangerous Diagnosis 1
Diagnosis: Neuroblastoma

Examination Findings
1. **Child looks unwell and miserable.** At the time of presentation most children with neuroblastoma have lost weight and are in discomfort due to the mass and/or circulating catecholamines
2. **Usually a flank mass.** Two-thirds of abdominal neuroblastomas arise from the adrenal glands. The mass is usually non-tender, firm and irregular, may cross the midline and may be ballotable. The remainder of abdominal neuroblastomas will arise from sympathetic nervous tissue elsewhere in the abdomen
3. **Check for neurological or ocular signs and closely examine the skin.** Neuroblastoma is associated with a wide variety of clinical findings based on the point of origin of the tumour, and these should be closely examined for

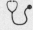

Box 5.2.17   Locations of Neuroblastoma

- Adrenal glands: 35%
- Retroperitoneum: 30–35%
- Mediastinum: 20%

- Neck: 1–5%
- Pelvis: 2–3%

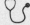

Box 5.2.18   Neuroblastoma: Signs Based on Tumour Site

Tumour location	Features
Abdomen	Abdominal mass, constipation, difficulty passing urine
Chest or neck	Palpable mass, breathlessness, difficulty in swallowing
Spinal cord	Weakness in the legs from cord compression

Dangerous Diagnosis 2
Diagnosis: Wilms' Tumour

Examination Findings
1. **Child looks well.** In contrast to neuroblastoma, despite often presenting with a very large mass, children with Wilms' tumour look surprisingly well
2. **Hypertension and haematuria.** Roughly a quarter of patients with Wilms' tumour have high blood pressure at diagnosis – be aware that there are age- and height-specific ranges for blood pressure. Painless macroscopic haematuria is often seen
3. **Flank mass, can get above and below it, does not cross the midline.** Unlike masses arising from the liver and spleen, you can usually feel the upper margin of a renal mass under the ribs, and the inferior margin may be palpated as low down as the pelvis
4. **Mass may be ballotable, but does not move with inspiration.** The mass will be felt to move upwards with bimanual palpation (balloting) of the abdomen, with one hand over the mass and the other at the renal angle gently pressing up

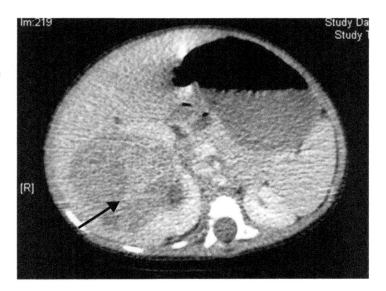

Figure 5.2.4 Wilms' tumour. Computed tomography (CT) abdomen showing a right-sided Wilms' tumour. Compare with the normal-sized left kidney. This child presented with a distended abdomen with no other symptoms. Note the obvious increase in abdominal girth from left to right. An ultrasound showed a renal mass suspicious of Wilms' and the CT gave more details, which until surgery and definitive histology were adequate to confirm the diagnosis.

Dangerous Diagnosis 3
Diagnosis: Other Malignancy

Examination Findings
1. **Non-mobile mass.** A fixed structure within the abdomen suggests invasion of local tissues and should raise alarm bells for malignancy
2. **Systemic features.** Cachexia, bruising, pallor, recurrent infections and bone pain are all systemic features associated with malignancy

---

Box 5.2.19   Special Considerations in Girls with Abdominal Masses   △△

- Ovarian cysts are common in neonates and are usually benign and undergo spontaneous regression
- In older girls, ovarian cysts may be associated with early puberty or malignancy
- In any girl with acute abdominal pain and a lower abdominal mass, consider ovarian torsion
- Ovarian tumours can occur in children

- In newborn girls, high levels of maternal circulating oestrogen result in cervical secretions, which can accumulate behind an intact hymen in the vaginal canal, causing a hydrometrocolpos
- Very rarely, in adolescent girls, menstrual blood can accumulate behind an imperforate hymen in the vaginal canal, resulting in cyclical abdominal pain and haematocolpos

Common Diagnosis 1
Diagnosis: Hydronephrosis

Examination Findings
1. **Flank mass.** It is possible to get above and below the mass and it should not cross the midline
2. **Mass may be ballotable.** A renal mass is ballotable and does not move with inspiration
3. **Unilateral or bilateral.** Depending on the pathology, hydronephrosis could be unilateral or bilateral. If there is obstruction low in the urinary tract, you may also feel a bladder mass

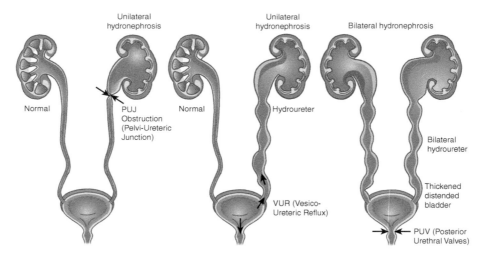

Figure 5.2.5 Different causes of hydronephrosis.

Common Diagnosis 2
Diagnosis: Constipation

Examination Findings
1. **Left lower quadrant mass.** The mass is usually palpated in the descending colon, although occasionally felt elsewhere in the abdomen with significant faecal loading
2. **Mobile mass.** The colon is considerably mobile and can often be rolled by the examiner's fingers
3. **Not tender.** Despite cramping abdominal pain associated with constipation, the mass itself is not tender

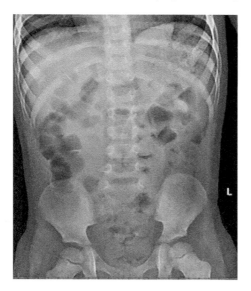

Figure 5.2.6 Faecal loading. Abdominal radiograph showing faecal loading in the rectum and all along the descending colon. Note the patchy fluffy appearance of stool compared to the emptier gas-filled bowel on the right. This child had a left-sided mobile mass and presented with abdominal pain. Soiling may give the false perception that bowel movements are regular. Normally, an x-ray is not indicated for constipation, but may be performed if there is diagnostic uncertainty.

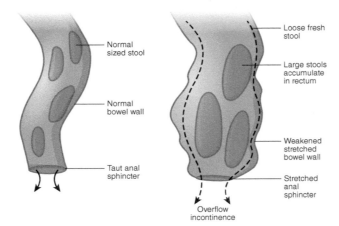

Figure 5.2.7 A depiction of a normal rectum showing normal stool collection (left). Chronic constipation leads to a distended rectum, with a weakened bowel wall, capable of holding larger quantities of stool (right). Propulsion of stools is limited by the weakened bowel wall. The stretched anal sphincter allows fresh loose stool to leak around impacted stool as overflow incontinence.

Common Diagnosis 3
Diagnosis: Splenomegaly

Examination Findings
1. **Cannot get above the mass.** The spleen is in the left upper quadrant and its superior margin is under the ribs so cannot be felt, though it can be percussed
2. **Moves diagonally toward the right iliac fossa with inspiration.** For this reason, begin your palpation for an enlarged spleen in the right iliac fossa. Additionally, the spleen has a notch that may be palpable
3. **Anaemia, jaundice, lymphadenopathy.** Anaemia and jaundice are consistent with underlying haemolysis, whereas lymphadenopathy may indicate an infectious, inflammatory or infiltrative aetiology
4. **Co-existing signs.** A targeted examination of other systems (e.g. cardiac, musculoskeletal) may reveal the underlying cause

Common Diagnosis 4
Diagnosis: Hepatomegaly

Examination Findings
1. **Cannot get above the mass.** The liver is in the right upper quadrant and its superior margin is under the ribs so cannot be felt, although it can be percussed
2. **Moves downwards toward the right iliac fossa with inspiration.** For this reason, begin your palpation for an enlarged liver in the right iliac fossa. Depending on the underlying pathology, the liver may be smooth or craggy
3. **Generalised lymphadenopathy, jaundice, ascites.** If you are confident you are feeling an enlarged liver, this will help you determine the underlying pathology

Common Diagnosis 5
Diagnosis: Abdominal wall hernia

Examination Findings
1. **Superficial mass, which should be reducible.** On palpation, this should be reducible. An irreducible (incarcerated) hernia should prompt an urgent surgical review
2. **Bowel sounds may be auscultated over the mass.** Most hernias contain bowel and auscultating is an easy way to confirm this
3. **May extend into the scrotum in boys.** Inguinal hernias in children are usually termed 'indirect' and result from congenitally patent processus vaginalis, the embryonic structure through which the testes descend. The hernia can follow this path and cause groin or scrotal swelling

5.2.7 KEY INVESTIGATIONS

Not all children will require invasive investigations; often diagnoses are made on clinical evidence from history and examination. Consider carefully which investigations are required for which patient.

Bedside

Table 5.2.1 Bedside tests of use in patients presenting with an abdominal mass

Test	When to perform	Potential result
Urine dipstick	Suspected: • Hydronephrosis with UTI • Renal mass, e.g. Wilms' tumour	• Nitrites and leukocytes suggest UTI • Haematuria may suggest Wilms' tumour
Urine culture	• If positive urine dipstick	• Positive culture indicates bacterial infection • Sensitivities guide antibiotic choice
Urine βHCG	• All post-pubertal girls	• Positive test confirms pregnancy
BP	Suspected: • Wilms' tumour • Hydronephrosis • Neuroblastoma	• ↑ BP seen in Wilms' tumour and neuroblastoma, or renal damage from hydronephrosis

BP, blood pressure; HCG, human chorionic gonadotropin; UTI, urinary tract infection

Blood Tests

Table 5.2.2 Blood tests of use in patients presenting with an abdominal mass

Test	When to perform	Potential result
FBC	Suspected: • Malignancy • Haematological disorders causing splenomegaly	• Pancytopenia: bone marrow failure, suggestive of malignancy • Anaemia with raised reticulocyte count consistent with haemolysis
Blood film	Suspected: • Malignancy • Haematological disorders causing splenomegaly	• Peripheral blasts indicate leukaemia • Abnormal red cell morphology may indicate underlying haematological disorder (e.g. SCD, HS)
U&E	Suspected: • Malignancy • Hydronephrosis	• ↑ Urea/creatinine suggests renal dysfunction in hydronephrosis or renal tumours
LFTs	Suspected: • Malignancy • Hepatomegaly • Splenomegaly	• Deranged liver enzymes in many of the listed causes of hepatomegaly • ↑ Bilirubin in haemolytic disorders
Blood culture	• Suspected sepsis (may be seen with appendix mass or UTI)	• Positive culture indicates bacterial infection • Sensitivities guide antibiotic choice
Urate and LDH	• Suspected malignancy	• ↑ Urate and LDH indicate high cell turnover
Viral serology	• Suspected viral cause of hepatomegaly or splenomegaly	• Positive result indicates infection (e.g. CMV, rubella, hepatitis A/B/C/D/E, EBV)
AFP	• Suspected hepatic malignancy	• ↑ Titres in hepatoblastoma and hepatocellular carcinoma
Autoimmune screen	• If strong clinical suspicion of autoimmune disorder as a cause for splenomegaly	• Autoantibodies such as ANA, anti-dsDNA, anti-Ro, anti-La may support the diagnosis of SLE, JIA

AFP, alpha-fetoprotein; ANA, antinuclear antibody; CMV, cytomegalovirus; dsDNA, double-stranded DNA; EBV, Epstein–Barr virus; FBC, full blood count; HS, hereditary spherocytosis; JIA, juvenile idiopathic arthritis; LDH, lactate dehydrogenase; LFTs, liver function tests; SCD, sickle cell disease; SLE, systemic lupus erythematosus; U&E, urea and electrolytes; UTI, urinary tract infection

Imaging

Table 5.2.3 Imaging modalities of use in patients presenting with an abdominal mass

Test	When to perform	Potential result
Abdominal/ pelvic/ renal ultrasound	• All children with abdominal mass unless evidence of constipation	• Characterisation and often diagnosis of abdominal masses, including cystic/solid components
Abdominal x-ray	• Consider in all children with abdominal mass unless evidence of constipation, if ultrasound non-diagnostic	• Bowel obstruction (hernia, appendix mass): dilated loops • Perforation (appendix mass): free air/fluid • Neuroblastoma: calcification may be seen • Constipation: x-ray should not be required to diagnose, but will demonstrate faecal loading
Chest x-ray	• Suspected malignancy	• Lymphadenopathy or metastases within the chest
CT abdomen or MRI abdomen	• To further evaluate masses after ultrasound	• Can provide an accurate diagnosis
MCUG in <1-year-old	• Suspected hydronephrosis to look for VUR	• Confirms VUR and grades severity
DMSA scan (nuclear medicine)	• Suspected hydronephrosis to determine renal function/scars	• Differential renal function will determine plan for surveillance or surgery
Mag 3 scan (nuclear medicine)	• Suspected hydronephrosis to assess the drainage of the kidneys/diagnose obstructions	• Will identify PUJ, VUJ obstructions, grade severity, to determine plans for surveillance or surgery

CT, computed tomography; DMSA, dimercaptosuccinic acid; MCUG, micturating cystourethrogram; MRI, magnetic resonance imaging; PUJ, pelvi-ureteric junction; VUJ, vesico-ureteric junction; VUR, vesico-ureteric reflux

Special

Table 5.2.4 Special tests of use in patients presenting with an abdominal mass

Test	When to perform	Potential result
Urine catecholamine studies	• Vanillylmandelic acid (VMA) and homovanillic acid (HVA) are products of catecholamine breakdown by neuroblastoma cells • Highly sensitive and specific for neuroblastoma	• Raised VMA or HVA in neuroblastoma

---

Box 5.2.20   Urinalysis in Children

- Babies and young children will not pass urine on demand
- Obtaining a urine sample is no small feat and requires patience and time
- It is important to ensure families understand the principles of a 'clean catch' to avoid contamination of the sample
- It may be appropriate to collect urine using an in/out catheter or by suprapubic aspiration

- Even when suffering from a urinary tract infection, babies may not reliably produce 'dipstick-positive' samples. Always ensure urine is sent for culture and request a 'forced culture', as they may not produce enough white cells to reach the threshold for culture in some labs

5.2.8 KEY MANAGEMENT PRINCIPLES

Diagnosis-specific management strategies are outlined here. It is expected that an 'ABCDE' approach to assessment and management is always undertaken (see Chapter 12.1, *The A to E Assessment*).

Dangerous Diagnosis 1
Diagnosis: Neuroblastoma

Management Principles
1. **Refer to tertiary paediatric oncology unit.** Further investigations and management will be undertaken in a tertiary centre
2. **Biopsy.** Biopsy confirms the diagnosis, either by incisional biopsy of the primary tumour or bone marrow aspiration if metastasis is suspected
3. **Staging of disease.** Staging is required to determine prognosis and treatment, using the International Neuroblastoma Risk Group Staging System. Further imaging includes computed tomography (CT), magnetic resonance imaging (MRI) with contrast and MIBG scan
4. **Risk stratification.** Risk stratification guides intensity of management and includes stage of disease, tumour ploidy, MYCN gene status, histopathological appearances and patient age
5. **Definitive treatment.** Treatment is complex, variable and beyond the scope of this chapter. It can involve surgery, radiation therapy, chemotherapy, stem cell rescue, autologous bone marrow transplantation, immunotherapy, isotretinoin and many other combinations. Overall survival at 5 years is roughly 80%, though in high-risk groups it is less than 50%

Box 5.2.21   MIBG Scan

- Radioisotope diagnostic nuclear medicine test
- MIBG (metaiodobenzylguanidine), a noradrenaline analogue, is labelled with radio-iodine

- Uptake by neuroblastoma cells is monitored with a gamma camera

---

Dangerous Diagnosis 2
Diagnosis: Wilms' tumour

Management Principles
1. **Nephrectomy.** If one kidney is affected, the whole kidney is surgically removed. If both kidneys are involved, then only the affected parts are removed. A nephrectomy allows for staging of the Wilms' and determination of further treatment
2. **Chemotherapy.** Neoadjuvant chemotherapy is usually given before the nephrectomy to reduce the size of the tumour. Post-operatively chemotherapy is also given. Duration depends on the stage and histology of the tumour
3. **Radiotherapy.** Not all patients require radiotherapy. However, if the histology is high risk, there is evidence of spread or the stage of the disease is high, then radiotherapy is usually indicated
4. **Prognostication.** Prognosis is good, with 5-year survival approaching 90%

Dangerous Diagnosis 3
Diagnosis: Other Malignancy

Management Principles
1. **Urgent referral to oncology.** Detailed initial blood tests may be required, for example viral screening. Hyperhydration, allopurinol and rasburicase may all be considered if tumour lysis is suspected

Common Diagnosis 1
Diagnosis: Hydronephrosis

Management Principles
1. **Ensure prompt treatment of UTI.** Families should be taught to identify the signs of UTI and the importance of sending urine for analysis if there is any suspicion of infection. If clinical suspicion arises in a child with known GU abnormalities, always send urine for culture regardless of the dipstick results and start antibiotics promptly

2. Specialist follow-up. Children with hydronephrosis and other GU tract abnormalities are at risk of recurrent infections, deteriorating renal function and hypertension. They should be referred to paediatric specialists who may consider:

- Antibiotic prophylaxis
- Imaging to detect the cause of hydronephrosis
- Surgery to prevent complications

Box 5.2.22   Indications for Surgery in Hydronephrosis

- Non-functioning kidney, e.g. multicystic dysplastic kidney
- Posterior urethral valves
- Marked ± persistent pelvi-ureteric junction (PUJ) obstruction

- Marked ± persistent vesico-ureteric junction (VUJ) obstruction
- Severe ± persistent vesico-ureteric reflux (VUR)

Figure 5.2.8 Micturating cystourethrogram (MCUG) done to evaluate the cause of left-sided hydronephrosis. The child is catheterised and a radio-opaque dye is inserted into the bladder. X-rays are taken as the child empties their bladder. Here, during urination there is backflow into the ureter and all the way up to the distended left kidney – this is grade 4 vesico-ureteric reflux (VUR). This (male) child also had an abnormal urinary stream due to phimosis and you can see urine pooling under the foreskin at the bottom of the image.

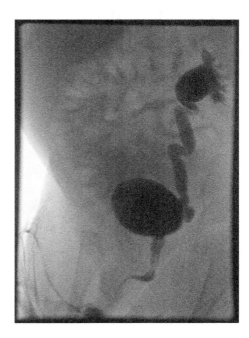

Figure 5.2.9 A dimercaptosuccinic acid (DMSA) scan was done to evaluate the same child's renal function. This is a nuclear medicine scan looking for renal uptake of an injected tracer. The left kidney has patchy uptake of the tracer, indicating renal scarring. Overall function of the left kidney was estimated at 36%.

Left   Right

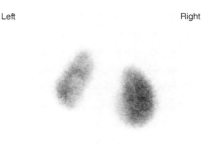

Common Diagnosis 2
Diagnosis: Constipation

Management Principles
1. **Disimpaction.** The presence of a faecal mass suggests there is faecal loading and possible impaction. Consider a disimpaction regime of laxatives. Rarely, hospital admission for disimpaction with stronger laxatives is needed. If there is no convincing faecal impaction, maintenance treatment for constipation is more appropriate
2. **Dietary and lifestyle advice.** Education is key and multidisciplinary input, especially from dieticians, can have a big impact. Incontinence services can help with behavioural modification and family support. Attention to fluid intake, a balanced diet and adequate daily exercise is beneficial. Online resources are useful to guide healthy diet and lifestyle choices

Box 5.2.23 Paediatric Movicol Disimpaction Regime and Ongoing Maintenance			
Age range	Child 1–5 years (Number of sachets)	Child 5–12 years (Number of sachets)	Child >12 years (Number of sachets)
Day 1	2	4	4
Day 2	4	6	6
Day 3	4	8	8
Day 4	6	10	8
Day 5	6	12	8
Day 6	8	12	8
Day 7	8	12	8

Note: Total daily dose should be taken over a 12-hour period. Disimpaction is achieved when type 7 stools on the Bristol Stool Chart are passed for at least 24 hours. Once achieved, reduce Movicol dose to maintenance dose - 2 sachets per day. Source: Adapted from National Institute for Health and Care Excellence (2017). Constipation in children and young people: diagnosis and management. Clinical guideline [CG99]. London: NICE. Movicol is a brand name for macrogol.

Common Diagnosis 3
Diagnosis: Splenomegaly

Management Principles
1. **Wide potential differential – management depends on cause.** An ultrasound can be a helpful starting point. Most causes will require discussion with haematology or oncology as appropriate

Common Diagnosis 4
Diagnosis: Hepatomegaly

Management Principles
1. **Wide potential differential – management depends on cause.** An ultrasound can be a helpful starting point. Discussion with a regional liver team can help guide further 'liver screen' tests

Common Diagnosis 5
Diagnosis: Abdominal wall hernia

Management Principles
1. **Inguinal hernias are likely to incarcerate, so warrant surgical referral.** The highest risk is in the first year of life, so refer babies with suspected inguinal hernias urgently. Older children in whom the hernia has always been reducible and asymptomatic can be referred routinely, but ensure families are aware of signs of incarceration
2. **Reassure parents of young children with umbilical hernias.** Umbilical hernias rarely incarcerate and usually close spontaneously by 4 years. Only consider referral to a surgical outpatient clinic if persisting beyond 4 years or if particularly large or troublesome
3. **Resuscitation and immediate surgical referral if signs of obstruction.** Tissues within a strangulated hernia can rapidly become non-viable and ischaemic. The bowel trapped can cause gastrointestinal obstruction. These children can become seriously unwell and need ABCDE assessment, intravenous access and often fluid resuscitation. Surgery is the definitive management
4. **Seek surgical advice for other hernias.** Incisional hernias may appear around previous surgical scars, and other possible hernias of the abdominal wall include epigastric and spigelian hernias

5.3 Vomiting

Samantha White

Department of Paediatrics, Wexham Park Hospital, NHS Frimley Health Foundation Trust, UK

CONTENTS

5.3.1 CHAPTER AT A GLANCE

Box 5.3.1   Chapter at a Glance

- Vomiting in children is not uncommon and is often not a serious sign
- The most common cause of vomiting in children is gastroenteritis, which is usually accompanied by diarrhoea

- More serious conditions can cause vomiting, however, and if the parents are concerned a thorough evaluation is necessary to rule these out

5.3.2 DEFINITION

- Vomiting is the expulsion of gastric contents from the mouth, which is usually forceful in nature
- Nausea is the unpleasant sensation of expecting to vomit; sometimes it precedes vomiting, but it can be an isolated symptom

Clinical Guide to Paediatrics, First Edition. Edited by Rachel Varughese and Anna Mathew. Series Editor: Christian Fielder Camm.
© 2022 John Wiley & Sons Ltd. Published 2022 by John Wiley & Sons Ltd.
Companion website: www.wiley.com/go/varughese/paediatrics

5.3.3 DIAGNOSTIC ALGORITHM

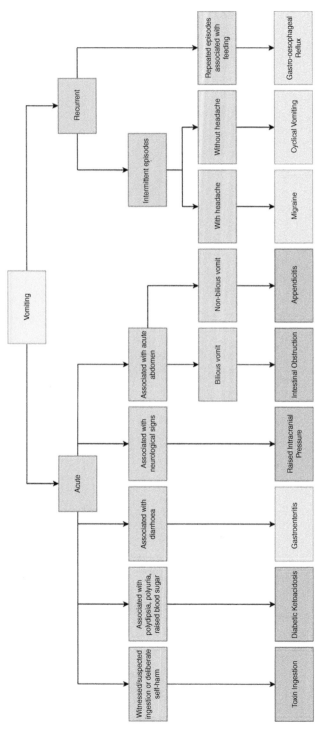

Figure 5.3.1 Diagnostic algorithm for the presentation of vomiting.

5.3.4 DIFFERENTIALS LIST

Dangerous Diagnoses

1. Intestinal Obstruction
- Obstruction along the gastrointestinal tract, which can be mechanical or functional
- The obstruction may be compressing the bowel from outside, lying within the bowel wall or within the lumen of the bowel
- Common symptoms are vomiting, abdominal pain and distension
- A surgical emergency requiring prompt evaluation to intervene before perforation of the bowel occurs
- The level of obstruction will dictate whether the vomiting is bilious
- Intussusception and volvulus are discussed separately in Chapter 5.1

2. Toxin Ingestion
- This can occur as a result of accidental ingestion by a toddler, deliberate ingestion by an older child or due to a medication error
- Overdose of some substances can be fatal and it is important to recognise and treat promptly
- Potential agents are opioids, non-steroidal anti-inflammatory drugs (NSAIDs), antibiotics, chemotherapy drugs, carbon monoxide, iron, paracetamol, antidepressants and ethanol. Also household items: cleaning fluids and solutions, and plants

---

Box 5.3.2   Causes of Intestinal Obstruction in Childhood   △△

Age of child	Causes
Infancy	• Hypertrophic pyloric stenosis • Duodenal atresia • Other bowel atresias: jejunal, ileal • Meconium ileus • Malrotation leading to volvulus • Hirschsprung disease
Older children	• Intussusception • Appendicitis • Incarcerated/strangulated hernias • Strictures (Crohn's disease) • Adhesions (post surgery) • Ileus • Foreign bodies, ingested (bezoars etc.) • Functional constipation • Distal intestinal obstruction syndrome

---

3. Raised Intracranial Pressure (ICP)
- Raised ICP may be secondary to a space-occupying lesion such as a brain tumour or bleed
- Meningitis, causing inflammation of the meninges, is another important cause of raised ICP to consider
- Vomiting can indicate an acute rise in ICP
- In babies whose cranial sutures have not fused, their skull can enlarge to accommodate rising pressure, but this is not the case in older children
- Raised ICP is covered in detail in Chapters 8.1 and 8.6. It will not be discussed further in this chapter

5. Diabetic Ketoacidosis (DKA)
- DKA occurs when cellular glucose uptake is impaired by insufficient insulin. The body switches to burning fatty acids, producing acidic ketone bodies
- Diagnostic triad of acidosis (pH <7.3), hyperglycaemia >11 mmol/L and ketonaemia >3 mmol/L
- Can be life-threatening. Must be managed with care to avoid cerebral oedema
- DKA is covered in detail in Chapter 7.2, and will not be discussed further in this chapter

6. Appendicitis
- Appendicitis is inflammation of the appendix, which is a small pouch connected to the colon at the level of the caecum
- May present as an 'acute abdomen'
- 75% of children with appendicitis have nausea and vomiting
- Appendicitis is covered in detail in Chapter 5.1, and will not be discussed further in this chapter

Box 5.3.3   Causes of Raised Intracranial Pressure in Childhood   △△

- Traumatic brain injury
- Meningitis/encephalitis
- Brain tumours
- Vascular malformations
- Intracerebral haemorrhage
- Pseudotumor cerebrii (idiopathic intracranial hypertension)

- Hydrocephalus
- Venous sinus thrombosis
- Systemic illness: systemic lupus erythematosus, Cushing's disease, adrenal insufficiency, renal and liver disease
- Craniosynostosis

Common Diagnoses

1. Gastroenteritis
- This is an acute cause of diarrhoea and vomiting in children
- 70% of cases are caused by viruses, which can be highly contagious, with the remainder caused by bacteria or parasites
- Illness is usually short-lived and self-resolving
- Mainstay of management is in preventing and treating dehydration, although antimicrobials are useful in bacterial and parasitic illnesses

2. Gastro-oesophageal Reflux (GOR)
- Affects around 40% of healthy infants, particularly before 1 year of age, and improves as the baby gets older
- Effortless regurgitation of milk into the oesophagus, which may then spill out of the mouth
- Simple GOR is benign, whereas gastro-oesophageal reflux disease (GORD) causes adverse effects and can be associated with faltering growth and persist into later childhood

3. Cyclical Vomiting
- Idiopathic episodic vomiting with symptom-free periods in between
- It should be a diagnosis of exclusion
- Can affect up to 2% of children, typically of school age
- Females are more commonly affected than males
- Episodes may be triggered by inter-current illness or psychological stressors

4. Cow's Milk Protein Allergy (CMPA)
- Most common food allergy in young children, caused by an immune reaction to cow's milk protein, which can be immunoglobulin (Ig) E or non-IgE mediated
- IgE-mediated reactions have immediate onset, whereas non-IgE-mediated reactions are usually delayed, sometimes by up to 48 hours
- If left undiagnosed, repetitive vomiting can lead to faltering growth

Box 5.3.4   Signs and Symptoms of Immunoglobulin (Ig) E versus non-IgE Cow's Milk Protein Allergy

	IgE		Non-IgE	
	Mild to moderate	Severe	Mild to moderate	Severe
Onset	Within 2 hours, often immediate		Within 48 hours	
Gastrointestinal	Vomiting Diarrhoea Abdominal pain/colic	Vomiting Diarrhoea Abdominal pain/colic	Reflux/vomiting Food refusal/aversion Abdominal pain/colic Diarrhoea Constipation Flatulence Blood/mucous in stools	Reflux/vomiting Food refusal/aversion Abdominal pain/colic Diarrhoea Constipation Flatulence Significant blood/mucous in stools Faltering growth
Skin	Pruritus Erythema Mild urticaria Mild angioedema Atopic eczema	Severe urticaria Severe angioedema	Pruritus Erythema Atopic eczema	Severe eczema

Box 5.3.4 (Continued)

	IgE		Non-IgE	
	Mild to moderate	**Severe**	**Mild to moderate**	**Severe**
Respiratory	Acute rhinitis Conjunctivitis	Cough Wheeze Shortness of breath Anaphylaxis	–	–

Source: Adapted from National Institute for Health and Care Excellence (2011). Food allergy in under 19s: assessment and diagnosis. Clinical guideline [CG116]. London: NICE.

5. Migraine
- Periodic episodes of headache that are usually one sided and can be associated with nausea, vomiting, photophobia and phonophobia
- There is a genetic preponderance and may be a positive family history
- Although classic migraines include an 'aura' with visual disturbances before the pain starts, migraines without an aura are more common
- Migraine is covered in detail in Chapter 8.1, and will not be discussed further in this chapter

Box 5.3.5 Non-gastrointestinal Infections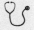

Vomiting can be a non-specific finding in children (particularly under-5s) and may be associated with non-gastrointestinal infections such as urinary tract infections, pneumonia, tonsillitis and otitis media

Diagnoses to Consider
1. Inborn Errors of Metabolism (IEM)
- Defects in metabolic enzymes lead to build-up of toxic metabolites
- Many IEMs cause faltering growth, due to an inability to utilise substrates in food, as a result of enzymatic defects
- Since correct treatment can be lifesaving, many are screened for on the day 5 newborn blood spot test
- IEMs are often autosomal recessive in inheritance and very rare, so the incidence increases in consanguineous families

When to consider: in a child who presents with hypoglycaemia in response to a minor illness. There may be a history of a sibling who died from a metabolic disease or an unknown cause

Box 5.3.6 Newborn Screening Programme (Blood Spot), UK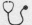

- Sickle cell disease
- Cystic fibrosis
- Congenital hypothyroidism
- Inherited metabolic disease:
- Phenylketonuria
- Medium-chain acyl-CoA dehydrogenase deficiency
- Maple syrup urine disease
- Isovaleric acidaemia
- Glutaric acidura type 1
- Homocystinuria (pyridoxine unresponsive)

Box 5.3.7 Pregnancy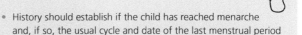

- Vomiting is associated with pregnancy, particularly in the first trimester
- It is classically described as morning sickness, but can occur at any time of the day
- This should always be considered in post-pubertal girls

- History should establish if the child has reached menarche and, if so, the usual cycle and date of the last menstrual period
- Questions about sexual activity might best be asked without parents present. Enquire about the age of the partner and establish whether there are safeguarding issues

5.3.5 KEY HISTORY FEATURES

Dangerous Diagnosis 1
Diagnosis: Intestinal obstruction

Questions
1. **What colour is the vomit?** Green bilious vomit suggests mechanical obstruction, at or distal to the duodenum. A proximal gastrointestinal obstruction above the level of the ampulla of Vater (where bile drains into the duodenum) will be non-bilious
2. **When did the child last open their bowels and are they passing flatus?** Children with intestinal obstruction will be unable to open bowels or pass flatus
3. **What is the character of the vomiting?** Projectile vomiting in babies around 6 weeks of age raises the likelihood of hypertrophic pyloric stenosis (note this vomiting is not bilious)
4. **Is there abdominal pain?** Abdominal pain is a cardinal sign of intestinal obstruction and is often colicky in nature, due to peristalsis at the site of obstruction
5. **How long after birth did they open their bowels?** Neonates should pass meconium within 48 hours of delivery. Delayed passage of meconium can be caused by Hirschsprung disease: an innervation disorder caused by absence of the ganglion cells in the myenteric and submucosal plexus, leading to functional obstruction
6. **Is there a history of previous abdominal surgery?** Patients who have previously undergone abdominal surgery are more likely to form adhesions. Adhesions allow the bowel to kink or twist, causing a total or partial obstruction of the intestine

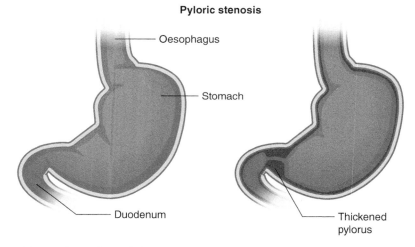

Pyloric stenosis

Oesophagus

Stomach

Duodenum

Thickened pylorus

Figure 5.3.2 Pyloric stenosis is a condition affecting babies at around 6 weeks. A thickened pyloric muscle prevents gastric emptying, and may be palpated as an olive-shaped mass in the epigastrium.

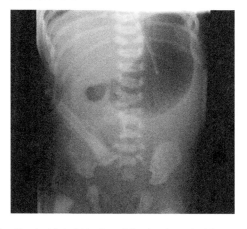

Figure 5.3.3 Abdominal x-ray demonstrating the double bubble sign of duodenal atresia. Many patients will also have associated anomalies. In this case, vertebral anomalies of the spine can also be seen.

Dangerous Diagnosis 2

Diagnosis: Toxin ingestion

Questions

1. **Has the child ingested a known substance?** Ingestion may be witnessed, or presumed, after finding a small child with empty medicine packets. It is important to know both the dose and the timing of the ingestion, where possible
2. **Does an older child have a history of low mood or self-harm?** Deliberate self-harm is seen mostly in teenagers and can be a cry for help or a suicide attempt. They may have left a note or may disclose self-poisoning. This should also be suspected in an unwell child with a background of mental health difficulties who does not make a disclosure

Common Diagnosis 1

Diagnosis: Gastroenteritis

Questions

1. **Has the child had diarrhoea?** Think about gastroenteritis in a child who suddenly develops vomiting and loose, watery stools. There may or may not be a history of fever
2. **How long have symptoms been present?** Gastroenteritis is usually an acute cause of vomiting and diarrhoea. The vomiting typically lasts between 1 and 2 days and usually resolves within 3. The diarrhoea may persist longer and in most children lasts for 5–7 days and usually resolves within 2 weeks
3. **Are any other family members also affected?** Viral gastroenteritis is highly contagious and may spread through a family. Food poisoning is also possible, and in the UK could be either bacterial or viral in origin (parasitic causes are more common in tropical countries). Infection is usually transmitted through ingesting undercooked meat, unpasteurised milk and untreated water
4. **Is there a history of foreign travel?** More likely to indicate a bacterial/parasitic cause of gastroenteritis and a stool sample should be considered

Box 5.3.8 Causes of Gastroenteritis		△△
Causative organism	**Incubation period**	**Duration of symptoms**
Campylobacter (most common in the UK)	2–5 days	Less than a week
Salmonella	12–72 hours	4–7 days
Listeria	Few days to several weeks	Within 3 days
Escherichia Coli (E. Coli)	1–8 days	Days to weeks
Shigella	Within 7 days	Up to a week
Viruses: rotavirus, norovirus	24–48 hours	Couple of days
Parasites: giardiasis, cryptosporidiosis, amoebiasis (uncommon in the UK)	Within 10 days	Weeks to months, depending on treatment

Common Diagnosis 2

Diagnosis: Gastro-oesophageal reflux

Questions

1. **How old is the child?** GOR is a very common symptom in infancy, with the majority of babies outgrowing this tendency by 1 year of age
2. **What is the character of the vomiting?** In GOR there is effortless regurgitation of feeds, which is not projectile. The vomit should not be bilious or blood stained and should consist of milk feeds
3. **When does the vomiting occur?** Usually the vomiting happens soon after feeding
4. **Is the baby otherwise well and thriving?** Simple GOR should not cause other symptoms and the infant should be thriving

Common Diagnosis 3

Diagnosis: Cyclical vomiting

Questions

1. **How old is the child?** Cyclical vomiting can present at any age, but frequently between 3 and 7 years

2. **What is the pattern of vomiting?** The typical pattern is recurrent cycles of vomiting with periods of being well in between. The episodes themselves typically last for 1–2 days and children can have around 12 episodes per year, remaining symptom free in between. Consider the diagnosis after three distinct episodes. Individual children will develop their own pattern

3. **Are there any other symptoms?** Cyclical vomiting is a diagnosis of exclusion and other causes of vomiting should be considered first before making this diagnosis. Episodes can be very severe and require hospitalisation, but should be self-terminating

4. **Is there a family history of migraine?** There appears to be an association between cyclical vomiting and migraine. Family history for migraine is often positive. Children with cyclical vomiting often grow out of these episodes as they get older, but up to 75% go on to suffer from migraines (with some going through an intermediate stage of abdominal migraine)

Common Diagnosis 4

Diagnosis: Cow's milk protein allergy

Questions

1. **Is cow's milk included in the diet?** Find out if the baby has recently started having cow's milk in their diet. If breastfed, find out if the mother has dairy in her diet

2. **How soon after ingesting cow's milk do the symptoms appear?** IgE-mediated CMPA reactions occur immediately after ingestion. Non-IgE-mediated reactions are delayed and may take up to 48 hours to present

3. **Is there blood or mucous in the stool?** CMPA can lead to enteropathy and proctitis, which may present as loose stools, diarrhoea or streaks of blood and mucous on opening bowels. Occult blood loss also leads to iron-deficiency anaemia

4. **Has their growth been falling off the centile lines?** Severe CMPA can lead to faltering growth, due to food aversion, diarrhoea, vomiting and colitis causing malabsorption

5. **Are there any associated respiratory symptoms?** Angioedema, upper respiratory tract symptoms of rhinorrhoea/congestion, and lower respiratory tract symptoms of difficulty in breathing, wheeze or cough are all associated with IgE-mediated reactions. There is a risk of anaphylaxis in these patients, and presence of these symptoms will direct investigations and management

5.3.6 KEY EXAMINATION FEATURES

Dangerous Diagnosis 1

Diagnosis: Intestinal obstruction

Examination Findings

1. **Abdominal tenderness and distension.** The child may have an acute abdomen with peritonism. The abdomen is distended and tender

2. **Hyperactive/absent bowel sounds.** Bowel sounds are initially hyperactive as an obstruction progresses due to accumulation of fluid and gas build-up in the intestinal tract with increased peristaltic movement. Later, bowel sounds become tinkling or absent. Important to listen for at least 2 minutes before concluding that bowel sounds are absent.

3. **Blood in the nappy.** 'Redcurrant jelly' stools, which contain fresh blood mixed with mucous, are the classic description seen in intussusception. This is a late sign and so is not always present

4. **Appears ravenously hungry.** The baby vomits immediately after feeds and then appears extremely hungry. This is a typical history of pyloric stenosis

Dangerous Diagnosis 2

Diagnosis: Toxin ingestion

Signs are extremely variable depending on the substance ingested. Examples of common signs, in addition to vomiting, are provided here.

Examination Findings

1. **Nausea, pallor, diaphoresis.** Paracetamol overdose may present with these or, alternatively, may have no signs at all. Very rarely, in late presentations there may be hypotension, abdominal pain and encephalopathy

2. **Altered mental status, slurred speech, loss of coordination, irregular breathing.** These are signs of alcohol poisoning. This is the leading of cause of toxin ingestion in the UK, especially among young people. Alcohol can often be smelt on the breath

3. **Low respiratory rate and pinpoint pupils.** These signs are suggestive of opiate toxicity. Clinical signs at presentation can vary depending on the dose and route of administration, but commonly include respiratory depression and pinpoint pupils

4. **Tachycardia, ataxia, delirium, urinary retention.** These signs may suggest tricyclic antidepressant overdose. A palpable bladder may be felt. In significant overdose there may be cardiac instability with arrhythmias, and neurological instability with coma and seizures

Common Diagnosis 1
Diagnosis: Gastroenteritis

Examination Findings
1. **Abdominal pain.** The child may have non-specific generalised abdominal discomfort on palpation. They should not have an acute abdomen and there should be no rebound tenderness or guarding
2. **Dehydration.** Depending on the preserved intake, volume losses and duration of illness, dehydration can range from mild to severe

Common Diagnosis 2
Diagnosis: Gastro-oesophageal reflux

Examination Findings
1. **Clinically well baby.** The baby should appear well with normal observations and no signs of dehydration or malnourishment. They are classically described as 'happy spitters' and should be thriving when plotted on an age-appropriate growth chart

Common Diagnosis 3
Diagnosis: Cyclical Vomiting

Examination Findings
1. **Dehydration.** Episodes can be severe and may lead to clinical dehydration or shock

Common Diagnosis 4
Diagnosis: Cow's milk protein allergy

Examination Findings
1. **Blood in the nappy.** Colitis often accompanies the enteropathy and fresh blood may be seen in the nappy
2. **Rash.** A variety of rashes can be seen, including erythema, atopic eczema or scratch marks from pruritus
3. **Faltering growth.** Plot on a growth chart to assess – this may demonstrate recent faltering growth

5.3.7 KEY INVESTIGATIONS

Not all children will require invasive investigations; often diagnoses are made on clinical evidence from history and examination. Consider carefully which investigations are required for which patient.

Bedside

Table 5.3.1 Bedside tests of use in patients presenting with vomiting

Test	When to perform	Potential result
Blood gas (capillary or venous)	• All children with significant vomiting	• ↑ pH, ↓ Cl, ↓K: hypochloraemic, hypokalaemic metabolic alkalosis indicates significant gastric losses, often seen in pyloric stenosis • ↓ pH, ↓ HCO₃, ↑ lactate: metabolic acidosis in sepsis, severe dehydration • pH 7.1–7.3: mild/moderate DKA • pH <7.1: severe DKA
Blood glucose	• All children with vomiting	• <2.6 mmol/L – hypoglycaemia in IEM, alcohol intoxication, ketotic hypoglycaemia, toxin ingestion • >10 – significant stress • >11 – consider DKA
Blood ketones	• All children with vomiting	• Ketones suggest catabolic state and need to be interpreted with blood glucose • Ketotic hypoglycaemia (↓ glucose, ↑ ketones) • DKA (↑ glucose, ↑ ketones)
Urine dip	• All children with vomiting	• Leucocytes, nitrites suggest urine infection • Glucose, ketones in DKA • Ketones in significant dehydration
Stool sample	• Suspected bacterial/parasitic gastroenteritis	• Identifies pathogens that need treating: *Campylobacter, Salmonella, Listeria, Escherichia Coli, Shigella, Giardia*
Urine βHCG	• All post-pubertal females	• Positive βHCG confirms pregnancy

Cl, chloride; DKA, diabetic ketoacidosis; HCG, human chorionic gonadotropin; HCO₃, bicarbonate; IEM, inborn errors of metabolism; K, potassium

Blood Tests

Table 5.3.2 Blood tests of use in patients presenting with vomiting

Test	When to perform	Potential result
FBC	• All patients with significant vomiting	• ↑ WCC, ↑ neutrophils: sepsis, appendicitis • ↑ Platelets: sepsis
CRP	• Patients with significant vomiting and suspected inflammatory cause	• Significant ↑ in bacterial infections • Less marked ↑ in viral infections
U&E	Patients with: • Signs of dehydration • DKA • Sepsis • Suspected toxin ingestion	• ↑ Urea/creatinine: acute kidney injury in dehydration, DKA, sepsis • ↑ Na: dehydration • ↓ K: gastric losses • ↓ Na: inappropriate ADH secretion (SIADH) in meningitis/encephalitis, sepsis • Various electrolyte disturbances in toxin ingestion
LFTs	• Suspected paracetamol overdose	• ↑ ALT is the most sensitive marker for liver injury
INR	• Suspected paracetamol overdose	• ↑ INR suggests liver impairment
Blood culture	• All systemically unwell children	• Positive culture confirms bacterial infection • Sensitivities guide antibiotic choice
RAST to CMP	• Suspected IgE-mediated milk allergy	• Specific IgE to CMP

ADH, antidiuretic hormone; ALT, alanine aminotransferase; CMP, cow's milk protein; CRP, C-reactive protein; DKA, diabetic ketoacidosis; FBC, full blood count; Ig, immunoglobulin; INR, international normalised ratio; K, potassium; LFTs, liver function tests; Na, sodium; RAST, radioallergosorbent test; SIADH, syndrome of inappropriate antidiuretic hormone; U&E, urea and electrolytes

Imaging

Table 5.3.3 Imaging modalities of use in patients presenting with vomiting

Test	When to perform	Potential result
Abdominal x-ray	• Suspected intestinal obstruction	• Obstruction: variety of signs including dilated loops proximally, absence of air distally, abnormal gas distribution (e.g. double bubble sign in duodenal atresia), soft tissue mass (e.g. intussusception) • Perforation: dilated bowel loops, fluid levels, free air
Abdominal ultrasound	Suspected: • Appendicitis if diagnostic uncertainty • Pyloric stenosis	• Appendicitis: inflamed appendix, free fluid in the peritoneum suggests rupture • Pyloric stenosis: thickened muscle with narrowed pyloric canal
CT head	• Suspected raised ICP • Usually quicker and easier to obtain than MRI, though involves radiation	• Identifies structural causes of ↑ ICP
MRI head	• Greater sensitivity than CT head at identifying causes of ↑ ICP • May require sedation	• Identifies causes of ↑ ICP, including structural causes and also some inflammatory and demyelinating lesions

CT, computed tomography; ICP, intracranial pressure; MRI, magnetic resonance imaging

Special

Table 5.3.4 Special tests of use in patients presenting with vomiting

Test	When to perform	Potential result
Upper GI contrast study	• Suspected upper GI obstruction	• Identification of obstruction
24-hour pH impedance monitoring	• Suspected significant GORD	• Reflux Index indicates severity of GORD
Drug screen, blood ± urine	• Blood paracetamol, alcohol, barbiturate levels • Urine for opiates, cocaine, methadone, benzodiazepines, amphetamines • Plasma paracetamol must be done 4 hours after ingestion, not before	• Presence and level of drugs will guide treatment

GI, gastrointestinal; GORD, gastro-oesophageal reflux disease

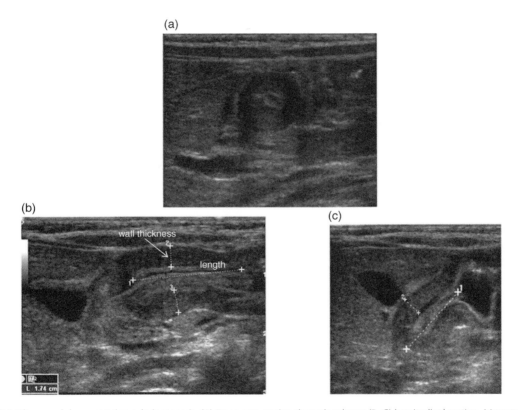

Figure 5.3.4 Ultrasound demonstrating pyloric stenosis. (A) Transverse section through pylorus; (B, C) longitudinal section. Measured layer should be <3 mm in thickness (one wall) and <15 mm in length (literature varies on this number – some say 17 mm). This patient had wall thickness of >4.1 mm and length of 17.4 mm.

5.3.8 KEY MANAGEMENT PRINCIPLES

Diagnosis-specific management strategies are outlined here. It is expected that an 'ABCDE' approach to assessment and management is considered standard practice (see Chapter 12.1, *The A to E Assessment*).

Management of dehydration with fluid replacement can be found in Chapter 12.3, *Tips for Fluid Prescribing*.

Dangerous Diagnosis 1

Diagnosis: Intestinal obstruction

Management Principles

1. **Nil by mouth and gastric decompression.** All patients should be kept nil by mouth and a nasogastric (NG) tube should be inserted to decompress the stomach and placed on free drainage. Output should be closely monitored, as NG losses may require replacement
2. **Fluid management and antibiotics.** Intravenous (IV) fluids for maintenance will be required as a minimum, with further fluids indicated as determined by clinical assessment of peripheral perfusion status and levels of hydration. The surgical team and local protocols will determine antibiotic administration
3. **Surgical intervention.** Referral should be made to the surgical team. Unstable patients may require emergency laparotomy

Dangerous Diagnosis 2

Diagnosis: Toxin ingestion

Management Principles

1. **Consult an appropriate poisons/toxicology resource (e.g. TOXBASE).** The national poisons database will give a detailed plan around which investigations and observations are required and can give advice on treatment. There may be a specific antidote to the ingested agent
2. **Manage electrolyte disturbances.** A variety of significant electrolyte disturbances can occur, as well as hypoglycaemia
3. **Inform the health visitor.** Parental education is important in the case of accidental ingestion of harmful substances by toddlers. Discuss locking medications away and keeping toxic substances out of children's reach. A home visit by the health visitor is likely to be beneficial to ensure a safe home environment for the child
4. **Child and Adolescent Mental Health Service (CAMHS) review.** Older children who have presented with deliberate self-poisoning should be reviewed by the CAMHS team prior to discharge to ensure that appropriate follow-up is in place, and that the child is safe for discharge.

Box 5.3.9   Management Principles for Paracetamol Overdose

- Treatment of paracetamol overdose can be complicated, and all hospitals should have a local guideline to follow, which will include a 'normogram' for interpreting paracetamol levels. General principles are included here
- Estimate dose ingested per kg and treat based on amount ingested, timing from overdose and whether it was single/staggered
- Baseline bloods = full blood count (FBC), international normalised ratio (INR), urea and electrolytes (U&E), liver function tests (LFTs), blood gas, paracetamol levels
- Discuss with local liver unit if raised alanine aminotransferase (ALT)/INR/creatinine, acidosis or signs of encephalopathy
- Full course of treatment is three consecutive intravenous infusions. Repeat bloods after treatment. If after treatment blood tests are abnormal, consider continuation of N-acetylcysteine (NAC) and discuss with local liver unit

Single overdose <8 hours	<ul><li>If < 1 hour since ingestion and >150 mg/kg, consider activated charcoal</li><li>Take baseline bloods at 4 hours</li><li>Plot paracetamol level on normogram and decide on NAC</li></ul>
Single overdose >8 hours	<ul><li>Take baseline bloods</li><li>If >150 mg/kg give NAC</li><li>If <150 mg/kg wait for bloods before NAC</li></ul>
Staggered overdose	<ul><li>Take baseline bloods</li><li>Give NAC</li></ul>

Common Diagnosis 1

Diagnosis: Gastroenteritis

Management Principles

1. **Assess dehydration.** A child who is not clinically dehydrated does not need to be admitted and can be managed at home with appropriate preventative measures to avoid dehydration. Children at risk of dehydration can take oral rehydration solution after a vomit or loose stool

2. **Fluid replacement.** Oral rehydration therapy should be attempted in a child who is clinically dehydrated. This can be via an NG tube if oral fluids are not tolerated. If the fluid challenge is unsuccessful, then the child will need to have IV fluids. If in shock, the child should receive fluid resuscitation
3. **Encourage good hand hygiene.** To prevent outbreaks of gastroenteritis, good hand hygiene should be encouraged for both children and their parents. Unwell children should not share towels and should be kept away from school or nursery until symptom free for 48 hours
4. **Antibiotic therapy.** This is not routinely required, but should be considered if there has been foreign travel or if sepsis is suspected. Organisms requiring antibiotics include *Clostridium difficile*, *Giardia*, *Shigella* or infants under 6 months with *Salmonella*

Common Diagnosis 2
Diagnosis: Gastro-oesophageal reflux

Management Principles
1. **Parental reassurance.** Reassure parents that this is a common problem that should get better in time and does not warrant further investigation or treatment
2. **Safety-netting advice.** Ensure the parents are aware that they should seek further advice if the child is developing red flag symptoms such as projectile or bilious vomiting
3. **Consider pharmacological intervention.** If the child is distressed by the reflux and has symptoms suggestive of GORD, consider using thickened feeds in a formula-fed baby or alginate therapy in a breastfed baby

Common Diagnosis 3
Diagnosis: Cyclical vomiting

Management Principles
1. **Fluid and electrolyte replacement.** Provide supportive management for acute episodes. Children often require hospitalisation with IV fluids and correction of electrolyte disturbance
2. **Anti-emetic therapy.** There may be some benefit in IV ondansetron during acute episodes
3. **Prophylaxis.** If episodes are severe, debilitating and affecting the child's quality of life, then prophylaxis with an anti-migraine therapy (such as amitriptyline) can be trialled. This is more likely to be successful if there is a positive family history of migraine

Common Diagnosis 4
Diagnosis: Cow's milk protein allergy

Management Principles
1. **Elimination trial of dietary cow's milk protein.** If the baby is breastfed, the mother should exclude cow's milk from her diet. If formula fed, hydrolysed formula is necessary. Elimination should be for 2–4 weeks. Home reintroduction is then advised to observe for return of symptoms
2. **Dietician.** Dieticians can advise on a balanced diet with sufficient calcium intake despite exclusion of cow's milk. They can also be very helpful in supporting reintroduction of dairy, as below
3. **Reintroduction of cow's milk.** In children with mild to moderate non-IgE-mediated CMPA, who have been well on a dairy-free diet for 6 months, gradual reintroduction of milk products should be advised. The 'milk ladder' is an evidence-based guideline for the home reintroduction of dairy and progresses from foods containing small amounts of well-cooked milk to uncooked dairy products and fresh milk

---

Box 5.3.10   Important Considerations in Non-Cow's Milk Protein Diets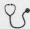

- Soya milk: not to be given before 6 months of age. Contains isoflavones, which may have oestrogenic effect. Cross-reactivity, with many children also reacting to soya
- Rice milk: not to be given <5 years of age, due to arsenic content

- Other mammalian milks: cross-reactivity, with many children also reacting to other animal milks

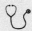

Box 5.3.11   The 'Milk Ladder'

Quantities of foods within each step are directed by a dietician. It is advised to remain on each step for at least 3 days before progressing to the next

- Step 1: Cookies/biscuits
- Step 2: Muffin
- Step 3: Pancake

- Step 4: Cheese
- Step 5: Yoghurt
- Step 6: Pasteurised milk/infant formula

Parents should be advised to look out for any recurrence of symptoms or reactions when progressing through the ladder. If reactions occur, they should revert to the previous step, which was successfully tolerated. Further attempts to progress will be guided by the severity of reaction

Source: Adapted from GP Infant Feeding Network (GPIFN) (2019). The milk allergy in primary care guideline. https://gpifn.org.uk/imap

5.4 Diarrhoea

Philippa Mikolajski

Department of Paediatrics, Oxford University Hospitals NHS Foundation Trust, Oxford, UK

CONTENTS

5.4.1 CHAPTER AT A GLANCE

> **Box 5.4.1 Chapter at a Glance**
>
> - Diarrhoea should be quantified in history: assessing frequency, consistency and stool volume
> - Although a common symptom in children, diarrhoea can be a sign of serious pathology and should not be ignored
> - Bloody diarrhoea should always be taken seriously and investigated

5.4.2 DEFINITION

Diarrhoea can be defined in two main ways:
- **Frequency and consistency:** three or more loose or liquid movements per day
- **Stool mass** (almost impossible to establish outside of a hospital): more than 20 g/kg/day in infants weighing <10 kg or a total of more than 200 g/day in children and teenagers

> **Box 5.4.2 Acute vs Persistent Diarrhoea**
>
> | Type of diarrhoea | Duration |
> | --- | --- |
> | Acute | Hours or days |
> | Persistent | >14 days |
> | Chronic | >30 days |
> | Recurrent | Recurs after 7 days |

Clinical Guide to Paediatrics, First Edition. Edited by Rachel Varughese and Anna Mathew. Series Editor: Christian Fielder Camm.
© 2022 John Wiley & Sons Ltd. Published 2022 by John Wiley & Sons Ltd.
Companion website: www.wiley.com/go/varughese/paediatrics

5.4.3 DIAGNOSTIC ALGORITHM

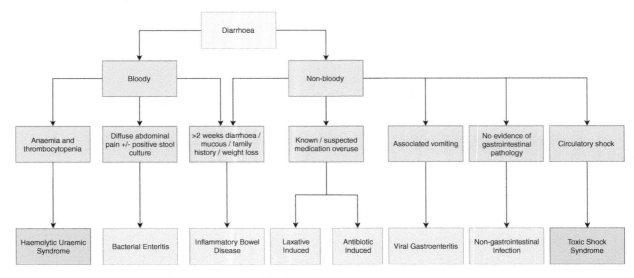

Figure 5.4.1 Diagnostic algorithm for the presentation of diarrhoea.

5.4.4 DIFFERENTIALS LIST

Dangerous Diagnoses

1. Haemolytic Uraemic Syndrome (HUS)

- Triad of haemolytic anaemia, thrombocytopaenia and acute kidney injury (AKI)
- Platelet microthrombi collect in the glomeruli, causing mechanical shearing of red blood cells, resulting in a microangiopathic haemolytic anaemia (MAHA)
- Renal impairment can be severe, requiring dialysis
- The most common cause is following infection with Shiga toxin producing *Escherichia coli* – *E. coli* 0157:H7
- *E. Coli* HUS is preceded by a diarrhoeal illness usually involving bloody diarrhoea, abdominal pain and vomiting
- Commonly acquired through contact with and then ingestion of contaminated material

Box 5.4.3 Haemolytic Uraemic Syndrome: Aetiology and Modes of Transmission of Escherichia coli 0157	
Aetiology	90% due to infection with Shiga toxin producing *E. coli*: *E. coli* 0157:H7 strain Less commonly: other bacterial or viral infections, medications, e.g. chemotherapy, inherited complement mutations
Transmission of *E. coli* 0157	Undercooked contaminated minced beef Direct contact with infected animals Unpasteurised milk Unwashed and contaminated fruit and vegetables Contaminated bodies of water Person-to-person spread

2. Toxic Shock Syndrome (TSS)

- TSS is rare but life-threatening
- It is caused by toxins produced by bacteria, most commonly by *Staphylococcus aureus* or *Streptococcus pyogenes*
- *S. aureus* TSS may be due to pneumonia, osteomyelitis, cellulitis or wound infection

- In children, the most common scenario for *S. pyogenes* TSS is in secondary bacterial infection of chickenpox
- Historically, TSS was primarily known as a complication of tampon use, but this has now reduced dramatically with patient education and manufacturing changes
- Presentation may be with profuse, watery, non-bloody diarrhoea, often accompanied by fever and rash
- Deterioration to shock can be rapid

Common Diagnoses

1. Viral Gastroenteritis
- Most common cause of diarrhoeal illness in children, which is often associated with vomiting
- Incubation period varies depending on the virus
- Illness is usually short-lived and self-limiting
- Since the introduction of rotavirus vaccination in the UK, norovirus is now the leading pathogen to cause infective diarrhoeal illness
- Mainstay of management is preventing and treating dehydration, although antimicrobials are useful in bacterial and parasitic illnesses

2. Bacterial Enteritis
- Spread is faeco-oral after exposure to farm animals, poultry or contaminated meat
- In contrast to viral gastroenteritis, high fever and crampy abdominal pain are significant symptoms
- Bloody diarrhoea (dysentery) is strongly suggestive of a bacterial cause, although not all bacteria cause dysentery
- Campylobacter is the most common cause of bacterial enteritis in the UK. See Chapter 5.3, *Vomiting*, Box 5.3.8 *Causes of Gastroenteritis*

3. Inflammatory Bowel Disease (IBD)
- Chronic inflammatory bowel change caused by a dysregulated mucosal immune response to intestinal microflora
- IBD is an umbrella term encompassing Crohn's disease and ulcerative colitis (UC). Both are characterised by unpredictable exacerbations and remissions
- The most common age of onset is during adolescence and there are very strong genetic and environmental influences, with higher prevalence in developed countries
- Diarrhoea is classically associated with blood and mucus
- There are a variety of extra-intestinal manifestations, more common in Crohn's disease

Box 5.4.4 Crohn's Disease and Ulcerative Colitis

	Crohn's disease	Ulcerative colitis
Symptoms	Cramping abdominal pain, typically right iliac fossa Blood in diarrhoea less common	Cramping abdominal pain, typically left iliac fossa Blood in diarrhoea very common Tenesmus and faecal urgency
Affected part of gastrointestinal (GI) tract	Anywhere along GI tract from mouth to anus	Large intestine
Distribution	'Skip lesions' typical, with areas of unaffected bowel between affected areas	Continuous disease from rectum upwards
Thickness of inflammation	Transmural inflammation	Mucosa/submucosal inflammation
Features on barium enema	'Cobblestone' appearance caused by fissures and ulcers, or 'string sign' caused by narrowing due to spasm or stricture	'Lead pipe' colon due to loss of haustra, causing a smooth, cylindrical appearance
GI complications	Strictures, fistulas, fissures, abscesses, perianal disease	Toxic megacolon, haemorrhage, marked increased risk of colon cancer
Extra-intestinal complications	Faltering growth, clubbing, aphthous ulcers, erythema nodosum, episcleritis, scleritis, uveitis, gallstones, peripheral arthritis	Primary sclerosing cholangitis, hepatitis, pyoderma gangrenosum, ankylosing spondylitis

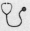

> **Box 5.4.5   Non-gastrointestinal Infections**
>
> Common infections of childhood such as otitis media, lower respiratory tract infections and urinary tract infections may initially present with non-specific symptoms such as diarrhoea and/or vomiting

Diagnoses to Consider

1. Laxative Induced
- Overuse of laxatives can cause diarrhoea
- Many children suffer with constipation and are prescribed paediatric Movicol®. Continued high-dose use once constipation has settled may cause diarrhoea
- Children with eating disorders may use laxatives as a method of losing weight

When to consider: in children where laxatives have been prescribed for constipation, or in teenagers with significant recent weight loss or where eating disorders are suspected

2. Antibiotic Induced
- Diarrhoea is a common side effect of antibiotic treatment, occurring in up to 25% of children, due to disruption of normal bowel microflora and mucosal integrity
- The most common culprits are penicillins, cephalosporins and clindamycin
- In more severe cases, screening for *Clostridium difficile* should be undertaken

When to consider: in those who have had oral antibiotics within the last few days

> **Box 5.4.6   Clostridium difficile**   ΔΔ
>
> *Clostridium difficile* is a Gram-positive, spore-forming, anaerobic bacillus, prone to overgrowth when bowel microflora are disrupted by antibiotics
> This occurs with prolonged duration of antibiotic use, multiple concurrent antibiotics, multiple courses of antibiotics and immunosuppression
>
> Diarrhoea is caused by the *Clostridium difficile* cytotoxin, and may progress to pseudomembranous colitis and toxic megacolon

5.4.5 KEY HISTORY FEATURES

Dangerous Diagnosis 1
Diagnosis: Haemolytic uraemic syndrome

Questions
1. **Has there been abdominal pain or vomiting?** Abdominal pain, vomiting and diarrhoea may represent a prodromal illness, 5–10 days prior to development of HUS. Ongoing abdominal pain should be noted, as severe HUS can cause serious gastrointestinal manifestations such as bowel necrosis, perforation and intussusception
2. **Has the child had bloody diarrhoea?** Children with HUS typically have a history of bloody diarrhoea following infection with *E. coli* 0157, the most common bacterial agent
3. **What is the urine output like?** Children very quickly progress into AKI, often passing an oral fluid challenge but remaining oliguric. Caution must be exercised to consider this before discharging home prematurely
4. **Has there been any contact with farm animals or ingestion of contaminated or unpasteurised foods?** *E. coli* are found normally in the intestines of animals, particularly cattle, and can be picked up from contaminated or uncooked meats and vegetables, or water contaminated with faeces containing *E. coli*
5. **Is there pallor?** The haemolysis, which is due to mechanical shearing of red cells, can be severe and rapid, causing acute pallor

Dangerous Diagnosis 2
Diagnosis: Toxic shock syndrome

Questions
1. **Has the child had any recent wounds or localised skin infections?** TSS often occurs secondary to *S. aureus* wound infection; some of these may not initially appear to be very significant. Secondary bacterial infection of chickenpox is a very important risk factor

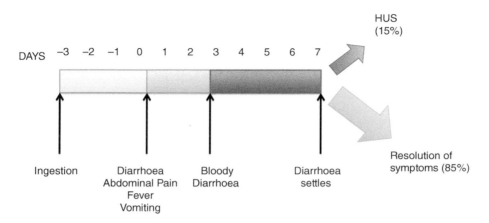

Figure 5.4.2 Typical pattern of *Escherichia coli* 0157 infection in children. Courtesy of Dr Ashish Patel.

2. **Is there a fever?** Fevers may have an abrupt onset and then remain persistently high
3. **Is the child lethargic, confused or drowsy?** Symptoms of altered mental state may indicate impending distributive shock

Common Diagnosis 1
Diagnosis: Viral gastroenteritis

Questions
1. **Has the child been around anyone with diarrhoea and vomiting?** Viral gastroenteritis is highly contagious and very quickly spread. If the child is at nursery or school, it is likely that is where they have picked up the virus. Incubation period is generally 12 hours to 5 days.
2. **How long have symptoms been present?** Gastroenteritis is usually an acute cause of vomiting and diarrhoea. Vomiting normally resolves within 3 days but diarrhoea lasts longer, typically for 5–7 days, but may persist for up to 2 weeks
3. **Is there blood or mucus in the stool?** Blood or mucus in the stool is unlikely to be a viral gastroenteritis and a different diagnosis should be considered

Common Diagnosis 2
Diagnosis: Bacterial enteritis

Questions
1. **Has the child had blood in their stool?** Blood in the stool raises the likelihood that there is a bacterial cause to the diarrhoea
2. **Has the child been abroad recently?** Some bacterial diarrhoeal illnesses are more prevalent outside the UK, particularly in developing countries, therefore travel history is always important
3. **Has the child eaten out recently?** As bacterial enteritis is associated with uncooked meats, asking if the child has eaten out is important. If there is a positive stool culture at a later date, Public Health authorities must be notified

---

Box 5.4.7   Bloody Diarrhoea Differentials   ΔΔ

Haemolytic uraemic syndrome	Inflammatory bowel disease
Bacterial enteritis	Sepsis
Intussusception	

Common Diagnosis 3

Diagnosis: Inflammatory bowel disease

Questions

1. **How long has diarrhoea been going on for?** IBD should be considered if there is a history of diarrhoea lasting more than 2 weeks or a history of intermittent, recurrent diarrhoea
2. **Is there a history of bloody diarrhoea?** Symptoms are usually insidious, starting with non-bloody diarrhoea, which then becomes bloody, with associated abdominal pain. Occasionally IBD can present with a more fulminant illness of severe, frequent bloody diarrhoea and acute severe abdominal pain. Patients may be anaemic
3. **Has the child's appetite altered?** Children with IBD often have reduced appetite or a fear of eating, as this can bring on symptoms of abdominal pain or tenesmus
4. **Has the child or parents noticed weight loss?** Patients with IBD struggle to maintain weight and frequently lose weight due to malabsorption. A common feature at presentation is a reduction in growth velocity, which can progress to short stature, delayed bone age and pubertal delay. IBD often has an insidious onset. To a clinician the child may look cachectic, but the parents may not have noticed the weight loss at first as it is often over a long period of time
5. **Is there a family history of IBD?** While IBD is multi-factorial, there is strong evidence to suggest a genetic component

5.4.6 KEY EXAMINATION FEATURES

See Chapter 12.3 for information on assessing hydration status.

Dangerous Diagnosis 1

Diagnosis: Haemolytic uraemic syndrome

Examination Findings

1. **Fluid overload, hypertension.** AKI causes impaired filtration leading to oliguria or anuria and fluid overload, with oedema. Hypertension is caused by fluid overload as well as renal impairment
2. **Pale.** The haemolysis leads to anaemia, which is clinically evident with the appearance of pallor. The low platelet count is not usually associated with bleeding, although petechiae can be noted
3. **Neurological symptoms.** Lethargy worsens over time as the combination of haemolysis, dehydration and uraemia progresses. Focal neurological deficits, or even seizures, can occur due to cerebral microvascular damage, though this is fortunately rare

---

Box 5.4.8   Clinical Presentation of Haemolytic Uraemic Syndrome

History	Diarrhoea in the last 2 weeks
General examination	Nausea and vomiting; signs of dehydration Diarrhoea: watery, ± bloody
Haematological	Pallor (microangiopathic haemolytic anaemia) Bleeding, rarely, from thrombocytopaenia
Renal	Acute kidney injury ± oliguria Hypertension Haematuria, proteinuria, raised creatinine
Neurological	Lethargy, irritable, seizures, coma, stroke

Dangerous Diagnosis 2

Diagnosis: Toxic shock syndrome

Examination Findings

1. **High fever.** Fever >38.8 °C is a key part of the TSS diagnosis
2. **Hypotension.** TSS can cause profound hypotension, which may be refractory to fluid replacement
3. **'Sunburn' rash.** A diffuse erythematous macular rash typically appears within a few hours of onset, with later desquamation. There may be hyperaemia of mucous membranes and conjunctivitis
4. **Altered mental status.** Cognitive or behavioural impairment suggests shock

Box 5.4.9   Diagnostic Criteria of Staphylococcal Toxic Shock Syndrome

All major and at least three minor criteria must be satisfied

	Diagnostic criteria
Major	Acute fever >38.8 °C Hypotension Rash: erythema with late desquamation
Minor	Vomiting/diarrhoea Mucous membrane inflammation: conjunctivae, pharynx, vagina Liver abnormalities: biochemical Renal abnormalities: oliguria/biochemical Severe muscle pain Central nervous system abnormalities: altered mental state Thrombocytopenia

Common Diagnosis 1
Diagnosis: Viral gastroenteritis

Examination Findings
1. **Abdominal pain.** The child may have non-specific generalised abdominal discomfort on palpation. They should not have an acute abdomen and there should be no rebound tenderness or guarding
2. **Dehydration.** Depending on the preserved intake, volume losses and duration of illness, dehydration can range from mild to severe

Common Diagnosis 2
Diagnosis: Bacterial enteritis

Examination Findings
1. **Dehydration.** Children can quickly become dehydrated; an accurate assessment is necessary to institute appropriate management. Remember, bacterial enteritis can progress to sepsis and many of these features can overlap
2. **Abdominal pain.** Due to vomiting and diarrhoea associated with the enteritis, children will often have quite severe abdominal pain, which can be diffuse

Common Diagnosis 3
Diagnosis: Inflammatory bowel disease

Examination Findings
1. **Abdominal tenderness.** The tenderness depends on the location of the active inflammation: Crohn's disease commonly causes right iliac fossa tenderness, while UC will more commonly cause left iliac fossa tenderness
2. **Oral ulcers to perianal disease.** Children with Crohn's may suffer with large painful aphthous mouth ulcers and can also have perianal disease (including perianal fistulae, skin tags and fissures) at the same time, as any part of the gut may be involved, unlike in UC
3. **Cachexia.** Children often have insidious weight loss and by the time of presentation are cachectic and malnourished with reduced fat and muscle mass. Faltering growth is more common in children with Crohn's
4. **Extra-intestinal manifestations.** There are a variety of extra-intestinal manifestations, many of which are more common in Crohn's than UC (see Box 5.4.4). Carefully examine joints, eyes and skin

5.4.7 KEY INVESTIGATIONS

Not all children will require invasive investigations; often diagnoses are made on clinical evidence from history and examination. Consider carefully which investigations are required for which patient.

Bedside

Table 5.4.1 Bedside tests of use in patients presenting with diarrhoea

Test	When to perform	Potential result
Blood gas (capillary or venous)	• Systemically unwell children	• ↓ pH, ↓ HCO$_3$, ↑ lactate: metabolic acidosis in sepsis, severe dehydration
Urinalysis	• Suspected HUS	• + Blood, + protein in HUS
Stool MC&S	Suspected: • Bacterial enteritis • HUS	• Identifies bacteria that need treating. *Campylobacter, Salmonella, Listeria, Escherichia Coli, Shigella* • Positive for *E. Coli* 0157 in HUS • Sensitivities guide antibiotic choice

HCO$_3$, bicarbonate; HUS, haemolytic uraemic syndrome; MC&S, microscopy, culture and sensitivity

Blood Tests

Table 5.4.2 Blood tests of use in patients presenting with diarrhoea

Test	When to perform	Potential result
FBC	Suspected: • HUS • TSS • Bacterial enteritis • IBD	• ↓ Hb, ↓ platelets: HUS • ↑ WCC, ↑ neutrophils: bacterial infection • ↑ Platelets: sepsis, chronic inflammation
Blood film	Suspected: • HUS • Bacterial infections	• Haemolysis (schistocytes, RBC fragments) and ↓ platelets in HUS • Left shift of neutrophils in infection • Hypochromic, microcytic anaemia in IBD
U&E	Suspected: • HUS • TSS • Bacterial enteritis • IBD	• ↑ Urea: mild dehydration • ↑ Urea, ↑ creatinine: AKI due to severe dehydration, severe sepsis, HUS • Na, K and HCO$_3$ disturbances in severe diarrhoea and dehydration
CRP	• Suspected bacterial infection	• Significant ↑ in bacterial infections • Less marked ↑ in viral infections
Clotting screen	• Suspected HUS or sepsis	• HUS: normal clotting screen • DIC (sepsis): (↑ PT and APTT, ↓platelets, fibrinogen, factor V and factor VIII)
Blood culture	• Suspected sepsis	• Positive culture confirms bacterial infection • Sensitivities will guide antibiotic treatment

AKI, acute kidney injury; APTT, activated partial thromboplastin time; CRP, C-reactive protein; DIC, disseminated intravascular coagulation; FBC, full blood count; Hb, haemoglobin; HCO$_3$, bicarbonate; HUS, haemolytic uraemic syndrome; IBD, inflammatory bowel disease; K, potassium; Na, sodium; PT, prothrombin time; RBC, red blood cell; TSS, toxic shock syndrome; U&E, urea and electrolytes

Imaging

Table 5.4.3 Imaging modalities of use in patients presenting with diarrhoea

Test	Justification	Potential result
Abdominal USS	• In suspected IBD	• Evaluates bowel wall thickness, extent of involvement, evidence of fistulas, abscesses
MRI	• In suspected IBD	• Imaging modality of choice for diagnosis, monitoring of disease activity and complications
Abdominal x-ray	• In suspected complicated colitis	• Toxic megacolon: a severe complication of both UC and *Clostridium difficile*

IBD, inflammatory bowel disease; MRI, magnetic resonance imaging; UC, ulcerative colitis; USS, ultrasound scan

Special

Table 5.4.4 Special tests of use in patients presenting with diarrhoea

Test	Justification	Potential result
Lower GI endoscopy	• In suspected IBD	• Macroscopic and histological appearance confirms diagnosis
Serology for *Escherichia coli* 0157	• In suspected HUS	• Positive serology supports HUS
Stool for ova and parasites	• If suspected parasitic cause of diarrhoea	• Identifies parasites that need treating e.g. *Giardia*, *Cryptosporidium*
Wound swab	• If wound infection and suspected TSS	• Isolates pathogen responsible for TSS • Sensitivities help guide antibiotic choice (particularly if methicillin-resistant staphylococcus aureus)

GI, gastrointestinal; HUS, haemolytic uraemic syndrome; IBD, inflammatory bowel disease; TSS, toxic shock syndrome

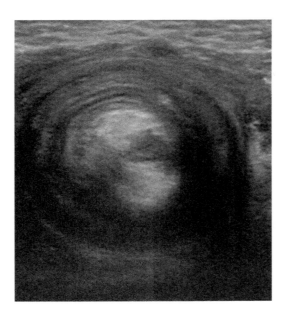

Figure 5.4.3 Ultrasound abdomen demonstrating intussusception. Note the classic 'target' appearance. The intussuscepted bowel is in the centre, with a circumferential sleeve of distal bowel around it.

5.4.8 KEY MANAGEMENT PRINCIPLES

Diagnosis-specific management strategies are outlined here. It is expected that an 'ABCDE' approach to assessment and management is always undertaken (see Chapter 12.1, *The A to E Assessment*).

Management of dehydration with fluid replacement can be found in Chapter 12.3, *Tips for Fluid Prescribing*.

Dangerous Diagnosis 1

Diagnosis: Haemolytic uraemic syndrome

Management Principles

1. **Maintain euvolaemic status.** It is important that children with HUS are kept euvolaemic to assist renal perfusion. They may require fluid replacement; however, due to the risk of renal failure, it is important to maintain a strict fluid balance to prevent volume overload. Weight should be monitored twice a day. In those with normal/increased intravascular volume and decreased urine output, fluid intake should be restricted to insensible losses plus urinary output

2. **Antibiotics.** If HUS is thought to be secondary to an infectious cause, antibiotics are vital. Use local policy to determine antibiotic choice. Ensure nephrotoxic medications are avoided
3. **Blood transfusion.** Packed red cell transfusion should be considered for haemoglobin (Hb) <60 g/L or if significantly symptomatic. The goal is to restore Hb to 80–90 g/L and not to normal, to avoid complications of fluid overload
4. **Antihypertensives.** Fluid overload can be associated with hypertension. Daily blood pressure should be recorded as a minimum. Renal impairment may aggravate renin-driven hypertension and require antihypertensive therapy with calcium channel blockers or angiotensin-converting enzyme (ACE) inhibitors. Seek senior/specialist advice
5. **Discussion with tertiary renal unit.** Fulminant renal failure can quickly develop with HUS, therefore it is important to discuss with the renal unit as the child may require dialysis

Dangerous Diagnosis 2
Diagnosis: Toxic shock syndrome

Management Principles
1. **Fluid resuscitation.** Children with TSS may become haemodynamically unstable with profound hypotension. Aggressive fluid replacement may be required to treat hypotension, renal failure and cardiovascular collapse
2. **Antibiotics.** High-dose anti-staphylococcal antibiotics are recommended. Addition of clindamycin may help terminate toxin production. Antibiotic administration should be within an hour of diagnosis, ideally earlier
3. **Vasopressors.** Refractory hypotension may require vasopressor/inotropic support and early discussion with the paediatric intensive care unit (PICU) is essential
4. **Corticosteroids + immunoglobulin.** Reserved for severe cases of TSS, to curb inflammatory response
5. **Regular monitoring.** Children with TSS can deteriorate very quickly even on treatment. It is therefore vital that they are monitored regularly, with strict fluid balance charts and regular observations

Common Diagnosis 1
Diagnosis: Viral gastroenteritis

Management Principles
1. **Hydration.** Most children can be managed at home, however a small number of children may require hospital admission for intravenous (IV) fluids. Unless severely dehydrated, the child should be started on an oral fluid challenge first. If they fail this, they may require admission for maintenance IV fluids. A small proportion may require IV fluid boluses for resuscitation if there are signs of shock

Box 5.4.10 Calculating Oral Fluid Challenge Volumes	
Daily fluid requirement	3–10 kg: 100 mL/kg = 100 × weight in kg 11–20 kg: additional 50 mL for every additional kg = 1000 + 50 × (weight – 10) >20 kg: additional 20 mL for every additional kg = 1500 + 20 × (weight – 20)
Oral fluid challenge: oral rehydration solution	Divide total volume by 24 hours Divide again by 6 to determine volume to be given every 10 minutes
Example	A child weighing 25 kg requires 1000 + 500 + 100 = 1600 mL in 24 hours This is 66.6 mL in 1 hour, which is 11.1 mL every 10 minutes

Common Diagnosis 2
Diagnosis: Bacterial enteritis

Management Principles
1. **Hydration.** An oral fluid challenge should be attempted. If not successful, IV fluids may be warranted. If there is bloody diarrhoea, it is important to check the patient does not have signs of early HUS
2. **Antibiotics.** In a well child, antibiotics may not be indicated. If systemically unwell, broad-spectrum antibiotics may be required. Discussion with local microbiology is useful if there are positive stool and blood cultures

Common Diagnosis 3

Diagnosis: Inflammatory bowel disease

Management Principles

1. **Multi-disciplinary team input.** Management of IBD is a specialist area and requires tertiary gastroenterology input. In addition, the involvement of dietetic support, clinical psychology, local paediatrician and GP are all required
2. **Inducing remission.** In Crohn's, first-line options are case dependent, but include glucocorticosteroids, e.g. prednisolone, enteral nutrition, budesonide and aminosalicylates. In UC, topical aminosalicylates are tried first, before oral treatment
3. **Add-on treatment.** For repeated or refractory cases in both UC and Crohn's, add-on treatment may be started. Options include immunosuppressive therapies such as azathioprine, mercaptopurine and methotrexate. Monoclonal antibodies, e.g. infliximab, may be considered in severe cases
4. **Maintaining remission.** This is a highly specialist area, and discussions with families will be required to decide whether maintenance treatment is recommended
5. **Surgery.** Surgery may be recommended either for those with localised disease, unacceptable side effects of medical management, refractory disease or for complications

5.5 Jaundice

Claire Roome

Department of Paediatrics, Stoke Mandeville Hospital, Buckinghamshire Healthcare NHS Foundation Trust, UK

CONTENTS

5.5.1 CHAPTER AT A GLANCE

> **Box 5.5.1 Chapter at a Glance**
>
> - This chapter considers the causes of jaundice (hyperbilirubinaemia) in children >1 year of age and adolescents
> - Jaundice is caused by raised levels of bilirubin, which is a by-product of the breakdown of haem
> - Jaundice can be conjugated, indicating decreased excretion of bilirubin by hepatic cells or biliary tract damage, or unconjugated, indicating increased production of bilirubin
> - Disorders resulting in unconjugated hyperbilirubinaemia are much more common; this distinction must be made early to institute appropriate management
> - Jaundice is common in the neonatal period and often has a very different aetiology, described in detail in Chapter 11.1

5.5.2 DEFINITION

Jaundice (icterus) is a yellow discoloration of the skin, sclera and mucous membranes as a result of hyperbilirubinaemia

Clinical Guide to Paediatrics, First Edition. Edited by Rachel Varughese and Anna Mathew. Series Editor: Christian Fielder Camm.
© 2022 John Wiley & Sons Ltd. Published 2022 by John Wiley & Sons Ltd.
Companion website: www.wiley.com/go/varughese/paediatrics

5.5.3 DIAGNOSTIC ALGORITHM

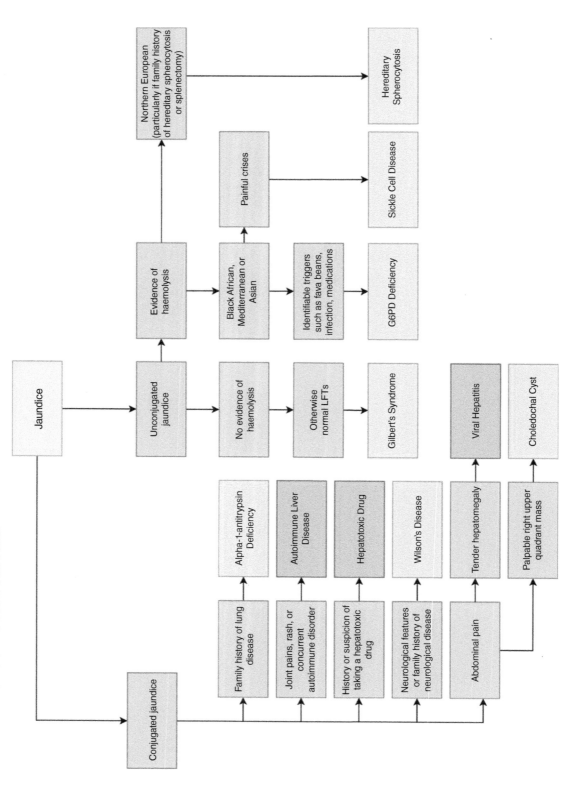

Figure 5.5.1 Diagnostic algorithm for the presentation of jaundice.

5.5.4 DIFFERENTIALS LIST

Dangerous Diagnoses

1. Viral Hepatitis
- There are five hepatitis viruses: A, B, C, D and E
- Hepatitis A and E are transmitted via the faecal-oral route, usually via contaminated water and food. They are the most common viral hepatitides in children
- Hepatitis B and C are transmitted sexually, parenterally or vertically
- Hepatitis D only affects those with hepatitis B, as it is an incomplete virus that requires the helper function of hepatitis B in order to replicate
- Other non-hepatotrophic viruses may cause hepatitis, including herpes simplex virus (HSV), Epstein–Barr virus (EBV), cytomegalovirus (CMV) and enteroviruses
- Typical prodrome includes lethargy, anorexia, nausea, abdominal pain, myalgia and sometimes fever
- Although most infections are self-limiting, fulminant liver failure can develop and carries a mortality of 70% without appropriate treatment

Box 5.5.2 Clinical Course in Hepatitis A, B and C

Hepatitis A	Transmission	Faeco-oral
	Duration of illness	Self-limiting; usually 2 weeks
	Risk of chronicity	Rare
	Complications	Rare
Hepatitis B	Transmission	Blood products, body fluids, vertical transmission
	Duration of illness	Icteric phase: 1–2 weeks, constitutional symptoms can last weeks to months
	Risk of chronicity	5–10%
	Complications	Chronic hepatitis, cirrhosis, liver failure, hepatocellular carcinoma
Hepatitis C	Transmission	Blood products, body fluids, vertical transmission Co-infection with hepatitis B/human immunodeficiency virus more likely
	Duration of illness	Uncertain, frequently subclinical
	Risk of chronicity	Higher with risk-taking behaviour, e.g. alcohol, intravenous drugs, tattoos
	Complications	Hepatic fibrosis, chronic hepatitis, cirrhosis, liver failure, hepatocellular carcinoma

2. Autoimmune Liver Disease
- Autoimmune hepatitis is a chronic disease, causing hepatic cell inflammation and necrosis leading to cirrhosis
- It is characterised by the presence of circulating autoantibodies and inflammatory changes on liver histology

3. Hepatotoxic Drugs
- A number of drugs can cause direct or indirect liver damage
- Paracetamol overdose has direct dose-dependent hepatotoxic effects and is the most common cause of drug-induced liver damage in developed countries
- Antimicrobials, oral contraceptive pill, anticonvulsants and non-steroidal anti-inflammatory drugs (NSAIDs) are also causes

---

Box 5.5.3   Reye's Syndrome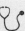

- Reye's syndrome is a progressive encephalopathy with acute liver failure
- Children present with drowsiness, confusion and seizures
- There is hypoglycaemia, raised ammonia and deranged liver function

- The liver is usually enlarged with fatty deposits
- Treatment is supportive, but mortality is high
- The link between Reye's syndrome and aspirin is the reason the latter is rarely used in children, the exception being in Kawasaki disease

Common Diagnoses

1. Gilbert Syndrome
- Gilbert syndrome is a benign autosomal recessive condition affecting 5% of the population
- Intermittent unconjugated jaundice can present in times of stress such as illness, vigorous exercise or fasting
- It is caused by a deficiency in the bilirubin-UGT (bilirubin–uridine diphosphate glucuronosyl transferase) enzyme. There is no underlying liver disease or haemolysis

2. Hereditary Spherocytosis (HS)
- This is the most common hereditary haemolytic anaemia in northern Europeans, inherited in an autosomal dominant manner
- HS is a disorder of spectrin, a structural component of the red cell membrane
- Red blood cells are spherocytic in shape and are destroyed by the spleen, causing a haemolytic anaemia, splenomegaly and gallstones

3. Glucose-6-Phosphate Dehydrogenase (G6PD) Deficiency
- An X-linked deficiency of the G6PD enzyme that is common in people of Mediterranean, Asian and Black African descent
- G6PD helps protect red blood cells from oxidative injury
- Most people with G6PD deficiency are asymptomatic
- Symptomatic patients can present with neonatal jaundice and episodes of acute haemolytic anaemia

---

Box 5.5.4   Causes of Haemolysis in Glucose-6-Phosphate Dehydrogenase (G6PD) Deficiency

- Infections: bacterial or viral
- Drugs: antibiotics, e.g. sulphonamides, antimalarials

- Fava beans: ingesting the beans or inhaling pollen from fava plants

---

4. Alpha-1-Antitrypsin (AAT) Deficiency
- Autosomal co-dominant condition associated with liver disease and chronic lung disease, with an incidence of 1:1600–2000 live births
- AAT is a protein released by the liver and has a role in preventing tissue damage
- Several subtypes with varying severity. Liver disease can occur in those who have the PiZZ genotype
- Liver disease can involve neonatal hepatitis, which may improve before diagnosis, followed by chronic hepatitis, cirrhosis or liver failure in later childhood or adulthood. There is a small risk of hepatocellular carcinoma
- Patients are predisposed to emphysema, but that tends to occur in adulthood
- There is a range of phenotypic severity

Diagnoses to Consider

1. Wilson Disease
- An autosomal recessive condition resulting in cumulative copper deposition in the liver, central nervous system and kidneys, with an incidence of 1:50000
- Hepatic presentation is usually in the first decade, with neurological symptoms in the second decade

When to consider: in any patient with jaundice and unexplained liver disease

2. Sickle Cell Disease (SCD)
- SCD is one of the most common autosomal recessive conditions seen globally that results in haemolytic anaemia
- SCD is most common in African and Mediterranean ethnicities and affects millions of people worldwide
- It is caused by mutations in the haemoglobin (Hb) beta gene
- The most common severe form is HbSS
- Haemolytic crises often present with pain, pallor, jaundice and lethargy

When to consider: when there is evidence of haemolytic anaemia and vaso-occlusive crises, or a known family history

3. Choledochal Cyst
- A congenital bile duct cyst that can cause obstruction of bile and present with jaundice with hepatomegaly
- Can cause intermittent pain and a palpable mass in older children
- Cholangitis and pancreatitis can occur as a result of the cyst

When to consider: in cases of intermittent obstructive jaundice with a palpable right upper quadrant mass and hepatomegaly, or recurrent bouts of pancreatitis

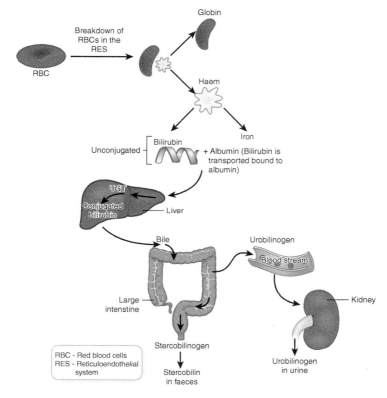

Figure 5.5.2 The metabolism of bilirubin. Red blood cells are degraded within the reticuloendothelial system (spleen, tissue macrophages and liver) into haem and globin. Haem is then further split into iron and bilirubin. Bilirubin is transported to the liver bound to albumin. It is in this form that bilirubin is insoluble and unconjugated. Once in the liver, uridine 5-diphospho-glucuronosyltransferase (UGT) converts insoluble bilirubin to conjugated water-soluble bilirubin. Normally the levels of unconjugated bilirubin remain low, but when the rate of bilirubin formation increases, such as in haemolysis, or when the conjugation rate decreases, an unconjugated hyperbilirubinaemia develops. Once conjugated, bilirubin is excreted from the liver into bile and converts to urobilinogen in the bowel. Some urobilinogen is reabsorbed into the portal system and some is then excreted into urine by the kidneys. Some, however, is made into stercobilin, which passes into faeces. Once conjugated, the bilirubin is water soluble. Therefore, dark urine and pale stools suggest biliary obstruction, from either intra- or extra-hepatic causes.

5.5.5 KEY HISTORY FEATURES

- Taking a thorough history is vital in cases of paediatric jaundice and can often give a clear indication as to the underlying pathology
- Asking about family history and ethnicity can be particularly helpful in identifying cases of haemolytic jaundice
- Clarifying the duration of illness can indicate chronic hepatitis or chronic liver disease, whereas prodromal flu-like symptoms or exposure to infected food, travel or affected individuals can indicate an infective hepatitis

Dangerous Diagnosis 1
Diagnosis: Viral hepatitis

Questions
1. **Any travel to endemic areas or ingestion of contaminated foods?** Hepatitis A and B in particular are more likely to be contracted in endemic areas such as Africa and South East Asia

2. **Any prodromal symptoms such as lethargy, fever, nausea, anorexia?** Flu-like symptoms can be present in the acute phase of hepatitis, although some patients may be completely asymptomatic
3. **Any abdominal pain?** There may be abdominal pain, particularly in the right upper quadrant, and diarrhoea
4. **Is the urine dark or faeces pale?** Although these are typically a feature of biliary obstruction, dark urine and pale stools can occur due to transient conjugated hyperbilirubinaemia in many acute hepatic illnesses
5. **Any contact with infected individuals?** Consider vertical transmission in the case of babies born to mothers infected with hepatitis B or C, or household contacts where infected individuals with hepatitis A may be in close contact

Dangerous Diagnosis 2
Diagnosis: Autoimmune liver disease

Questions
1. **Any other autoimmune conditions or family history of autoimmune conditions?** 30–50% of children diagnosed with autoimmune hepatitis have another autoimmune condition, such as autoimmune thyroid disease, type 1 diabetes mellitus or coeliac disease
2. **What age and gender is the child?** 75% of children with autoimmune hepatitis are female. The mean age of presentation is 7–10 years
3. **Any constitutional symptoms?** Lethargy, myalgia and nausea are commonly associated and onset is typically insidious

Dangerous Diagnosis 3
Diagnosis: Hepatotoxic drugs

Questions
1. **Any history of accidental or deliberate overdose?** Paracetamol is the drug most commonly associated with drug-induced liver injury. Hepatotoxicity due to paracetamol poisoning is dose dependent, with acute liver failure more likely with doses in excess of 150 mg/kg
2. **Any prescribed medications?** Certain antibiotics, anti-epileptics and oral contraceptive pills can cause hepatotoxicity
3. **Any use of herbal remedies or 'traditional' medicines?** Non-prescribed and herbal remedies can cause hepatotoxicity and can easily be missed without a thorough history
4. **Any vomiting?** Nausea and vomiting with paracetamol overdose typically peak 2–3 days after ingestion

Common Diagnosis 1
Diagnosis: Gilbert syndrome

Questions
1. **Any family history of jaundice?** Gilbert syndrome is an inherited condition, usually autosomal recessive
2. **Are there any identifiable triggers to the episodes of jaundice?** Fasting, surgery, dehydration, alcohol ingestion, illness, vigorous exercise and sleep deprivation may provoke jaundice
3. **Are there any other symptoms?** Gilbert syndrome is a benign condition and as such the child should be systemically well. Any other indication of illness should prompt a search for alternative diagnoses

Common Diagnosis 2
Diagnosis: Hereditary spherocytosis

Questions
1. **What ethnicity is the patient?** HS is the most common hereditary haemolytic anaemia in northern Europeans, affecting 1 in 2000 individuals
2. **Any family history of jaundice, anaemia or splenectomy?** Around 75% of cases of hereditary spherocytosis are dominantly inherited. Therefore, there may be a history of anaemia, jaundice or splenectomy in a sibling or parent
3. **Is there a history of jaundice in the neonatal period?** Approximately 30–50% of adults with HS had a history of jaundice during the first week of life

Common Diagnosis 3
Diagnosis: Glucose-6-phosphate dehydrogenase deficiency

Questions
1. **Any family history of jaundice?** G6PD deficiency is an X-linked recessive disorder, so ask about a history of affected males on the maternal side

2. **Any identifiable triggers?** Exposure to certain drugs (antimalarials and sulphonamides), infection, ketoacidosis or fava beans cause oxidant stress and acute episodic haemolytic anaemia
3. **What ethnicity is the patient?** Prevalence is high in persons of African, Mediterranean or Asian origin. This correlates with countries where malaria is endemic, as G6PD deficiency gives a selective advantage against severe malaria
4. **Is there a history of neonatal jaundice?** Jaundice can be very severe in some G6PD-deficient babies, especially in association with prematurity and infection

Common Diagnosis 4
Diagnosis: Alpha-1-antitrypsin deficiency

Questions
1. **Is there a family history of existing liver or respiratory disease?** AAT deficiency is inherited in an autosomal co-dominant pattern. There may be a family history of liver disease, or of emphysema in older relatives

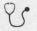

Box 5.5.5   What Is Autosomal Co-dominance?

- Co-dominance means that two different versions of the gene may be expressed, with both contributing to the phenotype. A typical example is blood group
- The SERPINA1 gene is responsible for alpha-1-antitrypsin (AAT), and has three main types of allele, M, S and Z:
  - M allele produces normal levels of AAT
  - S allele produces moderately low AAT
  - Z allele produces very little AAT

Genotype	Phenotype
MM	Normal AAT level
MS + SS	Subclinically reduced AAT level
SZ	Increased risk of developing lung disease, particularly if they smoke
MZ	Clinically moderate AAT deficiency, affecting lung and liver
ZZ	Clinically severe AAT deficiency, affecting lung and liver

5.5.6 KEY EXAMINATION FEATURES

- Physical examination in children should always include inspection of the urine and stools
- Dark urine and pale stools suggest biliary obstruction, from either intra- or extra-hepatic causes
- It is important to assess for signs of liver disease and evidence of anaemia

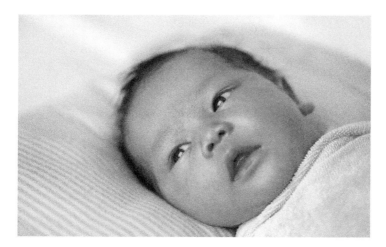

Figure 5.5.3 Scleral icterus in a baby with jaundice. Source: Reproduced with permission from Shutterstock.

Dangerous Diagnosis 1

Diagnosis: Viral hepatitis

Examination Findings: Note that examination findings vary according to the phase of infection.
1. **Tender hepatomegaly.** The liver may be tender and diffusely enlarged with a firm, sharp, smooth edge. 30% of patients also have splenomegaly
2. **Dark urine and pale stools.** Hepatobiliary disease can result in a conjugated hyperbilirubinaemia, causing acholic stools and dark urine
3. **Rashes.** Various rashes (urticarial, macular, maculopapular, purpuric) and even papular acrodermatitis (Gianotti–Crosti syndrome) may be present
4. **Signs of cirrhosis or fulminant liver failure.** Although most infections are self-limiting, some will progress to chronic liver failure or fulminant liver failure, so encephalopathy, evidence of coagulopathy, malaise, ascites and malnutrition may be evident. Those with chronic disease may develop finger clubbing

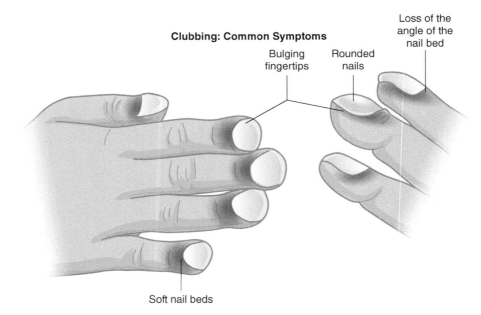

Clubbing: Common Symptoms

Bulging fingertips

Rounded nails

Loss of the angle of the nail bed

Soft nail beds

Figure 5.5.4 Signs of finger clubbing may be seen in chronic liver disease, characterised by widened, boggy nail beds, loss of the angle of the nail bed and increased curvature of the nails.

Box 5.5.6 West Haven Criteria for Grading of Hepatic Encephalopathy	
Severity	**Symptoms of hepatic encephalopathy**
Grade 1	• Mild confusion, anxiety or irritability • Disturbance of sleep pattern • Shortened attention span • Slowing of mental ability • May be difficult to recognise in children
Grade 2	• Excessive sleepiness and disorientation • Personality change and inappropriate behaviour • Inability to recognise or interact with parents
Grade 3	• Gross disorientation and confusion • Somnolence, but responsive to verbal stimuli • Hyperreflexia and positive Babinski sign
Grade 4	• Comatose

Dangerous Diagnosis 2
Diagnosis: Autoimmune liver disease

Examination Findings
1. **Hepatomegaly ± splenomegaly.** Hepatomegaly is a common finding, with a small number of cases also having splenomegaly
2. **Malnutrition and poor growth.** Autoimmune liver disease is a chronic condition, and as such growth and nutrition may be affected
3. **Evidence of autoimmunity.** Signs suggestive of thyroid dysfunction, type 1 diabetes mellitus, ulcerative colitis and coeliac disease may be evident
4. **Dark urine and pale stools.** Hepatobiliary disease results in a conjugated hyperbilirubinaemia, causing acholic stools and dark urine

Dangerous Diagnosis 3
Diagnosis: Hepatotoxic drugs

Examination Findings
1. **Change in conscious level.** Altered mental state may be secondary to drug ingestion or co-ingestion of other substances such as alcohol
2. **Evidence of liver failure.** Signs of liver failure such as encephalopathy, abdominal tenderness, coagulopathy and ascites may be evident, particularly in delayed presentation

Common Diagnosis 1
Diagnosis: Gilbert syndrome

Examination Findings
1. **Normal examination.** Other than mild jaundice, should be completely normal with no anaemia or signs of liver disease

Common Diagnosis 2
Diagnosis: Hereditary spherocytosis

Examination Findings
1. **Pallor.** Anaemia is frequently present. Concurrent parvovirus infection in children with HS can cause significant anaemia due to aplastic crisis
2. **Splenomegaly.** In most cases the spleen is enlarged in view of haemolysis
3. **Right upper abdominal tenderness.** This could be indicative of gallstones. Pigment gallstones are a common complication in HS

Common Diagnosis 3
Diagnosis: Glucose-6-phosphate dehydrogenase deficiency

Examination Findings: Note that examination is frequently normal between episodes of triggers by oxidant stress
1. **Dark urine, but normal stool colour.** 'Cola'-coloured urine secondary to haemoglobinuria from intravascular haemolysis can occur within 24 hours of exposure to an oxidant stress
2. **Pallor or other signs of anaemia.** Pallor, tachycardia and a systolic flow murmur can be evident secondary to haemolytic episodes

Common Diagnosis 4
Diagnosis: Alpha-1-antitrypsin deficiency

Examination Findings
1. **Hepatomegaly.** Hepatomegaly is common at presentation. Splenomegaly develops with cirrhosis and portal hypertension
2. **Pale stool and dark urine.** Hepatobiliary disease results in a conjugated hyperbilirubinaemia, causing acholic stools and dark urine
3. **Signs of chronic respiratory disease.** Consider these signs, but respiratory complications tend to occur in adulthood. Lung disease involves emphysematous changes, similar to chronic obstructive pulmonary disease (COPD). Dyspnoea, productive cough and wheeze are the main features
4. **Signs of liver disease.** Malnutrition, ascites and signs of portal hypertension may be evident

Box 5.5.7   Extra-pulmonary Manifestations of Alpha-1-Antitrypsin (AAT) Deficiency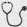

- **Necrotising panniculitis:** inflammation of subcutaneous adipose tissue causing raised red papules that break down to secrete an oily discharge
- **Granulomatosis with polyangiitis:** formerly known as Wegener's granulomatosis, this is a small to medium vessel vasculitis associated with granuloma formation

- **Rheumatoid arthritis:** chronic autoimmune inflammatory disorder affecting joints, with several extra-articular manifestations

5.5.7   KEY INVESTIGATIONS

Not all children will require invasive investigations; often diagnoses are made on clinical evidence from history and examination. Consider carefully which investigations are required for which patient.

Bedside

Table 5.5.1 Bedside tests of use in patients presenting with jaundice

Test	When to perform	Potential result
Blood sugar	• All children with jaundice • Those with acute/chronic liver disease may have impaired gluconeogenesis or impaired glucose tolerance • Sepsis, when it is a trigger for decompensation in SCD, HS and G6PD deficiency, causes impaired gluconeogenesis and glycogenolysis	• Blood sugar <2.6 mmol/L, >10 mmol/L (fasting), can indicate acute or worsening chronic liver disease • Blood sugar >10 mmol/L (fasting) can be seen in sepsis
Blood gas	• All children with new presentations of jaundice • Particularly important if paracetamol overdose is suspected, as a pH <7.25 has a 95% mortality and warrants emergency transplant	• pH <7.35 in combination with paracetamol overdose warrants urgent action (discuss with liver team) • pH <7.35, HCO_3 <22, BE <–2: indicate insufficient organ perfusion as in sepsis • Lactate >2 indicates poor perfusion, often seen in sepsis

BE, base excess; G6PD, glucose-6-phosphate dehydrogenase; HCO_3, bicarbonate; HS, hereditary spherocytosis; SCD, sickle cell disease

Blood Tests

Table 5.5.2 Blood tests of use in patients presenting with jaundice

Test	When to perform	Potential result
FBC and reticulocyte count	• Suspected haemolytic anaemia	• ↓ Hb and ↑ reticulocytes indicate haemolysis, as seen in SCD, G6PD and HS
LFTs	• All patients with jaundice • Helps distinguish between hepatocellular injury and cholestasis	• ↑ AST/ALT indicate hepatocellular injury • ↑ ALP suggests cholestasis, although this is not specific to liver disease
Split bilirubin level	• All patients with jaundice • An essential test to determine if the jaundice is conjugated or unconjugated in nature	• Unconjugated jaundice: conjugated fraction is <20% of the total • Conjugated jaundice: conjugated fraction is >20% of the total, or >17 µmol/L if the total level is <85 µmol/L
Blood film	• Suspected haemolysis in HS, SCD	• Howell–Jolly bodies in HS • Sickle-shaped cells in SCD
Albumin	• All patients with jaundice • Assesses the synthetic function of the liver	• ↓ Albumin in chronic liver disease

Table 5.5.3 Continued

Test	When to perform	Potential result
Clotting screen	• Suspected chronic liver disease • Assesses the synthetic function of the liver	• ↑ INR/PT in liver failure
Renal function	• Baseline test in all patients with jaundice	• Impaired renal function can be seen in cirrhosis or acute liver failure

ALP, alkaline phosphatase; ALT, alanine aminotransferase; AST, aspartate aminotransferase; FBC, full blood count; G6PD, glucose-6-phosphate dehydrogenase; Hb, haemoglobin; HS, hereditary spherocytosis; INR, international normalised ratio; LFTs, liver function tests; PT, prothrombin time; SCD, sickle cell disease

Imaging

Table 5.5.3 Imaging modalities of use in patients presenting with jaundice

Test	When to perform	Potential result
Abdominal ultrasound scan	• All new presentations of jaundice unless strong clinical evidence for Gilbert syndrome	• Characterises liver structure and size • Characterises spleen size • Gallstones • Choledochal cyst • Evidence of cirrhosis
Magnetic resonance cholangiopancreatogram (MRCP)	• Suspected obstructive jaundice • Particularly useful for assessing the biliary system	• Gallstones • Choledochal cyst • Other biliary system abnormalities

Special

Table 5.5.4 Special tests of use in patients presenting with jaundice

Test	When to perform	Potential result
Hepatitis serology	• Suspected viral hepatitis	• Positive hepatitis A/B/C (± D and E) serology
Autoantibodies	• Suspected autoimmune hepatitis	• Anti-ANA and anti-SMA associated with type 1 autoimmune hepatitis • Anti-LKM associated with type 2 autoimmune hepatitis
Amylase and lipase	• Suspected pancreatitis	• ↑ Amylase/lipase in pancreatitis that may be secondary to a choledochal cyst
LDH	Suspected: • Haemolytic disease • Hepatitis • Hepatocellular carcinoma	• ↑ LDH signifies increased cell turnover seen in haemolysis, hepatitis and malignancy
Immunoglobulins	• Suspected autoimmune hepatitis	• IgG typically >1.5 × normal limit in autoimmune hepatitis
Serum caeruloplasmin	• Suspected Wilson disease	• ↓ Caeruloplasmin in Wilson disease
Paracetamol levels	• Suspected paracetamol overdose	• ↑ In acute paracetamol overdose
G6PD enzyme or genetics	• Suspected haemolytic jaundice	• ↓ G6PD • Gene mutation of G6PD deficiency
AAT level and genetics	• Suspected AAT	• ↓ AAT • PiZZ genotype
Osmotic fragility	• Suspected HS	• ↑ Fragility in HS
Liver biopsy	• Suspected autoimmune hepatitis • Any other cause of jaundice with chronic features or diagnostic uncertainty	• Variety of changes depending on aetiology

AAT, alpha-1-antitrypsin; ANA, antinuclear antibody; G6PD, glucose-6-phosphate dehydrogenase; HS, hereditary spherocytosis; Ig, immunoglobulin; LDH, lactate dehydrogenase; LKM, liver-kidney microsomal; SMA, smooth muscle antibody

Box 5.5.8   Interpreting Hepatitis B Serology Results

Hepatitis B antigen/antibody	Status	Interpretation
HBsAg	Negative	Not immune
HBcAb	Negative	
HBsAb	Negative	
HBsAg	Negative	Past infection
HBcAb	Positive	
HBsAb	Positive	
HBsAg	Negative	Immune to hepatitis B vaccination
HBcAb	Negative	
HBsAb	Positive	
HBsAg	Positive	Acute/chronic infection
HBcAb	Positive	
HBsAb	Negative	

5.5.8 KEY MANAGEMENT PRINCIPLES

Diagnosis-specific management strategies are outlined here. It is expected that an 'ABCDE' approach to assessment and management is considered standard practice (see Chapter 12.1).

Box 5.5.9   Viral Hepatitis, a Notifiable Disease

Hepatitis A, B, C, D and E are notifiable diseases, and Public Health authorities should be notified

Box 5.5.10   Management of Acute Liver Failure

- Management of liver failure is directed at the complications that may develop
- Early discussion with a liver centre is important when managing these patients
- The mortality rate of acute liver failure or fulminant hepatitis without appropriate treatment is 70%

Complication of liver failure	Management principle
Hypoglycaemia	Maintain blood glucose >4 mmol/L with intravenous dextrose
Coagulopathy and increased risk of haemorrhage	Intravenous vitamin K, fresh frozen plasma (FFP) and H2 blockers
Encephalopathy and cerebral oedema	Fluid restriction and diuresis with mannitol Avoid sedation unless on assisted ventilation
Renal insufficiency	May require dialysis or haemofiltration
Liver transplant	Emergency liver transplant may be indicated in severe cases

Dangerous Diagnosis 1
Diagnosis: Viral hepatitis

Management Principles
1. **Symptomatic treatment.** Managing nausea, ensuring adequate hydration and nutrition, and rest are the mainstays of treatment. Avoidance of hepatotoxic drugs is essential. In older children, they must be advised to avoid alcohol
2. **Antiviral treatment.** No routine antivirals are indicated in viral hepatitis. The primary aim in chronic infection is to prevent progression to cirrhosis or liver failure. Chronic hepatitis B may be treated with pegylated interferon alfa and nucleoside or nucleotide analogues. Chronic hepatitis C may be treated with interferon alfa and ribavirin
3. **Liver transplant.** Liver transplant may be required in severe cases of liver failure

Box 5.5.11 Hepatitis A and B Immunisation Schedule in Children, UK

Vaccine	Aim	Schedule
Hepatitis B (newborn) Around 21% of newly acquired hepatitis B infection in the UK is through maternal–child transmission	Aim is to protect babies identified to be at risk through maternal screening from becoming chronically infected with hepatitis B All babies in the UK born after 1 August 2017 are given 3 doses; high-risk babies are given 6 doses	High risk: 6 doses Vaccine ± hepatitis B immunoglobulin at birth, 4 weeks and 12 months of age *and* Routine: all babies (3 doses as below) Vaccines at 8, 12 and 16 weeks of age with blood test at 12 months to exclude infection, confirm immune status
Hepatitis A	Travel to sub-Saharan Africa, Asia, the Middle East, South and Central America	Vaccine is a single initial dose, with a second dose 6–12 months later
Hepatitis B (older children)	Travel to sub-Saharan Africa, Asia, the Middle East and Southern and Eastern Europe	Vaccine is 3 doses spread over 3 weeks to 6 months

Dangerous Diagnosis 2

Diagnosis: Autoimmune hepatitis

Management Principles

1. **Long-term immunosuppressive therapy.** Steroids and azathioprine are commonly used, although efficacy is variable with relapses frequently occurring
2. **Monitoring.** Alanine aminotransferase (ALT) is used as a marker to monitor disease activity. Patients require monitoring for the long-term effects of steroid use
3. **Liver transplant.** Liver transplantation may be required in cases where medical treatment fails, or in fulminant liver failure

Dangerous Diagnosis 3

Diagnosis: Hepatotoxic drugs

Management Principles

1. **Removal of the offending drug.** Identifying and removing the hepatotoxic agent is important to prevent further damage
2. **Specific therapy.** In some cases a specific treatment exists, such as N-acetylcysteine in paracetamol hepatotoxicity
3. **Liver transplant.** Liver transplant may be required in fulminant liver failure

Common Diagnosis 1

Diagnosis: Gilbert syndrome

Management Principle

1. **Reassurance**. A clear explanation that there is no underlying liver disease is all that is required. Inform families that jaundice will likely reoccur during periods of stress or infection

Common Diagnosis 2

Diagnosis: Hereditary spherocytosis

Management Principles

1. **Folic acid.** Folic acid supports erythropoiesis as red blood cells are haemolysed
2. **Splenectomy.** Splenectomy is sometimes performed in moderate to severe cases to prevent haemolysis

Common Diagnosis 3

Diagnosis: Glucose-6-phosphate dehydrogenase deficiency

Management Principles

1. **Avoidance advice.** Parents and children should be provided with a list of drugs to avoid, including chemicals and foods that can cause oxidant stress and haemolysis
2. **Folic acid maintenance.** Folic acid supports erythropoiesis as red blood cells are haemolysed

Common Diagnosis 4
Diagnosis: Alpha-1-antitrypsin deficiency

Management Principles
1. **Smoking should be avoided.** Smoking has a pro-inflammatory impact on alveoli and patients with AAT deficiency should be strongly advised not to smoke
2. **Immunisation against hepatitis A and B**. Immunisation against viral hepatitis is recommended to prevent further hepatic insult
3. **Liver transplant.** Liver transplant may be required in fulminant liver failure

5.6 Faltering Growth

Rebecca Brown[1] and Helen Ratcliffe[2]

[1] *Department of Paediatrics, London School of Paediatrics, London, UK*
[2] *Oxford Vaccine Group, Centre for Clinical Vaccinology and Tropical Medicine, Oxford, UK*

CONTENTS

5.6.1 CHAPTER AT A GLANCE

Box 5.6.1   Chapter at a Glance

- Faltering growth, by definition, presents over time. It can therefore be a source of frustration and concern for parents
- It can be a marker of underlying chronic conditions, or of neglect
- The red book is a very useful tool for documenting weights and monitoring centiles
- This chapter will not cover neonatal weight loss, which tends to present over the first few days of life

5.6.2 DEFINITION

Faltering growth is where weight gain in childhood is significantly lower than expected for age and sex, resulting in measurements tracking down the centile lines.

5.6.3 DIAGNOSTIC ALGORITHM

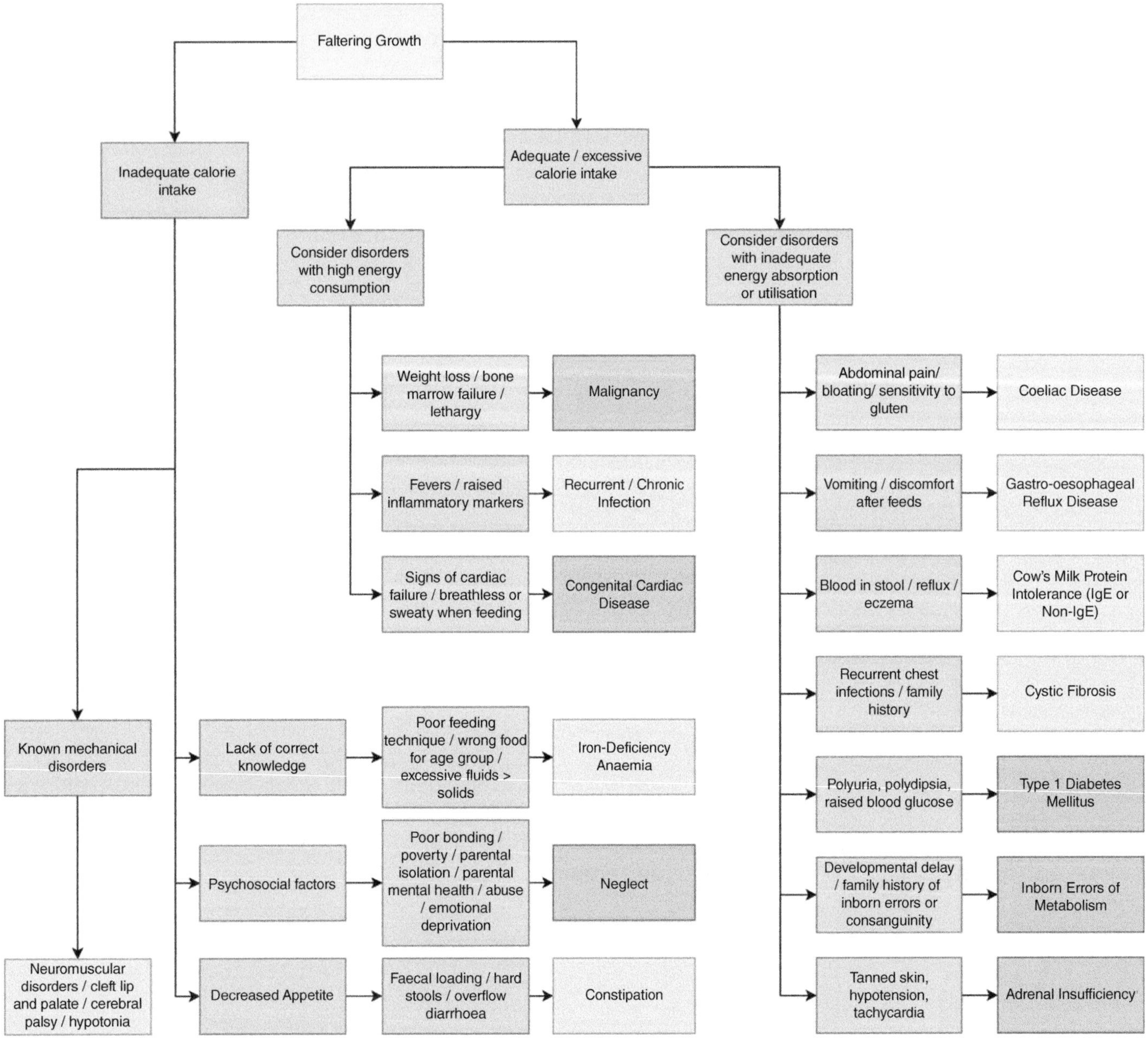

Figure 5.6.1 Diagnostic algorithm for the presentation of faltering growth.

5.6.4 DIFFERENTIALS LIST

Dangerous Diagnoses

1. **Type 1 Diabetes Mellitus (T1DM)**
   - Autoimmune condition caused by destruction of pancreatic beta cells. The body cannot synthesise insulin properly
   - Classic presentation is polyuria, polydipsia and weight loss, or failure to gain adequate weight
   - Presentation with diabetic ketoacidosis (DKA) is also common
2. **Adrenal Insufficiency**
   - Can be either primary or central
   - Primary: failure of adrenal cortex synthetic function. May affect glucocorticoid, mineralocorticoid and androgen hormone production
   - Central: dysfunction of either pituitary, affecting adrenocorticotropic hormone (ACTH) production, or hypothalamus, affecting corticotrophin-releasing hormone (CRH) production. This affects glucocorticoid (but not mineralocorticoid) production
3. **Inborn Errors of Metabolism (IEM)**
   - Defect or absence in an enzyme leads to either a deficiency or accumulation of a metabolite
   - Wide variety of categories and conditions
   - It is important to enquire about consanguinity, as most cases are inherited in an autosomal recessive manner
   - Detailed descriptions of congenital IEM are beyond the scope of this chapter
4. **Congenital Heart Disease (CHD)**
   - Many serious lesions will be picked up at the 20-week detailed anomaly scan. Others will be noted at either the newborn check or at the 6-week check
   - However, for some, first presentation will be due to cardiac failure. This might present as poor weight gain, associated with sweating and breathlessness when feeding
   - Faltering growth in heart failure is multifactorial. Reduced energy intake due to difficulty feeding is a main contributor. This is compounded by reduced exercise tolerance, malabsorption and end-organ dysfunction

---

Box 5.6.2   Malignancy   △△

- A common symptom of malignancy is weight loss
- Consider malignancy in any child who presents with weight loss, rather than faltering growth, particularly if other systemic symptoms are present, such as fever, bruising, recurrent infections, bone pain and pallor

---

Common Diagnoses

1. **Gastro-oesophageal Reflux Disease (GORD)**
   - Many babies have a degree of gastro-oesophageal reflux (GOR). This is a common presentation to both primary and secondary care
   - GORD is when there are pathological consequences, e.g. oesophagitis, aspiration pneumonia or poor weight gain
2. **Iron-Deficiency Anaemia (IDA)**
   - In infants under 6 months, anaemia may be physiological or due to an underlying haemoglobinopathy
   - In children over 6 months, an acquired anaemia such as IDA is more likely
   - Causes include low birth weight and poor iron supplementation, or early introduction of cow's milk below 1 year of age
   - 'Fussy eaters' often fall into this category, where they will frequently consume large amounts of milk to feel full instead of food. This leads to a spiral where they are not hungry and do not eat food. Cow's milk is low in iron, insufficient for requirements
3. **Cow's Milk Protein Allergy (CMPA)**
   - Most common food allergy in young children, caused by an immune reaction to cow's milk protein, which can be immunoglobulin (Ig) E or non-IgE mediated
   - Faltering growth is more commonly associated with the non-IgE-mediated subtype, due to food aversion, diarrhoea, vomiting and colitis causing malabsorption
   - CMPA is covered in detail in Chapter 5.3, and will not be discussed further in this chapter

4. Chronic Constipation

- Constipation affects up to 30% of children some time during childhood
- It is important to exclude serious underlying causes, which can cause faltering growth. These include spinal abnormalities, neuromuscular problems, Hirschsprung disease, bowel obstruction and pelvic malignancy
- Most cases are functional and lead to decreased appetite or may be a reflection of eating habits
- Constipation is covered in detail in Chapter 5.2, and therefore will not be discussed further in this chapter

---

Box 5.6.3   Mechanical Disorders   △△

- Children may have physical impairments to feeding. These are often known about long before faltering growth becomes apparent
- These include, but are not limited to:

- cleft lip and palate
- cerebral palsy
- hypotonia
- neuromuscular disorders

Diagnoses to Consider

1. Neglect

- There are many different psychosocial factors that may contribute to poor weight gain in a child, including poverty, poor parenting skills, poor understanding of nutrition and strong parental beliefs about certain restrictive diets
- It is important to remember that in cases of neglect there may be other elements of abuse, such as emotional, physical or sexual

When to consider: if there are concerns about the appearance of the child or interactions between child and carer

2. Cystic Fibrosis (CF)

- CF is a life-limiting genetic disorder that affects multiple body systems due to a mutation in the gene coding for the cystic fibrosis transmembrane conductance regulator (CFTR) protein
- This causes abnormal ion transport across the epithelium of the respiratory tract and pancreas, leading to increased viscosity of secretions
- Pancreatic insufficiency leads to malabsorption
- The majority of cases are diagnosed on routine newborn screening

When to consider: in those with recurrent chest infections or steatorrhoea, particularly if they did not undergo newborn screening

3. Coeliac Disease

- Coeliac disease is an autoimmune disorder of the small intestine caused by sensitivity to gluten in foods
- Exposure to dietary gluten leads to an enteropathy, with characteristic findings of villous atrophy on biopsy of the small intestine
- Presents with features of malabsorption such as abdominal pain, bloating, steatorrhoea and weight loss
- Children with Down syndrome and other autoimmune problems such as T1DM, selective IgA deficiency and autoimmune thyroiditis are at higher risk of developing coeliac disease

When to consider: in those whose growth falters once weaning is introduced after 6 months of age. In an older child, symptoms are more subtle, presenting with non-specific abdominal symptoms.

Box 5.6.4   Chronic and/or Recurrent Infections   △△

- Many children suffer from recurrent viral illnesses. This is often part of normal childhood and not indicative of underlying pathology
- In those with recurrent severe, atypical or chronic infections, there may be underlying immunodeficiency, which can be primary or secondary

- Regardless of aetiology, recurrent infections result in repeated episodes of reduced calorie intake and can lead to faltering growth

> **Box 5.6.5   Inflammatory Bowel Disease (IBD)**   △△
>
> - Consider IBD if there are insidious symptoms of non-bloody diarrhoea, which then becomes bloody, with associated abdominal pain
> - Patients with IBD struggle to maintain weight and frequently lose weight due to malabsorption. A common feature at
>
> presentation is a reduction in growth velocity, which can progress to short stature, delayed bone age and pubertal delay
> - IBD is covered in detail in Chapter 5.4

5.6.5 KEY HISTORY FEATURES

Dangerous Diagnosis 1
Diagnosis: Type 1 diabetes mellitus

Questions

1. **Is there a history of passing large volumes of urine? Has a previously continent child now started wetting the bed? If still in nappies, are the nappies heavier and need changing more frequently?** Urinary glucose excretion resulting from hyperglycaemia causes an osmotic diuresis. Nocturia or incontinence in a previously dry child or increased heavy/leaky wet nappies support polyuria
2. **Is there a history of increased thirst?** Polydipsia is caused by the increased serum osmolality from hyperglycaemia and hypovolaemia
3. **Is there a history of weight loss? Do clothes feel looser than they used to?** Weight loss is caused by fat and muscle breakdown due to impairment of glucose uptake from the blood. Ketosis leads to nausea and anorexia
4. **Is there a family history of T1DM?** Children have an increased susceptibility to developing T1DM if there is an affected family member, especially a parent
5. **Abdominal pain.** In DKA, abdominal pain can be associated with vomiting, which may be misleading, suggesting a surgical diagnosis

Dangerous Diagnosis 2
Diagnosis: Adrenal insufficiency

Questions

1. **Have there been any skin changes?** In primary adrenal insufficiency, hyperpigmentation arises from an increase in melanocyte-stimulating hormone (MSH), a breakdown product from an adrenocorticotrophic hormone (ACTH) precursor. Areas typically affected are the elbows, knees, palmar creases, axillae, tongue, palate, gums and scars
2. **Have there been any changes to weight or appetite?** Glucocorticoid deficiency causes weight loss. Mineralocorticoid deficiency (if primary adrenal insufficiency) causes urinary sodium loss. Children may complain of salt cravings and may have a reduced appetite
3. **Has there been vomiting or diarrhoea?** Nausea, vomiting and diarrhoea are features of glucocorticoid deficiency. There may also be generalised abdominal pain
4. **Have there been any problems with muscles or joints?** Glucocorticoid deficiency often leads to non-specific symptoms such as weakness, fatigue, myalgia and arthralgia

Dangerous Diagnosis 3
Diagnosis: Inborn errors of metabolism

Questions

1. **Have there been any concerns about the child's development?** A detailed developmental history is important. There may be a global deficit in achievement of developmental milestones, or it may be limited to one domain. Sometimes regression of previously achieved milestones may be reported
2. **Any problems with feeding?** Reduced gastrointestinal motility and other feeding issues are common
3. **Have you noticed any body odour or smell on their breath?** An abnormal breath/urine/perspiration/saliva odour could be a sign of organic acidaemias, amino acid disorders, urea cycle defects and fatty acid oxidation disorders

Dangerous Diagnosis 4
Diagnosis: Congenital heart disease

Questions
1. **Did the baby have any cardiac problems on antenatal scan?** Variable figures are documented, but up to 60% of CHD cases are detected on antenatal scans
2. **Any history of maternal diabetes?** 5% of infants of diabetic mothers are affected by CHD, compared to the background rate of around 1%. This is particularly raised in those with poor periconceptional glycaemic control
3. **Any family history of CHD?** Family history of a first-degree relative with CHD is a risk factor
4. **Does the child tire easily?** A baby may appear hungry, but tire quickly on feeding. Older children might be noted to have difficulty keeping up with peers when playing
5. **Is there a history of being sweaty with feeding?** Sweating, especially during feeding, can be a sign of cardiac failure

Common Diagnosis 1
Diagnosis: Gastro-oesophageal reflux disease

Questions
1. **How often and what volume does each feed contain?** Overfeeding is a common cause of vomiting. In bottle-fed babies, the volume of milk in mL/kg/day is easy to calculate. Babies with GORD may not settle well between feeds, may not lie flat and might display back arching after feeds (Sandifer syndrome)
2. **How often and how much does each vomit contain?** Frequent, large-volume vomits in GORD may be the reason the child is displaying faltering growth
3. **What colour is the vomit?** This is a screening question for emergencies. Bilious vomiting in a baby is a surgical emergency and requires prompt investigation. Vomiting in GORD should contain milky/gastric contents
4. **Are there any concerns about development?** Babies with underlying neurodisability or neuromuscular disease – with either hypotonia or hypertonia – often have reflux, and it is important to separate this from isolated GORD. Disordered swallowing with aspiration of fluids/food is also possible in this group of children

Common Diagnosis 2
Diagnosis: Iron-deficiency anaemia

Questions
1. **What does the child normally feed on?** Term babies are unlikely to become iron deficient unless they are being fed cow's milk or are breastfeeding from an iron-deficient mother. Once weaned, a diet of mostly cow's milk is a common cause, as it does not contain enough iron and reduces the appetite
2. **Has the child been tired?** Tiredness, lethargy and lack of concentration are typical symptoms of IDA
3. **In the older child, has there been any bleeding?** Nose bleeds and menstrual bleeds are often mistakenly overlooked in the history as considered insignificant bleeding
4. **Craving for non-food items?** This is known as pica, and is an uncommon phenomenon seen in IDA. Children with developmental delay are much more likely to be affected

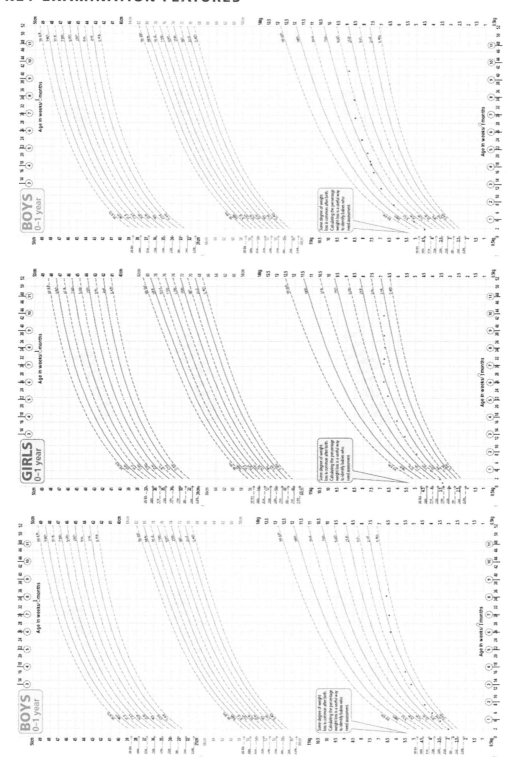

Figure 5.6.2 National Institute for Health and Care Excellence suggests thresholds for concern in faltering growth: (1) a fall across one or more weight centile spaces, if birthweight was below the 9th centile; (2) a fall across two or more weight centile spaces, if birthweight was between the 9th and 91st centiles; (3) a fall across three or more weight centile spaces, if birthweight was above the 91st centile. **Source:** Reproduced with permission of Royal College of Paediatrics and Child Health.

Dangerous Diagnosis 1
Diagnosis: Type 1 diabetes mellitus

Examination Findings
1. **Normal examination.** In children newly presenting with T1DM, not in DKA, there may be no findings beyond the classic history of polyuria, polydipsia and weight loss
2. **Dehydration.** In DKA, clinical signs of intravascular depletion include tachycardia and prolonged capillary refill due to poor perfusion
3. **Drowsiness.** In DKA, if the patient is significantly drowsy, airway patency can be compromised. This is related to the degree of acidosis. Cerebral injury due to cerebral oedema is an important cause of mortality

---

Box 5.6.6   Faltering Growth in Children with Known Type 1 Diabetes Mellitus (T1DM)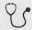

There are several reasons why children with T1DM may have ongoing issues with faltering growth:

- Non-compliance with medications
- Injecting insulin into the same site
- Incorrect administration technique
- Deliberate avoidance of insulin to achieve weight loss
- Development of associated autoimmune disorders, such as coeliac disease

---

Dangerous Diagnosis 2
Diagnosis: Adrenal insufficiency

Examination Findings:
1. **Hypotension.** Hypotension is more pronounced in primary adrenal insufficiency due to lack of aldosterone, leading to dehydration. Decreased cortisol contributes due to reduced adrenaline secretion. There will be a significant postural drop in blood pressure
2. **Hyperpigmentation.** Tanned skin results from excess melanin deposition, particularly on the face, neck, hands and buccal mucosa. This is accentuated at creases, folds and scars
3. **Tachycardia and shock.** There may be resting tachycardia. With delayed diagnosis, circulatory shock can develop, and can be accompanied by nausea and abdominal pain. Preexisting hypotension and tachycardia will become more marked and perfusion will be significantly compromised

Dangerous Diagnosis 3
Diagnosis: Inborn errors of metabolism
Each different inborn error has its own clinical features and examination findings. Some clinical features are common across many, which may help raise the index of suspicion.

Examination Findings
1. **Seizures.** IEMs should always be considered in first presentation of seizures, especially in infancy. It is important to note family history and consanguinity
2. **Organomegaly.** Hepatomegaly and/or splenomegaly are common features of many lysosomal storage disorders, glycogen storage disorders and mitochondrial disorders
3. **Dysmorphic features.** Can be present at birth or become more obvious with age

Dangerous Diagnosis 4
Diagnosis: Congenital heart disease

Examination Findings
1. **Respiratory distress.** In CHD, signs of respiratory distress include grunting, head bobbing, nasal flare, intercostal and sub-costal recession
2. **Tachycardia.** There may be tachycardia and cool peripheries indicate poor perfusion. On auscultation there may be a gallop rhythm
3. **Murmur.** In CHD, it is common to hear a heart murmur on auscultation, relating to the underlying defect. There may also be thrills or heaves palpable
4. **Crackles on auscultation.** Fine crepitations and wheeze may be heard on auscultation of the lungs, relating to pulmonary oedema
5. **Hepatomegaly.** If there is right heart failure, hepatomegaly results from hepatic congestion

Common Diagnosis 1
Diagnosis: Gastro-oesophageal reflux disease

Examination Findings
1. **Normal examination.** In the majority, diagnosis is based on history, and examination is normal
2. **Wheeze, cough or focal signs on auscultation.** Severe reflux can lead to aspiration, which causes inflammation of the airways and can present as chronic cough, wheezing and crackles in some areas of the chest

Common Diagnosis 2
Diagnosis: Iron-deficiency anaemia

Examination Findings
1. **Pallor.** Pallor, indicating anaemia, may be evident in conjunctivae or palmar creases
2. **Nail changes.** Prolonged IDA may cause spoon-shaped nails, known as koilonychia

5.6.7 KEY INVESTIGATIONS

Not all children will require invasive investigations; often diagnoses are made on clinical evidence from history and examination. Consider carefully which investigations are required for which patient.

Bedside

Table 5.6.1 Bedside tests of use in patients presenting with faltering growth

Test	When to perform	Potential result
Urine dip	• All children with faltering growth • Screens for infection and glycosuria • Subclinical UTIs can cause faltering growth	• +ve leucocytes, +ve nitrites in infection • Glycosuria suggests diabetes
Urine MC&S	• If positive urine dipstick	• Positive culture confirms bacterial infection • Sensitivities guide antibiotic choice
Blood sugar	Suspected: • T1DM • IEM	• <2.6 mmol/L: hypoglycaemia, consider IEM • >11 mmol/L: consider T1DM

IEM, inborn errors of metabolism; MC&S, microscopy, culture and sensitivity; T1DM, type 1 diabetes mellitus; UTI, urinary tract infection

Blood Tests

Table 5.6.2 Blood tests of use in patients presenting with faltering growth

Test	When to perform	Potential result
FBC	• All children with faltering growth	• ↓ Hb confirms anaemia • ↓ MCV, ↓ MCHC supports IDA • Pancytopenia suggests bone marrow failure in malignancy
Blood film	• If anaemia on FBC • Suspected malignancy	• Hypochromia, microcytosis in IDA • Peripheral blasts indicate leukaemia
Ferritin	• Suspected IDA	• ↓ Ferritin: IDA
ESR, CRP	• Suspected chronic/recurrent infection	• ↑ In infection and inflammation
U&E	• All children with faltering growth	• ↑ Urea and creatinine in dehydration, as seen in T1DM, severe GORD • ↓ Na and ↑ K in adrenal insufficiency
LFTs	• All children with faltering growth • Albumin is useful nutritional marker • LFTs deranged in IEM	• ↓ Albumin marker of chronic malnutrition • ↑ AST/ALT can be seen in IEM
Ammonia	• Suspected IEM	• ↑ Ammonia in IEM, particularly urea cycle defects
TFTs + thyroid antibodies	• All children with faltering growth	• ↑ TSH, ↓ T4 in hypothyroidism • Thyroid antibodies in autoimmune disease
Tissue transglutaminase – IgA	• Suspected coeliac disease	• >10 u/mL supports coeliac disease
Serum amino acids	• Suspected IEM	• High specific amino acids determine underlying IEM
GH	• Faltering growth with diagnostic uncertainty to rule out GH deficiency	• ↓ GH indicates deficiency and need for pituitary evaluation
Morning cortisol	• Suspected adrenal insufficiency • Does not discriminate between primary adrenal failure, ACTH deficiency, or an enzymatic defect in the production of cortisol	• ↓ Cortisol in adrenal insufficiency • May need a short synacthen test to further evaluate
Immunodeficiency screen	• Chronic/recurrent infections	• ↓ IgG/A/M ± IgG subclasses in isolation or combination

ACTH, adrenocorticotropic hormone; ALT, alanine aminotransferase; AST, aspartate aminotransferase; CRP, C-reactive protein; ESR, erythrocyte sedimentation rate; FBC, full blood count; GH, growth hormone; GORD, gastro-oesophageal reflux disease; Hb, haemoglobin; IDA, iron-deficiency anaemia; IEM, inborn errors of metabolism; Ig, immunoglobulin; K, potassium; LFTs, liver function tests; MCHC, mean corpuscular haemoglobin concentration; MCV, mean corpuscular volume; Na, sodium; T1DM, type 1 diabetes mellitus; TFTs, thyroid function tests; TSH, thyroid-stimulating hormone; U&E, urea and electrolytes

Imaging

Table 5.6.3 Imaging modalities of use in patients presenting with faltering growth

Test	When to perform	Potential result
Chest x-ray	Suspected: • CHD • CF • Aspiration due to GORD • Chronic/recurrent infections	• CHD: cardiomegaly ± perihilar changes • CF: evidence of bronchiectasis • Pneumonia: consolidation • Aspiration: right middle lobe consolidation

CF, cystic fibrosis; CHD, congenital heart disease; GORD, gastro-oesophageal reflux disease

Special

Table 5.6.4 Special tests of use in patients presenting with faltering growth

Test	When to perform	Potential result
Faecal elastase	• Suspected CF • Measure of exocrine pancreatic function	• ↓ In cystic fibrosis • Normal: >200 µg/g stool
Sweat test	• Gold standard when suspecting CF • Measures sweat chloride	• High Cl: >60 mmol/L • Borderline Cl: 30–60 mmol/L • Normal Cl: <30 mmol/L
Synacthen test	• Suspected adrenal insufficiency in those with low cortisol • Variation in practice as to whether low dose or short test is used	• Failure of cortisol to rise suggests adrenal problem • Appropriate rise of cortisol suggests pituitary deficiency of ACTH • Some evidence that 'short' test is less sensitive than 'low dose'
Upper GI endoscopy	• Suspected GORD	• Evidence of oesophagitis, gastritis
24-hour pH impedance monitoring	• Suspected GORD to assess RI	• ↑ RI in GORD
Urinary amino acids and organic acids	• Suspected IEM	• Specific high amino or organic acid concentrations determine underlying IEM
ECG	Suspected: • CHD • DKA • Adrenal insufficiency	• Tachycardia or ventricular hypertrophy in cardiac failure • Tall and tented T waves in hyperkalaemia
Interferon-gamma release assay	• If diagnostic uncertainty with TB contact history	• Positive result provides support for TB, but does not differentiate between active and latent

ACTH, adrenocorticotropic hormone; CF, cystic fibrosis; CHD, congenital heart disease; Cl, chloride; DKA, diabetic ketoacidosis; ECG, electrocardiogram; GI, gastrointestinal; GORD, gastro-oesophageal reflux disease; IEM, inborn errors of metabolism; RI, reflux index; TB, tuberculosis

5.6.8 KEY MANAGEMENT PRINCIPLES

Diagnosis-specific management strategies are outlined here. It is expected that an 'ABCDE' approach to assessment and management is always undertaken (see Chapter 12.1).

Dangerous Diagnosis 1
Diagnosis: Type 1 diabetes mellitus

Management Principles
1. **Management of acute presentations.** There will be local protocols for new diagnoses and DKA. These will address the need for fluid resuscitation, insulin administration and management of electrolyte disturbances
2. **Liaise with diabetic team and long-term insulin.** Close diabetic team supervision will help maintain good glycaemic control. Many different insulin regimes exist using daily injections or an insulin pump
3. **Liaise with dieticians, dietary and lifestyle changes.** Diet and exercise both have a major impact on glycaemic control. Education on these topics is a crucial part of the management of diabetes. Teenagers should be counselled on alcohol consumption

Dangerous Diagnosis 2
Diagnosis: Adrenal insufficiency

Management Principles
Acute
1. **Hydrocortisone.** Hydrocortisone should be given as an intravenous (IV) bolus. If no IV access within 15 minutes, this should be given intramuscularly (IM). Parents with children with known adrenal insufficiency are trained in giving IM hydrocortisone at home in an emergency. Hydrocortisone should then be continued 6 hourly
2. **IV fluids.** Adrenal crisis causes shock. Fluid resuscitation is as boluses of 20 mL/kg of isotonic solution, preferably 0.9% saline, followed by maintenance when stable

Ongoing
1. **Glucocorticoid supplementation.** Glucocorticoids, e.g. hydrocortisone, are used to supplement endogenous deficiency. Close monitoring of growth and bone age with dose adjustments will be required
2. **Mineralocorticoid supplementation.** If there is primary adrenal insufficiency, mineralocorticoid supplementation with fludrocortisone is also required
3. **Sick-day rules in stress conditions.** Additional glucocorticoids will be required in physiological stress to avoid adrenal crisis. Stress states include acute illness and surgery. If oral medication is not tolerated, then IM injection is required. Families should be educated to use IM hydrocortisone for emergency situations
4. **Adrenal insufficiency plan.** A written plan should be provided to families, including maintenance hydrocortisone dose, stress dose of oral, IM and IV hydrocortisone, and IM administration instructions. Ideally patients should carry a medical alert identification, indicating glucocorticoid dependency

Dangerous Diagnosis 3
Diagnosis: Inborn errors of metabolism
Management of IEMs will often require a quaternary-level discussion at a specialist metabolic centre. Specific management will depend on the specific IEM, but there are some general principles of how to manage a child who presents acutely unwell. Emergency treatment focuses on treating hypoglycaemia, hyperammonaemia and seizures.

Management Principles
1. **Prevent accumulation of metabolites.** Build-up of metabolites can cause permanent damage, so one of the first steps is to stop enteral feeds to prevent protein and carbohydrate intake until diagnosis is known
2. **Fluid resuscitation.** This is important to maintain circulating volume. It is worth remembering that fluid containing lactate should be avoided, as this could exacerbate a lactic acidosis
3. **Prevent catabolism.** IV dextrose should be given to prevent catabolism and maintain blood sugar levels

Dangerous Diagnosis 4
Diagnosis: Congenital heart disease

Management Principles
1. **Referral to cardiology.** Heart failure secondary to CHD will require referral to a tertiary cardiology centre to guide further investigation and management
2. **Optimise nutrition.** Faltering growth is due to increased metabolic demands, and poor intake due to breathlessness. Often, corrective surgery requires a target weight to be achieved. Consider concentrating feeds in bottle-fed infants, high-calorie supplementation or nasogastric (NG) feeds
3. **Initial management of cardiac failure.** Cardiac failure can be controlled through maintaining fluid balance, as noted above, and use of diuretic therapy such as furosemide, spironolactone or chlorothiazide. Advice should be sought from cardiology specialists
4. **Surgical correction.** The need and timing of corrective cardiac surgery depend on the underlying defect and can also vary in different tertiary centres

Common Diagnosis 1
Diagnosis: Gastro-oesophageal reflux disease

Management Principles
1. **Simple measures.** Upright positioning after feeds for 30 minutes or raising the head of the bed can be helpful. Smaller, more frequent or even thickened feeds might be considered
2. **Trial of cow's milk–free diet.** If GORD is a symptom of CMPA, symptoms may improve following exclusion
3. **Pharmacological and surgical management.** If conservative measures fail, it may be necessary to give a trial of acid-suppressing medication, usually a proton pump inhibitor (PPI) such as omeprazole, lansoprazole and esomeprazole. Surgical management – fundoplication with or without percutaneous endoscopic gastrostomy (PEG) or percutaneous endoscopic transgastric jejunostomy (PEG-J) insertion – may be necessary in very severe cases or those complicated by underlying conditions

Common Diagnosis 2
Diagnosis: Iron-deficiency anaemia

Management Principles
1. **Dietary iron.** Under 6 months: if bottle fed, ensure formula is fortified. If breastfed, consider a 3-month trial of iron supplements. Over 6 months: dietician can advise on iron-rich and fortified foods. Vitamin C aids with absorption. Limit cow's milk in the toddler age groups
2. **Supplemental iron.** If dietary measures alone are not enough, a 3-month trial of iron supplements can be tried, followed by re-checking the haemoglobin to guide cessation
3. **Transfusion.** Rarely necessary, as chronically low haemoglobin is often well tolerated. If evidence of haemodynamic compromise, then a blood transfusion is appropriate

6.1 Haematuria

Ashish Patel and Sally-Anne Hulton

Department of Paediatric Nephrology, Birmingham Women's and Children's NHS Foundation Trust, Birmingham, UK

CONTENTS

6.1.1 CHAPTER AT A GLANCE

Box 6.1.1 Chapter at a Glance

- Microscopic haematuria is a common problem in children, usually following viral illnesses
- Persisting microscopic haematuria or macroscopic haematuria warrants further clinical assessment and evaluation
- If there are associated abnormal features such as proteinuria, specialist tertiary review should be considered

6.1.2 DEFINITION

The presence of more than 5 red blood cells per millilitre in a sample of fresh uncentrifuged midstream urine, which can be macroscopic or microscopic in nature.

Clinical Guide to Paediatrics, First Edition. Edited by Rachel Varughese and Anna Mathew. Series Editor: Christian Fielder Camm.
© 2022 John Wiley & Sons Ltd. Published 2022 by John Wiley & Sons Ltd.
Companion website: www.wiley.com/go/varughese/paediatrics

6.1.3 DIAGNOSTIC ALGORITHM

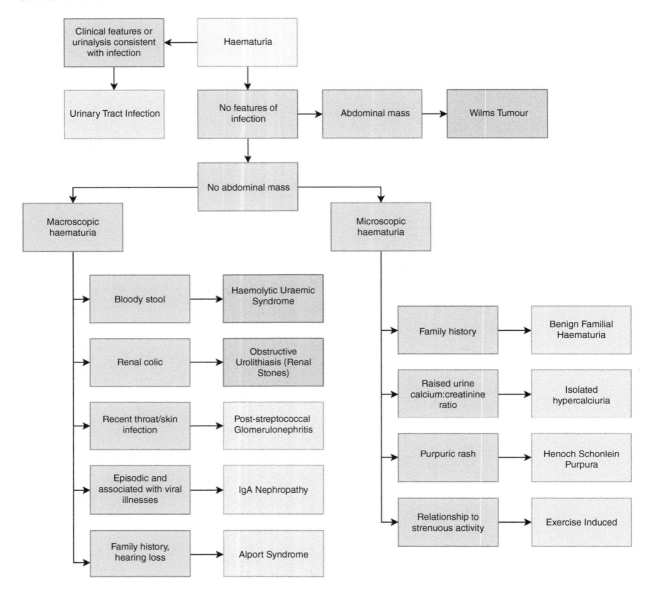

Figure 6.1.1 Diagnostic algorithm for the presentation of haematuria.

6.1.4 DIFFERENTIALS LIST

Dangerous Diagnoses

1. Obstructive Urolithiasis ('Renal Stones')

- Renal stones are less common in children than in adults
- Stones are caused by high levels of solutes that precipitate into crystals (calcium, oxalate, uric acid, cystine), or decreased levels of stone inhibitors (citrate, magnesium and pyrophosphate)
- The most common underlying contributor is hypercalciuria
- Flank or abdominal pain is the most common presenting symptom, but macroscopic haematuria can be present in up to 50% of children
- Can lead to obstruction of the urinary tract, leading to pelvic or ureteric obstruction

2. Wilms' Tumour
- Also called nephroblastoma, Wilms' tumour is an embryonal renal neoplasm
- Most cases are sporadic, but children with certain syndromes such as Beckwith–Weidemann syndrome are at increased risk
- Wilms' tumour typically presents aged 2–5 years and accounts for 5% of all childhood cancers
- Can present with an abdominal mass/incidental finding following a scan for haematuria
- Wilms' is rare >10 years, when a renal malignancy is more likely to be a renal cell carcinoma
- Haematuria is sometimes the only presenting complaint
- Wilms' tumour is covered in detail in Chapter 5.2 and will not be discussed further in this chapter

3. Haemolytic Uraemic Syndrome (HUS)
- Triad of haemolytic anaemia, thrombocytopenia and acute kidney injury often preceded by a diarrhoeal illness that is bloody
- The most common cause is following infection with Shiga toxin producing *Escherichia coli* – *E.coli* 0157:H7
- Commonly acquired through contact and then ingestion of contaminated material
- HUS causes progressive renal failure with oliguria or anuria
- Although microscopic haematuria may be a feature of renal involvement, red/dark urine is often a result of haemoglobinuria, due to intravascular haemolysis
- HUS is covered in detail in Chapters 4.2 and 5.4 and will not be discussed further in this chapter

Common Diagnoses

1. Urinary Tract Infection (UTI)
- Commonest cause for macroscopic haematuria in children
- More common in girls than boys, typical bacterial organism being *E. coli*
- Adenovirus can cause haemorrhagic cystitis in children with associated upper respiratory tract symptoms

2. Benign Familial Haematuria (Thin Basement Membrane Disease)
- Accounts for 1% of cases of persistent glomerular bleeding
- Caused by a mutation in type IV collagen in 50% of cases
- Persistent microscopic or episodic macroscopic haematuria with no other findings
- Need to exclude genetic conditions such as Alport syndrome
- No long-term associated renal complications

3. Idiopathic Hypercalciuria
- Excessive amounts of calcium in the urine in the setting of normal serum calcium levels
- Thought to be due to either tubular leakage of calcium from the kidneys or increased absorption of calcium from the gut
- Can be asymptomatic with only microscopic haematuria, or can go on to develop urolithiasis

4. Immunoglobulin (Ig) A Nephropathy
- IgA nephropathy is the most common underlying cause of primary glomerulonephritis in developed countries
- It is characterised by IgA deposition in the glomerulus, seen on renal biopsy
- There is a genetic preponderance, with East Asians and Caucasians most commonly affected
- IgA nephropathy is commonly asymptomatic for many years
- Haematuria is the most common presenting feature. Microscopic haematuria may be incidentally identified on urinalysis. Episodes of frank haematuria are associated with intercurrent infections
- Patients can develop progressive renal impairment

Box 6.1.2   Excessive Exercise and Haematuria (Apparent Haematuria)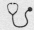

- Direct trauma to the flank or abdomen (e.g. in boxing) or perineum (e.g. cycling) can cause haematuria
- Higher-filtration pressures to the kidneys during exercise can lead to leakage of red blood cells into the urine
- Lactic acidosis may increase glomerular permeability, leading to increased excretion of red blood cells in the urine

- Myoglobinuria (red/brown urine) is a consequence of rhabdomyolysis
- March haemoglobinuria results from haemolysis due to direct impact on the vasculature of the feet
- Exercise-induced haematuria resolves with rest and does not cause any long-term complications

---

Diagnoses to Consider

1. Alport Syndrome
- Inherited glomerular disease characterised by haematuria, sensorineural hearing loss and ocular anomalies
- Most commonly inherited in an X-linked fashion, but may also be autosomal recessive, and rarely autosomal dominant

- Males tend to be more severely affected
- Progression to renal failure may occur in early adult life

When to consider: if there is family history of Alport syndrome, or a history of hearing/renal impairment in an adult relative

2. Post-streptococcal Glomerulonephritis

- Children have a preceding group A streptococcal infection of the skin or throat prior to onset of glomerulonephritis and macroscopic haematuria
- As the cause of the nephritis is glomerular in nature, the urine appears dark brown or 'cola' coloured, due to degradation of the red cells within the tubules
- Periorbital oedema, oliguria, hypertension and proteinuria may accompany the haematuria
- This condition is now uncommon in developed countries
- Long-term prognosis is usually good

When to consider: in those with a preceding history of throat or skin infection a few weeks prior to presentation

3. Henoch-Schönlein Purpura (HSP)

- HSP is a systemic IgA vasculitis affecting the skin, mucosal membranes, joints and kidneys
- Palpable purpura are a key aspect of diagnosis, which may be associated with petechiae and ecchymoses. These are usually symmetrical, typically affecting gravity-dependent areas such as the lower limbs and buttocks
- Purpura is accompanied by arthritis in 50–75%, abdominal pain in 50% and renal involvement in 25–50% of children
- May be precipitated by infection, classically haemolytic streptococci
- HSP is covered in detail in Chapters 9.2 and 10.2

When to consider: in children with palpable purpura over lower limbs and buttocks

---

Box 6.1.3 Causes of Visibly Red Urine without Evidence of Haematuria   ΔΔ

It is important to remember that urine that appears visibly red may not be haematuria

- Haemoglobinuria
- Myoglobinuria
- Drugs, e.g. rifampicin, doxorubicin, nitrofurantoin
- Foods, e.g. beetroot, food dyes, berries
- Inborn errors of metabolism, e.g. porphyria, tyrosinaemia
- Factitious illness
- Urate crystals in neonates
- Menstruation

Box 6.1.4 Common Neonatal Causes of Haematuria   ΔΔ

- Urinary tract infection
- Coagulopathy, e.g. thrombocytopaenia, haemorrhagic disease of the newborn
- Thrombosis – renal artery or renal vein thrombosis
- Trauma
- Acute tubular necrosis – due to hypotension, sepsis or drugs
- Medications – non-steroidal anti-inflammatory drugs
- Nephrocalcinosis
- Structural anomalies, e.g. posterior urethral valves
- Genetic causes, e.g. polycystic kidney disease

Conditions that cause neonatal haematuria are not otherwise discussed in this chapter

---

6.1.5 KEY HISTORY FEATURES

Dangerous Diagnosis 1

Diagnosis: Obstructive urolithiasis

Questions

1. **Is there any associated abdominal pain?** The pain associated with renal colic pain is typically described as severe and spasmodic, radiating between the loin and groin
2. **Is there associated vomiting?** Unlike most other causes of haematuria, there can be a significant history of nausea and vomiting
3. **Is there a history of renal structural abnormalities or urinary infections?** Structural urinary tract abnormalities increase the likelihood of renal stones. In addition, recurrent UTIs, particularly with urease-producing organisms, such as *Proteus* or *Klebsiella*, promotes formation of phosphate salts
4. **Is there a history of malabsorption or a ketogenic diet?** Malabsorptive conditions (e.g. coeliac disease or short gut) may result in hyperoxaluria. A ketogenic diet, used in epilepsy, leads to hypercalciuria (due to chronic metabolic acidosis), hypocitraturia (citrate being a stone inhibitor) and uric acid crystal formation (due to lowered urinary pH)

5. **What is the medication history?** Several medications can predispose to urinary calculi. These include nasal decongestants (e.g. ephedrine), loop diuretics, acetazolamide, antiepileptics (e.g. topiramate) and some antibiotics (e.g. ciprofloxacin and sulfonamides)

Common Diagnosis 1
Diagnosis: Urinary tract infection

Questions
1. **Are there associated urinary symptoms?** Older children with UTIs may have urinary symptoms such as increased frequency and dysuria, sometimes associated with haematuria. In infants, irritability and an altered urinary stream may be noted
2. **Is there a known structural abnormality of the renal tract**? Children with structural anomalies are more prone to developing UTIs
3. **Has there been a history of fever?** Infants and children with UTIs usually present with fevers. If there is no focus for a fever in a child, a urine sample should be obtained, dipped for testing using dipsticks, and then sent for microscopy and culture. See Chapter 3.1, *Fever*, Box 3.1.15, *Categorising Urinary Tract Infections (UTIs)*

Common Diagnosis 2
Diagnosis: Benign familial haematuria (thin basement membrane disease)

Questions
1. **Is there a family history of haematuria?** There is likely to be a family history of microscopic or episodic macroscopic haematuria
2. **Is the child otherwise well?** Urinalysis is often done for other reasons, and the microscopic haematuria incidentally picked up

Common Diagnosis 3
Diagnosis: Idiopathic hypercalciuria

Questions
1. **Is there a family history of nephrolithiasis?** There may be a family history of renal stones
2. **Was the patient born prematurely?** Children who are born prematurely are more likely to develop hypercalciuria and nephrolithiasis
3. **Is there any pain on passing urine?** Occasionally, dysuria, urgency and frequency are reported. Enuresis is a rare complaint

Common Diagnosis 4
Diagnosis: Immunoglobulin A nephropathy

Questions
1. **When does the macroscopic haematuria occur?** Intercurrent illnesses such as upper respiratory tract infections are often triggers
2. **What is the pattern of haematuria?** The haematuria is macroscopic during the intercurrent infection and becomes microscopic or is absent between episodes

6.1.6 KEY EXAMINATION FEATURES

Dangerous Diagnosis 1
Diagnosis: Obstructive urolithiasis

Examination Findings
1. **Discomfort/distress with bouts of abdominal pain.** During bouts of renal colic, patients are unable to lie still or get comfortable. Often there is very little else to find on examination
2. **Signs of sepsis.** Fever, tachycardia or hypotension associated with the colicky abdominal pain and a urine dipstick positive for leukocytes and nitrites could suggest an infected obstructed urolithiasis, which is a surgical emergency

Common Diagnosis 1
Diagnosis: Urinary tract infection

Examination Findings
1. **Suprapubic/loin tenderness.** Tenderness on palpation over the lower abdomen or suprapubic region may suggest cystitis. Tenderness on balloting the kidney might indicate a pyelonephritis

2. **Fever.** Fevers are common. UTIs are difficult to diagnose in infants and toddlers due to non-specific symptoms and signs, with fever often the only sign of note

Common Diagnosis 2

Diagnosis: Benign familial haematuria

Examination Findings

1. **Otherwise well.** This is a diagnosis of exclusion. All other differentials should be considered first. Examination will be normal, with a normal blood pressure, but with isolated persistent microscopic haematuria

Common Diagnosis 3

Diagnosis: Idiopathic hypercalciuria

Examination Findings

1. **Otherwise well.** This diagnosis cannot be determined on examination. Non-specific flank or lower abdominal tenderness is noted on occasion. The diagnosis can only be confirmed by assaying urinary calcium

Common Diagnosis 4

Diagnosis: Immunoglobulin A nephropathy

Examination Findings

1. **Coryza.** In 80% of cases there is a history of a synchronous upper respiratory infection associated with the onset of macroscopic haematuria
2. **Episodic macroscopic haematuria.** The haematuria is macroscopic, sometimes with clots, and settles when the child recovers

6.1.7 KEY INVESTIGATIONS

Not all children will require invasive investigations; often diagnoses are made on clinical evidence from history and examination. Consider carefully which investigations are required for which patient.

Bedside

Table 6.1.1 Bedside tests of use in patients presenting with haematuria

Test	When to perform	Potential result
BP	• All patients with haematuria	• ↑ BP: suggests glomerular cause
Urine dipstick	• All patients with haematuria	• Leucocytes and nitrites: UTI • Blood: confirms haematuria • Protein: requires further investigation for causes of proteinuria
Urine protein:creatinine ratio (early morning)	• All patients with 1+ proteinuria on dipstick for quantification of proteinuria	• ↑ Ratio identifies glomerular disease as cause of proteinuria
Urine MC&S	• All patients with haematuria for examination of red cell morphology, and to identify infection	• Dysmorphic or red cell casts suggest bleeding is glomerular in origin; normal red cell morphology suggests lower tract sources • Positive culture confirms bacterial infection and sensitivities guide antibiotic choice
Urine calcium:creatinine ratio (best as second morning urine sample)	• Suspected idiopathic hypercalciuria	• ↑ Calcium:creatinine ratio suggests hypercalciuria
Stool MC&S	• Suspected HUS	• Positive for *Escherichia Coli* 0157 in HUS

BP, blood pressure; HUS, haemolytic uraemic syndrome; MC&S, microscopy, culture and sensitivity; UTI, urinary tract infection

Blood Tests

Table 6.1.2 Blood tests of use in patients presenting with haematuria

Test	When to perform	Potential result
FBC	• All patients with significant/persistent haematuria	• ↓ Hb, ↓platelets: consider HUS • ↓ Hb: common in chronic renal disease
U&E	• All patients with haematuria	• ↑ Urea, ↑ creatinine: acute or chronic kidney injury
Serum calcium	• Suspected idiopathic hypercalciuria	• ↔ Calcium required for diagnosis
Complement levels	• Suspected post-streptococcal glomerulonephritis	• ↓ C3, ↔ C4: classical of post-streptococcal glomerulonephritis
ASO titres	• Suspected post-streptococcal glomerulonephritis	• ↑ Titres: support diagnosis of post-streptococcal glomerulonephritis
Serum immunoglobulins	• Suspected IgA nephropathy	• ↑ IgA: seen in up to 30% of patients with IgA nephropathy

ANA, antinuclear antibody; ASO, antistreptolysin-O; FBC, full blood count; Hb, haemoglobin; HUS, haemolytic uraemic syndrome; Ig, immunoglobulin; U&E, urea and electrolyte

Imaging

The requirement to image the renal tract following a diagnosis of a UTI is determined by age, mode of presentation and causative organism. In the UK, the National Institute for Health and Care Excellence (NICE) guidelines for the management of UTI provide the necessary recommendations. See Chapter 3.1, *Fever*, Box 3.1.20, *Investigations Following Urinary Tract Infection (UTI)*.

Table 6.1.3 Imaging modalities of use in patients presenting with haematuria

Test	When to perform	Potential result
Renal and urinary tract ultrasound	• Consider in all patients with haematuria	• Structural abnormalities • Tumours • Renal calculi

Special

Table 6.1.4 Special tests of use in patients presenting with haematuria

Test	When to perform	Potential result
Renal biopsy	• To obtain tissue diagnosis if persisting macroscopic or microscopic haematuria, associated proteinuria or abnormal renal function	• Can identify glomerular causes of haematuria
Genetic assessment	• Suspected genetic cause for haematuria	• Familial causes, e.g. Alport syndrome

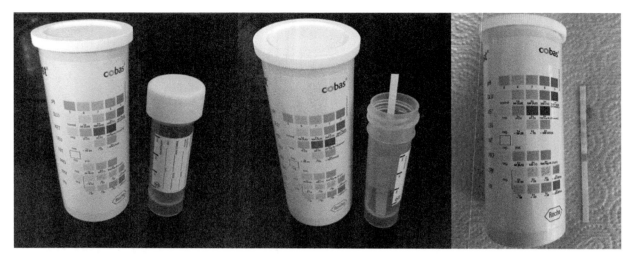

Figure 6.1.2 How to perform and interpret a urine dipstick. 1. Ensure urine dipsticks are in date. 2. Remove a testing strip from the container and insert fully into the urine sample. 3. Remove the strip from the urine sample, remove excess urine and place horizontally onto kitchen paper. 4. Interpret findings against the dipstick analysis guide on the urine dipstick container after 60 seconds.

6.1.8 KEY MANAGEMENT PRINCIPLES

Diagnosis-specific management strategies are outlined here. It is expected that an 'ABCDE' approach to assessment and management is considered standard practice (see Chapter 12.1, *The A to E Assessment*).

Dangerous Diagnosis 1
Diagnosis: Obstructive urolithiasis

Management Principles
1. **Prepare for surgery/make nil by mouth.** If acute ureteric obstruction occurs, surgery may be indicated, and a paediatric urologist should be informed. The obstructed stone may be removed surgically via ureterorenoscopy with or without lithotripsy. If surgery is planned, make the child nil by mouth
2. **Analgesia.** Obstructive urolithiasis can be very painful and therefore prompt analgesia should be provided

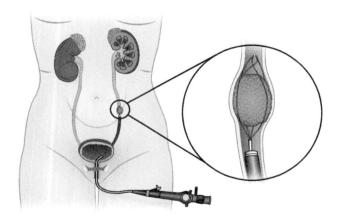

Figure 6.1.3 A ureterorenoscopy is performed under general anaesthetic and involves the passage of a small endoscope through the bladder and into the ureter in order to retrieve the stone.

3. **Intravenous (IV) fluids.** To maintain adequate hydration following vomiting, and to facilitate passage of the stone, children should be commenced on IV fluids. Caution is required if anuria has been caused by bilateral obstruction until surgical relief is obtained. After surgical intervention, fluid requirements may increase due to post-operative diuresis.

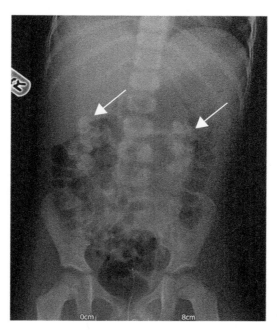

Figure 6.1.4 Renal calculi as seen on an abdominal x-ray.

Common Diagnosis 1
Diagnosis: Urinary tract infection

Management Principles
1. **Antibiotics.** Antibiotics should be commenced based on local guidelines. Urine microscopy, culture and sensitivity (MC&S) identification of the causative organism can help tailor antibiotic therapy. Antibiotics can be given orally, but IV antibiotics may be indicated if there are signs of sepsis, pyelonephritis or in young infants. Remember that children already receiving antibiotic prophylaxis for renal structural problems should be treated with an alternative antibiotic in the acute phase, or until urine sensitivities are obtained
2. **High fluid intake.** Advice should be given to parents to ensure their child is drinking adequate amounts
3. **Undertake imaging following treatment.** This should be undertaken as recommended by NICE guidelines, based on age/mode of presentation and organism isolated
4. **Lifestyle measures.** Constipation can increase the risk and recurrence of UTIs through poor bladder emptying, and dietary modification may be required (See Chapter 3.1, *Fever*, Box 3.1.20, *Investigations Following Urinary Tract Infection (UTI)*). Appropriate hygiene measures should be recommended, including preference for showers over bubble baths, toilet paper wiping from front to back only and wearing cotton pants.

Common Diagnosis 2
Diagnosis: Benign familial haematuria

Management Principle
1. **Reassurance.** Thin basement membrane disease is a generally benign condition and a diagnosis of exclusion. Reassurance is provided through the general practitioner, who can review the patient every 2 years with an early-morning urine sample to check for proteinuria, which would prompt referral to a nephrologist

Common Diagnosis 3

Diagnosis: Idiopathic hypercalciuria

Management Principles

1. **High fluid intake.** Fluid intake is encouraged to lower urine calcium levels
2. **Monitor dietary intake of sodium.** Low calcium intake in the diet is not recommended in children, but a low-salt diet is important in the management of hypercalciuria. This is because sodium increases the amount of calcium in the urine and can trigger renal calculi formation
3. **Diuretics.** If urine calcium levels remain high despite conservative measures and there is a high risk of nephrolithiasis, thiazide diuretics may be used to help with renal calcium excretion

Common Diagnosis 4

Diagnosis: Immunoglobulin A nephropathy

Management Principles

1. **Close monitoring.** With evidence of isolated microscopic haematuria without proteinuria, monitoring is recommended. Renal function, blood pressure and urinalysis should be monitored 6-monthly to screen for proteinuria, as this suggests disease progression, and would prompt a referral to a nephrologist
2. **Reduce proteinuria.** If proteinuria develops, a renal biopsy may be necessary. Angiotensin-converting enzyme (ACE) inhibitors or angiotensin receptor blockers (ARBs) are recommended as first line to reduce the proteinuria
3. **Manage hypertension.** Developing hypertension is a risk factor. Lifestyle modification to reduce weight and a low-salt diet are recommended for prevention. If antihypertensives are required, seek specialist advice

---

Box 6.1.5   Indications for Renal Biopsy in Haematuria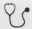

- Persistent microscopic haematuria with diagnostic uncertainty
- Associated proteinuria
- Associated hypertension
- Associated abnormal renal function
- Persisting low complement levels
- Positive autoantibodies

6.2 Oedema

Simon Mattus[1] and Rachel Varughese[2]
[1]Department of Paediatrics, Wexham Park Hospital, Frimley Health NHS Foundation Trust, Slough, UK
[2]Department of Paediatrics, Oxford University Hospitals NHS Foundation Trust, Oxford, UK

CONTENTS

6.2.1 CHAPTER AT A GLANCE

> **Box 6.2.1 Chapter at a Glance**
>
> - Oedema has a wide differential diagnosis and may be a sign of a serious underlying medical condition
> - An unwell-looking child with generalised oedema warrants emergency assessment and treatment
> - A well-appearing child ought to be seen urgently, often the same day, for a diagnostic work-up
> - Understanding of the pathophysiology will quickly help narrow down the differential diagnoses
> - Oedema can be localised or generalised, and this chapter will primarily focus on generalised oedema

6.2.2 DEFINITION

Oedema is the excessive accumulation of fluid in the body tissues.

6.2.3 DIAGNOSTIC ALGORITHM

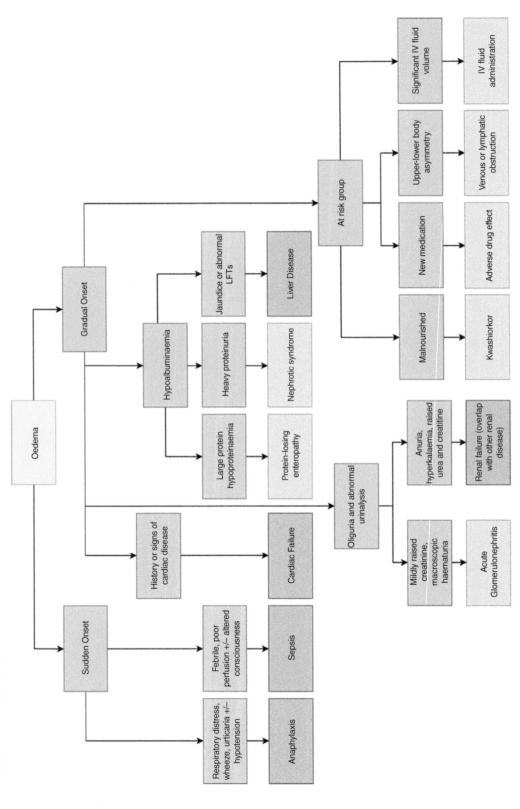

Figure 6.2.1 Diagnostic Algorithm for the Presentation of Oedema.

Box 6.2.2 Physiological Mechanisms Underlying Oedema

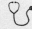

Mechanism	Explanation
Reduced oncotic pressure	• This occurs in low-protein states, either due to reduced synthesis or increased loss • A reduction in albumin in the intravascular space leads to decreased plasma oncotic pressure. Water is drawn from the intravascular space to the interstitium • This results in a reduction in intravascular volume. The response to this is activation of the renin-angiotensin-aldosterone (RAA) pathway and antidiuretic hormone (ADH) release • These pathways promote water and sodium retention, further decreasing plasma oncotic pressure
Increased hydrostatic pressure	• This occurs when there is increased intravascular pressure in the capillary beds • If venous pressure is increased, the increased capillary hydrostatic pressure forces water from the intravascular space into the interstitium • Venous pressure is increased in states of increased intravascular volume (often driven by excess sodium and water retention) or venous obstruction causing back pressure
Increased vascular permeability	• If capillaries are damaged by injury or pro-inflammatory mediators, endothelial cell junctions widen • This results in a 'leaky' capillary, which allows increased fluid and macromolecules (such as albumin and globulins) to leave the vessel
Decreased lymphatic drainage	• Under normal circumstances, the lymphatic system absorbs fluid from the interstitium and returns it to the venous system. Impairment will result in oedema

6.2.4 DIFFERENTIALS LIST

Dangerous Diagnoses

Box 6.2.3 Two Emergency Causes of Oedema

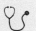

Sepsis and anaphylaxis are two life-threatening causes of oedema, although they rarely present with oedema as their primary feature. As such they will not be discussed further in this chapter.

Condition	Definition	Mechanism of oedema
Sepsis	Life-threatening organ dysfunction caused by a dysregulated host response to infection	• Increased vascular permeability due to pro-inflammatory mediators • Reduction in oncotic pressure, due to increased catabolism of albumin, and albumin loss to the extravascular space • Renal retention of sodium and water in response to decreased renal perfusion
Anaphylaxis	Life-threatening allergic reaction	• Markedly increased vascular permeability due to histamine and platelet activating factor • Renal retention of sodium and water in response to decreased renal perfusion

1. Cardiac Failure
- Heart failure in children is usually due to structural heart disease, such as a congenital cardiac abnormality or cardiomyopathy. Acquired causes include myocarditis, rheumatic fever, arrhythmias and metabolic diseases
- Oedema is primarily due to increased hydrostatic pressure, through two main mechanisms:
  - Reduced cardiac output stimulates the renin-angiotensin-aldosterone system (RAA), which causes renal retention of sodium and water
  - Impaired ventricular function causes venous back pressure
- Extent and site of oedema depend on the nature of ventricular dysfunction:
  - Left ventricular dysfunction – pulmonary oedema
  - Right ventricular dysfunction – peripheral (mainly lower-extremity) oedema
- Peripheral oedema due to cardiac failure is unusual in infants

2. Liver Disease
- Oedema may be a feature of both chronic liver disease and acute liver failure
- Oedema is due to increased hydrostatic pressure and reduced oncotic pressure
  - Cirrhosis causes increased venous resistance, effectively acting as an obstruction to venous flow, resulting in lower-limb oedema. The same mechanism leads to portal hypertension, which can cause ascites
  - Disruption in hepatic synthetic function results in reduced albumin levels
- Overall, this is an uncommon cause of oedema in children, but is important to exclude

---

Box 6.2.4   Causes of Liver Disease in Children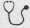

- Infection (viral hepatitis)
- Biliary tree structural abnormalities (atresia or Alagille syndrome)

- Intrinsic genetic liver disease (alpha-1 antitrypsin deficiency, Wilson disease, cystic fibrosis)

Box 6.2.5   Renal Failure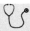

- Both acute and chronic renal failure can cause generalised oedema
- Oedema is due to increased capillary hydrostatic pressure, due to renal retention of sodium and water

- Causes can be divided into pre-renal, intra-renal and post-renal
- Two common renal diseases of childhood, acute glomerulonephritis and nephrotic syndrome, are included in this chapter as their own diagnoses, since both cause oedema in their own right

---

Common Diagnoses

1. Nephrotic Syndrome
- Nephrotic syndrome is one of the most common renal diseases seen in childhood, with 1 in 50,000 children diagnosed in the UK each year
- It is characterised by a tetrad of generalised oedema, proteinuria, hyperlipidaemia and hypoalbuminaemia, due to increased glomerular filtration membrane permeability to proteins
- Oedema is caused both by reduced oncotic pressure, due to renal excretion of protein, and subsequent sodium and water retention in response to reduced intravascular volume
- Nephrotic syndrome usually affects children aged 2–5 years, but can occur at any age
- Specific types are dependent on biopsy appearances. The most common type is minimal change disease
- Most respond well to treatment, with no long-term sequelae, but there is a risk of renal failure, particularly in those who relapse

2. Acute Glomerulonephritis (AGN)
- AGN is a result of glomerular injury and inflammation, resulting in reduced glomerular filtration, with sodium and water retention
- AGN typically affects children 2–15 years old and presents with a tetrad of haematuria, proteinuria, oedema and hypertension
- Most cases are due to an autoimmune response. In children, this usually follows a streptococcal infection of the skin or throat
- It is characterised by an abrupt onset of inflammation and proliferation of the glomeruli
- Oedema is primarily due to increased hydrostatic pressure due to renal sodium and water retention

Box 6.2.6   Cause of Nephrotic Syndrome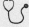

Primary nephrotic syndrome

- Occurs in the absence of an underlying cause
- Idiopathic nephrotic syndrome is the most common type, accounting for >90% of cases between 1 and 10 years of age
- Renal biopsy shows minimal changes, known as 'minimal change disease', and most children are steroid responsive

Secondary nephrotic syndrome

- Defined as nephrotic syndrome associated with underlying systemic or renal disease
- These often cause a mixed picture, with nephrotic and nephritic features
- Causes include systemic lupus erythematosus, post-infective glomerulonephritis, Henoch–Schönlein purpura and haemolytic uraemic syndrome

---

Box 6.2.7   Causes of Acute Glomerulonephritis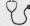

Primary glomerulonephritis

- Immunoglobulin A nephropathy
- Membranoproliferative glomerulonephritis
- Anti-glomerular basement membrane disease

Secondary glomerulonephritis

- Post-streptococcal glomerulonephritis
- Vasculitis: Henoch–Schönlein purpura
- Systemic lupus erythematosus

---

3. Protein-Losing Enteropathy (PLE)

- PLE is characterised by severe protein loss from the gastrointestinal tract
- Oedema is caused by reduction in plasma oncotic pressure due to hypoproteinaemia
- There are several causes, including inflammatory bowel disease, coeliac disease, primary intestinal lymphangiectasia and infectious enteropathy, with treatment and prognosis depending on the underlying aetiology
- There is emerging evidence that occult PLE may be responsible for more low-protein states than is currently recognised

---

Box 6.2.8   Protein-Losing Enteropathy (PLE) Causes and Mechanisms

There are three broad categories of PLE:

- Diseases damaging gastrointestinal epithelium without causing erosions

- Diseases causing gastrointestinal erosions or ulceration
- Diseases involving increased lymphatic pressure

Box 6.2.9   Intravenous (IV) Fluid Administration   △△

- IV fluids are a common iatrogenic cause of oedema
- IV fluids cause oedema through increased plasma hydrostatic pressure and reduction of oncotic pressure by dilution

- Pay particular attention to this in high-dependency units, unwell surgical patients and patients on hyperhydration regimes (e.g. oncology wards, sickle cell disease)
- The key to this is in the history, as the examination is generally non-specific

---

Diagnoses to Consider

1. Venous Obstruction

- Venous obstruction can be broadly split into three categories: extrinsic venous compression, thrombosis or congestion
- Oedema develops distal to the site of obstruction
- If the obstruction is in a large central vein (e.g. the inferior vena cava, IVC), this may look like generalised oedema
- There are numerous causes, which include indwelling vascular access, medications, immobilisation, malignancy and thrombophilia

When to consider: when the oedema is predominantly in one distal vascular territory

2. Lymphatic Dysfunction or Obstruction

- This typically involves lower limbs and may be primary or secondary
- Congenital causes include congenital lymphoedema (Milroy disease), Turner syndrome and Noonan syndrome
- Trauma, cellulitis, cancer and its treatment can injure the lymphatics to the point where their function is disrupted. Filariasis (parasitic lymph infection) is uncommon in the developed world, but is particularly common in the tropics

- Obstruction is uncommon, but pelvic tumours should always be considered

When to consider: in an at-risk patient when the oedema is predominantly in one or more limbs

---

Box 6.2.10   Kwashiorkor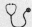

- Kwashiorkor describes oedema due to severe malnutrition
- Depending on location, this may be anywhere from the most common cause of oedema (developing countries) to vanishingly rare (developed countries)
- Total calorie intake may be normal, but made up entirely of carbohydrate

- The aetiology and pathophysiology are incompletely understood, but are likely to involve:
  - Severe protein malnutrition causing insufficient albumin synthesis, resulting in oedema through reduced plasma oncotic pressure
  - Cellular dysfunction and glycosaminoglycan disruption, causing release of water into the extracellular space

---

Box 6.2.11   Medications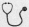

- A number of medications have the ability to cause oedema
- In particular, vasodilatory antihypertensive agents cause salt and water retention, thereby increasing hydrostatic pressure. Examples are calcium channel blockers such as nifedipine or amlodipine
- Toxic drugs, such as chemotherapy, can also precipitate other causes of oedema, e.g. cardiac failure or glomerulonephritis

- It may be difficult to remember a complete list of medications capable of causing oedema. If the oedema appears following the addition of a new medication, see whether it is a known adverse effect of that drug

---

Box 6.2.12   Localised Oedema

Oedema that affects one region of the body is known as localised oedema

Cause	Details
Angioedema	Facial oedema that can either be hereditary, due to anaphylaxis or angiotensin-converting enzyme (ACE) inhibitors
Superior vena cava obstruction	Acute facial oedema associated with upper limb swelling and plethora due to venous back pressure
Dactylitis	Swollen and painful digits due to sickle cell anaemia
Insect bite	Localised inflammatory reaction caused by an insect or snake bite leads to oedema, induration and erythema
Thrombophlebitis	Inflammation of vasculature leads to localised swelling
Deep vein thrombosis	Most commonly affects leg veins, with oedema distal to obstruction, causing unilateral swelling
Burns	Direct capillary damage causes capillary leak

6.2.5 KEY HISTORY FEATURES

Dangerous Diagnosis 1
Diagnosis: Cardiac failure

Questions

1. **Is the child known to have a cardiac anomaly?** Over half of congenital heart disease is identified antenatally or in the postnatal check (25% and 30%, respectively)

2. **In a younger child: is feeding difficult or is there faltering growth?** Infants in cardiac failure do not feed normally. There is prolonged feeding time, with decreased volume intake. This is accompanied by irritability with feeding, sweating, stop–start and even refusal of feeds, followed by waking up ravenous. Over time this leads to insufficient weight gain

3. **In the older child: do they get breathless with exertion?** Exertional dyspnoea is a predominant symptom of heart failure, due to pulmonary oedema and impaired systemic organ perfusion as a result of reduced cardiac output

Dangerous Diagnosis 2
Diagnosis: Liver disease

Questions
1. **Has there been a prodromal infection?** Hepatitis viruses are a common cause of liver injury. A prodromal viral-like illness days to weeks before liver failure is also typical in cases that end up classified as indeterminate paediatric acute liver failure

2. **Is behaviour normal?** Encephalopathy may be subtle and only noticed by those most familiar with the child. Ask the caregivers if they have noticed any unusual behaviours

3. **Is there a personal or family history of a liver or biliary tree condition?** This should make hepatic failure top of the differentials in an oedematous child

Common Diagnosis 1
Diagnosis: Nephrotic syndrome

Questions
1. **Have parents noticed periorbital oedema?** 'Puffy eyes' is a common presenting complaint in nephrotic syndrome. Oedema is more noticeable in low-resistance areas, affecting eyes and genitals initially. Periorbital oedema is more noticeable in the morning, after lying down all night

2. **Have clothes been noticeably tighter?** Oedema in nephrotic syndrome is generalised, and change in the fit of clothes and shoes may be a subtle sign of fluid retention. Children may look as though they have gained weight. Pedal oedema is worse at the end of the day, due to gravity

3. **Has urine output changed?** Parents may comment that children are passing less urine than normal

4. **Has there been a preceding infection?** For reasons not fully understood, nephrotic syndrome seems more common in the weeks after an infection, particularly an upper respiratory tract infection

Common Diagnosis 2
Diagnosis: Acute glomerulonephritis

Questions
1. **Is the child's urine dark-coloured or bloody?** As the cause of the nephritis is glomerular in nature, the urine appears dark brown or 'cola' coloured, due to degradation of the red cells within the tubules

2. **Are they passing less urine than normal?** Glomerulonephritis typically causes oliguria

3. **Has the child had a recent infection?** Post-infectious glomerulonephritis is the most common subtype. Post-streptococcal glomerulonephritis presents 2–6 weeks after a streptococcal pharyngitis or cellulitis

4. **Has there been complaint of abdominal pain?** Abdominal pain is a frequent symptom associated with AGN

Common Diagnosis 3
Diagnosis: Protein-losing enteropathy

Questions
1. **Has the child been losing or failing to gain weight?** Protein-losing enteropathies are a feature of chronic gastrointestinal disease. There will usually be a preceding history suggesting problems with intestinal absorption

2. **Does the child have diarrhoea or other altered stools?** Bloody, diarrhoeal or mucous stools point towards an intestinal pathology

3. **Is there associated abdominal pain or discomfort?** Although this is not specific, it is often a feature of enteropathies. Note that intestinal oedema itself can be painful

6.2.6 KEY EXAMINATION FEATURES

Box 6.2.13 Common Examination Features in Patients with Oedema

Generalised oedema is associated with fluid shifts throughout body tissues. When it is clinically apparent in superficial tissues, it is also likely found elsewhere. These are some common examination findings that may be seen irrespective of the cause of oedema

Examination findings	Details
Eyelid and/or scrotal/vulval swelling	Generalised oedema is most readily apparent in areas of low tissue resistance, e.g. periorbital, labial and scrotal regions
Dependent oedema	Gravity means that oedema settles in dependent areas – lower limbs for mobile children, or the torso if lying down. Palpate over a bony prominence to assess for pitting
Respiratory distress	Fluid shifts into the pleural space cause pleural effusion. This may result in respiratory distress. Examination features include reduced air entry and stony dullness to percussion
Abdominal distension	Ascites is a common manifestation of generalised oedema. Examination features include abdominal distension and shifting dullness

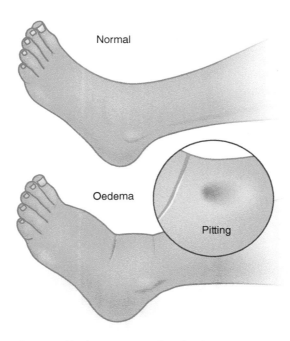

Figure 6.2.2 Oedema can be visually assessed by the appearance of swollen dependent areas and shiny skin. Pressing on a bony prominence and then releasing may leave an indentation known as 'pitting oedema'.

Dangerous Diagnosis 1

Diagnosis: Cardiac failure

Examination Findings

1. **Heart murmur.** This may be an indicator of an underlying structural cardiac anomaly
2. **Crackles on lung auscultation.** Crackles indicate pulmonary oedema, typically a complication of left-sided heart failure. This may be accompanied by tachypnoea
3. **Raised jugular venous pulse (JVP) or pulsatile hepatomegaly.** These signs of right-sided back pressure are typical of cardiac failure. Whether you can see a JVP or not is highly dependent on the patient's anatomy and is difficult in most young children. Hepatomegaly is more reliable
4. **Poor distal perfusion.** Pulses may be difficult to feel, with increased capillary refill time and cool peripheries
5. **Faltering growth.** Heart failure causes poor weight gain, and in the long term may cause problems with growth

Dangerous Diagnosis 2

Diagnosis: Liver disease

Examination Findings

1. **Easy bruising or bleeding.** Coagulopathy is a feature of hepatic synthetic failure. This is an extremely complex process that that affects pro- and anticoagulant factors as well as pro- and antifibrinolytic factors
2. **Jaundice.** Jaundice is a common sign of liver and biliary tree disease due to an abnormality in the metabolism of bilirubin
3. **Signs of portal hypertension.** Liver cirrhosis can cause portal hypertension. Venous congestion can lead to oesophageal varices, which may present with upper gastrointestinal bleeding or melaena. Cutaneous vascular changes include distended veins on the abdomen due to collateral shunting through superficial vessels. There may also be splenomegaly and ascites
4. **Features of encephalopathy.** This may manifest as irritability or lethargy in infants. Older children present with drowsiness, confusion or behavioural change

Common Diagnosis 1

Diagnosis: Nephrotic syndrome

Examination Findings

1. **Marked oedema.** Except for oedema and its complications, the rest of the examination is normal, and the child usually looks otherwise well. Periorbital and pitting pedal oedema is usually particularly significant

Box 6.2.14   Complications of Nephrotic Syndrome

Complication	Details
Increased risk of infections	Due to hypogammaglobulinaemia and loss of complement factors. In addition, oedema fluid is a good medium for bacterial growth, predisposing to peritonitis and empyema
Venous thromboembolism	Postulated to be as a result of renal loss of antithrombotic factors and increased production of prothrombotic factors by the liver
Renal insufficiency	Due to hypovolaemia from intravascular compartment fluid shift into interstitium, or due to the underlying glomerular pathology
Anasarca	Massive oedema may lead to an inability to walk (scrotal, vulval or leg pain), tissue breakdown, or respiratory distress from significant pleural effusions and/or ascites

Common Diagnosis 2

Diagnosis: Acute glomerulonephritis

Examination Findings

1. **Haematuria.** Macroscopic 'cola'-coloured urine is typical of AGN

2. **Hypertension.** AGN is associated with hypertension due to glomerular involvement and sodium retention, leading to fluid overload
3. **Otherwise asymptomatic.** Glomerulonephritis may be insidious, with few specific exam features
4. **Fever and rash.** These indicate secondary glomerulonephritis due to vasculitis or other systemic illness

Common Diagnosis 3
Diagnosis: Protein-losing enteropathy

Examination Findings
1. **Low weight for age.** Enteropathy causing protein loss is often associated with faltering growth
2. **Normal examination.** Examination is otherwise normal

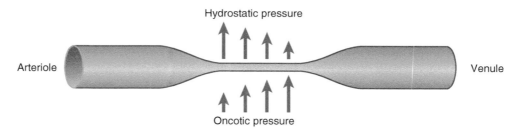

Figure 6.2.3 Starling's hypothesis helps explain fluid shifts between the intravascular space and the interstitium. Hydrostatic pressure drives fluid out of capillaries, but decreases as blood traverses the capillary from arteriole to venule. Meanwhile, oncotic pressure increases as the filtering fluid leaves behind impermeable proteins, drawing fluid back into the intravascular space. Vascular permeability and lymphatic drainage will both affect this balance.

6.2.7 KEY INVESTIGATIONS

Not all children will require invasive investigations; often diagnoses are made on clinical evidence from history and examination. Consider carefully which investigations are required for which patient.

Bedside

Table 6.2.1 Bedside tests of use in patients presenting with oedema

Test	When to perform	Potential result
Urine dipstick	• All children with oedema	• ↑↑ Protein: markedly raised in nephrotic syndrome • ↑↑ Blood, ↑ protein: acute glomerulonephritis
VBG	• All children with oedema	• Lactic acidosis: poor perfusion, e.g. sepsis/cardiac failure • Other metabolic acidosis or ↑ K: renal failure • ↑ Cl: Excess IV saline administration • ↑ Glucose: stress response, sepsis, liver failure
Throat swab	• All children with oedema	• Group A streptococcus suggests post-streptococcal AGN
ECG	• Suspected cardiac failure	• Likely to be normal, but may provide clues to numerous potential causes of cardiac failure • Axis deviation or bundle branch block: congenital heart disease • Large QRS voltages: ventricular hypertrophy • ST segment changes: myo/pericarditis • Arrhythmias may be captured

AGN, acute glomerulonephritis; Cl, chloride; ECG, electrocardiogram; IV, intravenous; K, potassium; VBG, venous blood gas

Blood Tests

Table 6.2.2 Blood tests of use in patients presenting with oedema

Test	Justification	Potential result
FBC	• Suspected sepsis	• ↓ Hb: chronic conditions, particularly renal failure • ↑ WCC: sepsis (WCC may also be low) • ↓ Lymphocytes: seen in PLE
U&E	• All children with oedema	• ↑ Urea, ↑ creatinine, ± ↑ potassium: renal failure, acute kidney injury from intravascular fluid loss
Albumin	• All children with oedema • Albumin is the major determinant of intravascular oncotic pressure	• ↓: Protein-losing states (nephrotic syndrome, enteropathies) or reduced synthesis (liver failure) • Normal: eliminates oncotic pressure as a cause for oedema
LFTs	• Suspected liver disease	• Elevated liver enzymes: liver injury • Elevated bilirubin: liver disease, or biliary tree pathology
Clotting screen	• Suspected liver disease	• ↑ PT ± ↑ APTT: coagulopathy due to liver disease
Immunoglobulins A/G/M, thyroglobulin, caeruloplasmin, fibrinogen and transferrin	• All children with oedema • Large molecules are lost through the gut in protein-losing states	• ↓: Protein-losing enteropathy • Normal in renal protein loss
Lipids and triglycerides	Suspected: • Nephrotic syndrome • AGN	• ↑: Often markedly so in nephrotic syndrome
ASOT	• Suspected AGN	• ↑ Titres suggest group A streptococcal infection
Anti-DNAse B	• Suspected AGN	• ↑ Antibodies in group A streptococcal infection
Complement C3 and C4	• Suspected AGN	• ↓ C3, ↓ C4 in AGN and atypical nephrotic syndrome
Blood culture	• Suspected sepsis	• Positive culture confirms bacterial infection • Sensitivities guide antibiotic choice

AGN, acute glomerulonephritis; APTT, activated partial thromboplastin time; ASOT, anti-streptolysin O titre ; FBC, full blood count; Hb, haemoglobin; LFTs, liver function tests; PLE, protein-losing enteropathy; PT, prothrombin time; U&E, urea and electrolytes

Imaging

Table 6.2.3 Imaging modalities of use in patients presenting with oedema

Test	When to perform	Potential result
Chest x-ray	Suspected: • Cardiac failure • Any child with oedema and respiratory distress	• Pleural effusions and pulmonary oedema: common lung manifestations of generalised oedema – not necessarily diagnostically useful, but may help evaluate the burden of fluid accumulation • Cardiomegaly: cardiac disease • Pathognomic cardiac contour: various congenital heart defects
Abdominal ultrasound	• Sometimes a useful adjunct in investigating kidneys/liver/ gastrointestinal tract	• May demonstrate renal abnormalities, post-renal obstruction, cirrhosis, hepatomegaly, biliary tree abnormalities, focal intestinal inflammation or masses, depending on the cause of oedema

Special

Table 6.2.4 Special tests of use in patients presenting with oedema

Test	When to perform	Potential result
Urine protein:creatinine ratio	• Suspected hypoalbuminaemia	• >200 mg/mmol in nephrotic syndrome • May be elevated to a lesser degree in non-nephrotic renal disease
Urine microscopy	• Suspected AGN	• Presence of red cell casts is suggestive of AGN
Renal biopsy	• Suspected renal disease other than typical nephrotic syndrome	• Minimal change disease is the most common finding of typical idiopathic nephrotic syndrome, although biopsy is not usually warranted • Many other specific diagnostic features of renal disease can be identified
Stool alpha-1 antitrypsin	• Suspected PLE	• ↑ In PLE – a 24-hour collection is more accurate than a spot sample
Upper and lower gastrointestinal endoscopy	• Suspected PLE • Enables intestinal biopsy	• Mucosal erythema, loss of vascularity, erosions in ulcerative colitis • Classic skip lesions, cobblestones, or mouth ulcers in Crohn's disease

AGN, acute glomerulonephritis; PLE, protein-losing enteropathy

---

Box 6.2.15 Transudate or Exudate

- An abnormal collection of fluid within a compartment (e.g. pleural effusion or ascites) may require needle aspiration for diagnostic or therapeutic purposes
- The contents of the fluid can be analysed, allowing categorisation as a transudate or exudate
- Transudates, resulting from filtration across the capillary wall, are characterised by low protein content, low cellularity and low specific gravity. Exudates, caused by local inflammation, are rich in protein, cells and have a high specific gravity
- The conditions leading to generalised oedema discussed in this chapter should give rise to a transudate. Exudates are usually caused by infection or malignancy

---

6.2.8 KEY MANAGEMENT PRINCIPLES

Diagnosis-specific management strategies are outlined here. It is expected that an 'ABCDE' approach to assessment and management is always undertaken (see Chapter 12.1, *The A to E Assessment*).

All patients with oedema should have careful fluid balance monitoring, with input–output measures, and daily weights.

Dangerous Diagnosis 1

Diagnosis: Cardiac failure

Management Principles

1. **Refer to cardiology and establish the underlying cause.** Treatment of cardiac failure varies drastically depending on the cause. Refer early to cardiology, who can provide specialist assessment and echocardiography in order to identify underlying structural problems
2. **Treat oedema.** Diuretics are used to promote renal excretion of sodium and water, to reduce pulmonary and systemic congestion. Loop diuretics, such as furosemide, are widely used for both acute and chronic management. Other options for chronic control include spironolactone and thiazide diuretics
3. **Specialist treatment.** For heart failure refractory to simple medical therapy, specialist escalation will be required. Device therapy includes a pacemaker, cardiac resynchronisation therapy and ventricular assist devices. In very unwell children with reversible cardiac disease, extracorporeal membrane oxygenation (ECMO) can be considered. Cardiac transplant is the treatment of choice for end-stage heart failure

Dangerous Diagnosis 2

Diagnosis: Liver disease

Management Principles

1. **Establish the underlying cause.** There are multiple potential causes of liver failure and early treatment can be organ saving. Focus on ruling in or out treatable causes first

2. **Transfer to a specialist unit.** Paediatric liver failure is an uncommon and challenging medical emergency, due to multisystem involvement and the potential for rapid neurological deterioration. Management requires specialist input and early referral to a specialist liver unit is recommended

3. **Monitor electrolytes.** Metabolic and electrolyte disturbances are common and frequent monitoring is required. Hypoglycaemia, hyponatraemia and hypokalaemia need to be promptly recognised and treated

4. **Treat complications.** Complications involve cardiovascular dysfunction, respiratory failure, relative adrenal insufficiency, renal failure, infection, nutritional deficits, coagulopathy, hepatic encephalopathy and cerebral oedema. Management will require intensive care input

Common Diagnosis 1

Diagnosis: Nephrotic syndrome

Management Principles

1. **Treatment for hypovolaemia.** Most children will appear otherwise well, but if there is evidence of hypovolaemia, 10 mL/kg bolus of 4.5% albumin can be given. Furosemide should be given during the infusion unless clinically shocked

2. **Prednisolone.** Children with typical features of nephrotic syndrome should be started on steroids. Refer to local protocol. Currently, an 8-week initial course is recommended. This involves prednisolone 60 mg/m^2/day (maximum 80 mg) for 4 weeks, reduced to 40 mg/m^2 on alternate days for 4 weeks (maximum 60 mg)

3. **Gastric protection.** For the duration of steroid treatment, gastric protection with ranitidine or omeprazole should be given

4. **Penicillin V prophylaxis.** Infection is the main cause of death in children with nephrotic syndrome, and risk for encapsulated organisms is particularly increased. Although evidence is limited, it is reasonable to give penicillin V prophylaxis while proteinuria is present

5. **Dietary modifications.** A low-salt diet is recommended to minimise oedema and reduce thirst and fluid intake

6. **Investigate further if recurrent or steroid non-responsive**. Most children will not need more than the first-line work-up, as nephrotic syndrome is common and resolves in due course. At 4 weeks, persistent proteinuria suggests steroid-resistant disease. This, as well as recurrence, is indicative of more significant pathology that warrants discussion with a specialist renal unit. Renal biopsy should be considered

---

Box 6.2.16   Typical and Atypical Features of Nephrotic Syndrome

Typical	Atypical
• 1–10 years old	• <1 year old or >10 years old
• Normal blood pressure	• Hypertension
• Normal renal function	• Raised creatinine
• Haematuria absent or microscopic	• Macroscopic haematuria
• Normal complement levels	• Low C3/C4

Features of typical disease are consistent with minimal change disease. Any features of atypical disease warrant an early paediatric nephrology referral for consideration of renal biopsy

---

Box 6.2.17   Definitions Commonly Used in Nephrotic Syndrome

Condition	Definition
Nephrotic syndrome	Early-morning urine protein:creatinine ratio >200 mg/mmol and plasma albumin <25 g/L
Remission	Dipstick protein negative or trace for 3 consecutive days
Relapse	After having been in remission, recurrence of ≥3+ proteinuria, either for 3 consecutive days or with oedema
Frequent relapses	After having been in remission, ≥2 relapses within 6 months or ≥3 within any 12-month period
Steroid dependence	2 relapses occurring during corticosteroid therapy or within 14 days of stopping corticosteroids
Steroid resistance	Failure to achieve complete remission after 8 weeks of prednisolone at 60 mg/m^2/day

Common Diagnosis 2

Diagnosis: Acute glomerulonephritis

Management Principles

1. **Antibiotics.** Since the majority of paediatric cases follow a group A streptococcal infection, phenoxymethylpenicillin is recommended for 10 days
2. **Salt and fluid restriction.** This will manage oedema and help reduce symptoms while renal function is impaired
3. **Manage hypertension.** Calcium channel blockers, angiotensin-converting enzyme (ACE) inhibitors or sometimes hydralazine are typically used
4. **Referral to specialist renal unit in atypical cases.** In general, the prognosis for post-streptococcal AGN is good, with 95% of children making a full recovery. A small proportion will develop rapidly progressive glomerulonephritis and should be referred to a specialist unit for consideration of renal biopsy and immunosuppression. Options include pulsed methylprednisolone and/or prednisolone followed by cyclophosphamide and/or plasmapheresis. Long-term treatment with tacrolimus or mycophenolate mofetil may be required

Common Diagnosis 3

Diagnosis: Protein-losing enteropathy

Management Principles

1. **Identify and treat the underlying cause.** Gastrointestinal (GI) endoscopy – oesophago-gastro-duodenoscopy (OGD) and colonoscopy – will be required. Cross-sectional abdominal imaging or laparoscopy may be useful when endoscopy and biopsy do not yield a diagnosis. The mainstay of PLE treatment is to address the underlying cause
2. **Provide high-protein and low-fat nutrition.** A high-protein diet may help ameliorate GI protein loss. Low fat content reduces stimulation of the lymphatic system, thereby decreasing protein loss
3. **Consider octreotide.** Octreotide provides splanchnic vasoconstriction and therefore theoretically reduces gut fluid and protein loss in several conditions. Its use is not well established

6.3 Scrotal Swelling

Emma Hughes

Department of Paediatrics, Great Western Hospitals NHS Foundation Trust, Swindon, UK

CONTENTS

6.3.1 CHAPTER AT A GLANCE

> **Box 6.3.1   Chapter at a Glance**
>
> - Scrotal swelling in children should always be assessed as soon as possible following onset
> - This chapter will also include scrotal masses
> - Testicular torsion and strangulated inguinal hernias are both time-critical surgical emergencies
> - Unilateral swelling or pain is often associated with underlying testicular pathology

6.3.2 DEFINITION

Localised or generalised swelling of the scrotal sac, with or without pain.

6.3.3 DIAGNOSTIC ALGORITHM

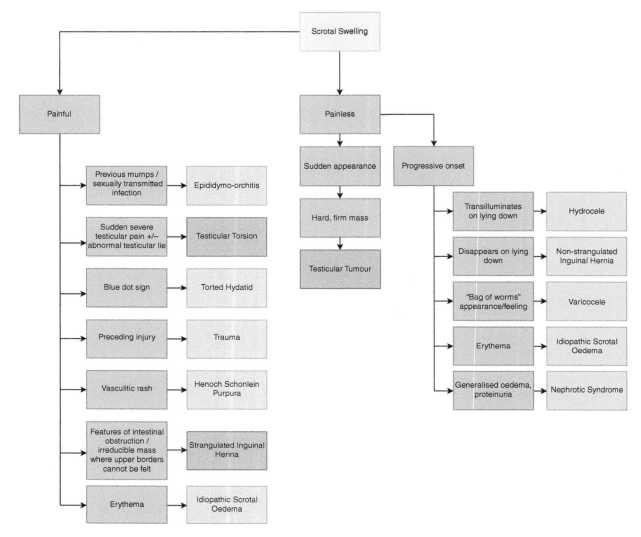

Figure 6.3.1 Diagnostic algorithm for the presentation of scrotal swelling.

6.3.4 DIFFERENTIALS LIST

All cases of scrotal swelling in children are treated as emergency assessments until potentially testes-compromising causes have been ruled out.

Dangerous Diagnoses

1. **Testicular Torsion**
   - The spermatic cord, which contains both the testicular vein and artery, twists within the scrotum, thereby causing ischaemia of the testicle
   - Requires rapid diagnosis and surgical exploration to avoid necrosis and loss of the respective testicle
   - Irreversible damage can occur in as little as 4 hours following torsion
2. **Testicular Tumours**
   - Most testicular tumours are germ cell tumours, which are rare in pre-pubertal boys
   - Testicular tumours are the most common solid tumour in adolescent and young adult males
   - Caucasians are most commonly affected

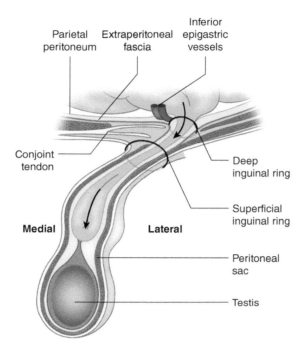

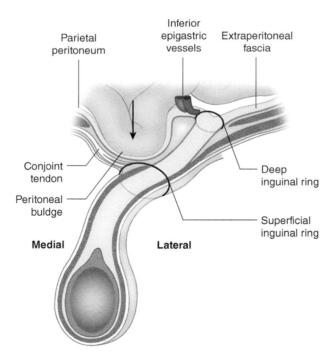

Figure 6.3.2 (A) An indirect hernia is caused by abdominal contents that pass through the deep inguinal ring, through the inguinal canal and through the superficial ring. (B) A direct hernia is caused by a weakness in the posterior wall of the inguinal canal, where abdominal contents pass through this defect, emerging in the inguinal canal, medial to the deep ring.

- Germ cell tumours can be malignant or benign, or contain malignant and benign elements within the same tumour
- Presentation is usually with painless testicular swelling, or an incidentally noticed mass, although rapidly growing tumours may cause acute pain

3. Inguinal Hernia
- A protrusion of abdominal contents through the inguinal canal into the scrotum
- Occurs in up to 5% of full-term infants and up to 30% of pre-term infants
- More common in males
- There are two main types: indirect and direct. Extension into the scrotum usually indicates an indirect hernia
- Complications include incarceration, where the bowel becomes entrapped and the hernia is not able to be reduced, risking intestinal obstruction. A strangulated hernia occurs when the entrapped bowel suffers from vascular compromise, risking bowel necrosis.

Common Diagnoses

1. Hydrocele
- A collection of fluid between the parietal and visceral layers of the tunica vaginalis
- Can occur adjacent to the testis or along the spermatic cord
- Congenital simple hydroceles usually resolve spontaneously within the first year of life

2. Varicocele
- Classically described as feeling like a 'bag of worms' on palpation and caused by dilatation of the internal spermatic veins and the pampiniform venous plexus
- Uncommon in pre-pubertal boys
- Occurs in 15% of adolescent boys and is often asymptomatic, with 90% occurring on the left and 10% bilaterally
- An isolated right-sided varicocele is rare

3. Epididymo-orchitis
- Sometimes referred to as either 'epididymitis' (inflammation of the epididymis) or 'orchitis' (inflammation of the testicle)
- Pain and inflammation tend to start in the spermatic cord and spread to include the testicle
- Isolated orchitis is rare, but it is important to consider mumps and other viral infections
- In painless swelling, consider tuberculous orchitis (epididymis hard and irregular with thickened spermatic cord)

4. Torted Hydatid
- The hydatid of Morgagni is a foetal remnant of the Mullerian duct located at the upper pole of the testis

5. Nephrotic Syndrome
- Nephrotic syndrome is one of the most common renal diseases seen in childhood, usually affecting children between 2 and 5 years of age
- Increased glomerular filtration membrane permeability to proteins leads to a tetrad of generalised oedema, proteinuria, hyperlipidaemia and hypoalbuminaemia
- Oedema often appears first in areas of low tissue resistance, e.g. periorbital, labial and scrotal regions. As such, scrotal swelling may be an initial presenting feature
- Nephrotic syndrome is discussed in detail in Chapter 6.2 and will not be discussed further in this chapter

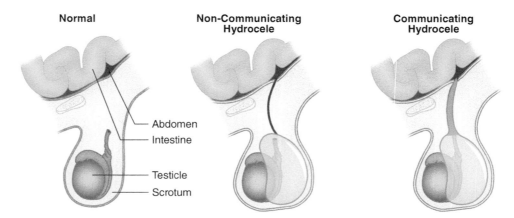

Figure 6.3.3 The difference between a non-communicating and a communicating hydrocele. When the hydrocele is transilluminated, the fluid portion is lit up, confirming the hydrocele clinically.

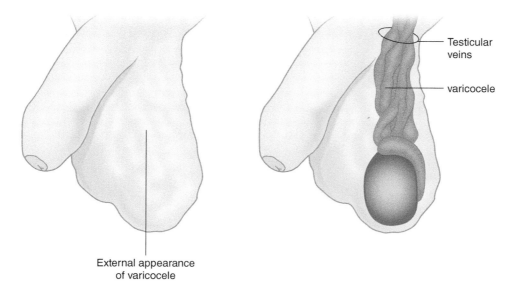

Testicular veins

varicocele

External appearance
of varicocele

Figure 6.3.4 A varicocele involves abnormal distension of the pampiniform venous plexus in the scrotum. The external appearance and feel are often described as like a bag of worms.

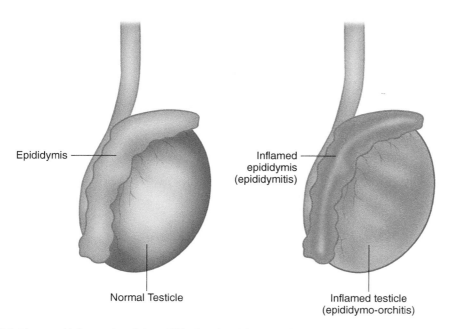

Epididymis

Normal Testicle

Inflamed
epididymis
(epididymitis)

Inflamed testicle
(epididymo-orchitis)

Figure 6.3.5 Diagram of inflammation of the epididymis and testicle in epididymo-orchitis.

Diagnoses to Consider

1. Trauma

- Injuries sustained during contact sports as well as non-accidental injury should be considered
- Trauma can occasionally cause secondary torsion

When to consider: in a patient who has any history of trauma, but also consider it as a mode of non-accidental injury, especially in pre-verbal boys

2. Henoch–Schönlein Purpura (HSP)

- HSP is a systemic immunoglobulin (Ig) A vasculitis affecting the skin, mucosal membranes and kidneys
- HSP can present with an acute abdomen and acute intussusception should be considered
- The typical presentation is with a purpuric rash on the lower half of the body and arthralgias/arthritis affecting knees, ankles and wrists
- Painful scrotal oedema may be present in affected boys
- Other vasculitic illnesses can cause scrotal swelling, such as Kawasaki disease and polyarteritis nodosa
- HSP is covered in detail in Chapters 9.2, *Non-blanching Rash* and 10.2, *Swollen Joint*

When to consider: in children with palpable purpura affecting lower limbs and buttocks

---

Box 6.3.2   Idiopathic Scrotal Oedema

- Idiopathic scrotal oedema is a rare cause of scrotal swelling and erythema, often considered to be a diagnosis of exclusion, most common in children under 10 years old
- There is acute-onset oedema of skin and dartos fascia without involvement of deeper layers or testes
- Pathology is unclear, but thought to be related to a hypersensitivity reaction, similar to that seen in angioedema, with eosinophilia in two-thirds of cases
- The condition is benign and self-limiting, resolving in 3–5 days. Non-steroidal anti-inflammatory drugs (NSAIDs) can be used for symptomatic relief

---

6.3.5 KEY HISTORY FEATURES

Box 6.3.3   Preparation for Theatre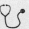

In situations where urgent surgical input may be required, it is sensible to establish the following from the start of your assessment until a management plan has been made:

- Check when the patient last ate or drank
- Ensure they are nil by mouth

Dangerous Diagnosis 1

Diagnosis: Testicular torsion

Questions

1. **What was the nature of the onset of pain?** Onset of testicular pain is sudden and severe. Testicular torsion may present with generalised abdominal pain
2. **Is there a history of scrotal trauma?** Scrotal trauma can predispose to testicular torsion. A contusion may cause the spermatic cord to twist
3. **Are there any associated symptoms?** Often boys with testicular torsion will have associated nausea and vomiting

Dangerous Diagnosis 2

Diagnosis: Testicular tumours

Questions

1. **When did the swelling start?** There is a gradual onset over weeks or months, with a slowly progressive swelling
2. **Is there any pain?** Testicular tumours are normally painless, but a dragging or heavy sensation may be described
3. **Any other associated symptoms?** There may be weight loss, gynaecomastia, lower back or abdominal pain. Also consider symptoms associated with possible metastasis, e.g. breathlessness
4. **Any relevant medical history?** Risk factors include cryptorchidism, previously undescended testis, Klinefelter syndrome and a positive family history

Dangerous Diagnosis 3

Diagnosis: Inguinal hernia

Questions

1. **Is it painful?** Incarcerated and strangulated hernias cause pain, particularly on straining or lifting, whereas inguinal hernias that are reducible will be painless. If bowel ischaemia is present, pain will be severe.
2. **Does it disappear on lying flat?** Reducible hernias can disappear on lying flat; incarcerated and strangulated hernias will not
3. **When was the last time the bowels were opened? Any vomiting?** Incarcerated and strangulated hernias can present with features of intestinal obstruction, including nausea, vomiting, abdominal pain and failure to pass stool or flatus
4. **Any past medical or family history?** There is an increased risk in those with connective tissue disorders and a positive family history of inguinal hernias

Common Diagnosis 1

Diagnosis: Hydrocele

Questions

1. **When was the swelling first noted?** Hydroceles can be congenital, therefore will be present from birth. This will usually spontaneously resolve within the first 2 years. In older boys, it might be precipitated by trauma, infection, surgery or tumour
2. **Is it painful?** Hydroceles are generally painless. Sometimes a heavy or dragging sensation is described

Common Diagnosis 2

Diagnosis: Varicocele

Questions

1. **What was the nature of the onset?** Varicoceles usually present chronically over a period of time and, similar to a hydrocele, are usually painless, but might cause a heavy sensation
2. **Any impairment in testicular growth?** This can be a complication of varicocele, with the testicle on the affected side at risk of being smaller

Common Diagnosis 3

Diagnosis: Epididymo-orchitis

Questions

1. **What was the nature of the onset?** Onset is usually relatively rapid, over hours. In milder infections there can be a more gradual onset, over days
2. **Any other recent illnesses?** Orchitis usually occurs 4–8 days following parotitis in mumps infection. Urinary tract infections can also cause orchitis
3. **Are they sexually active?** In pubertal boys, a full sexual history should be obtained and sexually transmitted infections considered. There might be associated discharge

Common Diagnosis 4

Diagnosis: Torted hydatid cyst

Questions

1. **What was the nature of the onset?** Onset tends to be insidious and unilateral
2. **Is it painful?** A torted hydatid cyst can be acutely painful, often meaning testicular torsion is considered as a differential to be excluded

6.3.6 KEY EXAMINATION FEATURES

Box 6.3.4   General Considerations for Examination of Scrotal Swelling

- Always examine the patient in the presence of a chaperone
- Ask older boys if they would like their parents to leave the room if they are present
- Explain to the child and parent what the examination will involve and ask permission as appropriate
- Often examination in both the lying and standing positions is useful
- Include the groin and lower abdomen in the examination

Dangerous Diagnosis 1
Diagnosis: Testicular torsion

Examination Findings
1. **Significant pain.** The child will be in significant pain and unwilling to allow anyone to palpate the scrotum. They might be vomiting or retching with the pain and are likely to be tachycardic
2. **Erythema ± scrotal elevation.** Swelling and redness are noted unilaterally. There might be a degree of elevation of the scrotum on the affected side
3. **Abnormal testis lie.** The testis may have an abnormal transverse lie. There is likely to be an absent cremasteric reflex and usually no relief of pain on elevation of the testicle. Undescended testes can predispose to torsion, so examination of the inguinal region and abdomen is also important

Dangerous Diagnosis 2
Diagnosis: Testicular tumour

Examination Findings
1. **Hard, painless mass.** Compare the size of both testes; the affected testis is usually hard and painless to palpation
2. **Lymphadenopathy.** There may be inguinal lymphadenopathy
3. **Unilateral limb swelling.** Venous engorgement and subsequent lymphoedema of the ipsilateral limb may occur

Dangerous Diagnosis 3
Diagnosis: Inguinal hernia

Examination Findings
1. **Cough impulse.** A positive cough impulse will usually be displayed in reducible hernias. The patient is asked to cough, and the increase in intra-abdominal pressure forces an increase in the volume of the hernia in the scrotum
2. **Erythematous or dusky skin.** A visual inspection is important as any appearance of red or dusky skin is concerning for a possible strangulated hernia
3. **Unable to get above the swelling.** Since the origin of the mass is abdominal, it is not possible to get above the swelling. This means that during palpation, the mass continues up into the inguinal canal
4. **Reducible or irreducible.** This is an essential evaluation to determine whether the hernia is incarcerated or strangulated. Attempts to reduce the hernia should be made – if difficult or impossible, the hernia may be incarcerated or strangulated, and urgent surgical opinion should be sought
5. **Tenderness.** The degree of pain is important; reducible hernias are usually non-tender, incarcerated hernias are likely to be uncomfortable or painful, and strangulated hernias may cause severe pain due to bowel necrosis
6. **Disappears with lying.** Reducible hernias will often disappear when lying down and reappear on standing

Common Diagnosis 1
Diagnosis: Hydrocele

Examination Findings
1. **Fluctuant, painless swelling.** There will be a soft, non-tender, fluctuant swelling surrounding the testis or further up the spermatic cord. It is usually possible to get above it on palpation. Attempts to reduce the mass will be unsuccessful
2. **Transilluminates.** The mass will transilluminate when a torch is shone through the swelling. This means that when a torch is held up to the scrotal skin, the whole scrotum lights up orange

Common Diagnosis 2
Diagnosis: Varicocele

Examination Findings
1. **Bag of worms.** The mass feels like a 'bag of worms' above the testis (most often the left) within the spermatic cord
2. **Testicular size.** Assess symmetry of testes, as the varicocele may impair growth
3. **Increase with Valsalva manoeuvre.** Valsalva manoeuvre will increase the size, and some cases will demonstrate a positive cough impulse
4. **Reduction on lying down.** Since it is dependent on gravity, a varicocele will reduce when lying down

Common Diagnosis 3

Diagnosis: Epididymo-orchitis

Examination Findings

1. **Fever.** There is usually pyrexia, and patients often look unwell
2. **Erythema and oedema.** There can be erythema as well as oedema of the scrotum
3. **Painful palpable swelling.** Epididymo-orchitis causes a painful palpable swelling that is usually unilateral (although bilateral cases do exist, for example due to mumps). It can be difficult to distinguish from torsion. However, in contrast to torsion, pain is usually relieved by elevation, and the cremasteric reflex is usually present

Common Diagnosis 4

Diagnosis: Torted hydatid

Examination Findings

1. **Pain.** Tender, particularly at the upper pole of the testis
2. **Blue dot.** The 'blue dot' sign is seen in up to a third of cases. This is a dark blue discoloration at the upper pole of the testis

6.3.7 KEY INVESTIGATIONS

Not all children will require invasive investigations; often diagnoses are made on clinical evidence from history and examination. Consider carefully which investigations are required for which patient.

Bedside

Table 6.3.1 Bedside tests of use in patients presenting with scrotal swelling

Test	When to perform	Potential result
Urine dip and MC&S	Suspected: • Epididymo-orchitis • HSP • Nephrotic syndrome • Trauma	• Nitrites, leucocytes: UTI causing epididymo-orchitis • Haematuria, proteinuria: HSP • Proteinurina: nephrotic syndrome • Haematuria: may be seen in trauma
Urethral swabs and culture	• Suspected epididymo-orchitis if obvious urethral discharge	• Sexually transmitted infection identified with antibiotic sensitivities

HSP, Henoch–Schönlein purpura; MC&S, microscopy, culture and sensitivity; UTI, urinary tract infection

Blood Tests

Table 6.3.2 Blood tests of use in patients presenting with scrotal swelling

Test	When to perform	Potential result
FBC	Suspected: • Epididymo-orchitis • Testicular tumours • HSP (to evaluate platelets in non-blanching rash)	• ↑ WCC, ↑ neutrophils: bacterial infection • ↓ Hb: may be seen in malignancy • Normal platelets are seen in HSP
CRP	• Suspected epididymo-orchitis	• Significant ↑ in bacterial infections
U&E	Suspected: • Nephrotic syndrome • HSP	• ↑ Urea, ↑ creatinine if renal impairment in nephrotic syndrome or HSP
Albumin and cholesterol	• Suspected nephrotic syndrome	• ↓ Albumin and ↑ cholesterol in nephrotic syndrome
Blood cultures	• If systemically unwell and pyrexial	• Positive culture confirms bacterial growth • Sensitivities guide antibiotic choice
Tumour markers (AFP and βHCG)	• Suspected testicular tumour	• ↑ AFP, ↑ βHCG in testicular tumours

AFP, alpha-fetoprotein; CRP, C-reactive protein; FBC, full blood count; Hb, haemoglobin; HCG, human chorionic gonadotropin; HSP, Henoch–Schönlein purpura; U&E, urea and electrolytes

Imaging

Table 6.3.3 Imaging modalities of use in patients presenting with scrotal swelling

Test	When to perform	Potential result
Ultrasound scan of scrotum with Doppler	• All children with scrotal swelling	• Evaluation of scrotum, testes and surrounding structures • Extremely valuable in diagnosis of all causes of scrotal swelling • If index of suspicion for torsion low, can be considered prior to surgical exploration • Waiting for ultrasound should not delay surgical referral in testicular torsion or strangulated inguinal hernia

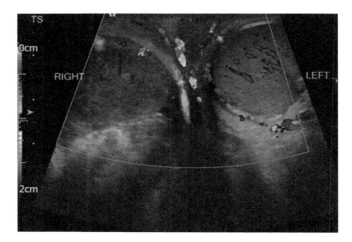

Figure 6.3.6 A testicular ultrasound demonstrating a testicular torsion. Normal echotexture and blood flow within testis on left. Right testis slightly hypoechoic compared to left, no blood flow within testis and increased blood flow surrounding. Note that the ultrasound can be normal if scanned early on in the process or if torsion is intermittent.

6.3.8 KEY MANAGEMENT PRINCIPLES

Diagnosis-specific management strategies are outlined here. It is expected that an 'ABCDE' approach to assessment and management is always undertaken (see Chapter 12.1, *The A to E Assessment*).

Box 6.3.5   Analgesia

For all painful scrotal swellings, administer appropriate analgesia. This will not 'mask' significant pain but will aid in examination, allowing the scrotum to be palpated more thoroughly

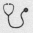

Dangerous Diagnosis 1
Diagnosis: Testicular torsion

Management Principles
1. **Urgent surgical referral.** If torsion is strongly suspected, urgent surgical exploration is required, with untwisting and orchidopexy of the affected side and orchidopexy of the unaffected side. An unsalvageable testis can be removed. Severe damage can occur in as little as 4 hours following torsion
2. **External manipulation.** An experienced surgeon might attempt external manipulation to untwist the testis – this can provide some relief pending exploration, but should never replace definitive surgery

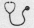

> **Box 6.3.6   Indications for Surgical Referral of Hydroceles in Children**
>
> - Underlying pathology, e.g. torsion, tumour
> - Suspicion of an inguinal hernia, as this can be difficult to distinguish sometimes from a hydrocele
> - Localised to the spermatic cord
> - Suggestion of an abdomino-scrotal hydrocele
> - Persistent beyond 2 years

Dangerous Diagnosis 2

Diagnosis: Testicular tumour

Management Principles

1. **Refer to oncology.** Further investigations and management will be guided by a tertiary oncology service. Adjuvant chemo-therapy ± radiotherapy will be required in malignant cases. There should be consideration of long-term effects of treatment, as well as the need for follow-up into adolescence and adulthood
2. **Surgery.** Referral to the urology team will usually be made as part of the oncology multi-disciplinary team, once the diag-nosis is confirmed. Orchidectomy is likely and prostheses are available

Dangerous Diagnosis 3

Diagnosis: Inguinal hernia

Management Principles

1. **Urgent surgical referral: if features of strangulation or incarceration.** Urgent admission to hospital under surgical care is needed and the patient made nil by mouth. Intravenous (IV) access should be obtained, and a naso-gastric tube sited if features of intestinal obstruction
2. **Outpatient surgical referral: if features of reducible hernia.** Refer to paediatric surgeons urgently as an outpatient

Common Diagnosis 1

Diagnosis: Hydrocele

Management Principles

1. **Watch and wait: in congenital cases.** Spontaneous resolution is likely in children under 2 years old. Referral to paediatric surgeon will be required otherwise
2. **Consider surgical referral: in non-congenital cases.** Consider possible underlying causes and refer appropriately. Idiopathic hydroceles can be managed with reassurance and scrotal support. Large hydroceles causing discomfort can be referred to paediatric surgeons

Common Diagnosis 2

Diagnosis: Varicocele

Management Principles

1. **Surgical referral.** Referral is indicated if there is impaired testicular growth, the varicocele does not drain on lying down or if it has appeared acutely and is painful. Varicocelectomy will be required to preserve fertility
2. **Further investigations.** Right-sided varicoceles are very rare, and if noted may indicate the presence of an abdominal or retroperitoneal mass

Common Diagnosis 3

Diagnosis: Epididymo-orchitis

Management Principles

1. **Antibiotics.** Treat according to the likely cause and reassess after 3 days with microbiology results if no improvement. If immunocompromised or with signs of severe infection, consider admission
2. **Sexual health referral.** Referral to a sexual health specialist should be made in pubertal boys if sexually transmitted infec-tions are suspected

Common Diagnosis 4
Diagnosis: Torted hydatid

Management Principles
1. **Conservative.** If the 'blue dot' sign is present, or pain is mild and resolving, it would be reasonable to reassure and discharge home on simple analgesia
2. **Surgical referral.** If diagnosis is uncertain and there is any suspicion of a testicular torsion, urgent surgical exploration should be considered

7.1 Hypoglycaemia

Rachel Varughese

Department of Paediatrics, Oxford University Hospitals NHS Foundation Trust, Oxford, UK

CONTENTS

7.1.1 CHAPTER AT A GLANCE

> **Box 7.1.1 Chapter at a Glance**
>
> - Glucose is the preferred fuel of the brain
> - Hypoglycaemia is a medical emergency that can be life-threatening, but is reversible with prompt recognition and treatment
> - It can lead to collapse, coma, seizures or long-term neurological damage and death
> - Young children are more susceptible to hypoglycaemia due to higher glucose utilisation rates with larger relative brain volume and lower muscle mass
>
> - Hypoglycaemia is frequently seen as a complication in patients with known diabetes mellitus. This will not be discussed in this chapter, as it does not usually pose a diagnostic challenge
> - Neonatal hypoglycaemia (first 2–3 days of life) is a different entity and will not be discussed

7.1.2 DEFINITION

Hypoglycaemia describes low-plasma glucose. Definitions vary depending on age and patient population.
In general, hypoglycaemia is defined as:
- Most children: <2.6 mmol/L
- Diabetic patients: <4 mmol/L

Clinical Guide to Paediatrics, First Edition. Edited by Rachel Varughese and Anna Mathew. Series Editor: Christian Fielder Camm.
© 2022 John Wiley & Sons Ltd. Published 2022 by John Wiley & Sons Ltd.
Companion website: www.wiley.com/go/varughese/paediatrics

7.1.3 DIAGNOSTIC ALGORITHM

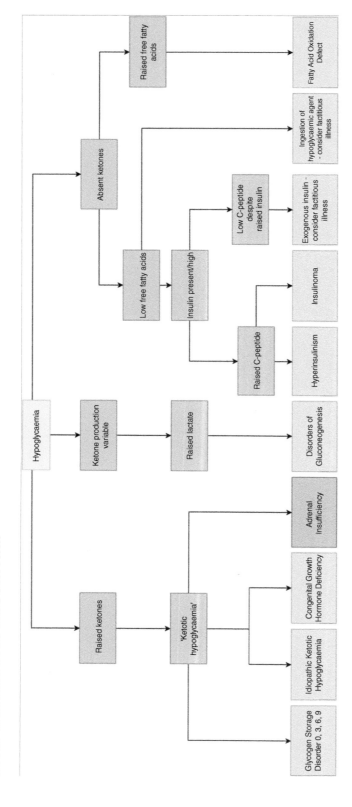

Figure 7.1.1 Diagnostic algorithm for the presentation of hypoglycaemia.

7.1.4 DIFFERENTIALS LIST

Hypoglycaemia of any cause can be dangerous if profound or prolonged. The differential diagnosis is broad and an exhaustive list of causes is beyond the scope of this chapter.

Box 7.1.2   Normal Glucose Homeostasis

Glucose is obtained from:

- Intestinal absorption of food
- Glycogenolysis
- Gluconeogenesis

During fasting:

- Insulin is suppressed

- There is increased glucagon, cortisol and growth hormone leading to:

  - Glucose production, by glycogenolysis and gluconeogenesis
  - Alternate fuel synthesis, by lipolysis and ketogenesis

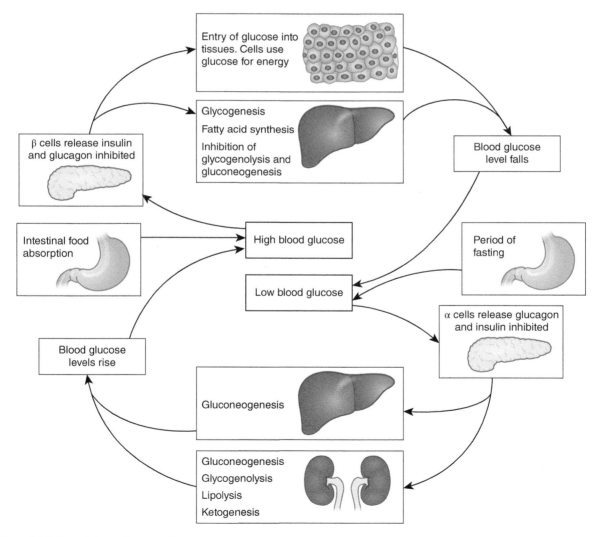

Figure 7.1.2 Normal glucose homeostasis.

Dangerous Diagnoses
1. Adrenal Insufficiency
- Adrenal insufficiency can be primary or secondary
- Primary insufficiency is caused by adrenal cortex dysfunction, often leading to mineralocorticoid and androgen deficiency in addition to cortisol insufficiency
- Secondary insufficiency is due to inadequate pituitary adrenocorticotropic hormone (ACTH) or hypothalamic corticotropin-releasing hormone (CRH), causing decreased cortisol levels alone
- Key features are hypoglycaemia, hypotension and hyponatraemia
- Underlying causes can be extensive and a high index of suspicion must be used to identify new cases

---

Box 7.1.3   Causes of Adrenal Insufficiency   △△

The causes of adrenal insufficiency are extensive. In general, causes are either primary adrenal or secondary hypothalamic/pituitary in origin

	Congenital	Acquired
Primary	• Congenital adrenal hyperplasia • Congenital adrenal hypoplasia • Metabolic: adrenoleukodystrophy • Mitochondrial: Kearns–Sayre	• Autoimmune: Addison disease • Infection: cytomegalovirus/tuberculosis • Infiltrative: haemochromatosis, sarcoidosis, malignancy • Medication: ketoconazole, phenytoin • Surgery: bilateral adrenalectomy
Secondary	• PROP1 mutation • Pituitary aplasia/hypoplasia • Isolated adrenocorticotropic hormone (ACTH) deficiency • Holoprosencephaly • Corticotropin-releasing hormone (CRH) deficiency	• Corticosteroid withdrawal after high-dose/prolonged use • Radiation therapy • Trauma • Surgery • Tumours: craniopharyngioma

---

2. Sepsis
- Although inherently dangerous, hypoglycaemia is very unlikely to be the presenting sign of sepsis
- If present, it is associated with a poor prognosis
- Sepsis is discussed in detail in Chapters 3.1 and 13.1, and will not be discussed further in this chapter

Common Diagnoses
1. Idiopathic Ketotic Hypoglycaemia
- The commonest cause of hypoglycaemia in children beyond the neonatal period, characterised by reduced tolerance to fasting
- Typically seen in children between 18 months and 5 years, with spontaneous remission by 8–9 years
- Diagnosis of exclusion
2. Hyperinsulinism
- Transient hyperinsulinism is common in the neonatal period, particularly in infants born to diabetic mothers, due to increased endogenous insulin production in utero. Perinatal stress can also induce hyperinsulinism
- Congenital hyperinsulinism is persistent and can be due to genetic mutations or in association with syndromes such as Beckwith–Wiedemann syndrome.

Box 7.1.4   Differential Diagnosis of Ketotic Hypoglycaemia   △△

- Idiopathic – most common, diagnosis of exclusion
- Hormone deficiencies: growth hormone, cortisol (adrenal insufficiency)
- Glycogen storage disorders – 0, 3, 6, 9
- Ketone utilisation defects

Diagnoses to Consider

1. Congenital Growth Hormone Deficiency
- Growth hormone is synthesised in the anterior pituitary gland
- It is an important counter-regulatory hormone, defending against hypoglycaemia
- More likely to cause hypoglycaemia in infancy with congenital deficiency than in older children with acquired deficiency
- There may be severely low growth velocity or prolonged jaundice in the neonatal period
- There may be accompanying deficiencies of other anterior pituitary hormones, particularly if there are midline defects (panhypopituitarism)

When to consider: in persistent or recurrent hypoglycaemia in a young child, particularly if there are midline defects

2. Fatty Acid Oxidation Defect (FAOD)
- Inborn error of metabolism leading to failure of mitochondrial beta-oxidation or carnitine-based mitochondrial transport of fatty acids
- Several types affecting different chains – most common is medium-chain acyl-CoA dehydrogenase deficiency (MCADD)
- Fatty acid oxidation defects are tested for in the UK routine 5-day newborn blood spot
- The severe neonatal form presents with rapidly progressive cardiomyopathy
- Acute illness can lead to recurrent hypoketotic hypoglycaemia, liver dysfunction, myopathy or rhabdomyolysis

When to consider: in infants with hypotonia, liver dysfunction or encephalopathy, particularly if there is a family history of infant death

---

Box 7.1.5   Three Types of Fatty Acid Oxidation Defects (FAODs)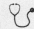

There are many types of FAODs. In general, they can be divided by their age of onset:

- **Neonatal onset:** frequently fatal, presenting within the first weeks of life, with cardiomyopathy, hypoketotic hypoglycaemia and liver dysfunction
- **Infantile onset:** presents in infancy or childhood. Intercurrent illnesses trigger episodic lethargy and vomiting, leading to

hepatic dysfunction, hypoketotic hypoglycaemia, encephalopathy or sudden death
- **Adolescent or adult onset:** presents with episodic muscle weakness, muscle pain, rhabdomyolysis and kidney injury

---

3. Glycogen Storage Disorders (GSD)
- Glycogen is the stored form of glucose in the liver, which can be used as a source of energy in times of glucose need, during fasting
- Glycogen is also a form of energy for high-intensity muscle activity
- These disorders are a large heterogenous group, with 15 variants described. They all involve some problem with the storage of glycogen, meaning glucose cannot be released at times of fasting, causing hypoglycaemia. Severity varies – in general, types 1 and 3 tolerate shorter durations of fasting (3–4 hours) than others
- Most are autosomal recessive mutations affecting glycogenolysis or gluconeogenesis

When to consider: in infants or young children with failure to thrive and liver dysfunction

4. Other Disorders of Gluconeogenesis
- Many disorders lead to impaired gluconeogenesis – see Box 7.1.6

When to consider: in infants presenting unwell with lactic acidosis after fasting, particularly if parents are consanguineous. There may be a rapid onset and deterioration, but there might be a history of faltering growth or developmental delay

---

Box 7.1.6   Disorders of Gluconeogenesis   ∆∆

Galactosaemia	• Autosomal recessive condition where the enzyme galactose-1-phosphate uridyl transferase for the metabolism of galactose to glucose is missing or defective • Develops on ingestion of galactose, e.g. in lactose-containing milk – may present with jaundice, hepatosplenomegaly and hypoglycaemia
Hereditary fructose intolerance	• Deficiency of aldolase B enzyme, which is essential in fructose metabolism, impairing gluconeogenesis
Fructose-1,6-bisphosphatase deficiency	• Enzyme essential in fructose metabolism, impairing gluconeogenesis
Pyruvate carboxylase deficiency	• Enzyme essential in gluconeogenesis
Phosphoenolpyruvate carboxykinase deficiency	• Extremely rare • Two forms: PEPCK1 and PEPCK2

5. Ingestion of Hypoglycaemic Agents/Insulin
- Ingestions may be intentional or unintentional and may include oral hypoglycaemic agents or insulin administration
- Consider factitious illness in severe hypoglycaemia with an abrupt onset and no clear trigger
- Ethanol, salicylates and beta blockers may also cause hypoglycaemia. Be aware that history might be obscured in factitious illness. Rarely, unripe lychees cause hypoglycaemia

When to consider: in hypoglycaemia of rapid onset with no identified medical trigger

6. Insulinoma
- An insulin-secreting neuroendocrine tumour causing non-ketotic hypoglycaemia
- Most commonly benign, but can be malignant
- Very rare in children, but may be seen in the setting of multiple endocrine neoplasia (MEN1), which causes tumours in parathyroid, pancreas and pituitary

When to consider: in older children with persistent and recurrent hypoglycaemia that is not necessarily triggered by fasting

---

Box 7.1.7   Whipple's Triad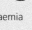

Whipple's triad typically manifest in older children, and may indicate insulinoma:

- Episodic hypoglycaemia
- Neuroglycopaenic symptoms/signs

- Immediate resolution of symptoms/signs when hypoglycaemia corrected

---

Box 7.1.8   Organic Acidaemias

- Organic acidaemias are a type of inborn error of metabolism, resulting from defects in amino acid breakdown
- Many are tested for in the UK newborn blood spot screening programme
- There are a wide variety of types and severity ranges from life-threatening to asymptomatic

- Metabolic acidosis is a hallmark of presentation and children may be mistaken for having sepsis. Metabolic decompensation is often triggered by a stressful episode of illness, trauma or surgery
- Some types of organic acidaemias affect ketone metabolism as well as that of proteins, and are known as ketogenic or ketolytic. This sub-type is associated with hypoglycaemia, which usually presents on fasting

---

7.1.5 KEY HISTORY FEATURES

Box 7.1.9   Symptoms of Hypoglycaemia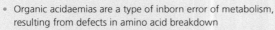

	Neurogenic (autonomic)	**Neuroglycopenic**
Cause of symptom	Sympathetic neural response to hypoglycaemia	Brain dysfunction from insufficient glucose supply
Symptoms	• Sweating • Tremor • Anxiety • Tachycardia • Palpitations • Hunger	• Confusion • Behavioural changes/irritability • Visual changes • Lethargy • Loss of consciousness • Seizures

Infants and young children may be asymptomatic, but it is still important to determine any symptoms prior to presentation

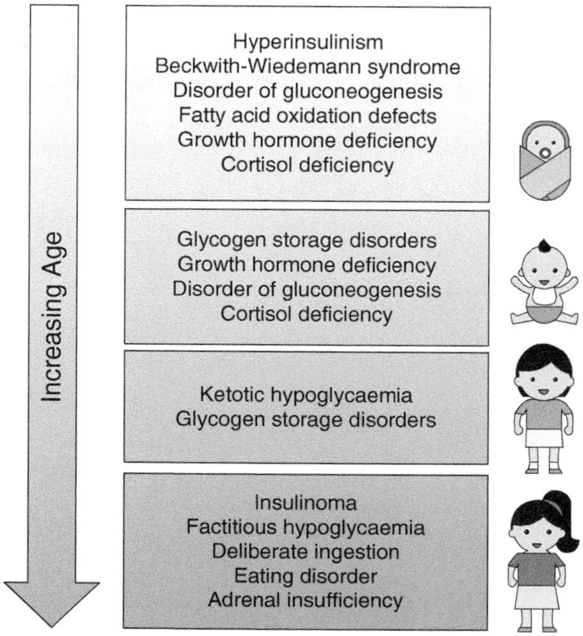

Hyperinsulinism
Beckwith-Wiedemann syndrome
Disorder of gluconeogenesis
Fatty acid oxidation defects
Growth hormone deficiency
Cortisol deficiency

Glycogen storage disorders
Growth hormone deficiency
Disorder of gluconeogenesis
Cortisol deficiency

Ketotic hypoglycaemia
Glycogen storage disorders

Insulinoma
Factitious hypoglycaemia
Deliberate ingestion
Eating disorder
Adrenal insufficiency

Increasing Age

Figure 7.1.3 Causes of hypoglycaemia according to age. Age is an important indicator of underlying diagnosis and can narrow down the differential to likely options. While there are always exceptions, some conditions are more likely to present as a neonate, infant, young child or older child.

Dangerous Diagnosis 1
Diagnosis: Adrenal insufficiency

Questions
1. **Have there been any skin changes?** In primary adrenal insufficiency, hyperpigmentation arises from an increase in melanocyte-stimulating hormone (MSH), a breakdown product from an adrenocorticotrophic hormone (ACTH) precursor. Areas typically affected are the elbows, knees, palmar creases, axillae, tongue, palate, gums and scars
2. **Have there been any changes to weight or appetite?** Glucocorticoid deficiency causes weight loss. Mineralocorticoid deficiency (if primary adrenal insufficiency) causes urinary sodium loss. Children often complain of salt cravings and may have a reduced appetite
3. **Has there been vomiting or diarrhoea?** Nausea, vomiting and diarrhoea are features of glucocorticoid deficiency. There may also be generalised abdominal pain
4. **Have there been any problems with muscles or joints?** Glucocorticoid deficiency often leads to non-specific symptoms such as weakness, fatigue, myalgia and arthralgia

---

Box 7.1.10   Hyperpigmentation in Addison Disease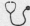

- Primary adrenal insufficiency results from reduced cortisol production from the adrenal glands
- Decreased negative feedback stimulates the hypothalamus to produce corticotropin-releasing hormone (CRH) and the pituitary to produce adrenocorticotropic hormone (ACTH). ACTH is derived from a precursor molecule called pro-opiomelanocortin (POMC), which is also the precursor for melanocyte-stimulating hormone (MSH)
- Therefore, stimulation of more POMC leads to more MSH, resulting in increased melanin

Common Diagnosis 1

Diagnosis: Ketotic hypoglycaemia

Questions

1. **How old is the child?** Children with ketotic hypoglycaemia are usually 18 months to 5 years old, due to higher glucose utilisation rates with larger relative brain volume and lower muscle mass. Slim children are particularly at risk
2. **Has there been an intercurrent illness?** Common triggers include fasting (e.g. tonsillitis), acute illness (e.g. gastroenteritis) or strenuous exercise

Common Diagnosis 2

Diagnosis: Hyperinsulinism

Questions

1. **Was there a history of maternal diabetes or perinatal stress?** Transient hyperinsulinism usually occurs in babies of mothers with diabetes or those who have experienced perinatal stress
2. **When was the first episode?** Neonatal transient hyperinsulinism presents in the first day or two of life, usually resolving within 1 week–6 months of life. In congenital hyperinsulinism, approximately 60% of infants experience a hypoglycaemic episode within the first month of life, and the rest by early childhood
3. **When does the hypoglycaemia occur?** Unlike most hypoglycaemia, episodes may occur at any time, even post prandial
4. **What was the birth weight?** Babies with congenital hyperinsulinism or Beckwith–Wiedemann syndrome may be large for gestational age. Babies with perinatal stress-induced hyperinsulinism may have had intrauterine growth restriction

---

Box 7.1.11   Hypoglycaemic-Associated Autonomic Failure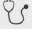

Repeated hypoglycaemia can blunt neurogenic symptoms to hypoglycaemia, which can lead to delayed awareness until blood glucose is very low

---

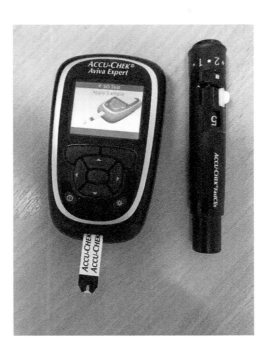

Figure 7.1.4 There are a variety of point-of-care blood sugar monitors that give instant blood glucose readings from a capillary blood sample.

7.1.6 KEY EXAMINATION FEATURES

Dangerous Diagnosis 1
Diagnosis: Adrenal insufficiency

Examination Findings
1. **Hypotension.** Hypotension is more pronounced in primary adrenal insufficiency due to lack of aldosterone, leading to dehydration. Decreased cortisol contributes due to reduced adrenaline secretion. There will be a significant postural drop in blood pressure
2. **Hyperpigmentation.** Tanned skin results from excess melanin deposition, particularly on the face, neck, hands and buccal mucosa. This is accentuated at creases, folds and scars
3. **Tachycardia and shock.** There may be resting tachycardia. With delayed diagnosis, circulatory shock can develop, and can be accompanied by nausea and abdominal pain. Preexisting hypotension and tachycardia will become more marked and perfusion will be significantly compromised

Common Diagnosis 1
Diagnosis: Ketotic hypoglycaemia

Examination Findings
1. **Low muscle mass.** Children are typically small and slim
2. **Symptomatic hypoglycaemia with absence of other features.** There should be no other associated features such as short stature, jaundice or hepatomegaly

Common Diagnosis 2
Diagnosis: Hyperinsulinism

Examination Findings
1. **Signs of associated syndromes.** Transient or congenital hyperinsulinism does not have specific features, but syndromic hyperinsulinism may. See Box 7.1.12

Box 7.1.12   Signs in Syndromes Associated with Hypoglycaemia

Syndrome	Signs
Turner syndrome	• Short stature • Webbed neck • Low hairline at back of neck • Lymphoedema of hands and feet • Coarctation of aorta/bicuspid aortic valve • Skeletal abnormalities • Premature ovarian failure
Beckwith–Wiedemann syndrome	• Abdominal wall defects, e.g. exomphalos • Macroglossia • Macrosomia • Hemihyperplasia (asymmetrical overgrowth) • Anterior ear lobe creases • Renal anomalies • Association with embryonal tumours, e.g. Wilms' tumour
Kabuki syndrome	• Distinctive facial features: long palpebral fissures, broad nose, large ears • Faltering growth • Short stature • Speech delays • Skeletal abnormalities • Hypotonia • Feeding difficulty • Limb and spinal abnormalities • Ventricular septal defect/atrial septal defect

7.1.7 KEY INVESTIGATIONS

Not all children will require invasive investigations; often diagnoses are made on clinical evidence from history and examination. Consider carefully which investigations are required for which patient.

Bedside

Table 7.1.1 Bedside tests of use in patients presenting with hypoglycaemia

Test	When to perform	Potential result
Blood sugar	• Once hypoglycaemia has been identified, regular repeat tests should continue throughout treatment and afterwards	• Resolution or recurrence of hypoglycaemia
Blood ketones	• All children with hypoglycaemia to identify ketotic from non-ketotic hypoglycaemia	• Raised ketones indicates ketotic hypoglycaemia
Blood gas	• All children with hypoglycaemia	• ↓ pH, ↓ bicarbonate (HCO_3), ↑lactate indicate metabolic acidosis: seen in inborn errors of metabolism, alcohol intoxication and salicylate poisoning

In ketotic hypoglycaemia with strong clinical evidence of idiopathic ketotic hypoglycaemia, further investigations may not be immediately warranted.

Further blood tests require obtaining samples *at the time of hypoglycaemia*. Collectively, these are known as a hypoglycaemia screen.

Blood Tests

Table 7.1.2 Blood tests of use in patients presenting with hypoglycaemia

Test	When to perform	Potential result
Plasma glucose	• To confirm hypoglycaemia	• Confirmation of hypoglycaemia
Insulin	• Insulin should be suppressed in hypoglycaemia	• Any detectable insulin is abnormal in the presence of hypoglycaemia
C-peptide	• Measure of endogenous insulin production	In the setting of detectable insulin: • C-peptide detectable: consistent with endogenous insulin excess • C-peptide undetectable: suggests exogenous insulin administration
Beta-hydroxybutyrate	• Type of ketone, therefore, should be elevated in hypoglycaemia	• Inappropriately ↓ level consistent with insulin excess or FAOD
FFA	• To indicate FAOD	• Inappropriately ↓ level consistent with insulin excess • ↑ FFA with ↓ ketones suggest FAOD
Lactate	• Raised in some metabolic conditions	• ↑ In disorder of gluconeogenesis or glycogen storage disorder
Ammonia	• Raised in some metabolic conditions	• ↑ in FAOD, organic acidaemias, some congenital hyperinsulinism and some disorders of gluconeogenesis
Cortisol	• To screen for primary or secondary adrenal insufficiency	• Inappropriately ↓ level consistent with adrenal insufficiency. Not diagnostic – prompts further tests
GH	• To look for GH deficiency	• ↓ GH: confirms deficiency – needs further tests
Acylcarnitine profile	• To identify FAOD – acylcarnitines are intermediary metabolites used in fatty acid oxidation	• Specific acylcarnitine profile help identify type of FAOD
Free and total carnitines	• To identify FAOD – carnitines essential in transport of fatty acids into mitochondria for oxidation	• ↑ or ↓ levels, interpreted with acylcarnitine profile, help identify type of FAOD

FAOD, fatty acid oxidation defect; FFA, free fatty acids; GH, growth hormone

Imaging

Table 7.1.3 Imaging modalities of use in patients presenting with hypoglycaemia

Test	When to perform	Potential result
CT/MRI/PET-CT	• Only if high suspicion of insulinoma, which is rare	• Identification of insulinoma

CT, computed tomography; MRI, magnetic resonance imaging; PET-CT, positron emission tomography–computed tomography

Special

Table 7.1.4 Special tests of use in patients presenting with hypoglycaemia

Test	When to perform	Potential result
Urine organic acids	• Screening for inborn errors of metabolism	• Abnormal in some types of fatty acid oxidation defect (FAOD) • Organic acidaemias
Urine-reducing substances	• Screening for inborn errors of metabolism	• Positive test indicates disorder of carbohydrate metabolism, e.g. galactosaemia
Urine ketones	• Only if blood ketones not possible	• Non-ketotic hypoglycaemia will require further investigation
Diagnostic fast	• To induce hypoglycaemia if hypoglycaemia screen not obtained previously • Only to be done under specialist conditions • FAOD must be excluded, as prolonged fasting can lead to life-threatening complications	• Hypoglycaemia induced • Symptoms of neuroglycopaenia • Ability to conduct hypoglycaemia screen (as already listed)
Glucagon stimulation test	• To look for excess glycogen reserves in hyperinsulinism	• Glycaemic response to glucagon is excessive in hyperinsulinaemia due to excess glycogen reserves from insulin suppression of hepatic glycogenolysis

7.1.8 KEY MANAGEMENT PRINCIPLES

Diagnosis-specific management strategies are outlined here. It is expected that an 'ABCDE' approach to assessment and management is always undertaken (see Chapter 12.1).

Dangerous Diagnosis 1
Diagnosis: Adrenal insufficiency

Management Principles
Acute
1. **Hydrocortisone.** Hydrocortisone should be given as an intravenous (IV) bolus. If no IV access within 15 minutes, it should be given intramuscularly (IM). Parents with children with known adrenal insufficiency are trained in giving IM hydrocortisone at home in an emergency. Hydrocortisone should then be continued 6 hourly
2. **IV fluids.** Adrenal crisis causes shock. Fluid resuscitation is as boluses of 20 mL/kg of isotonic solution, preferably 0.9% saline, followed by maintenance when stable

Ongoing
1. **Glucocorticoid supplementation.** Glucocorticoids, e.g. hydrocortisone, are used to supplement endogenous deficiency. Close monitoring of growth and bone age with dose adjustments will be required
2. **Mineralocorticoid supplementation.** If there is primary adrenal insufficiency, mineralocorticoid supplementation with fludrocortisone is also required
3. **Sick-day rules in stress conditions.** Additional glucocorticoids will be required in physiological stress to avoid adrenal crisis. Stress states include acute illness and surgery. If oral medication is not tolerated, then IM injection is required. Families should be educated to use IM hydrocortisone for emergency situations

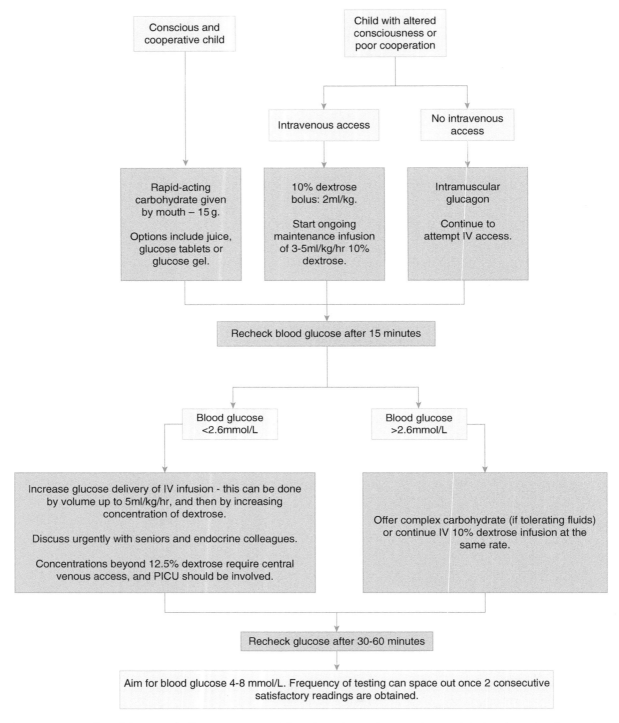

Figure 7.1.5 Regardless of the cause, significant or symptomatic hypoglycaemia must be promptly treated. Options depend on the conscious level of the patient.

4. **Adrenal insufficiency plan.** A written plan should be provided to families, including maintenance hydrocortisone dose, stress dose of oral, IM and IV hydrocortisone, and IM administration instructions. Ideally patients should carry a medical alert identification, indicating glucocorticoid dependency

Common Diagnosis 1
Diagnosis: Ketotic hypoglycaemia

Management Principles
1. **Supportive treatment.** Treatment involves avoidance of fasting, with supplementation of a carbohydrate drink during periods of reduced eating or acute illness. There are various types of carbohydrate solution, which tend to come as a powder to make up with water
2. **Reassurance.** Ketotic hypoglycaemia is usually outgrown by 8–10 years of age

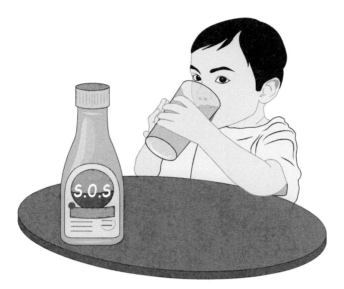

Figure 7.1.6 There are variety of powdered carbohydrate drink mixes for use as a rescue treatment in dietary management of children with propensity for fasting hypoglycaemia, e.g. ketotic hypoglycaemia and glycogen storage disorders.

Common Diagnosis 2
Diagnosis: Hyperinsulinism

Management Principles
1. **Supportive treatment.** Hypoglycaemia will often require high concentration IV maintenance replacement. Transient hyperinsulinism may resolve on its own
2. **Diazoxide.** Diazoxide blocks sulfonylurea receptors on beta pancreatic cells, decreasing insulin release. Children with certain genetic mutations are less likely to respond. Side effects include hypertrichosis and water retention
3. **Somatostatin analogues.** Analogues of somatostatin, e.g. octreotide, may be used as second line

7.2 Hyperglycaemia

Caroline Taylor

Department of Paediatrics, Buckinghamshire Healthcare NHS Trust, Aylesbury, UK

CONTENTS

7.2.1 CHAPTER AT A GLANCE

Box 7.2.1   Chapter at a Glance

- Hyperglycaemia is an excess of glucose in the bloodstream, often associated with diabetes mellitus
- Hyperglycaemia is also a stress response, frequently seen in severely ill children, due to impaired glucose metabolism, peripheral insulin resistance and relative insulin deficiency

- Administration of exogenous catecholamines, glucocorticoids and dextrose infusions tends to worsen hyperglycaemia
- Although this is not strictly a presenting complaint, bedside blood glucose testing is a common part of triage and hyperglycaemia may be picked up incidentally

---

7.2.2 DEFINITION

- A fasting blood glucose level above 7 mmol/L is considered to be hyperglycaemia
- A random blood glucose level above 11 mmol/L is also considered to be hyperglycaemia

---

Clinical Guide to Paediatrics, First Edition. Edited by Rachel Varughese and Anna Mathew. Series Editor: Christian Fielder Camm.
© 2022 John Wiley & Sons Ltd. Published 2022 by John Wiley & Sons Ltd.
Companion website: www.wiley.com/go/varughese/paediatrics

7.2.3 DIAGNOSTIC ALGORITHM

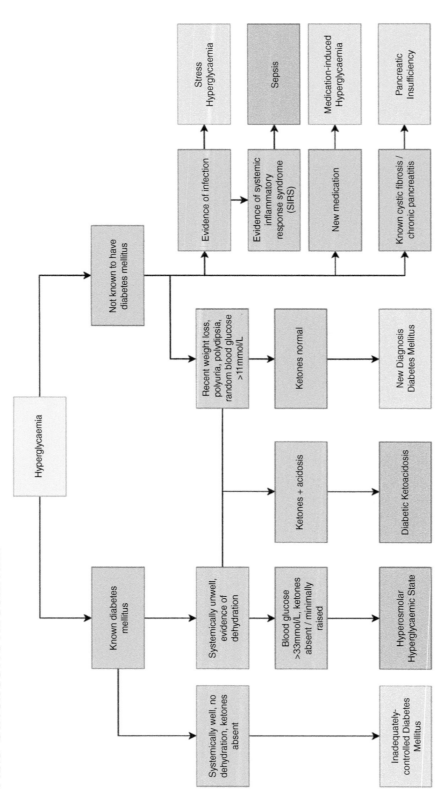

Figure 7.2.1 Diagnostic algorithm for the presentation of hyperglycaemia.

7.2.4 DIFFERENTIALS LIST

Dangerous Diagnoses

1. Diabetic Ketoacidosis (DKA)

- DKA occurs when cellular glucose uptake is impaired by insufficient insulin. The body switches to burning fatty acids, producing acidic ketone bodies
- It is characterised by high glucose and high ketones in the urine or blood
- DKA is potentially life-threatening. If untreated, it can lead to cerebral oedema, coma and eventually death

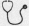

Box 7.2.2   Precipitating Factors in Diabetic Ketoacidosis (DKA)

- Inadequate insulin
  - Known diabetics, on insufficient insulin treatment
  - The first presentation of diabetes mellitus may be in DKA (around 30% of cases)
- Intercurrent infections
- Non-compliance of insulin in known diabetics (accounts for up to 45% of cases)
- Poor adherence to 'sick-day rules'

2. Hyperosmolar Hyperglycaemic State (HHS)

- HHS was previously called hyperglycaemic hyperosmolar non-ketotic coma (HONK) due to the characteristic lack of ketone production
- It is almost exclusively found in type 2 diabetics and often preceded by an intercurrent illness
- HHS is potentially life-threatening due to the risk of cerebral oedema

3. Sepsis

- Sepsis is a life-threatening condition that arises due to a dysregulated host response to infection
- Hyperglycaemia may be an early sign of evolving sepsis
- Fever, tachycardia and hypotension are commonly seen along with hyperglycaemia
- Prompt treatment with fluid resuscitation, intravenous (IV) antibiotics and other supportive measures may prevent serious complications, mortality and long-term morbidity
- Sepsis is covered in detail in Chapter 3.1 and will not be discussed further in this chapter

Common Diagnoses

1. New Diagnosis of Diabetes Mellitus

- New-onset diabetes mellitus is an important and common cause of hyperglycaemia
- There is often a preceding history of polyuria, polydipsia, weight loss/faltering growth, weakness and lethargy
- Classically, type 1 is associated with childhood diabetes, and type 2 with adult diabetes
- However, type 2 diabetes is now becoming increasingly prevalent due to rising childhood obesity

2. Drug Induced

- Steroids, beta blockers, diuretics and antipsychotic drugs have all been found to cause hyperglycaemia
- When prescribing one of these drugs, there needs to be an awareness of the potential side effect of hyperglycaemia. The risks and benefits, drug dose and duration should be considered with this in mind

Box 7.2.3   Stress Hyperglycaemia

- Stress is an important cause of hyperglycaemia
- Infection and pain are the most common causes
- Hyperglycaemia is a consequence of multiple factors, including release of cortisol and catecholamines
- There is transient hyperglycaemia due a state of temporary insulin resistance in response to the stress of illness
- It is often discovered incidentally following bedside blood glucose testing and usually resolves spontaneously once the initial 'stressor' has resolved

Diagnoses to Consider

1. Pancreatic Insufficiency

- Although not common, diabetes can develop in children and young people with cystic fibrosis, a condition termed cystic fibrosis–related diabetes (CFRD), or following chronic pancreatitis
- Progressive destruction of the islets of Langerhans may occur in the second decade, and the beta cells are replaced with fibrous tissue, leading to insulin deficiency
- The incidence of CFRD in childhood is very low, but can rise to around 20% in adolescence

When to consider: in patients who have known pancreatic insufficiency, such as those with cystic fibrosis or previous pancreatitis

2. Monogenic Diabetes

- Monogenic diabetes was formerly referred to as maturity-onset diabetes of the young (MODY)
- Monogenic diabetes is an autosomal dominant condition that frequently presents in adolescence or early adulthood
- In contrast to type 1 and type 2 diabetes, which have a polygenic inheritance pattern, mutations in a single gene account for this rare form of diabetes mellitus
- In most cases, the gene mutation is inherited from a parent, although spontaneous mutations have also been noted. Genetic testing is required to make a diagnosis
- There are two main forms, neonatal diabetes mellitus (NDM), and MODY, which is much more common
- In MODY, the ability of the pancreas to produce insulin is limited, which leads to hyperglycaemia and over time the complications associated with diabetes, including retinopathy, nephropathy, neuropathy and cardiovascular disease
- Treatment may be with either insulin or oral hypoglycaemic agents

When to consider: monogenic diabetes is usually an inherited disease that develops due to a single gene mutation. Box 7.2.4 describes some key features

---

Box 7.2.4   When to Consider Monogenic Diabetes

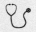

- When diabetes is diagnosed in the first 6 months of life (type 1 diabetes is rarely diagnosed this early)
- In adolescence when there is a strong family history of diabetes
- In non-insulin-dependent diabetes, with absence of predisposing features of type 2 diabetes, such as obesity

- With mild hyperglycaemia, which is noted incidentally on blood testing
- With associated extra-pancreatic features such as renal cysts

---

7.2.5 KEY HISTORY FEATURES

Dangerous Diagnosis 1
Diagnosis: Diabetic ketoacidosis

Questions
1. **Is the child a known diabetic?** Always consider that DKA may be the first presentation of a child with new onset of diabetes mellitus. In known cases of diabetes, DKA must always be the top differential
2. **Has the child been able to eat?** Symptoms of abdominal pain and vomiting may stop the child from eating their regular meals and lead to disturbances in glycaemic control. If unrecognised, dehydration, laboured breathing and an altered mental state may herald DKA
3. **Have the parents changed the usual insulin regime?** When a child becomes unwell, parents can sometimes omit or lower doses of insulin for fear that their child's blood glucose may fall dangerously low. Patients with diabetes will have a detailed plan of 'sick-day rules' to follow when they are unwell or have reduced oral intake. This should determine any changes to insulin dose and when to seek medical help
4. **Is the child old enough to administer their own insulin and are they compliant?** Teenagers may rebel against having to comply with their dietary and insulin regime and may omit doses as a result. Omitting medication is also sometimes seen in teenage girls with concerns about body image, who may choose not to take their insulin in an attempt to lose weight. These behaviours may trigger DKA
5. **Has the young teenager started drinking alcohol or taking illicit substances?** Indulging in excessive alcohol intake and substance misuse are other reasons for hyperglycaemia and DKA in known diabetics

---

Box 7.2.5   Sick-Day Rules for Diabetes

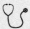

- Children with diabetes, and their parents, must have a comprehensive understanding of how to manage insulin during intercurrent illnesses
- Parents may intuitively think that an unwell child with reduced oral intake should have insulin omitted
- In fact, cortisol release during periods of stress or illness can result in hyperglycaemia and ketone production

- Insulin requirements can be significantly higher, even if oral intake is reduced
- Children should be advised to never stop insulin, even if not eating, and to always check for ketones regardless of blood glucose. A detailed written plan is provided to all diabetics, with instructions of how to respond to different blood glucose and ketone levels, and when to seek help

Dangerous Diagnosis 2

Diagnosis: Hyperosmolar hyperglycaemic state

Questions

1. **Does the patient have a diagnosis of type 2 diabetes?** HHS is almost exclusively found in type 2 diabetic children. Due to these children still having some intrinsic insulin production, ketone production and acidosis are less likely to occur
2. **Has the child become increasingly thirsty or are they passing large volumes of urine?** Polyuria and polydipsia usually develop over several days
3. **Has there been confusion, disorientation or altered mental state?** As diagnosis is often delayed, severe dehydration may result in headache, disorientation and decreased levels of consciousness
4. **Is the child overweight or have they been drinking large quantities of carbonated sugar-rich drinks?** Obesity is a particular risk for developing HHS, and drinking sugar-rich drinks as polydipsia progresses has been noted as a risk factor for severe hyperglycaemia

Common Diagnosis 1

Diagnosis: New diagnosis of diabetes mellitus

Questions

1. **Has there been increased thirst or urinary frequency?** Diabetes commonly presents with the triad of polyuria, polydipsia and weight loss
2. **Has there been a recent history of bedwetting?** This is a common symptom and is a reflection of the large volumes of urine produced
3. **Has there been any recent weight loss despite a good appetite?** Parents are often concerned that despite a good appetite, the child seems to be losing weight
4. **Is there a family history of type 1 diabetes?** The risk of developing diabetes is significantly increased if there is a genetic susceptibility in the family. If both parents are affected, the risk to offspring can be up to 30%

Common Diagnosis 2

Diagnosis: Drug induced

Questions

1. **Is the child on any regular medication?** Several drugs can cause hyperglycaemia as a side effect, including steroids, beta blockers, diuretics and antipsychotic drugs
2. **When was the medication started?** Some children may only need a short course of a particular medication, but that might be sufficient to precipitate hyperglycaemia and glycosuria

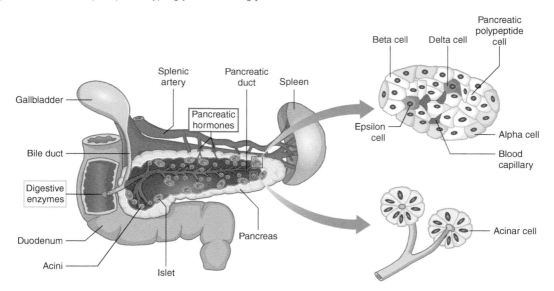

Figure 7.2.2 The pancreas has both exocrine and endocrine functions. Exocrine function is delivered through the acinar cells, through synthesis of digestive enzymes, secreted into the pancreatic duct and then the duodenum. Endocrine function occurs in collections of cells known as the islets of Langerhans. Synthesis of hormones occurs in the islet cells, and includes alpha cells (glucagon), beta cells (insulin) and delta cells (somatostatin).

3. **Is there a plan in place to monitor for potential side effects of medication?** Monitoring urine dipsticks for glycosuria, checking blood pressure regularly and watching for Cushingoid signs are necessary when children are started on long-term steroid courses. Similar screening measures may be necessary for other medications

7.2.6 KEY EXAMINATION FEATURES

Dangerous Diagnosis 1
Diagnosis: Diabetic ketoacidosis

Examination Findings
1. **Signs of dehydration.** Prolonged capillary refill, reduced skin turgor and dry mucous membranes indicate dehydration. Hypotension is suggestive of decompensated hypovolaemic shock
2. **Acidotic breathing.** Hyperventilation and 'Kussmaul' deep breathing are commonly seen to compensate for metabolic acidosis, which is often quite marked
3. **Altered mental state.** Lethargy, drowsiness, confusion and disorientation may be present, depending on the severity of DKA. This is usually a result of the acidosis, although cerebral oedema must always be considered
4. **Abdominal tenderness.** There may be generalised abdominal pain on palpation

Dangerous Diagnosis 2
Diagnosis: Hyperosmolar hyperglycaemic syndrome

Examination Findings
1. **Obesity.** Obesity is a common factor predisposing to development of type 2 diabetes in children. Accurate assessments of dehydration may be more difficult as a result
2. **Acanthosis nigricans.** This is velvety darkening of the skin, particularly in skin folds, and is an indicator of insulin resistance
3. **Profound dehydration.** Children with HHS often have a delayed diagnosis as their symptoms of polyuria and polydipsia increase gradually. As a result, they may present with severe dehydration
4. **Altered mental state.** In the later stages, there may be a headache, with disorientation and decreased level of consciousness, as a result of severe dehydration
5. **Neurological dysfunction.** Neurological examination may reveal blurred vision, depressed tendon reflexes, tremors or fasciculation of muscles

Common Diagnosis 1
Diagnosis: New diagnosis of diabetes mellitus

Examination Findings
1. **Signs of dehydration.** There may be varying degrees of prolonged capillary refill, reduced skin turgor and dry mucous membranes, depending on the duration of the illness prior to presentation
2. **Faltering growth.** It is common for children with newly diagnosed diabetes to have a history of recent weight loss, as the lack of insulin prevents glucose metabolism
3. **Normal examination.** The child may be relatively well at presentation, with no clinical signs

Common Diagnosis 2
Diagnosis: Drug induced

Examination Findings
1. **Normal examination.** There may be no specific examination findings, so history is key
2. **Side effects of medications.** There may be side effects of the causative medications. For example, if hyperglycaemia is steroid induced, there may be Cushingoid features, including weight gain, a rounded face, easy bruising, purple striae, interscapular fatty hump and thin hair

7.2.7 KEY INVESTIGATIONS

Not all children will require invasive investigations; often diagnoses are made on clinical evidence from history and examination. Consider carefully which investigations are required for which patient.

Bedside

Table 7.2.1 Bedside tests of use in patients presenting with hyperglycaemia

Test	When to perform	Potential result
Blood gas (venous)	Suspected: • DKA • HHS	• DKA: pH <7.3, HCO_3 <15 mmol/L (varies depending on severity) • HHS: pH normal or borderline low, HCO_3 >15 mmol/L
Blood glucose and ketones	Suspected: • DKA • HHS • New diagnosis of diabetes mellitus	• DKA: ↑ Glucose, but not usually as high as in HHS, ketones >3.0 mmol/L • HHS: glucose >33 mmol/L, ketones normal or minimally raised • Diabetes mellitus: random blood glucose >11 mmol/L, ketones normal
Urine ketones	Suspected: • DKA • HHS	• DKA: markedly raised • HHS: normal or minimally raised
ECG monitoring	• In DKA and HHS, electrolyte imbalance can be seen at presentation, and develops during treatment	• Early detection of changes consistent with electrolyte imbalance

DKA, diabetic ketoacidosis; ECG, electrocardiogram; HCO_3, bicarbonate; HHS, hyperosmolar hyperglycaemic state

Blood Tests

Table 7.2.2 Blood tests of use in patients presenting with hyperglycaemia

Test	When to perform	Potential result
FBC	• Suspected sepsis	• ↑ WCC, ↑ neutrophils indicate bacterial infection
CRP	• Suspected sepsis	• ↑ CRP, higher in bacterial than viral infections
Serum osmolality	Suspected: • DKA • HHS	• Raised in DKA • Markedly raised in HHS >330 mOsmol/kg
U&E	Suspected: • DKA • HHS	• ↑ Urea, ↑ creatinine raised in dehydration due to DKA • K level useful to guide management, especially if insulin required
Calcium, magnesium, phosphate	Suspected: • DKA • HHS	• ↓ Levels of phosphate, magnesium, calcium can be seen
HbA1C	Suspected: • Diabetes mellitus • DKA • HHS	• Level indicates long-term glucose control, and guides further management
Islet cell antibodies	• New diagnosis of diabetes mellitus	• Positive test supports diagnosis of type 1 diabetes
Blood culture	• Suspected sepsis	• Positive culture confirms bacterial infection • Sensitivities guide antibiotic choice

CRP, C-reactive protein; DKA, diabetic ketoacidosis; FBC, full blood count; HbA1C, haemoglobin A1C; HHS, hyperosmolar hyperglycaemic state; K, potassium; U&E, urea and electrolytes

Special

Table 7.2.3 Special tests of use in patients presenting with hyperglycaemia

Test	When to perform	Potential result
Thyroid function tests	• Useful screening test in new diagnosis of diabetes mellitus	• Autoimmune thyroid disease (associated with type 1 diabetes)
Coeliac screen	• Useful screening test in new diagnosis of diabetes mellitus	• Coeliac disease (associated with type 1 diabetes)
Genetic testing	• Suspected monogenic diabetes	• Gene identification confirms diagnosis

Box 7.2.6   Differentiating Diabetic Ketoacidosis (DKA) and Hyperosmolar Hyperglycaemic State (HHS)   ΔΔ

Feature	DKA	HHS
Type of diabetes	Type 1 predominantly	Type 2 predominantly
Endogenous insulin levels	Very low	May be normal
Blood glucose	Raised	Markedly raised
Serum osmolality	Variable	Markedly raised
Ketosis	Marked	Absent or very mild
Metabolic acidosis	Marked	Absent or very mild

7.2.8 KEY MANAGEMENT PRINCIPLES

Diagnosis-specific management strategies are outlined here. It is expected that an 'ABCDE' approach to assessment and management is always undertaken (see Chapter 12.1).

Dangerous Diagnosis 1

Diagnosis: Diabetic ketoacidosis

DKA management is very specific. It is essential to consult a local or national guideline in order to direct management.

Management Principles

1. **Fluid resuscitation.** If there are clinical signs of shock, IV fluid resuscitation should be initiated with boluses of 0.9% sodium chloride. There are specific rules as to how much to give, and guidelines should be followed closely. Maintenance fluid is dependent on the degree of dehydration, which is estimated by the degree of acidosis
2. **Potassium.** 20 mmol of potassium should be added to every 500 mL of normal saline once the child has started passing urine, or potassium levels are below the higher range of normal
3. **Start IV insulin infusion.** Start insulin infusion 1–2 hours after starting IV fluids. An insulin infusion is usually started at 0.05–0.1 units/kg/hr. The lower dose is thought to be adequate in most children
4. **Dextrose.** Dextrose is added to IV fluids once the blood glucose levels are less than 14 mmol/L. Change fluids to 0.9% saline with 5% glucose and 20 mmol potassium chloride in every 500 mL bag
5. **Regular observations and senior review.** Strict input–output charts, hourly neuro-observations, monitoring of vital signs, continuous electrocardiogram (ECG), and regular blood gas and electrolyte monitoring are essential, with senior review undertaken at each stage
6. **Monitor blood glucose and ketones.** These should be checked hourly once treatment has commenced. Blood ketone concentration should fall by 0.5 mmol/L per hour and glucose concentration by 3 mmol/L per hour
7. **Seek senior advice.** Should the child not respond to treatment as expected, senior advice should always be sought early
8. **Establish subcutaneous therapy.** Once controlled, subcutaneous insulin therapy will be commenced (if new diagnosis) or recommended (if known diabetic), on advice of the diabetic team

Box 7.2.7   Categorising Severity of Diabetic Ketoacidosis

	Venous pH	Bicarbonate	% dehydration
Mild	7.2–7.29	<15 mmol/L	Assume 5%
Moderate	7.1–7.19	<10 mmol/L	Assume 7%
Severe	<7.1	<5 mmol/L	Assume 10%

Source: Adapted from British Society for Paediatric Endocrinology and Diabetes (2020). Integrated care pathway for the management of children and young people with diabetic ketoacidosis. https://www.bspe d.org.uk/media/1742/dka-icp-2020-v1_1.pdf

Dangerous Diagnosis 2

Diagnosis: Hyperosmolar hyperglycaemic state

Management Principles

1. **Fluid resuscitation and correction of dehydration.** Patients are often severely dehydrated and may require a 20 mL/kg bolus of 0.9% saline. Fluid deficits of 12–15% are often assumed. Maintenance fluids should be 0.45–0.9% saline. Plasma glucose should fall by around 4–6 mmol/L per hour. If decreasing by more than 5 mmol/L per hour, then consider adding 5% glucose to maintenance fluids
2. **Start IV insulin infusion.** Early insulin infusion is often unnecessary, as ketosis is usually minimal. Fluid resuscitation alone results in a steady decline in serum glucose levels. The hyperglycaemia helps maintain the intravascular volume, so a rapid drop can lead to circulatory collapse. Low dose IV insulin infusion (0.025–0.05 units/kg/hr) should be started once the blood glucose level is no longer falling with IV fluids alone
3. **Regular observations and senior review.** Strict input–output charts, hourly neuro-observations, monitoring of vital signs, continuous ECG, and blood gas and electrolyte monitoring are essential, with senior review undertaken at each stage
4. **Electrolyte replacement.** Electrolyte imbalance of potassium, phosphate and magnesium are more frequently seen than in DKA. Potassium is often required, especially if insulin infusion is started. Phosphate and magnesium replacement is also advised if levels are low; seek senior advice, as replacement is controversial
5. **Treat underlying cause.** Often HHS develops secondary to illness, so antibiotics should be started if there is clinical evidence of infection

Common Diagnosis 1

Diagnosis: New diagnosis of diabetes mellitus

Management Principles

1. **Fluid replacement.** If dehydrated, fluid replacement may be required
2. **Insulin therapy.** Exogenous insulin therapy will be required, and the local diabetic team will decide on either subcutaneous injections several times a day or an insulin pump
3. **Patient and parent education**. Diabetes is a long-term illness where patient and parental engagement is critical to gaining control and preventing complications. Detailed education from the diabetes team, including the dietician, doctor and specialist nurse, is essential
4. **Sick-day rules.** The diabetes team will give advice on how to manage fluctuating glucose levels during intercurrent illnesses when reduced oral intake and the stress of the infection can cause temporary insulin resistance. Closer blood glucose monitoring with adjustment of insulin dose will be advised to manage any hyperglycaemia and ketones

Common Diagnosis 2

Diagnosis: Drug induced

Management Principles

1. **Consider benefits of medication.** This will be a risk–benefit analysis. Hyperglycaemia may be an acceptable risk if the treatment is essential. Otherwise, alternative treatment should be considered

8.1 Headache

Dora Steel

Department of Paediatrics, London School of Paediatrics, London, UK

CONTENTS

8.1.1 CHAPTER AT A GLANCE

Box 8.1.1   Chapter at a Glance

- Most childhood headaches are benign, but serious conditions such as a brain tumour need to be excluded
- Headaches are a common presenting complaint in childhood, with a high prevalence rate: 80% of children will experience at least one bout by age 16

- Assessment of headache relies heavily on history and examination, with neuroimaging and other investigations required only in specific circumstances
- It is unusual for a child under 4 years old to complain of headache, so this should always be taken seriously

---

8.1.2 DEFINITION

The sensation of pain located in or around the head.

Clinical Guide to Paediatrics, First Edition. Edited by Rachel Varughese and Anna Mathew. Series Editor: Christian Fielder Camm.
© 2022 John Wiley & Sons Ltd. Published 2022 by John Wiley & Sons Ltd.
Companion website: www.wiley.com/go/varughese/paediatrics

8.1.3 DIAGNOSTIC ALGORITHM

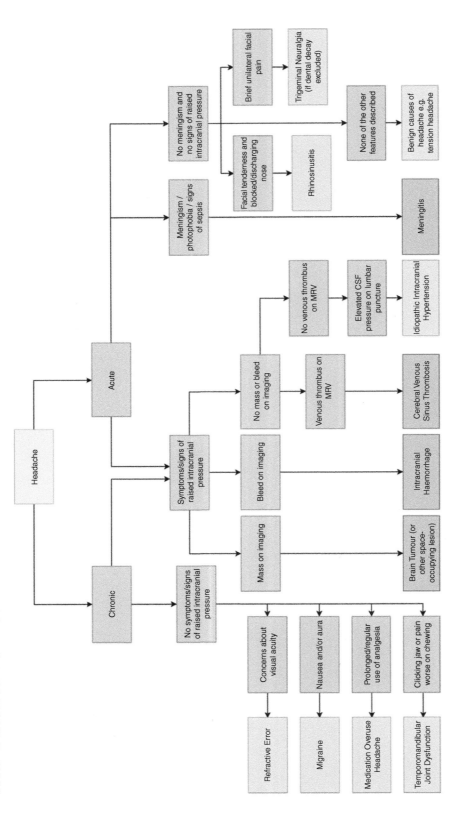

Figure 8.1.1 Diagnostic algorithm for the presentation of headache.

8.1.4 DIFFERENTIALS LIST

Dangerous Diagnoses

1. Meningitis/Encephalitis

- Meningitis refers to an inflammation of the meninges. Encephalitis refers to an inflammation of the brain
- Meningitis may be caused by a bacterial, viral or (more rarely) tubercular or fungal infection
- Meningococcal disease (caused by *Neisseria meningitidis*) is less common in the UK since it was introduced into the routine childhood vaccination programme
- Other bacteria (e.g. *Haemophilus influenzae* and *Streptococcus pneumoniae*) can also cause meningitis, but their prevalence in the UK has also reduced since the introduction of the *H. influenzae* B (Hib) and pneumococcal vaccines in infancy
- Bacterial meningitis carries a significant risk of death or permanent disability
- In encephalitis, viral causes predominate, with herpes simplex being the most common. It can however occur as a consequence of bacterial, fungal and parasitic infections, as well as systemic conditions such as autoimmune diseases
- The clinical presentation can overlap with meningitis, so they are treated similarly in the acute setting

---

Box 8.1.2   Causes of Bacterial Meningitis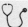

Age	Organisms
Birth to 3 months	Group B *Streptococcus* *Escherichia coli* *Listeria monocytogenes*
3 months–5 years	*Neisseria meningitidis* *Streptococcus pneumoniae* *Haemophilus influenzae*
5 years and above	*Neisseria meningitidis* *Streptococcus pneumoniae*
Other bacteria	Syphilis Tuberculosis

---

2. Space-Occupying Lesion (SOL)

- This includes tumours, intracranial vascular malformations and abscesses
- Brain tumours are the commonest solid tumours in childhood, and account for 1 out of 4 childhood cancers
- Headache may be accompanied by signs of raised intracranial pressure (ICP) and vomiting
- Focal neurological deficits may not appear until the tumour is quite large
- The child may appear systemically well

Box 8.1.3   Differentials for a Space-Occupying Lesion

- Brain tumour
- Metastasis of an extracranial cancer
- Vascular malformation
- Haematoma
- Abscess
- Tuberculoma

---

3. Cerebral Venous Sinus Thrombosis (CVST)

- Sinuses provide venous drainage from the brain. They may become thrombosed, most commonly the superior sagittal sinus or cavernous sinus
- Usually triggered by a subdural empyema (pus around the brain from an ear or sinus infection), mastoiditis, meningitis or an underlying abnormal clotting tendency (thrombophilia)

4. Intracranial Haemorrhage

- Non-traumatic bleeds are usually due to rupture of a congenital arteriovenous malformation leading to subarachnoid or intraparenchymal haemorrhage

- Very severe, sudden headache accompanied by nausea and sometimes seizures, focal neurological deficit and/or loss of consciousness
- Immediate neurosurgical assessment is required

Common Diagnoses
1. Idiopathic Intracranial Hypertension (IIH)
- Also known as pseudotumor cerebri
- Previously described as 'benign intracranial hypertension'
- ICP is raised (>20 cmH$_2$O) in the absence of a space-occupying lesion
- Most common in teenage girls, especially if overweight, but can occur at any age
- Can lead to disabling visual loss in up to 10%
2. Tension-Type Headache
- Commonest type of headache
- Classical description of the headache is of a tight band-like pain around the head
- Should only be diagnosed where other causes have been ruled out
3. Migraine
- Recurrent headaches with associated nausea and often photophobia and phonophobia
- Although classic migraines include an 'aura' of visual disturbance before the pain starts, migraines without aura are more common
4. Rhinosinusitis
- Infection of the facial sinuses can cause facial pain, sometimes associated with headache
5. Refractive Error
- Undiagnosed refractive error is a common cause of headache as eyes strain to compensate for the inability to focus

Diagnoses to Consider
1. Trigeminal Neuralgia
- Attacks of sharp, severe pain involving one side of the face, which is often described as 'stabbing' or 'shooting', lasting for a few seconds up to a few minutes
- Not fully understood, but believed to be related to dysfunction of the trigeminal nerve
- Triggers can include chewing, touching the area or cold wind. Remember, facial pain worse on chewing could also indicate dental decay
- When treatment is required, anticonvulsant medications such as carbamazepine or gabapentin may be used

When to consider: in children with a history of severe, short-lasting attacks of pain
2. Temporomandibular Joint (TMJ) Dysfunction
- Pain arising from the TMJ, which is involved in chewing, typically felt in the jaw and face, but it can also be referred to the head, neck or ear
- Dental review is often required to confirm the diagnosis
- Management is supportive, with analgesia, ice, massaging the affected area and eating soft food

When to consider: in children with pain worse on eating, particularly if jaw clicking or locking on chewing.
3. Medication Overuse Headache
- Chronic headache caused by prolonged frequent use of simple analgesia
- Diagnosis of exclusion

When to consider: in children with frequent or recurrent analgesia use

8.1.5 KEY HISTORY FEATURES

Dangerous Diagnosis 1
Diagnosis: Meningitis/encephalitis

Questions
1. **Has the child had a fever or preceding illness?** Fever in an unwell child who has a headache should lead to the consideration of meningitis. Sinusitis and otitis media can lead to intracranial infection through direct spread of infection
2. **Is there any neck stiffness or photophobia?** This is the classic symptom triad of meningism, i.e. meningeal irritation. Younger children will not complain of these symptoms, so a high index suspicion is required in this age group
3. **Is there vomiting/nausea?** Vomiting is a common non-specific symptom of bacterial meningitis and may indicate raised ICP
4. **Is the child sleepy, irritable or 'not themselves'?** Both excessive irritability (especially with a high-pitched, inconsolable cry) and excessive drowsiness are worrying signs. If the parent reports a young child is very unlike their normal self, take this seriously.

5. **Is the child fully vaccinated?** The UK infant vaccination schedule includes vaccinations against *Meningococcus* B and C, *Pneumococcus*, Hib and measles, but infections can occur even in fully vaccinated children
6. **Is there any history of herpetic lesions or suspected contact with herpes simplex?** Ask about vesicular lesions in the recent history or exposure to herpetic lesions elsewhere, e.g. from kissing a parent affected with a cold sore

Dangerous Diagnosis 2
Diagnosis: Space-occupying lesion

Questions
1. **What time of day is the headache worst?** Headaches caused by raised ICP are generally worse in the morning, as ICP rises during the night. This is both a positional effect and due to vasodilatation secondary to increased nocturnal blood carbon dioxide (CO_2) levels
2. **Has the child been vomiting or suffering from nausea?** Classically raised ICP causes nausea, with the headache partially relieved after vomiting
3. **Has there been any change in the child's personality, abilities or balance?** Any suggestion that a child's development, school performance or motor skills have deteriorated is strongly suggestive of a serious underlying pathology.

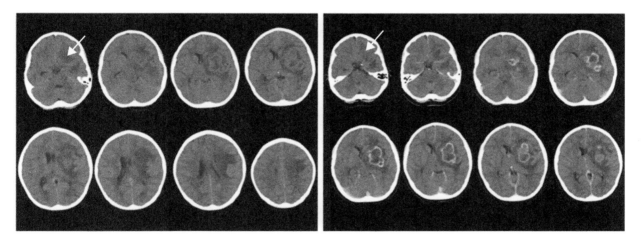

Figure 8.1.2 Pre- and post-contrast computed tomography of a glioma in a 12-year-old girl presenting with headache, vomiting and bilateral papilloedema.

Box 8.1.4   When There Is No Headache: Signs of Brain Tumours in Children Too Young to Complain

- Head circumference crossing centiles upwards
- Unexplained persistent vomiting
- Developmental regression
- Head tilt
- Abnormal eye movements (especially nystagmus or paralytic squint)
- Behavioural change
- Focal seizures

Box 8.1.5   Symptoms and signs of a brain tumour in older children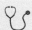

- Headache, can wake from sleep or particularly early morning
- Unexplained nausea and vomiting
- Visual disturbances, e.g. double vision, temporary loss of vision, squint
- Slurred speech
- Stiff neck, head tilt
- Behavioural change
- Confusion and irritability
- Memory problems, deterioration in schoolwork
- Seizures
- Gait disturbance
- Weakness on one side of face, arms, legs

Dangerous Diagnosis 3
Diagnosis: Cerebral venous sinus thrombosis

Questions
1. **Is there a history of recent ear or upper respiratory tract infection?** Many cases of CVST are triggered by subdural empyema, which is usually the result of a sinus or ear infection, including mastoiditis
2. **What time of day is the headache worst?** As with space-occupying lesions, CVST causes raised ICP and therefore headaches are typically worse in the morning
3. **Does the child have a significant past medical history?** Other causative conditions can include inherited thrombophilias, leukaemia, nephrotic syndrome and sickle cell disease

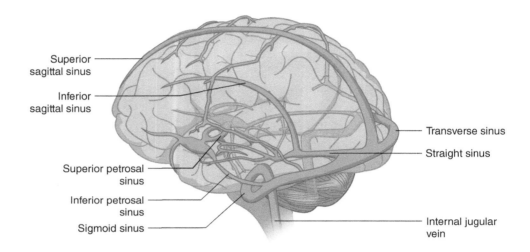

Superior sagittal sinus

Inferior sagittal sinus

Superior petrosal sinus

Inferior petrosal sinus

Sigmoid sinus

Transverse sinus

Straight sinus

Internal jugular vein

Figure 8.1.3 Layout of the dural venous sinuses of the brain (simplified): a thrombus can occur in any of these.

Dangerous Diagnosis 4
Diagnosis: Intracranial haemorrhage

Questions
1. **How rapid was the onset of the headache?** Subarachnoid or intraparenchymal haemorrhage usually causes very sudden, severe pain, with onset over seconds
2. **Did any associated symptoms of raised ICP or neurological deficit develop at or around the same time?** The sudden increase in ICP may cause vomiting or seizures. Subarachnoid or intraparenchymal haemorrhage can also cause sudden unilateral weakness of the limbs and/or face
3. **Is there a history of trauma or suspicion of non-accidental injury (NAI)?** A history of trauma is relevant to understanding the pathology. You must also consider NAI, and take a detailed history of the mechanism of injury. Consider if history is consistent with signs and remember details may be purposely obscured

Common Diagnosis 1
Diagnosis: Idiopathic intracranial hypertension

Questions
1. **What time of day is the headache worst? Are there any signs of raised ICP?** As with other causes of raised ICP, IIH typically causes morning headaches. Nausea and vomiting also suggest raised ICP, but are not helpful in distinguishing the exact cause

2. **Have there been any disturbances of hearing or vision?** Many children with IIH report a 'rumbling' or 'machinery' noise in their ears. In severe cases visual impairment starts to develop due to pressure on the optic nerves
3. **Are there any risk factors present for IIH?** Being female, overweight, excessive Vitamin A, the combined oral contraceptive pill and certain antibiotic usage (e.g. tetracyclines) are known risk factors for developing IIH

Common Diagnosis 2
Diagnosis: Tension-type headache

Questions
1. **Is the headache described as a tight band around the head?** Tension headaches are typically described as a squeezing, tight or band-like pain around the head
2. **Has the child been under any particular stress at home or at school?** Although stress is a risk factor for tension headaches and should always be explored, in some children there may not be an obvious stressor
3. **Are there any features to suggest other causes of headache?** Tension headache should only be diagnosed where other dangerous causes of headache have been ruled out

Common Diagnosis 3
Diagnosis: Migraine

Questions
1. **What does the child do when they get the headache?** Migraines typically cause photophobia (light aversion) and phonophobia (noise aversion). The child is likely to seek out a dark, quiet place, look pale and miserable, and lie down if possible
2. **When they were younger, were they a colicky baby, or a child who had tummy-aches?** In young children and babies, migraines often present as attacks of abdominal pain or unexplained crying, with headaches often not appearing until late childhood or adolescence
3. **Are any family members affected with migraines?** There is also often a family history of migraines
4. **Can the child describe the location and character of the pain?** Children may describe a pulsating or hammering pain associated with nausea. Although classically migraine (from the Greek word 'hemikrania') is unilateral, many cases are actually bilateral

---

Box 8.1.6   Migraine Auras

Migraine auras can be highly variable and sometimes quite dramatic – but remember, at least two-thirds of migraine sufferers never experience one

Aura category	Aura symptoms
Visual	• Flashing lights (scintilla) • Zigzag lines (fortification spectra) • Blind spots (scotomas) • Visual loss in part of one eye, or both eyes
Sensory	• Tingling • Pins and needles in face, body, hands (paraesthesia) • Hyperacusis • Tinnitus
Speech	• Aphasia • Slurring or mumbling words
Focal neurology/brainstem	• Hemiplegia • Dysarthria • Vertigo • Ataxia

> **Box 8.1.7   Diagnostic Criteria for Migraine: 5-4-3-2-1**
>
> - At least **five** attacks (or two if aura is present)
> - Attacks last from **four** hours to **three** days
> - Pain has at least **two** of the following characteristics: unilateral, pulsatile, at least moderate in severity, worse on physical activity
>
> - At least **one** is present out of nausea and photophobia/phonophobia
>
> Source: Adapted from International Headache Society (2018). *The international classification of headache disorders*, 3rd edn. https://ichd-3.org

Common Diagnosis 4
Diagnosis: Rhinosinusitis

Questions
1. **Has the child had a cold or a feverish illness?** Rhinosinusitis usually occurs in the context of an upper respiratory tract infection: the child may report cough and/or sore throat
2. **Does the nose feel blocked or stuffy?** There may also be thick greenish or purulent discharge from the nose, and sense of smell is often impaired
3. **Is the pain worse on leaning forwards?** Pain will also be worsened by Valsalva manoeuvres, including coughing or straining. It is important to note that this can be seen with raised ICP as well

Common Diagnosis 5
Diagnosis: Refractive error

Questions
1. **When did the child last have an eye test?** Although routine eye testing is offered in the UK when children start primary school, refractive errors can develop at any age. Only a minority of children actually attend the recommended 2-yearly eye test
2. **Does the child have difficulty reading the whiteboard at school?** Other signs of visual difficulties include wanting to sit close to the television and holding books or toys very close to the face
3. **Is there any focal neurological deficit?** Although benign eye problems such as refractive errors are common, be careful not to miss more serious causes. Rapid deterioration of vision, new double vision, nystagmus or a new squint are always concerning, and in such instances other neurological causes including an SOL should be considered

8.1.6 KEY EXAMINATION FEATURES

Varying levels of consciousness may accompany some of these diagnoses, which can be assessed using the Glasgow Coma Scale (see Chapter 12.2).

Dangerous Diagnosis 1
Diagnosis: Meningitis/encephalitis

Examination Findings
1. **Bulging fontanelle.** In children whose cranial sutures are yet to fuse, i.e. those under 12 months of age, there may be a bulging fontanelle
2. **Meningism.** Meningism causes restriction of neck flexion: a child who can put their chin on their chest is not meningitic. Reduction in neck movement is not a reliable sign in babies; look for irritability (a high-pitched or moaning, inconsolable cry) instead
3. **Photophobia.** If the child is truly photophobic, they will probably either keep their eyes closed or ask for the lights to be turned off
4. **Altered mental status.** This includes confusion, delirium, drowsiness and impaired consciousness
5. **Appears systemically unwell.** Children with infective meningitis nearly always appear systemically unwell and may have signs consistent with sepsis. The exception is tuberculous meningitis, which can be more insidious
6. **Non-blanching purpuric rash.** Meningococcal septicaemia may lead to disseminated intravascular coagulation (DIC), causing a purpuric rash (normally in the setting of circulatory collapse). Absence of a rash does not rule out meningitis
7. **Herpetic skin lesions.** Assess for any herpetic lesions – groups of vesicular lesions on an erythematous base

Figure 8.1.4 Detecting meningism on clinical examination: Kernig's sign (inability to passively extend knee with hip in 90° flexion) and Brudzinski's sign (passive neck flexion leads to flexion of knees and hips).

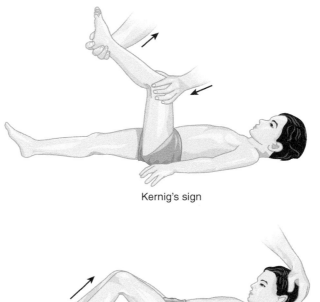

Kernig's sign

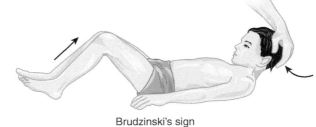

Brudzinski's sign

Dangerous Diagnosis 2
Diagnosis: Space-occupying lesion

Examination Findings
1. **Papilloedema.** Papilloedema is a strong indicator of raised ICP, but paediatric fundoscopy is challenging. Always consider referring to an ophthalmologist for review
2. **Abducens (6th) nerve palsy.** The abducens nerve emerges from the brainstem. High ICP may stretch it along the bony clivus and cause a 6th nerve palsy. Since this is an effect of generalised raised ICP, it is called a 'false localising sign'
3. **Focal neurological signs.** The majority of paediatric brain tumours involve the posterior fossa (brainstem and cerebellum) so always check for cerebellar signs. Other focal neurological deficits, though rarer, are also significant

Figure 8.1.5 Papilloedema (right) compared with a normal optic disc (left).

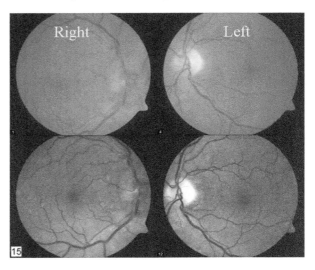

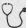

Box 8.1.8   Clinical Signs of Cerebellar Dysfunction, Using the Acronym DANISH

D – Dysdiadochokinesia, dysmetria
A – Ataxia (broad-based, unsteady gait; wobbly when standing still, with feet together)
N – Nystagmus
I – Intention tremor (check for this and past-pointing with the finger-nose test)
S – Slurred/staccato speech
H – Hypotonia (not always easy to detect)

Dangerous Diagnosis 3

Diagnosis: Cerebral venous sinus thrombosis

Examination Findings

1. **Papilloedema.** Always consider referring to an ophthalmologist for review
2. **Focal neurological signs.** The 3rd, 4th, 5th and 6th nerves all pass through the cavernous sinus, so their function may be impaired by a cavernous sinus thrombus – causing a partial or complete ophthalmoplegia. With thrombi in other locations, limb weakness, facial droop or aphasia can sometimes develop

Dangerous Diagnosis 4

Diagnosis: Intracranial haemorrhage

Examination Findings

1. **Signs of severely elevated ICP.** With this diagnosis, you may not have time to look for papilloedema. Be aware of Cushing's triad
2. **Focal neurological deficits.** Focal deficit can occur due to mass effect from the bleed, or secondary ischaemia. Look for focal limb or facial weakness and check plantar reflexes

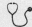

Box 8.1.9   Cushing's Triad: Late Signs of Raised Intracranial Pressure

• Hypertension
• Bradycardia
• Irregular respiration

Common Diagnosis 1

Diagnosis: Idiopathic intracranial hypertension

Examination Findings

1. **Papilloedema.** As above – ask an ophthalmologist if unable to visualise the optic disc
2. **Abducens (6th) nerve palsy.** The abducens nerve emerges from the brainstem. High ICP may stretch it along the bony clivus and cause a 6th nerve palsy. Since this is an effect of generalised raised ICP, it is called a 'false localising sign'. Its absence does not rule this diagnosis out
3. **Is the child overweight with a high Body Mass Index (BMI)?** While being overweight is a risk factor, a normal body mass does not rule this diagnosis out

Common Diagnosis 2

Diagnosis: Tension-type headache

Examination Findings

1. **Scalp tenderness.** The scalp may be sore and tender, as may the muscles of the neck and trapezius
2. **The rest of the examination is likely to be normal.** A full general and neurological examination will be reassuringly normal

Common Diagnosis 3
Diagnosis: Migraine

Examination Findings
1. **Pallor.** During an attack, children tend to look pale and miserable
2. **Occasionally unilateral neurological deficits.** A small minority of migraines present with auras that, rather than visual disturbances, involve unilateral weakness or aphasia. In these cases, neuroimaging might be required to rule out other disorders before the diagnosis of migraine can be confirmed

Common Diagnosis 4
Diagnosis: Rhinosinusitis

Examination Findings
1. **Facial tenderness.** Local tenderness over the sinuses is highly suggestive of sinusitis
2. **Nasal discharge.** Greenish or purulent nasal discharge is typical
3. **Halitosis.** Likely to be present in chronic sinusitis

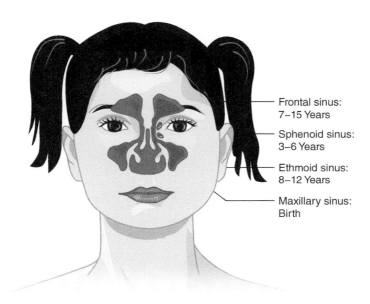

Frontal sinus:
7–15 Years

Sphenoid sinus:
3–6 Years

Ethmoid sinus:
8–12 Years

Maxillary sinus:
Birth

Figure 8.1.6 Position of the sinuses with approximate age at pneumatisation.

Common Diagnosis 5
Diagnosis: Refractive error

Examination Findings
1. **Check visual acuity.** Conduct a preliminary screening check, either using a Snellen chart, or recognition of small pictures in younger children. If you suspect an eye disorder, refer the child on to an optometrist and/or ophthalmologist
2. **Check eye movements.** Although a chronic squint can cause headaches in itself, a new paralytic squint indicates a new focal cranial nerve deficit, suggestive of potential serious underlying pathology
3. **Perform fundoscopy.** Papilloedema can present with visual disturbances. Once again, consider asking an ophthalmologist to assess if the optic disc is not clearly visualised

8.1.7 KEY INVESTIGATIONS

Not all children will require invasive investigations; often diagnoses are made on clinical evidence from history and examination. Consider carefully which investigations are required for which patient.

Bedside

Table 8.1.1 Bedside tests of use in children presenting with headache

Test	When to perform	Potential result
Blood pressure	• Suspected raised ICP	• Hypertension could be due to raised ICP, but is a late sign and only occurs with severely elevated ICP
Blood gas (capillary or venous)	• If systemically unwell	• ↓ pH, ↓ HCO$_3$, ↑ lactate indicate metabolic acidosis, suggestive of circulatory compromise • ↑/↓ Glucose may occur in sepsis

HCO$_3$, bicarbonate; ICP, intracranial pressure

Blood Tests

Blood tests do not form part of the routine assessment of headache unless dangerous diagnoses are suspected.

Table 8.1.2 Blood tests of use in children presenting with headache

Test	When to perform	Potential result
FBC	• If systemically unwell • Normal platelet count should be confirmed before performing a lumbar puncture in an *unwell* child (not routinely necessary in a well child)	• ↑ WCC, ↑ neutrophils: bacterial infection • ↓ Platelets: DIC in meningitis/sepsis • ↓ Hb: in intracranial haemorrhage, may be falsely reassuring in acute haemorrhage • Pancytopenia: malignancy with bone marrow involvement
CRP	• If systemically unwell	• Significant ↑ in bacterial infections
U&E	• If systemically unwell	• ↓ Na: meningitis associated with syndrome of inappropriate ADH secretion
Clotting screen + fibrinogen	• If systemically unwell • Normal coagulation should be confirmed before lumbar puncture in an *unwell* child (not routinely necessary in a well child)	• ↑ PT, ↑ APTT: severely septic children may have deranged clotting, varying from mild coagulopathy to fulminant DIC • ↓ Fibrinogen: consumption in DIC
Meningococcal PCR	• Suspected meningitis • More sensitive than blood culture in identifying meningococcal infection	• Most labs will not routinely test for bacteria other than *Neisseria meningitidis*.
Blood culture	• If systemically unwell	• Positive culture confirms bacterial infection • Sensitivities guide antibiotic choice

ADH, antidiuretic hormone; APTT, activated partial thromboplastin time; CRP, C-reactive protein; DIC, disseminated intravascular coagulation; FBC, full blood count; Hb, haemoglobin; Na, sodium; PCR, polymerase chain reaction; PT, prothrombin time; U&E, urea and electrolytes; WCC, white cell count

Imaging

Table 8.1.3 Imaging modalities of use in children presenting with headache

Test	When to perform	Potential result
CT head	• Suspected meningitis, as a preliminary to lumbar puncture • Rapidly progressing neurological deficit or reduced level of consciousness, for rapid evaluation	• CT is good at identifying hydrocephalus, acute intracranial bleeding, some space-occupying lesions • Can be normal: meningitis, some space-occupying lesions without hydrocephalus, CVST, IIH
CT angiography	• Suspected intracranial haemorrhage	• Can help identify where the bleeding point is and guide surgical intervention
CT venography	• Suspected CVST where MRI is unavailable or impractical	• Can diagnose CVST

Table 8.1.3 (Continued)

Test	When to perform	Potential result
MRI head	• Preferred modality in most settings, if time allows	• Accurate assessment of brain parenchyma including tumours, abscesses or bleeds
MRI with contrast	• Suspected space-occupying lesion	• Improved accuracy in identifying brain tumours
MR angiography	• Usually used in subacute settings, for example to follow up after a subarachnoid haemorrhage	• Can identify aneurysms, arteriovenous malformations, vasculopathies and arterial thrombi
MR venography	• Suspected CVST	• Can reliably rule CVST in or out • Remember that in some cases CVST is associated with subdural empyema, which may require draining

Note: MRA and MRV do *not* necessarily require contrast, whereas CTA/CTV always do
CT, computed tomography; CVST, cerebral venous sinus thrombosis; IIH, idiopathic intracranial hypertension; MRI, magnetic resonance imaging

Special

Table 8.1.4 Cerebrospinal fluid (lumbar puncture) tests of use in children presenting with headache

Test	When to perform	Potential result
CSF MC&S	• Suspected meningitis • Cell count helps diagnose meningitis and distinguish bacterial and viral cases • NB: Xanthochromia testing is not routinely used to diagnose subarachnoid haemorrhage in children	• Occasionally, organisms visible on Gram staining • Bacterial culture takes up to 48 hours; positive result confirms infection and guides antibiotic choice • White cell count is raised (>20 × 10^6/L in neonates, or >5 × 10^6/L in older infants and children) in meningitis • Typically, polymorphs predominate in bacterial meningitis and lymphocytes in viral meningitis • If the sample is heavily blood-stained, white cell count is unreliable • CSF PCR for meningococcus and pneumococcus may also be available
CSF viral PCR	• Suspected meningitis/encephalitis • Confirming viral meningitis can rationalise antimicrobial choice	• Panels vary between different laboratories: HSV1 and 2 are always included, and most panels include varicella zoster virus, parechovirus and enterovirus
CSF glucose (paired with blood glucose)	• Suspected meningitis	• In bacterial (but not viral) meningitis, CSF glucose is often reduced: <40% of the blood glucose is abnormal
CSF protein	Suspected: • Meningitis • IIH	• ↑ In healthy newborns • ↑ In bacterial, fungal and mycobacterial meningitis • Often ↓ in IIH • Usually ↑ in CVST (if LP done as part of general work-up)
CSF acid-fast bacilli staining and mycobacterial culture	• Suspected mycobacterial meningitis	• If acid-fast bacilli are not identified on initial staining, culture may take several weeks
CSF manometry	• Suspected IIH (after excluding a space-occupying lesion)	• ↑ (>20 cmH_2O) in IIH • Usually ↑ in CVST

CSF, cerebrospinal fluid; CVST, cerebral venous sinus thrombosis; HSV, herpes simplex virus; IIH, idiopathic intracranial hypertension; LP, lumbar puncture; MC&S, microscopy, culture and sensitivity; PCR, polymerase chain reaction

---

Box 8.1.10 Contraindications to Lumbar Puncture

• Child instability, e.g. shock, respiratory compromise or immediately after a convulsion
• Abnormal coagulation suspected, or platelets <100 x 10^9/L
• Extensive or spreading purpuric rash
• Infection of the tissue overlying the lumbar puncture site

• Fluctuating or impaired consciousness (Glasgow Coma Score <9, or 3 points below child's baseline)
• Signs of raised intracranial pressure: relative hypertension and bradycardia, papilloedema, abnormal posturing, abnormal 'doll's eye' movements*
• Pupils unequal, dilated or poorly responsive*
• Focal neurological signs*

*These are relative contraindications. Once obstructive hydrocephalus has been excluded, lumbar puncture in the presence of raised intracranial pressure can be sight-saving. Always discuss with a consultant (or most senior clinician available) first

8.1.8 KEY MANAGEMENT PRINCIPLES

Diagnosis-specific management strategies are outlined here. It is expected that an 'ABCDE' approach to assessment and management is always undertaken (see Chapter 12.1, The A to E Assessment)

Dangerous Diagnosis 1
Diagnosis: Meningitis/encephalitis

Management Principles
1. **Urgent broad-spectrum antibiotics.** In the community setting, intramuscular benzylpenicillin should be given. In hospital a third-generation cephalosporin is used, usually high-dose intravenous (IV) ceftriaxone. Cefotaxime is often used in children <6 weeks old due to the risk of jaundice with ceftriaxone (see Chapter 13.1, Sepsis Management)
2. **Consider adjuvant antimicrobials:**
   - **Amoxicillin:** to cover for *Listeria monocytogenes* in children <3 months of age
   - **Anti-staphylococcal antibiotics:** if intracerebral shunts are in situ
   - **Aciclovir:** if a herpes simplex meningoencephalitis is suspected
   - **Vancomycin:** in those who have recently travelled outside the UK or with prolonged, multiple exposure to antibiotics
3. **Management of raised ICP.** See Chapter 13.5, Raised Intracranial Pressure Management
4. **Dexamethasone.** In children over 3 months of age, dexamethasone is recommended if any of the following cerebrospinal fluid (CSF) findings are present:
   - Frankly purulent CSF
   - CSF white cell count (WCC) >1000/μL
   - Protein concentration >1 g/L in the context of raised CSF WCC
   - Bacteria present on Gram stain

Dexamethasone should be given at the time of, or as soon as possible after, the first dose of antibiotics. This can reduce the risk of hearing impairment and other long-term neurological damage
5. **Monitor for deterioration.** Very close monitoring for signs of deterioration is required, with respiration, pulse, blood pressure, oxygen saturations and Glasgow Coma Scale score. Rapid deterioration is possible, regardless of initial severity
6. **Audiology follow-up.** All patients with confirmed bacterial meningitis should undergo audiology follow-up due to the risk of associated sensorineural deafness
7. **Alert public health authorities.** Confirmed bacterial meningitis is a public health concern and the appropriate authorities should be informed. Contact tracing might be required with prophylactic antibiotics provided to high-risk contacts

Dangerous Diagnosis 2
Diagnosis: Space-occupying lesion

Management Principles
1. **Urgent neurosurgical specialist input.** Time-critical transfer to a neurosurgical unit may need to be arranged. Hydrocephalus/raised ICP will require emergency procedures such as ventriculostomy/external ventricular drain and shunt placement
2. **Manage raised ICP.** Medical treatment of raised ICP may be required prior to surgical management. Involvement of intensive care colleagues is essential, as children may require intubation and ventilation. See Chapter 13.5, Raised Intracranial Pressure Management
3. **Tertiary oncology.** Management of paediatric brain tumours is complex and often involves surgery, radiotherapy (conventional or proton beam) and chemotherapy. Many children have lasting impairments of physical or cognitive ability, behaviour, hearing or vision, and will need long-term multidisciplinary support

Dangerous Diagnosis 3
Diagnosis: Cerebral venous sinus thrombosis

Management Principles
1. **Anticoagulation.** Unless there is a contraindication such as an associated intracranial haemorrhage, anticoagulation with treatment-dose low molecular weight heparin should be commenced
2. **Antibiotics.** CVST in children may be triggered by sinus or ear infections complicated by subdural empyema. If this is the case, treat with appropriate broad-spectrum IV antibiotics and consider surgical drainage
3. **Manage complications.** Complications can include seizures, which should be managed with anticonvulsant medication, and raised ICP, which may need to be treated with acetazolamide and/or therapeutic lumbar puncture. See Chapter 13.5, Raised Intracranial Pressure Management

Dangerous Diagnosis 4

Diagnosis: Intracranial haemorrhage

Management Principles

1. **Urgent neurosurgical review.** Unless you are located in a neurosurgical centre, this is likely to be a time-critical transfer as per your local policy
2. **Acute management of raised ICP.** Seizures are also common and anticonvulsant medication may be required, as advised by tertiary neurology specialists. See Chapter 13.5, Raised Intracranial Pressure Management
3. **Further management.** Surgical management, for example craniectomy, surgical clipping or endovascular coiling, might be warranted

Common Diagnosis 1

Diagnosis: Idiopathic intracranial hypertension

Management Principles

1. **Exclude an SOL first.** It is not safe to perform a lumbar puncture until obstructive hydrocephalus has been ruled out (by scanning), as this could lead to coning and death
2. **Therapeutic lumbar puncture (LP).** This is usually the quickest way to reduce the pressure and therefore protect the child's vision. This may need to be done in a graduated manner with more than one LP, depending on how high the initial opening pressure is
3. **Consider acetazolamide and/or surgical intervention.** The child's progress can be monitored by their symptoms (especially visual acuity and headache), but most children will need further treatment

---

Box 8.1.11   Further Management Options for Idiopathic Intracranial Hypertension (IIH)

- Serial therapeutic lumbar punctures: children do not always tolerate this well
- Acetazolamide: this carbonic anhydrase inhibitor reduces the production of cerebrospinal fluid. Side effects include nausea, electrolyte disturbances and metabolic acidosis

- Some children will require a neurosurgical shunt (usually ventriculoperitoneal or lumboperitoneal)
- For many children, the safest and most effective way to manage IIH is by weight loss, but other measures may be required in the meantime

---

Box 8.1.12   Cerebrospinal Fluid (CSF) Manometry: How to Do It

- Standard manometers may only go up to 40 cmH$_2$O: open two in case the pressure is very high
- Make sure you have worked out how to fit the manometer together, and which end attaches to the spinal needle, before going near the child
- The child should be lying on their side. If manometry is performed upright, pressures will be higher
- If the child is under general anaesthesia, note the value of the end-tidal carbon dioxide (CO$_2$). Raised CO$_2$ raises the intracranial pressure

- Once the needle is in place, extend the child's hips enough that there is no pressure on the abdomen. Not doing this could also lead to a falsely high reading
- Check opening pressure first, before any other tests
- It is usually easiest to leave the manometer in place while you collect your samples
- If reducing the pressure by draining CSF, only reduce it down to 20 cmH$_2$O, no lower. If the opening pressure is over 40, then only reduce it by half (e.g. for an opening pressure of 60 cmH$_2$O, reduce to 30 cmH$_2$O)

Common Diagnosis 2

Diagnosis: Tension-type headache

Management Principles

1. **Reassurance.** Tension headaches are painful and annoying, but not dangerous. Sometimes, all the child and their family really need is reassurance that they do not have a brain tumour
2. **Analgesia.** Offer simple painkillers such as paracetamol or ibuprofen. Advise that these should not be used too frequently, to avoid development of medication overuse headache. It is never advisable to take painkillers to prevent headaches, and opioids should not be prescribed

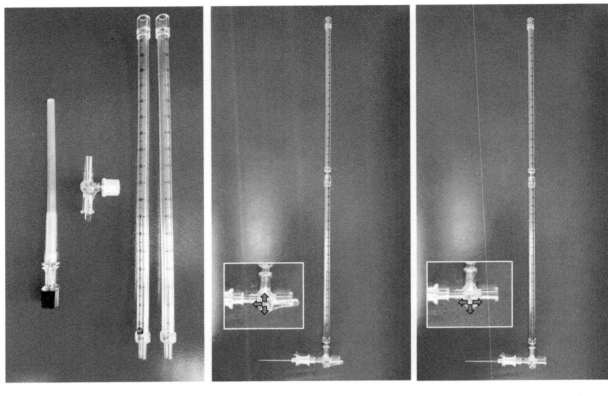

Figure 8.1.7 Cerebrospinal fluid (CSF) manometry for use in idiopathic intracranial hypertension. (A) Equipment required includes lumbar puncture needle, three-way tap and CSF manometer. (B) Equipment assembled, with three-way tap positioned to allow CSF pressure measurement. (C) Equipment assembled, with three-way tap positioned to allow CSF collection and drainage.

3. **Non-pharmacological measures.** Asking the family to keep a headache diary may help to identify patterns or triggers, which can then be addressed. Staying well hydrated, getting plenty of sleep and, if possible, reducing stress will all be helpful

Common Diagnosis 3
Diagnosis: Migraine

Management Principles
1. **Analgesia.** For many children, pain can be adequately controlled by simple analgesia – paracetamol and/or ibuprofen – and if required anti-emetics. Taking analgesia early is more effective at aborting the headache. If oral medications are not tolerated due to vomiting, buccal anti-emetics such as prochlorperazine may be used for older children
2. **Consider triptans.** Triptans are specific anti-migraine agents. Most are not licensed in young children, but in adolescents sumatriptan or zolmitriptan, orally or as a nasal spray, can be very helpful
3. **Consider prevention.** Frequent migraines impact severely on a child's school attendance and quality of life

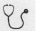

Box 8.1.13   Measures for Prevention of Migraine

- Identify triggers – suggest the patient keeps a headache diary. Some older girls may notice that migraines coincide with their menstrual cycle
- Avoid triggers – commonly the 5Cs (caffeine, chocolate, cheese, citrus, colourings), strawberries and Marmite. Some children are sensitive to strong smells and exposure to strong sunlight

- Ensure adequate sleep and discuss sleep hygiene
- Optimise hydration and avoid skipping meals
- Where these measures are inadequate, a trial of prophylactic medication can be given: either pizotifen, propranolol or topiramate as first line

Common Diagnosis 4
Diagnosis: Rhinosinusitis

Management Principles
1. **Analgesia.** Simple analgesia such as paracetamol and/or ibuprofen will usually be adequate
2. **Consider intranasal corticosteroids.** Steroids delivered as a nasal spray, for up to 2 weeks, may help unblock the nose. They are only recommended in children over 12
3. **Antibiotics are not usually required.** Sinusitis is usually caused by viruses and will not be helped by antibiotics. However, if there is suspicion that complications such as meningitis, involvement of the orbit or Pott's puffy tumour (osteomyelitis of the frontal bone) are developing, then the child needs urgent IV antibiotics

Common Diagnosis 5
Diagnosis: Refractive error

Management Principle
1. **Refer to optometry.** Only quite a basic assessment of visual acuity is possible in primary care, paediatric clinic or A&E. For further testing and appropriate glasses, the child should see an optometrist

8.2 Suspected Seizures

Geetha Anand

Department of Paediatrics, John Radcliffe Hospital, Oxford University Hospitals NHS Foundation Trust, Oxford, UK

CONTENTS

8.2.1 CHAPTER AT A GLANCE

> **Box 8.2.1   Chapter at a Glance**
>
> - The differential diagnoses are challenging when a child presents with a suspected seizure
> - The first challenge is differentiating a true seizure from an alternative event, such as syncope or another type of 'funny turn'
> - A careful history is the key to diagnosis. Keeping an open mind is important if there is uncertainty
>
> - Obtaining a video record of an event also helps in making a correct diagnosis
> - This chapter will explore both the differentials for a seizure as well as diagnoses that are underlying causes of seizures
> - Any child that is experiencing a prolonged seizure, or recurrent seizures in keeping with status epilepticus, should be promptly treated (see Chapter 13.4, *Prolonged Seizure Management*)

8.2.2 DEFINITION

- A seizure is a transient clinical event due to abnormal excessive or synchronous neuronal activity in the brain
- A seizure may also be referred to as an 'epileptic' seizure. This does not mean the child has epilepsy, which is a disease involving increased predisposition to recurrent epileptic seizures

Clinical Guide to Paediatrics, First Edition. Edited by Rachel Varughese and Anna Mathew. Series Editor: Christian Fielder Camm.
© 2022 John Wiley & Sons Ltd. Published 2022 by John Wiley & Sons Ltd.
Companion website: www.wiley.com/go/varughese/paediatrics

8.2.3 DIAGNOSTIC ALGORITHM

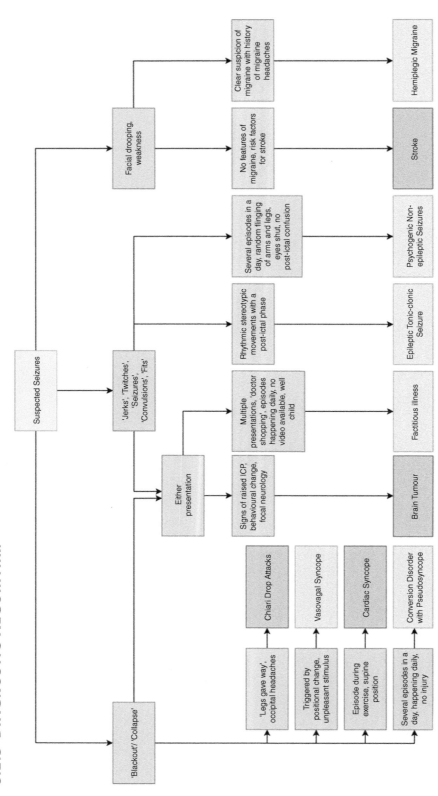

Figure 8.2.1 Diagnostic algorithm for the presentation of suspected seizures.

8.2.4 DIFFERENTIALS LIST

Dangerous Diagnoses

1. Cardiac Syncope
- Cardiac syncope is transient loss of consciousness due to decreased cerebral blood flow as a result of a sudden decrease in cardiac output secondary to an intrinsic cardiac issue
- This could be as a result of left or right ventricular outflow tract obstruction and/or arrhythmia
- It is a rare cause of syncope in children, but one that needs prompt specialist input
- Cardiac syncope is also discussed in more detail in Chapter 2.3, *Syncope*

2. Brain Tumour
- Funny turns that are as a result of an underlying brain tumour can take the form of epileptic seizures, posturing from raised intracranial pressure (ICP) or sometimes loss of consciousness
- Epileptic seizures can be focal, which may or may not progress to bilateral convulsive seizures
- Sudden obstruction to cerebrospinal fluid (CSF) flow can also present with loss of consciousness. This can happen with colloid cysts of the third ventricle
- There are usually other associated signs and symptoms attributable to the tumour other than just the 'funny turn' (e.g. focal neurology, signs of raised ICP), but the younger the child, the more non-specific (and possibly overlooked) are the associated symptoms

3. Stroke
- Strokes can cause epileptic seizures or other funny turns associated with raised ICP or focal neurological deficit
- The three main types of stroke include arterial ischaemic strokes (AIS), cerebral venous sinus thrombosis (CVST) and haemorrhagic stroke
- Can affect a child at any age, including infancy
- There are several risk factors depending on the background medical history, the age of the child and the presence of infection
- Signs and symptoms can be difficult to recognise, and a high index of suspicion is required. Can be mistaken for Todd's paresis, which is transient abnormal focal neurology following a seizure

4. Chiari Drop Attacks
- A Chiari malformation is characterised by downward displacement of brain tissue through the foramen magnum into the upper cervical canal, which may cause impaired CSF flow
- There are four types. Type 1, involving herniation of the cerebellar tonsils, is the most common and may be accompanied by syringomyelia. It can only be diagnosed on neuroimaging
- Very rarely, syncope may be the primary presenting symptom, a phenomenon termed 'Chiari drop attack'
- The precise mechanism is not known. It has been postulated that it is secondary to dysautonomia caused by hindbrain compression

Figure 8.2.2 Magnetic resonance image showing type 1 Chiari malformation, with herniation of cerebellar tonsils through the foramen magnum.

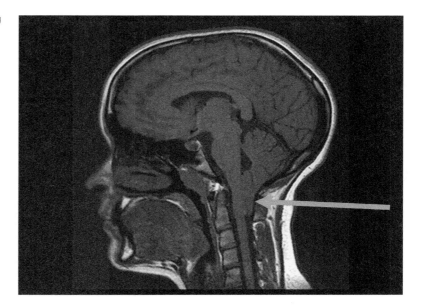

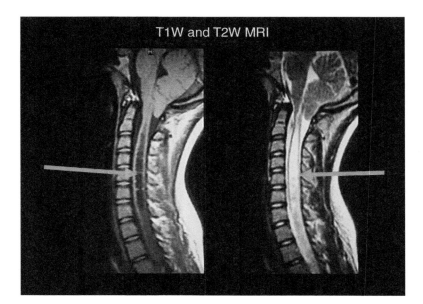

Figure 8.2.3 Magnetic resonance image of Chiari malformation with syringomyelia. Syringomyelia involves a cystic cavity within the spinal cord 'syrinx', which may or may not communicate with the CSF pathways. Communicating syringomyelia is frequently associated with type 1 Chiari malformations.

Common Diagnoses
1. Epileptic Seizures
- These arise as a result of hypersynchronous electrical activity of the neurons of the brain
- They can be broadly classified as focal or generalised based on the point of origin of the seizure
- Common seizure types include tonic, clonic, tonic–clonic, atonic, myoclonic, absences and focal seizures
- Tonic–clonic seizures, especially those that last longer than 5 minutes, are the most common seizure to present to the emergency department
- Underlying aetiology is often idiopathic, but causes can include genetic, structural, infectious, metabolic and immune disorders

Box 8.2.2 Classification of Seizures in Childhood

Type of seizure	Type of epilepsy	Description
Generalised seizures	Tonic–clonic	• Sudden-onset, rhythmical tonic–clonic jerking of all limbs • Breathing may be affected • Variable duration • May/may not have tongue biting or urine incontinence • Post-ictal phase
	Tonic	• Sudden-onset episodes of increased tone of all limbs, leading to posturing • Variable duration
	Clonic	• Sudden-onset episodes of generalised rhythmical jerking of all limbs • Variable duration
	Atonic	• Sudden paroxysmal loss of postural tone associated with falls or head drops
	Myoclonic	• Sudden brief, isolated jerking of limbs • May happen in clusters
	Absence	• Sudden onset and offset • Brief interruption of consciousness associated with arrest in motor activity • Automatisms involving eye, mouth or limb may be observed

Box 8.2.2   (Continued)

Type of seizure	Type of epilepsy	Description
Focal seizures	Frontal	• Motor disturbance associated with fearful behaviour at times
	Temporal	• Most common form of focal epilepsy • Auras, feelings of fear and panic, nausea, auditory, visual, or olfactory hallucinations, associated with variable motor movements • Can last minutes
	Occipital	• Motor movements of the eyes and head • Visual disturbance with possible headache and vomiting
	Focal with secondary generalisation	• Motor disturbance of one part of the body, spreading to involve all limbs
Combined generalised and focal seizures		• Frequently associated with an epilepsy syndrome, e.g. Dravet, Lennox Gastaut
Unknown	Unknown	• Unable to determine whether the seizure is generalised or focal, even after investigation

2. Psychogenic Non-epileptic Seizures (PNES)

- These are generally caused by emotional or mental stress, considered to be part of the spectrum of conversion disorders. The term pseudo-seizures should no longer be used
- They resemble epileptic seizures outwardly, but are not as a result of hypersynchronous electrical discharges from the neurons of the brain
- There are different types, including dissociative seizures, panic attacks and factitious seizures
- Another term used for this group of seizures is non-epileptic attack disorder (NEAD)

3. Vasovagal Syncope

- This is the most common form of syncope and it is mediated by the vasovagal reflex
- May occur with sudden change in posture or with exposure to emotional stress or pain
- Triggering the vasovagal reflex leads to hypotension and/or bradycardia
- Loss of consciousness is often preceded by pallor, blurred vision, dizziness, sweating, nausea and feeling warm
- Frequently followed by fatigue
- Vasovagal syncope is covered in detail in Chapter 2.3, *Syncope*, and will not be discussed further in this chapter

Box 8.2.3   Jerking Movements with Vasovagal Syncope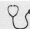

- It is very important to note that involuntary myoclonic jerking movements can commonly occur with vasovagal syncope
- Sometimes these can be very prominent
- It is important to understand that parents and caregivers may interpret these movements as seizures and reassurance is often necessary

Diagnoses to Consider
1. Psychogenic Pseudosyncope (PPS)

- PPS is considered to be part of the spectrum of conversion disorders
- In this presentation, there is the appearance of loss of consciousness in the absence of true loss of consciousness
- Many children experience preceding symptoms of light-headedness, shortness of breath and tingling
- Affected individuals generally do not sustain injury and can recall events from during the episode

When to consider: in children having numerous episodes a day of sudden transient slumping to the ground, which can last minutes to hours

2. Fabricated or Induced Illness (FII)

- This is a rare safeguarding issue in which a parent (usually the mother) fabricates illness in their child. One of the commonest false presenting symptoms is 'seizure'
- Generally, these events are only witnessed by the perpetrator (often a parent)
- There may be repeated attendances with unusual symptoms in a 'well child'
- Parents will frequently seek advice from multiple professionals and hospitals, remaining unconvinced and dissatisfied by the advice given

When to consider: in children with multiple hospital presentations with symptoms that do not 'add up'

3. Hemiplegic Migraine

- This can be confused with stroke. Patients experience transient hemiplegia. The migraine headache typically follows the weakness, but can precede it or even be absent
- There are two types of hemiplegic migraine: familial and sporadic
- Migraines are discussed in detail in Chapters 8.1, *Headache* and 8.3, *Acute Hemiparesis*

When to consider: in children with personal or family history of migraines

8.2.5 KEY HISTORY FEATURES

History taking is essential in formulating a likely diagnosis. The key questions that must be answered are:
- Was the concerning event truly a seizure?
- What type of seizure was it?
- Is there a likely cause for the seizure?
- If the concerning event was not a seizure, what is the alternative diagnosis?

General Questions
- Is there a history of previous seizures? Were these febrile seizures or otherwise unprovoked? How many and how often have previous seizures occurred?
- Is there a family history of seizures?
- Take a full birth, medical, developmental and medication history

Further questions can be divided into 'before', 'during' and 'after'. Both the child and witnesses should be asked for their recollection of events.

Before
- Has the child been well, or is there an intercurrent febrile illness or other new/evolving symptoms?
- What was the child doing before the event?
- Was the child asleep or awake prior to the event?
- Were they sleep deprived?
- Was there any warning ('aura') before the event? If so, what was it?
- Were there any observed triggers for the event?

During
- How long did the event last?
- Were there any observed abnormal body movements?
- Was consciousness preserved or impaired?
- What did the child look like during the event? Were there any changes in skin colour?
- Was there any loss of continence?

After
- What was the behaviour like following the event?
- How long after the event ceased did it take for return to normal behaviour?
- Does the child have memory of the event?

Dangerous Diagnosis 1

Diagnosis: Cardiac syncope

Questions

1. **What was the patient doing just before the syncope?** If syncope happens in the standing position or during exercise (i.e. in a state of increased cardiac output), there is a greater possibility of its being of cardiac origin
2. **Does the patient have known cardiac disease?** Congenital or acquired heart disease that causes right or left outflow tract obstruction, or an increased risk of arrhythmias, could be the underlying cause, e.g. severe aortic stenosis, hypertrophic cardiomyopathy
3. **Is there a family history?** There is often a family history of cardiac structural/conduction abnormalities, sudden death or early use of pacemakers
4. **Was there a prodrome?** Very frequently there is only a very brief prodrome with palpitations or no prodrome at all

Dangerous Diagnosis 2

Diagnosis: Brain tumour

Questions

1. **If the patient presented with seizures, ascertain carefully how the seizures started.** Focal-onset seizures with or without progression to bilateral convulsive seizures may indicate an underlying space-occupying lesion. However, focal epilepsy can also occur independently of an underlying structural lesion

2. **If the patient has presented with syncope, ask for specific triggers.** Was the patient leaning forward just prior to the syncope? 'Ball-valve' obstruction of the foramen of Munro by third ventricle cysts/tumours can cause acute hydrocephalus and loss of consciousness. Triggering the syncope in such instances is positional

3. **Are there any symptoms of raised intracranial pressure?** Ask about headaches (especially nocturnal and early morning), vomiting, clumsiness and deterioration in skills. In a young child, the signs and symptoms can be non-specific such as irritability (can manifest as personality change), sleep disturbance and weight loss

Dangerous Diagnosis 3
Diagnosis: Stroke

Questions
1. **Was any focal weakness noticed?** The main symptoms of stroke can be remembered using the well-advocated acronym FAST: Face–Arms–Speech–Time. Focal weakness is more likely to be seen in older children
2. **How old is the child and how sudden was the presentation?** The younger the child, the more non-specific their symptoms, and in many instances they may present like sepsis, with lethargy, apnoea, behavioural change and irritability. Older children are more likely to present with sudden-onset severe headache, vomiting, altered conscious levels, focal seizures and focal neurological deficits. Other possible symptoms include new-onset ataxia, dizziness and sudden-onset neck pain or neck stiffness
3. **Are there any risk factors?** Has there been a preceding infection, especially varicella, underlying congenital heart disease, family history etc.? Risk factors vary depending on the specific type of stroke

Box 8.2.4   Risk Factors Associated with Stroke

System	Details
Cardiac disease	Cardiac repair/catheterisation, cyanotic heart disease, cardiomyopathies, prosthetic valves, rheumatic heart disease
Haematologic	Sickle cell disease, prothrombotic disorders, protein C and S deficiency, factor 7 and 8 deficiency, iron-deficiency anaemia
Infection	Systemic: varicella, human immunodeficiency virus (HIV), mycoplasma, chlamydia, tuberculosis (TB)
	Head and neck: bacterial and viral meningitis/encephalitis, mastoiditis, periorbital cellulitis
Vascular	Arteriovenous malformations, Sturge Weber disease, neurofibromatosis, von Hippel–Lindau syndrome, Moyamoya
Syndromic and metabolic disease	Marfan syndrome, tuberous sclerosis, homocystinuria, folic acid and vitamin B_{12} deficiency
Vasculitis	Kawasaki, Henoch–Schönlein purpura, polyarteritis nodosa, systemic lupus erythematosus, juvenile rheumatoid arthritis, inflammatory bowel disease, sarcoidosis, Sjögren syndrome, Behçet disease
Oncology	Complication of intracranial tumour: leukaemia, lymphoma
Trauma	Traumatic arterial dissection
Drugs	Oral contraceptive pill, amphetamines, ecstasy, cocaine, glue sniffing, heroin

Box 8.2.5   FAST Acronym for Recognition of Stroke

- **Face** – the face may have dropped on one side, the person may not be able to smile, or their mouth or eye may have dropped
- **Arms** – the person may not be able to lift both arms and keep them there because of arm weakness or numbness in one arm
- **Speech** – their speech may be slurred or garbled, or the person may not be able to talk at all, despite appearing to be awake
- **Time** – it is time to dial 999 immediately if you see any of these signs or symptoms

Dangerous Diagnosis 4
Diagnosis: Chiari drop attacks

Questions
1. **Is there a history of headache?** Headaches in Chiari malformation are usually occipital headaches that are made worse by coughing, sneezing or straining (Valsalva). Often short-lived and relieved when activity stops
2. **Are there any suggestive symptoms?** Patients can be asymptomatic, but may also have a combination of symptoms, such as neck pain, tingling, numbness, weakness, poor coordination, gait disturbance, vomiting and swallowing difficulty

Common Diagnosis 1
Diagnosis: Epileptic seizure

Questions
1. **What happened first and what was the patient doing when the event happened?** It is very important to get as much detail as possible about the events leading up to the onset of the seizure in order to identify any triggers, the presence of auras or change in behaviour, and to exclude alternative diagnoses
2. **What happened next?** A detailed history about how the episode evolved is crucially important, including whether consciousness was preserved or not, whether the child displayed any signs such as head turning to one side, chewing, mouthing movements, eyelid blinking, fumbling with clothes etc. Did the child lose tone and fall to the ground?
3. **Did the seizure start on one side or were all limbs affected?** This is to establish whether there was a focal or generalised seizure, or whether there was a combination of both
4. **If there is an eye-witness, ask for a description (obtaining a video of an event is ideal).** Getting an eye-witness account describing the seizure and its duration is central to making the correct diagnosis. In epileptic seizures, additional features such as rolling of eyes, 'frothing' from the mouth, biting the tongue or inside of the cheek, and loss of bowel/ bladder control are commonly seen
5. **What happened after the event?** Was there a post-ictal phase? Not all seizures have this, but when present it can include drowsiness, confusion or unresponsiveness for a short period, often followed by sleep
6. **Is there an intercurrent febrile infection?** Children between 6 months and 5 years are at risk of febrile convulsions, in association with a rapid rise in temperature during an intercurrent illness

---

Box 8.2.6   Preservation of Consciousness in Epileptic Seizures

Generalised seizures
- Awareness is always impaired with loss of consciousness
- Any seizure type may present in isolation, or can be associated with other seizure types

- The presence of several seizure types in the same patient can often lead to the diagnosis of an epilepsy syndrome, especially when combined with electroencephalogram and neuroimaging features

Focal seizures
- Awareness may or may not be impaired: 'focal-aware' and 'focal-impaired awareness'
- Focal-aware seizures were previously known as simple partial seizures. Consciousness and memory are preserved

- Focal-impaired awareness seizures were previously known as complex partial seizures. Consciousness and memory are impaired, although they may be limited rather than absent

---

Common Diagnosis 2
Diagnosis: Psychogenic non-epileptic seizure

Questions
1. **Describe the episode (obtaining a video of an event is ideal).** Jerking of limbs is seen in a random fashion (as opposed to the rhythmic, synchronised tonic–clonic jerks of an epileptic fit). Pelvic movements/pelvic thrusts predominate, eyes remain shut and there is no post-ictal confusion
2. **What are the age and sex of the child?** This picture is seen more often in females and in adolescence
3. **Are there any life events that may be a trigger?** Close questioning may reveal a life event that may be a stressor and contributor to this presentation

4. How often does it happen? Could be quite frequent. There will be no serious injuries in-spite of the often dramatic presentation

8.2.6 KEY EXAMINATION FEATURES

Varying levels of consciousness may accompany some of these diagnoses, which can be assessed using the Glasgow Coma Scale (GCS; see Chapter 12.2, *Assessment of Consciousness*). Many diagnoses involve transient events, and examination may be normal in the interim.

Dangerous Diagnosis 1
Diagnosis: Cardiac syncope

Examination Findings
1. **May be normal.** Once the child has recovered from the syncopal episode, as is usually the case by the time they are brought to the Emergency Department, examination can be normal
2. **Signs of underlying cardiac disease.** Auscultate for a cardiac murmur. Look for scars that indicate previous cardiac surgery. Monitor for arrhythmias. Feel the pulse to confirm it is regular

Dangerous Diagnosis 2
Diagnosis: Brain tumour

Examination Findings
1. **Focal neurological signs.** Examine carefully for weakness and cranial nerve palsies
2. **Signs of raised ICP.** Examination findings of raised ICP may present very late. 'Red flags' include hypertension, relative bradycardia, papilloedema (may require dilatation and ophthalmology opinion) and 6th nerve palsy
3. **Gait.** The child may be generally clumsy and may display a hemiplegic or broad-based ataxic gait
4. **Weight.** Is there weight loss or excessive recent weight gain (as is the case with some tumours such as a craniopharyngioma)?
5. **Head circumference.** In an infant, it is important to measure and plot head circumference, as cranial sutures will not have fused

Dangerous Diagnosis 3
Diagnosis: Stroke

Examination Findings
1. **Focal neurological deficits.** These can sometimes be subtle. Examine carefully for cranial nerve palsies and hemiplegia
2. **Speech.** There may be dysarthria or aphasia
3. **Mental status.** The child may display agitation or confusion, which may be a change to baseline, or an indication of being post-ictal. There may be a decrease in the level of consciousness and GCS should be quantified
4. **Cardiac examination.** Look for evidence of heart murmurs that could point to congenital heart disease, which could predispose to thromboembolic events, or bleeds if on anticoagulation
5. **Non-specific signs.** In the very young, lethargy, apnoea and hypotonia may be the only signs

Dangerous Diagnosis 4
Diagnosis: Chiari malformation
1. **Examination can be normal.** Most children will have a normal examination
2. **Neurological examination.** Examine for deficits in power and sensation of the upper torso, hand and arms (as a result of possible associated syrinx). These will respect the spinal level of the syrinx. Look for scoliosis and gait disturbance
3. **Developmental delay.** In infants, the symptoms can be non-specific, such as generalised hypotonia, gross motor delay, swallowing difficulties/failure to thrive and opisthotonic posturing (state of severe hyperextension with back arching)

Common Diagnosis 1
Diagnosis: Epileptic seizure

Examination Findings
1. **Normal examination.** Examination can be normal if the patient has fully recovered
2. **Focal neurology.** Post-ictal focal neurological deficit can indicate Todd's paresis

3. **Post-ictal period.** Depending on the type of seizure, children may or may not be drowsy at initial assessment if the seizure was within the last hour
4. **Ask bystanders to mimic the event or show a video clip, if available.** Viewing a video of an event is invaluable to supplement information from history
5. **Clinical evidence of a source of infection in a child aged 6 months–5 years.** Children with febrile convulsions should be examined for a source of infection to support this diagnosis (rather than considering serious infections such as meningitis). Upper respiratory tract infections, tonsillitis, otitis media or urinary tract infections may be evident

---

Box 8.2.7   Febrile Convulsions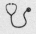

A febrile convulsion is an epileptic seizure occurring in a child aged from 6 months to 5 years, precipitated by rapidly rising fever arising from infection outside the nervous system in a child who is otherwise neurologically normal.

	Simple febrile convulsion	Complex febrile convulsion
Duration	Less than 15 minutes	More than 15 minutes
Seizure type	Generalised tonic–clonic seizures	Focal features
Post-ictal	Complete recovery within 1 hour	Incomplete recovery within 1 hour, prolonged drowsiness or transient hemiparesis (Todd's paresis)
Recurrence	No recurrence within 24 hours	Recurrence within 24 hours

- Prolonged febrile convulsions will require rescue medication
- A complex febrile seizure could indicate an alternative underlying cause, which may require further investigation

Advice for parents

- Febrile convulsions can affect 1 in 20 children
- Febrile seizures are not epilepsy and do not increase the risk of epilepsy
- There is a 30% chance of having another febrile seizure
- Antipyretics should be given regularly and early during further febrile illnesses, and remove extra clothing
- In the event of a further febrile seizure, stay with the child, seek help and place them on their side
- Children tend to grow out of febrile seizures, which usually cease after the age of 5 years

---

Common Diagnosis 2
Diagnosis: Psychogenic non-epileptic seizure

Examination Findings
1. **Examination is usually normal.** Teenage girls are most commonly affected
2. **'Affect' could reflect an underlying anxiety.** It is important to note the demeanour and general mood of the child
3. **Episodes can be provoked through suggestion.** This is quite a common finding and a useful way to witness an episode

8.2.7 KEY INVESTIGATIONS

Not all children will require invasive investigations; often diagnoses are made on clinical evidence from history and examination. Consider carefully which investigations are required for which patient.

Bedside

Table 8.2.1 Bedside tests of use in patients presenting with suspected seizures

Test	When to perform	Potential result
Blood sugar	• All children with syncope/suspected seizures	• <2.6 mmol/L: hypoglycaemia • <3: in suspected stroke, this is the treatment threshold
ECG	• All children with syncope/suspected seizures	• Brady/tachyarrhythmia, prolonged QTc, Wolff–Parkinson–White syndrome
Lying/standing BP	• All children with syncope	• A drop in systolic BP of 20 mmHg, or diastolic BP of 10 mmHg, is diagnostic of orthostatic hypotension

BP, blood pressure; ECG, electrocardiogram

Blood Tests

Table 8.2.2 Blood tests of use in patients presenting with suspected seizures

Test	When to perform	Potential result
U&E, calcium, magnesium	• All children with suspected seizures	• ↓ Ca, ↓/↑ Na, ↓ Mg: may cause seizures
FBC, CRP, blood cultures	• Prolonged febrile convulsions to investigate for sepsis	• ↑ WCC, ↑ neutrophils, ↑ CRP suggest bacterial infection • Positive blood culture confirms organism
Clotting screen, fibrinogen	• Suspected stroke	• Deranged clotting may increase risk of haemorrhagic stroke • Ischaemic stroke may cause haemostatic abnormalities
Thrombophilia screen (seek advice)	• Only in suspected venous thrombotic stroke	• Deficiency in many factors increases the risk of thrombotic strokes

Ca, calcium; CRP, C-reactive protein; FBC, full blood count; Mg, magnesium; Na, sodium; U&E, urea and electrolytes

Imaging

Table 8.2.3 Imaging modalities of use in patients presenting with suspected seizures

Test	When to perform	Potential result
CT brain/CT angiography	Suspected: • Stroke (within 1 hour of Emergency Department admission) • Brain tumour • Raised ICP of any cause	• Stroke: haemorrhage, ischaemic change, artery occlusion • Tumour: identifies mass • May identify other causes of raised ICP
MRI brain/spinal cord, MR angiography/MR venography brain	Children with: • Focal seizures • Drop attacks • Brain tumour • To further evaluate CT findings as above	• Identifies structural abnormalities: space-occupying lesions, Chiari malformation, bleeds, ischaemic change, infection, congenital malformations

CT, computed tomography; ICP, intracranial pressure; MRI, magnetic resonance imaging

Special

Table 8.2.4 Special tests of use in patients presenting with suspected seizures

Test	When to perform	Potential result
Echocardiogram	• Suspected cardiac syncope	• Structural cardiac abnormalities, e.g. outflow tract obstruction
Holter/loop recording	• Suspected cardiac syncope	• Paroxysmal arrhythmias
EEG	• Children with a clinical diagnosis of epilepsy	• Features defining specific epilepsy types and syndromes
Video telemetry	• May be needed in some difficult cases of PNES, especially when families do not accept the diagnosis	• No EEG correlates suggestive of an epileptic event identified at the time of the event

EEG, electroencephalogram; PNES, psychogenic non-epileptic seizures

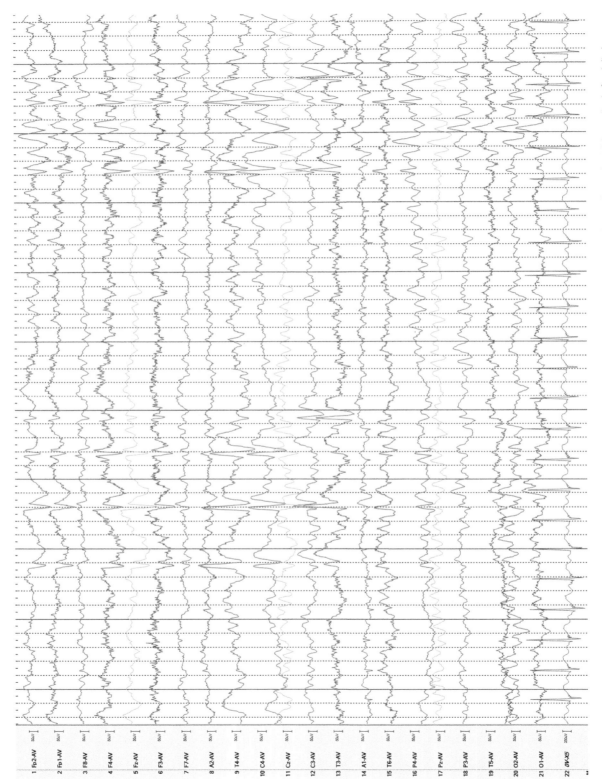

Figure 8.2.4 Electroencephalogram from a 3-year-old girl who presented with nocturnal seizures associated with facial twitching and a gurgling noise. High-amplitude focal discharges (sharp and slow waves) are seen independently over the right and left centro-temporal regions. The morphology and distribution of the discharges would be in keeping with childhood epilepsy with centro-temporal spikes.

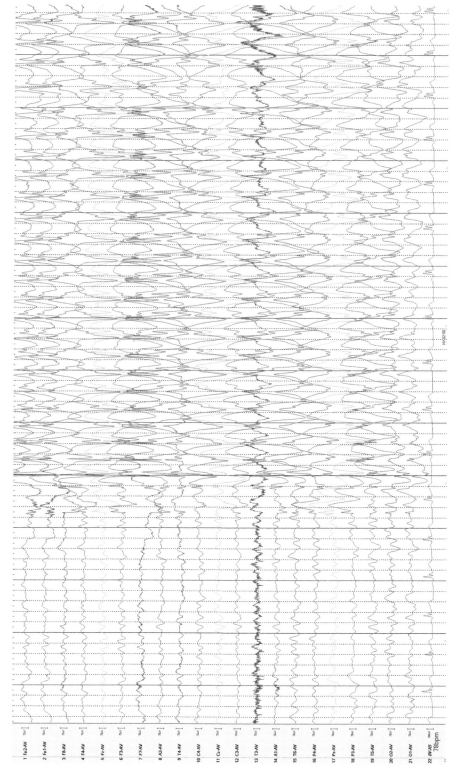

Figure 8.2.5 Electroencephalogram of a 7-year-old boy with childhood absence epilepsy. During hyperventilation, there was a burst of generalised high-amplitude 3 Hz spike wave discharges, which was clinically associated with behavioural arrest (cessation of hyperventilation) and loss of awareness (unable to recall the colour called out during the event).

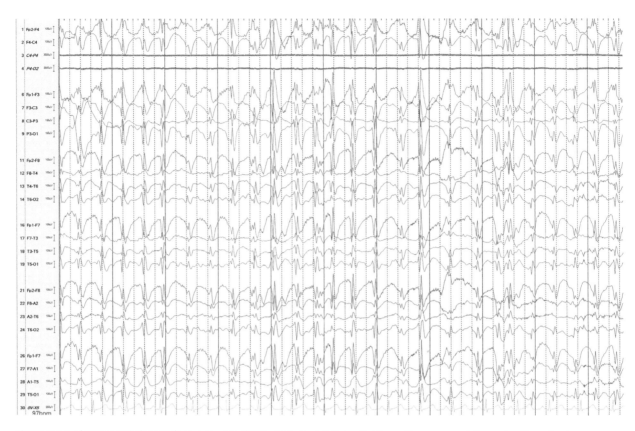

Figure 8.2.6 Electroencephalogram from a 11-year-old boy in absence status epilepticus with a presumed diagnosis of juvenile absence epilepsy. During this time, it was noted that he was not his usual self and was unable to answer simple questions.

8.2.8 KEY MANAGEMENT PRINCIPLES

Diagnosis-specific management strategies are outlined here. It is expected that an 'ABCDE' approach to assessment and management is always undertaken (see Chapter 12.1, *The A to E Assessment*).

For management of prolonged epileptic seizures, see Chapter 13.4, *Prolonged Seizure Management*.

Dangerous Diagnosis 1
Diagnosis: Cardiac syncope

Management Principles
1. **Urgent referral to cardiology.** Any patient with red flags for cardiac syncope in history, family history or electrocardiogram (ECG) should be referred to cardiology, who will determine investigations and management. If clinically well, may not need inpatient admission, but seek clarification from specialists
2. **Safety advice.** Advice should centre around supervision in situations that will put the patient at risk if they were to have a syncopal episode. In cases where there is strong suspicion of cardiac syncope, suggest avoidance of high-intensity exercise until cardiac review

Dangerous Diagnosis 2
Diagnosis: Brain tumour

Management Principles
1. **Urgent neurosurgical specialist input.** Time-critical transfer to a neurosurgical unit may need to be arranged. Hydrocephalus/raised ICP will require emergency procedures such as ventriculostomy/external ventricular drain and shunt placement

2. **Manage raised ICP.** Medical treatment of raised ICP may be required prior to surgical management. Involvement of intensive care colleagues is essential, as children may require intubation and ventilation (see Chapter 13.5, *Raised Intracranial Pressure Management*)

3. **Tertiary oncology.** Definitive management will be guided by tertiary oncology specialists. Specific treatment modalities will be a combination of surgery, radiation therapy and/or chemotherapy

Dangerous Diagnosis 3
Diagnosis: Stroke

Management Principles
Haemorrhagic Stroke
1. **Urgent referral to neurosurgery.** Time-critical transfer to a neurosurgical centre is imperative for definitive management
Ischaemic Stroke
1. **Urgent referral to neurology and neurosurgery.** Emergency surgical treatments such as thrombectomy and decompressive craniectomy should be considered. Further management is specialist and will be guided by neurology
2. **Aspirin.** Aspirin should be administered within 1 hour, unless there are contraindications such as intracranial bleeding. If thrombolysis is being considered, aspirin may be delayed
3. **Thrombolysis.** Thrombolysis is a specialist decision and will be determined by radiological and clinical examination, using the Pediatric National Institutes of Health Stroke Scale (see Chapter 8.3, *Acute Hemiparesis*, Box 8.3.13, *Thrombolysis*)

Dangerous Diagnosis 4
Diagnosis: Chiari drop attacks

Management Principles
1. **Refer to neurosurgeons.** If the patient is well, this can be a non-urgent referral for consideration of foramen magnum decompression surgery

Common Diagnosis 1
Diagnosis: Epileptic seizures

Management Principles
1. **Safety advice.** Advise supervision in situations (water, heights, while crossing roads, around fire etc.) that will put the child at risk if they were to have a seizure. Advise them to always wear a helmet when cycling and avoid cycling by the side of roads
2. **Plan actions for potential further seizure management.** Discuss recovery position. Call for an ambulance if the seizure lasts for longer than 5 minutes
3. **Anti-epileptic drugs (AEDs).** If the child has had more than two epileptic fits, commencement of AED will need to be considered, preferably after an electroencephalogram (EEG); seek advice from a senior member of the team. If already on AED and presenting with a 'breakthrough fit', the dose may need to be increased; again, seek advice from a senior member of the team
4. **Rescue medication.** In children who have had tonic/tonic–clonic seizures that have lasted longer than 5 minutes, consider prescribing a rescue medication such as buccal midazolam for use at home/school
5. **Epilepsy Action is a useful website for families/carers.** www.epilepsy.org.uk provides free help and advice to families about coping with epilepsy
6. **Follow up in clinic, and involve the epilepsy nurse.** Follow-up by a senior paediatrician will need to be arranged after discussion. Epilepsy nurses provide a crucial role in supporting the child and family, and are important members of the multidisciplinary team

Common Diagnosis 2
Diagnosis: Psychogenic non-epileptic seizure

Management Principles
1. **Choose words carefully.** Avoid using the phrase 'There is nothing wrong with you'. Do not offer a 'trial' of anti-epileptic medication
2. **Psychotherapy.** Psychotherapy is essential to explore underlying stressors. Treatment is targeted towards the underlying emotional needs of the child

8.3 Acute Hemiparesis

Samyami S. Chowdhury

Department of Paediatric Neurology, John Radcliffe Hospital, Oxford University Hospitals NHS Foundation Trust, Oxford, UK

Acknowledgement: Dr Sithara Ramdas, Dr Robin Joseph, Consultant Paediatric Neuroradiologist, Oxford University Hospital, UK

CONTENTS

8.3.1 CHAPTER AT A GLANCE

> **Box 8.3.1   Chapter at a Glance**
>
> - Acute hemiparesis can be life-threatening, depending on the underlying pathophysiology, and therefore dangerous diagnoses must be excluded
> - Contacting a paediatric neurologist is encouraged at an early stage, especially where neurological signs and symptoms are challenging or fluctuating
>
> - Clinical evaluation coupled with neuroimaging is needed for accurate diagnosis and subsequent management

8.3.2 DEFINITION

Sudden-onset motor weakness along one side of the body.

8.3.3 DIAGNOSTIC ALGORITHM

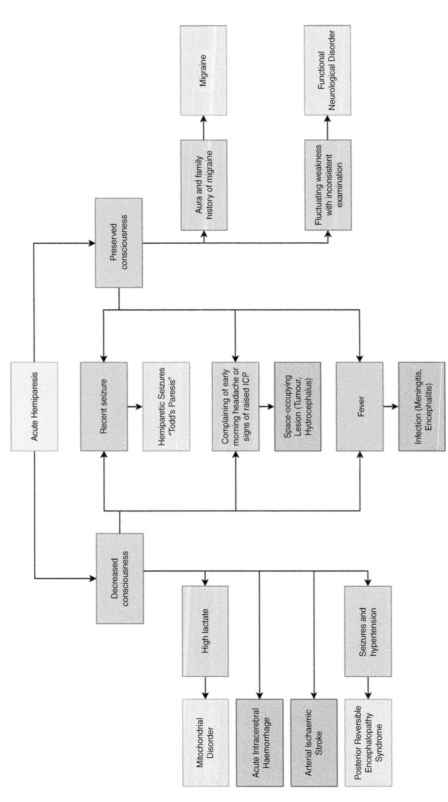

Figure 8.3.1 Diagnostic algorithm for the presentation of acute hemiparesis.

8.3.4 DIFFERENTIALS LIST

Dangerous Diagnoses

1. Acute Intracranial Haemorrhage

- All types of intracranial haemorrhage can present with acute hemiparesis
- These can occur at any age and the common causes include accidental and non- accidental trauma, arteriovenous (AV) malformations and tumours
- Headache will be accompanied by nausea and sometimes seizures, focal neurological deficit and/or loss of consciousness
- In addition to hemiparesis, children may have signs of raised intracranial pressure (ICP), which will need urgent attention

Figure 8.3.2 Computed tomography brain showing an acute left-sided subdural collection (orange arrow). There is significant mass effect with midline shift from left to right. There is compression of the ipsilateral lateral ventricle with dilatation of the contralateral lateral ventricle.

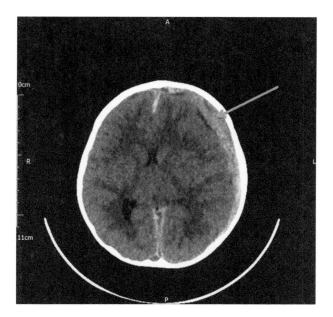

Figure 8.3.3 Computed tomography brain showing a large acute right frontal intraparenchymal haematoma (orange arrow) with distortion and mass effect on surrounding structures.

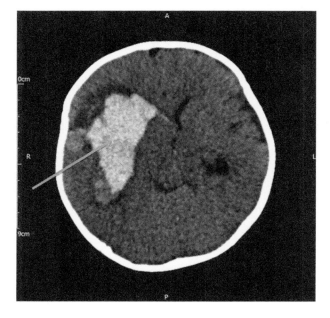

Box 8.3.2   Types of Intracranial Haemorrhage

Type	Anatomical location	Likely aetiology
Intracerebral haemorrhage	Bleeding into the parenchyma of the brain	Non-traumatic
Subarachnoid haemorrhage	Bleeding into the space between the pia and the arachnoid membranes	Non-traumatic rupture of cerebral aneurysms, arteriovenous malformations (AVMs), tumours, vasculitis
Subdural haemorrhage	Bleeding into the space between the dura and arachnoid membranes	Likely traumatic
Epidural haemorrhage	Bleeding between the dura membrane and the skull bone	Likely traumatic

2. Arterial Ischaemic Stroke (AIS)

- Stroke can present with acute-onset focal neurological deficit, often hemiparesis
- Additional features typically include facial weakness, speech disturbances (if dominant hemisphere involved) and visual field defect (hemianopia). Depending on the arterial territory involved, other focal deficits may be present
- The most common site of occlusion is the middle cerebral artery

(A)   (B)

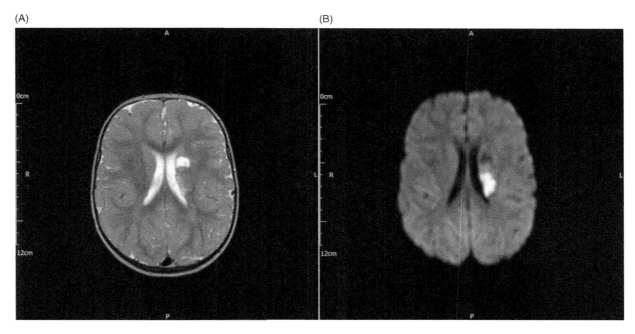

Figure 8.3.4 (A) T2-weighted axial magnetic resonance imaging (MRI). (B) Diffusion-weighted imaging (DWI) MRI. There is acute infarct in the corona radiata posteriorly, extending to the margin of the left lateral ventricle, which is evident on DWI (B) as an area of bright signal. In addition, there is an established infarct more anteriorly, which shows a bright signal on T2 (A) similar to cerebrospinal fluid, but does not show a bright signal on DWI, indicating it is chronic.

Box 8.3.3   Risk Factors for Ischaemic Stroke

Risk factor	Description
Sex/ethnicity	Black, Asian, male sex
Vasculitis	Inflammatory arteritis
Cardiac disorders	Cardiomyopathy, congenital heart disease, right-to-left shunts, prosthetic valves
Hypercoagulable states	Sickle cell disease, prothrombin/factor V Leiden thrombophilia, protein C/S deficiency
Infection	Varicella zoster
Trauma	Cranio-cervical arterial dissection
Metabolic disorders	Mitochondrial myopathy, encephalopathy, lactic acidosis and stroke-like episodes (MELAS), mitochondrial disease, homocystinuria
Genetic/syndromic disorders	NF1, hereditary haemorrhagic telangiectasia, Moyamoya

3. Brain Tumour

- Acute hemiparesis is usually from haemorrhage into or around the tumour. Additional features may be present, including headache, seizures, cranial nerve abnormalities or signs of raised ICP
- Haemorrhage may mask the tumour on computed tomography (CT) scan and magnetic resonance imaging (MRI) head is required
- Tumours may be hemispheric, middle fossa or posterior fossa in location

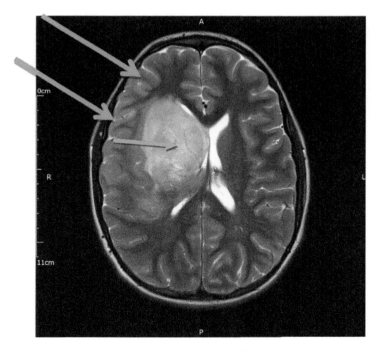

Figure 8.3.5 T2-weighted magnetic resonance imaging. There is a large right-sided intra-axial mass centred on the basal ganglia (blue arrow). Note that the frontal lobe more superficially is also abnormal (orange arrow), being thickened and too bright. Appearances are in keeping with a very large intrinsic glioma.

4. Acute Hydrocephalus

- Hydrocephalus is due to an excessive volume of intracranial cerebrospinal fluid (CSF)
- It can rarely present as hemiparesis with other features of raised ICP
- May be *communicating* or *non-communicating*, depending on whether the CSF communicates between the ventricular system and subarachnoid space
- Causes of acquired hydrocephalus include brain tumours, intracranial haemorrhage or infection. It may develop due to direct obstruction to CSF flow or raised ICP due to cerebral oedema and subsequent impaired venous return
- Beware of the child with a ventriculo-peritoneal (VP) shunt in situ and consider shunt malfunction

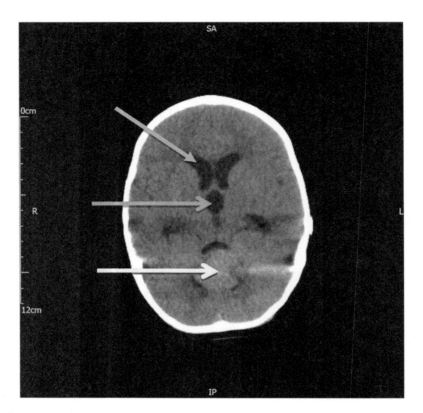

Figure 8.3.6 Computed tomography brain showing a mass in the 4th ventricle (yellow arrow) causing acute obstructive hydrocephalus. Note the dilatation of the temporal horns of the lateral ventricles (blue arrow) and the rounded distended 3rd ventricle (orange arrow). This is a neurosurgical emergency and requires urgent referral/transfer for consideration of cerebrospinal fluid diversion.

5. Meningitis/Encephalitis

- Hemiparesis may be a feature at presentation or evolve during the course of bacterial or viral meningitis
- Infection, associated inflammation or a combination of both can cause hemiparesis due to vasculitis, venous thrombosis or parenchymal necrosis
- Additional features such as seizures are likely to be present
- Meningitis/encephalitis is covered in detail in Chapters 3.1, *Fever* and 8.1, *Headache*, and will not be discussed further in this chapter

Common Diagnoses
1. Hemiplegic Migraine

- Hemiparesis can be seen in complicated migraine or familial hemiplegic migraine (FHM)

- Complicated migraine: hemiparesis lasts up to 24 hours, causing unilateral weakness of the arm and face, often less pronounced in the leg. Contralateral throbbing frontotemporal headache. Function recovers after a period of sleep
- FHM: family history of hemiplegic migraine is essential for diagnosis. Autosomal dominant. Symptoms last 2–3 days. Usually the neurological deficit fully recovers after the attack is over
- Both these types are diagnoses of exclusion in a child with a first presentation of hemiparesis

2. Hemiparetic Seizures

- 'Todd's paresis' is hemiparesis that lasts for minutes to hours following a focal or generalised seizure
- Most commonly, but not exclusively, occurs after a prolonged seizure caused by an underlying structural abnormality

Diagnoses to Consider

1. Posterior Reversible Encephalopathy Syndrome (PRES)

- Also known as reversible posterior leukoencephalopathy syndrome
- Diagnosis relies on clinical and radiological features, which are reversible
- Presents with rapid onset of symptoms with headache, visual disturbance, seizures and encephalopathy
- Due to oedema affecting the occipital lobe, there can be a range of visual loss from blurred vision to blindness. This may present as a post-ictal phenomenon after a seizure
- Classic radiological findings include white matter vasogenic oedema affecting bilateral occipital and parietal lobes seen on MRI
- Although there are several risk factors for PRES, most cases are attributed to hypertension, with some theories describing it as a variant of hypertensive encephalopathy
- Severe hypertension causes interruption to brain autoregulation and vasospasm

When to consider: in children with headache or behavioural changes evolving over a matter of hours, particularly if on neurotoxic medications such as cyclosporin A, methotrexate, cyclophosphamide and tacrolimus

---

Box 8.3.4   Risk Factors for Posterior Reversible Encephalopathy Syndrome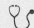

- Acute or chronic kidney disease
- Hypertension
- Autoimmune vascular disease

- Immunosuppressant drugs: tacrolimus, cyclosporin A
- Chemotherapy drugs: cyclophosphamide
- Infections/sepsis/shock

---

2. Mitochondrial Disorders

- There are many types of mitochondrial disease, of varying phenotypes and severity, which are associated with hemiparesis
- One example is MELAS (mitochondrial myopathy, encephalopathy, lactic acidosis and stroke-like episodes)
- Signs and symptoms often appear after a period of normal development, with a wide range of onset from 2 to 15 years of age
- Early symptoms are non-specific and can include myalgia, recurrent headaches, anorexia and vomiting
- Stroke-like episodes occur, including temporary hemiparesis, altered consciousness, visual disturbances, seizures and headaches, with focal acute inflammatory ischaemic changes on MRI, which are not confined to a single vascular territory. These can be triggered by intercurrent illness
- Stepwise neurodevelopmental deterioration with incomplete recovery between deterioration is often the presenting picture. Ask about hearing problems, as sensorineural deafness is associated with MELAS

When to consider: in children who present with non-specific central nervous system (CNS) symptoms with multisystem involvement. Can present at all ages, commonly early infancy and teenage years

3. Functional Neurological Disorder

- Fluctuating weakness with a disproportionate effect on function
- Inconsistent neurological examination findings are the hallmark
- Symptoms cannot be attributed to a structural or organic cause
- Over time, underlying psychological and stress factors may become apparent
- This is a diagnosis of exclusion

When to consider: in children with fluctuating weakness in whom serious organic pathology has been ruled out

Box 8.3.5 DSM-5 Criteria for Functional Neurological Disorders

- One or more symptoms of altered voluntary or sensory function
- Incompatibility between symptoms and neurological or medical conditions
- Symptoms or deficits not better explained by another medical or mental condition
- Symptoms or deficits cause significant distress or impairment in social/occupational functioning

Box 8.3.6 Transient Hemiplegia in Children with Diabetes

- Children with type 1 diabetes mellitus are at risk of hypoglycaemia
- Hypoglycaemia is a rare cause of transient hemiplegia in some individuals
- Underlying mechanism is unknown, with theories including vasospasm, cerebral oedema or reversible brain cell injury
- Hemiplegic attacks most commonly occur during sleep, often associated with an intercurrent respiratory illness
- They usually last 3–24 hours, with complete recovery
- There may be other autonomic and neuroglycopenic features of hypoglycaemia

8.3.5 KEY HISTORY FEATURES

Dangerous Diagnosis 1
Diagnosis: Acute intracranial haemorrhage

Questions
1. **Is there abrupt onset?** Subarachnoid or intraparenchymal haemorrhage usually causes very sudden, severe pain, with onset over seconds
2. **Is there a history of sudden onset of severe headache and/or vomiting?** This is a sign of raised ICP. The child may also be confused, irritable or drowsy
3. **Is there a history of trauma or suspicion of non-accidental injury (NAI)?** Trauma is relevant to understanding the pathology. You must also consider NAI, take a detailed history of mechanism of injury and consider if this is plausible to explain the symptoms and clinical signs
4. **Is there a past medical history consistent with increased bleeding risk?** Children may have known vascular or bleeding disorders, putting them at high risk for haemorrhage. It is important to find out if they take anticoagulant medications

Box 8.3.7 Risk Factors for Intracranial Haemorrhage

Category	Risk factor
Vascular	- Arteriovenous malformation - Cavernous sinus malformations - Cerebral arterial aneurysms - Moyamoya
Haematological	- Functional platelet disorders - Thrombocytopenia - Severe inherited bleeding disorders, e.g. haemophilia - Anticoagulant medication - Severe vitamin K deficiency - Sickle cell disease
Illicit drug use	- Amphetamines - Cocaine
Gender/ethnicity/age	- Age 15–19 years - Black ethnicity - Male gender

Dangerous Diagnosis 2
Diagnosis: Arterial ischaemic stroke

Questions
1. **Is there a history of acute onset of focal neurological deficit?** Sudden hemiparesis is a typical feature. Consciousness is often preserved
2. **Are there other neurological features?** There may be visual deficits or, if the dominant hemisphere is involved, aphasia with speech difficulties. Abrupt onset favours haemorrhagic or embolic stroke. A stuttering onset favours a thrombotic event
3. **Is there a history of seizures?** Focal seizures are not uncommon, especially in neonates. This may precede the hemiparesis
4. **Did a headache accompany the onset of neurological deficits?** Older children may complain of severe headache with the onset of symptoms

Dangerous Diagnosis 3
Diagnosis: Brain tumour

Questions
1. **Have headaches been present for a while?** Headache can be a sign of raised ICP, depending on the type and location of the tumour. Red flags include waking at night with headaches and early-morning headaches
2. **Is there a history of seizures? Are they focal?** With cerebral hemispheric tumours, focal seizures are a common feature
3. **Any change in behaviour or school performance?** Parents will frequently report that their child's behaviour has changed. Red flags include lethargy, irritability and/or decreased school performance
4. **Any vision and gait abnormalities?** The child may complain of blurred vision or double vision, and observers may comment that there is a lack of eye movement. Ataxia is a symptom of a posterior fossa tumour

Dangerous Diagnosis 4
Diagnosis: Acute hydrocephalus

Questions
1. **Is there an increasing head size?** In early infancy, prior to cranial suture fusion, there may be accelerated head growth, which can be quantified by measuring the head circumference
2. **Does the child complain of a headache?** The headache is typically worse when supine. In young children and babies, headache may present as crying when lying down or at night-time. Vomiting and sitting up improve the pain
3. **Are there any visual disturbances?** Reports of the child always looking down, 'sun setting' and divergent squint are possible if the hydrocephalus has progressed. In older children, blurred vision, diplopia and loss of vision may be noted
4. **Are there any risk factors?** Underlying pathology includes tumours, infection, myelomeningocele and intracranial haemorrhage

Common Diagnosis 1
Diagnosis: Hemiplegic migraine

Questions
1. **Is there concomitant visual or speech/language disturbance?** Blind spots, flashing lights, double vision and/or speech and language difficulties may be present, known as 'aura'. See Chapter 8.1, *Headache*, Box 8.1.6, *Migraine Auras*.
2. **Is there sensory loss on the same side as hemiplegia?** Numbness or paraesthesia is frequently experienced on the same side as the motor deficit
3. **Family history of hemiplegic migraine.** There are two types of hemiplegic migraine, familial and sporadic. A family history is essential to diagnose the familial variety: a first-degree relative with at least one hemiplegic attack. Genetic testing is possible for four genes, the most common being *CACNA1A*
4. **Have there been previous episodes? Do they resolve within 72 hours?** Neurological deficits commonly last around 1 hour, but complete resolution can take up to 72 hours. There should be no deficits between episodes.

Common Diagnosis 2

Diagnosis: Hemiparetic seizures

Questions

1. **Did a seizure precede the weakness?** It is essential to the diagnosis that a seizure occurred prior to the onset of weakness
2. **Has this happened before and, if so, how long did the weakness last?** Weakness lasts minutes to hours after a focal or generalised seizure (most commonly a prolonged seizure) with full recovery
3. **Is consciousness impaired?** After the post-ictal phase, where the child may be lethargic or confused, consciousness should return to normal

8.3.6 KEY EXAMINATION FEATURES

General Considerations

Varying levels of consciousness may accompany most of these diagnoses, which can be assessed using the Glasgow Coma Scale (GCS; see Chapter 12.2, *Assessment of Consciousness*).

Box 8.3.8	Medical Research Council Grading Scale for Muscle Strength	
0	Nil	
1	Flicker of movement	
2	Movement with gravity eliminated	
3	Sustained antigravity power	
3+	Momentarily against resistance	
4/4+	Movement against resistance	
5–	Unsure if weak	
5	Normal	

Dangerous Diagnosis 1

Diagnosis: Acute intracerebral haemorrhage

Examination Findings

1. **Decreased level of consciousness.** The level of consciousness should be assessed using the GCS
2. **Focal neurological signs.** Varying signs may be present including aphasia, dysarthria (indicates dominant hemisphere affected), hemianopia, visual loss, hemiparesis, gait disturbance or ataxia
3. **Cushing's triad.** This is the triad of hypertension, bradycardia and irregular respiratory pattern. It is a late sign indicating brainstem compression due to raised ICP and should prompt emergency treatment. See Chapter 8.1, *Headache*, Box 8.1.9, *Cushing's Triad: Late Signs of Raised Intracranial Pressure*

Dangerous Diagnosis 2

Diagnosis: Arterial ischaemic stroke

Examination Findings

1. **Decreased levels of consciousness.** Assess the level of consciousness using the GCS. Younger children are more likely to present with an encephalopathy
2. **Focal neurological signs.** Younger children may present with subtle motor deficits; however, asymmetry of movement, posture and tone should be evident. Older children may meet the 'FAST' criteria with face, arm and speech problems (see Chapter 8.2, *Suspected Seizures*, Box 8.2.5, *FAST Acronym for Recognition of Stroke*). Increased tone and brisk reflexes are late signs and their absence should not detract from considering a central cause
3. **Systems examination assessing risk factors.** Neck trauma increases the possibility of dissection. Various underlying diagnoses may be the cause

Box 8.3.9   Risk Factors for Arterial Ischaemic Stroke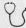

System	Conditions
Cardiac	Right-to-left shunts, infective endocarditis
Skin	Neurofibromatosis, connective tissue disorders
Infections	Chickenpox (*Varicella Zoster*)
Trauma	Head and neck injuries

Dangerous Diagnosis 3

Diagnosis: Brain tumour

Examination Findings

1. **Upper motor neuron signs.** Examine carefully for loss of power, increased tone, hyperreflexia, upgoing plantar reflexes and clonus, and signs of supratentorial tumours
2. **Gait.** There may be either a hemiplegic (supratentorial tumour) or ataxic (infratentorial tumour) gait
3. **Papilloedema.** Papilloedema is swelling of the optic disc caused by raised ICP
4. **Ophthalmoplegia.** Depending on the location of the tumour, there may be ophthalmoplegia from direct tumour effect or a false localising cranial nerve palsy (commonly 6th), indicating raised ICP. Fixed dilated pupils, from 3rd nerve compression, is a very ominous, late sign of raised ICP
5. **Altered mental state.** Tumours causing rapidly rising ICP, either due to the mass itself or obstructive hydrocephalus, may lead to an altered sensorium, with lethargy, irritability and confusion.
6. **Cerebellar signs.** Infratentorial tumours may present with ataxia and tremor. See Chapter 8.1, *Headache*, Box 8.1.8, *Clinical Signs of Cerebellar Dysfunction, Using the Acronym DANISH* for other cerebellar signs.

Dangerous Diagnosis 4

Diagnosis: Acute hydrocephalus

Examination Findings

1. **Signs of raised ICP – sutures open.** In babies, there may be a bulging anterior fontanelle, with prominent scalp veins and accelerated head growth. In older infants, there may be macrocephaly
2. **Signs of raised ICP – sutures fused.** 'Sun setting' is a persistent downward gaze, a sign of raised ICP in young children. There may be papilloedema. Cushing's triad is a late sign
3. **Upper motor neuron signs.** Stretching and disruption of corticospinal fibres lead to upper motor neuron signs, with loss of power, increased tone, hyperreflexia, upgoing plantar reflexes and clonus
4. **VP shunt in situ.** In a child with a known shunt and new neurological signs, shunt malfunction, disconnection or blockage should be the top differential diagnosis

Box 8.3.10   Symptoms Associated with Ventricular Shunt Malfunction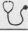

Shunt malfunction	Features
Over-drainage	Headache is worse on standing up and relieved by lying down
Under-drainage	Signs of raised intracranial pressure

Box 8.3.11   Risk Factors for Developing Hydrocephalus

- Tumour: brain, spinal cord
- Haemorrhage: intracranial haemorrhage, head injury
- Infection: bacterial or viral meningitis

Common Diagnosis 1

Diagnosis: Hemiplegic migraine

Examination Findings

1. **Hemiplegia with sensory loss.** This is an essential finding. Weakness is more severe in the face and arm than the leg. The weakness outlasts the headache. Hemianaesthesia, numbness and paraesthesia of the face or limb are prominent features of familial hemiplegic migraine

2. **Alterations of conscious level, visual disturbance, aphasia.** These are frequently noted; aphasia is observed when the dominant hemisphere is affected
3. **Complete recovery.** Recovery is usually complete and by the time the patient arrives in the emergency department, examination may be normal

Common Diagnosis 2
Diagnosis: Hemiparetic seizure

Examination Findings
1. **Unilateral weakness of limb.** Weakness ranges from partial to complete, but is self-limiting, usually resolving within 24 hours (often before)
2. **Preserved consciousness.** After the post-ictal phase, the child will be alert and well
3. **Brisk tendon reflexes.** Reflexes may be unusually brisk in the immediate post-seizure period

8.3.7 KEY INVESTIGATIONS

Not all children will require invasive investigations; often diagnoses are made on clinical evidence from history and examination. Consider carefully which investigations are required for which patient.

Bedside

Table 8.3.1 Bedside tests of use in patients presenting with acute hemiparesis

Test	When to perform	Potential result
Blood gas (capillary or venous)	• All children with acute hemiparesis	• ↓ pH, ↓ HCO_3, ↑ lactate indicate metabolic acidosis, suggestive of circulatory compromise • ↑/↓ Glucose may occur in sepsis
BP	• All children with acute hemiparesis	• Normal BP: rules out hypertensive encephalopathy • ↑BP: PRES, raised ICP
Glucose	• All children with acute hemiparesis	• Hypoglycaemia may cause transient hemiparesis

BP, blood pressure; HCO_3, bicarbonate; ICP, intracranial pressure; PRES, posterior reversible encephalopathy syndrome

Blood Tests

Table 8.3.2 Blood tests of use in patients presenting with acute hemiparesis

Test	When to perform	Potential result
FBC	• All children with acute hemiparesis	• ↑ Hb: Polycythaemia may be seen in preexisting right-to-left cardiac shunt • ↑ WCC, ↑ neutrophil: bacterial infection • ↓ Platelets: severe sepsis • ↓ Hb important in management of SCD with AIS
CRP	• All children with acute hemiparesis	• ↑ In infection
Lactate	• All children with acute hemiparesis	• ↑ In mitochondrial disease, meningitis, encephalitis, sepsis
HbSS	• Known or suspected sickle cell disease	• HbSS status significantly increases the risk of stroke • %HbS important in management of SCD with AIS
Thrombophilia screen (seek advice)	• Suspected thrombotic stroke	• Deficiency in many factors increase the risk of thrombotic strokes

AIS, arterial ischaemic stroke; CRP, C-reactive protein; FBC, full blood count; Hb, haemoglobin; SCD, sickle cell disease

Imaging

Table 8.3.3 Imaging modalities of use in patients presenting with acute hemiparesis

Test	Justification	Potential result
CT head (± CT angiogram, CT venogram)	• All children with acute hemiparesis unless strong clinical evidence for migraine	• Radiological finding will determine underlying reason for presentation, including structural abnormalities, brain tumour, hydrocephalus, intracranial haemorrhage, cerebral oedema, arterial ischaemic stroke, venous infarction
MRI head with stroke sequences (seek advice from radiology)	• More sensitive for ischaemic injury than CT	• May confirm ischaemic stroke
MRA circle of Willis and neck vessels (from aortic arch)	• Suspected haemorrhagic stroke	• May confirm intracerebral aneurysms, arteriovenous malformations or reveal craniocervical arterial dissection
Trans-oesophageal echo (discuss with cardiology)	• To look for cardiac lesions/source of embolic stroke	• Right-to-left shunt • Embolic source • Patent foramen ovale

CT, computed tomography; MRA, magnetic resonance angiography; MRI, magnetic resonance imaging

Special

Lumbar puncture should only be performed once raised ICP has been excluded.

Table 8.3.4 Special tests of use in patients presenting with acute hemiparesis

Test	Justification	Potential result
CSF MC&S	• In suspected meningitis/encephalitis	• Cell count: ↑ neutrophils (bacterial infection), ↑ lymphocytes (viral infection) • Positive culture confirms bacterial infection • Sensitivities guide antibiotic choice
CSF viral PCR	• In suspected meningitis/encephalitis • Confirming viral meningitis can rationalise antimicrobial choice	• Panels vary between different laboratories: HSV1 and 2 are always included, and most panels include varicella zoster virus, parechovirus and enterovirus
CSF protein, glucose	• In suspected meningitis/encephalitis	• ↑ Protein, ↓ glucose in bacterial meningitis
CSF lactate	• In suspected mitochondrial disease	• ↑ Lactate in mitochondrial disease
Conventional angiography	In suspected: • Haemorrhagic stroke, as more sensitive than MRA for identification of posterior circulation stroke • CNS vasculitis	• Identify AVM • Posterior circulation stroke • May show small vessel disease, better visualised than MRA
EEG	• In suspected hemiparetic seizures	• Epileptiform discharges in contralateral hemisphere may be seen in interictal EEG
Genetic testing	• Familial hemiplegic migraine • Mitochondrial disease	• Familial hemiplegic migraine: *CACNA1A* mutation • Mitochondrial disease: *POLG* mutation

AVM, arteriovenous malformation; CNS, central nervous system; CSF, cerebrospinal fluid; EEG, electroencephalogram; HSV, herpes simplex virus; MC&S, microscopy, culture and sensitivity; PCR, polymerase chain reaction

---

Box 8.3.12   Thrombophilia Screen for Inherited Causes of Hypercoagulable States

- Factor V Leiden
- Protein C and S
- Prothrombin 20210 mutation
- Antithrombin III

- Antiphospholipid antibodies (anticardiolipin and lupus anticoagulation)
- Consider von Willebrand factor antigen, factor VIII and XII

8.3.8 KEY MANAGEMENT PRINCIPLES

Diagnosis-specific management strategies are outlined here. It is expected that an 'ABCDE' approach to assessment and management is always undertaken (see Chapter 12.1, *The A to E Assessment*).

Dangerous Diagnosis 1
Diagnosis: Acute intracerebral haemorrhage

Management Principles
1. **Manage signs of raised ICP.** For management of raised ICP, see Chapter 13.5, *Raised Intracranial Pressure Management*
2. **Urgent neurosurgical evaluation.** May require surgical clipping of aneurysms, endovascular occlusion with coils or glue, or evacuation of large haematoma to alleviate ICP
3. **Discuss with a paediatric haematologist.** If there is a known underlying bleeding disorder, or for any abnormal clotting results, coagulation management options must be discussed urgently with haematology
4. **Minimise risk of secondary ischaemia/infarct.** Following haemorrhage there is a risk of arterial vasospasm, which may lead to secondary ischaemia or infarct. Maintain cerebral perfusion pressure, support blood pressure and give intravenous (IV) fluids. Consider nimodipine to prevent vasospasm

Dangerous Diagnosis 2
Diagnosis: Arterial ischaemic stroke

Management Principles
Thrombotic Stroke
1. **Aspirin.** Aspirin at 5 mg/kg should be administered within 1 hour, unless there are contraindications such as intracranial bleeding. If thrombolysis is being considered, aspirin may be delayed. Aspirin should not routinely be given to those with sickle cell disease
2. **Urgent referral to neurology and neurosurgery.** Emergency surgical treatments such as thrombectomy and decompressive craniectomy should be considered. All further management should be directed by neurology specialists
3. **Discuss with haematology.** If pro-thrombotic state found (e.g. factor V Leiden), discuss with haematologist, as prolonged antiplatelet agents will be required
4. **Thrombolysis.** Thrombolysis is a specialist decision and will be determined by radiological and clinical examination, using the Pediatric National Institutes of Health Stroke Scale

Embolic Arterial Stroke
1. **Low molecular weight (LMW) heparin.** If an embolic mechanism is proven, medium-term anticoagulation with LMW heparin should be used. Use for 3 months in dissection or until source of emboli is removed

Vasculopathic Arterial Ischaemic Stroke
1. **Neurosurgical referral.** Neurosurgical intervention for underlying cause (correction of large vessel disease, surgical bypass and revascularisation in Moyamoya syndrome)
2. **Medical management.** In vasculitis due to active chickenpox, 3 weeks' high-dose IV aciclovir. Consider aspirin in vasculopathy, such as post-varicella stroke

---

Box 8.3.13   Thrombolysis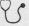

- Tissue plasminogen activator (tPA) is off-label in children, but can be considered in some children presenting with arterial ischaemic stroke (AIS), if >2 years of age. This is a specialist decision and is made on a case-by-case basis, using computed tomography (CT)/CT angiography findings or magnetic resonance (MR) imaging/MR angiography findings. Treatment must be able to be administered within 4.5 hours of symptom onset

- Treatment should be commenced at the location of AIS diagnosis, which may be a secondary care emergency department or paediatric ward

Box 8.3.14   Special Considerations in Arterial Ischaemic Stroke

- In children with cardiac disease, a multi-disciplinary decision, involving paediatric neurologists, cardiologists and haematologists, will be required regarding choice of antiplatelet or anticoagulation therapy, on a risk–benefit basis

- In children with sickle cell disease, urgent blood transfusion (usually exchange transfusion) is required to reduce haemoglobin (Hb) S to <30% and increase Hb to >110 g/L. If the exchange transfusion is likely to be delayed, a top up transfusion should be given to increase Hb to 100 g/L.

Dangerous Diagnosis 3
Diagnosis: Brain tumour

Management Principles
1. **Manage raised ICP.** Medical treatment of raised ICP may be required prior to surgical management. Involvement of intensive care colleagues is essential, as children may require intubation and ventilation (see Chapter 13.5, *Raised Intracranial Pressure Management*)
2. **Reduce cerebral oedema.** Dexamethasone is given on oncology advice, to reduce vasogenic cerebral oedema
3. **Urgent neurosurgical specialist input.** In children with raised ICP due to tumour or hydrocephalus, urgent neurosurgical referral and time-critical transfer to a neurosurgical unit should be arranged. Surgical debulking may be required to relieve raised ICP. Hydrocephalus may require an urgent insertion of ventriculo-peritoneal shunt or external ventricular drain
4. **Multi-disciplinary approach with neurosurgeons and oncologists.** Further decisions regarding biopsy, staging, resection, adjuvant chemotherapy and radiotherapy will be taken by neurosurgeons and oncologists. Many children have lasting impairments of physical or cognitive ability, behaviour, hearing or vision, and will need long-term multi-disciplinary support

Dangerous Diagnosis 4
Diagnosis: Acute hydrocephalus

Management Principles
1. **Urgent neurosurgical referral.** Urgent discussion with neurosurgeons is needed, to determine the need for a ventriculo-peritoneal shunt/endoscopic 3rd ventriculostomy/ external ventricular drain
2. **Manage signs of raised ICP.** See Chapter 13.5, *Raised Intracranial Pressure Management*

Common Diagnosis 1
Diagnosis: Hemiplegic migraine

Management Principles
1. **Analgesia, nurse in a quiet environment.** For many children, pain can be adequately controlled by simple analgesia – paracetamol and/or ibuprofen – and if required anti-emetics
2. **Acetazolamide if confirmed *CACNA1A* positive.** Acetazolamide is a preventative treatment, and should only be initiated after discussion with a paediatric neurologist. See Chapter 8.1, *Headache*, Box 8.1.13, *Measures for Prevention of Migraine*

Common Diagnosis 2
Diagnosis: Hemiparetic seizures

Management Principles
1. **Watch and wait.** Todd's paresis is a self-limiting condition, so weakness will resolve spontaneously
2. **Anti-epileptic medication for seizures.** Anti-epileptics may be required for seizures – class to be decided depending on type of seizure

8.4 Acute Lower-Limb Weakness

Samyami S. Chowdhury

Department of Paediatric Neurology, John Radcliffe Hospital, Oxford University Hospitals NHS Foundation Trust, Oxford, UK

Acknowledgement: Dr Sithara Ramdas, Dr Robin Joseph, Consultant Paediatric Neuroradiologist, Oxford University Hospital, UK

CONTENTS

8.4.1 CHAPTER AT A GLANCE

> **Box 8.4.1 Chapter at a Glance**
>
> - Acute lower-limb weakness can be extremely distressing for both child and parent
> - Clinical presentation is variable, ranging from minor neurological deficits to complete paralysis
> - Causes should be considered neuroanatomically from muscle, neuromuscular junction, peripheral nerve, anterior horn cell and spinal cord
>
> - Timing is critical for assessment and management in order to preserve neurological function where cord compression is suspected

8.4.2 DEFINITION

Weakness or acute flaccid paralysis, with rapid progression and clinical onset in less than 5 days.

Clinical Guide to Paediatrics, First Edition. Edited by Rachel Varughese and Anna Mathew. Series Editor: Christian Fielder Camm.
© 2022 John Wiley & Sons Ltd. Published 2022 by John Wiley & Sons Ltd.
Companion website: www.wiley.com/go/varughese/paediatrics

8.4.3 DIAGNOSTIC ALGORITHM

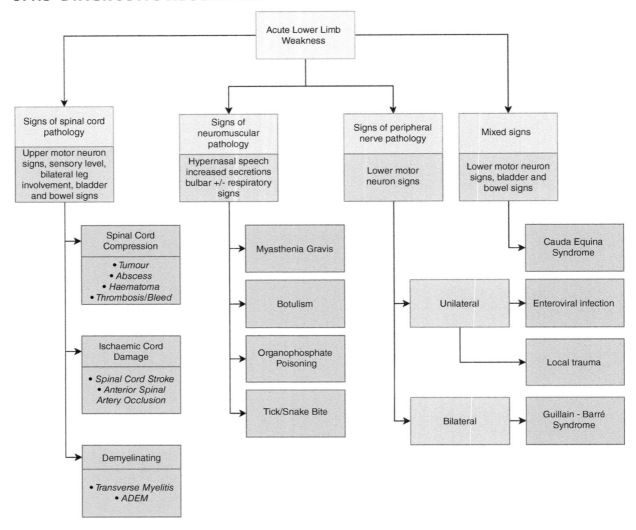

Figure 8.4.1 Diagnostic algorithm for the presentation of acute lower-limb weakness.

8.4.4 DIFFERENTIALS LIST

Dangerous Diagnoses

All cases of acute lower limb weakness must be assessed urgently to rule out a neurological or neurosurgical emergency.

1. Spinal Cord Compression
- There are many causes of spinal cord compression, including trauma, neoplasm and infection
- Spinal cord injuries are rare before adolescence. The majority are due to road traffic accidents or sporting injuries
- Traumatic spinal cord injury can result in varying degrees of damage to the spinal cord with different prognostic outcomes
- In neonates, spinal cord trauma can result from umbilical cord catheterisation or from neck injury during delivery
- Extramedullary lesions are not the only emergency but all cord compressions are neurosurgical emergencies
- Intramedullary lesions can mimic acute transverse myelitis
- Prompt diagnosis with early appropriate management has better long-term neurological outcomes

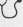

Box 8.4.2   Consequences of Traumatic Spinal Cord Injuries

- Spinal cord swelling
- Spinal cord contusion/oedema
  - Cord oedema only: favourable prognosis
  - Cord oedema and contusion: intermediate prognosis
  - Cord contusion only: worse prognosis
- Intramedullary haemorrhage
- Extrinsic compression, e.g. from fracture fragment or disc herniation
- Spinal cord transection

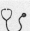

Box 8.4.3   Spinal Space-Occupying Lesions

- Space-occupying lesions of the spine can be primary tumours or metastatic
- Spinal pathology can cause symmetrical neurological deficit below the lesion, according to anatomical location
- Onset of symptoms can often be insidious
- Spinal abscess can also produce neurological deficits along with systemic symptoms
- Pathologies can be divided according to their preferred location within the spinal cord

Location	Causes
Epidural	Leukaemia, lymphoma, neuroblastoma, abscess, metastasis
Intradural	Neurofibroma, sarcoma, lipoma, meningioma, metastasis
Intramedullary	Astrocytoma, ependymoma, arteriovenous malformation, metastasis

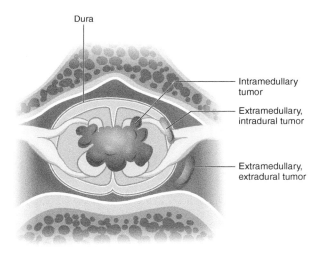

Figure 8.4.2 Spinal space-occupying lesions can be divided into intramedullary, intradural and extradural.

2. Transverse Myelitis

- Local inflammation of the spinal cord with cerebrospinal fluid (CSF) pleocytosis (↑ white cell count, WCC), demyelination and cord swelling
- There is often a non-specific preceding upper respiratory tract infection
- Signs and symptoms are usually bilateral, but not always symmetrical
- There may be a defined sensory level on examination
- Causes include infection, post- or para-infectious conditions, and immune-mediated responses
- Infectious agents can cause spinal cord dysfunction by directly infecting the spinal cord parenchyma or by triggering an immune-mediated response
- Can occur in isolation, in various connective tissue conditions such as systemic lupus erythematosus (SLE), juvenile rheumatoid arthritis (JRA), sarcoidosis, vasculitis or with other central nervous system (CNS)-demyelinating conditions, such as acute demyelinating encephalomyelitis (ADEM) or optic neuritis

Box 8.4.4   Cauda Equina Syndrome

- The cauda equina is the bundle of nerve roots that emerge from the end of the spinal cord
- Cauda equina syndrome occurs when these nerves become severely compressed

- Symptoms may start as sciatica, progressing to weakness or numbness in both legs, saddle anaesthesia and bowel/bladder disturbance

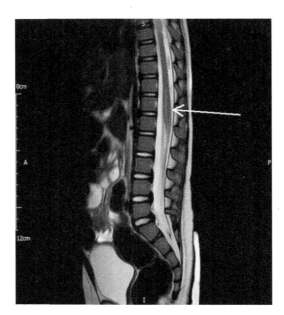

Figure 8.4.3 Magnetic resonance imaging of the spine showing an ill-defined increased T2 signal in the cord substance involving the distal cord and conus (arrow). The abnormality extends for more than two vertebral levels and fits with a radiological picture of transverse myelitis.

3. Guillain–Barré Syndrome (GBS)
- GBS is the most common cause of acute lower-limb generalised weakness
- It is an acute immune-mediated ascending demyelinating polyradiculoneuritis, causing mixed motor and sensory deficits
- It is often preceded by a non-specific infection, such as an upper respiratory tract infection or gastroenteritis
- Classical triad is of ascending weakness, areflexia and elevated CSF protein without raised white cell count

4. Myasthenic Crisis
- Life-threatening complication of myasthenia gravis (MG)
- Disorder of neuromuscular transmission due to either reduction or dysfunction of acetylcholine receptors (AChRs)
- Can present at any age
- Myasthenic crisis can be seen in transient neonatal MG (infants born to mothers with MG), juvenile MG and congenital myasthenia syndromes
- Respiratory failure requiring intubation and ventilation may be seen in severe cases
- Precipitated by intercurrent illness, surgery, stress, under-medication and menstruation
- Beware of cholinergic crisis due to over-medication with acetylcholinesterase inhibitors, which are used as treatment

5. Acute Disseminated Encephalomyelitis
- Post-infectious encephalomyelitis, which can be seen days to weeks after a mild viral illness or immunisation
- Caused by antibodies to the virus crossreacting with myelin surface proteins
- Behavioural change or encephalopathy must be present for diagnosis
- Multifocal white matter lesions on neuroimaging (magnetic resonance imaging) are seen
- Spinal cord inflammation can be associated
- There can be rapid clinical progression to coma

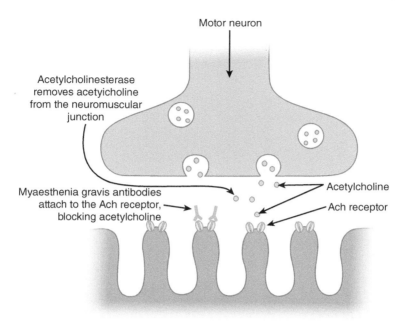

Figure 8.4.4 The motor neuron functions when an action potential reaches a neuromuscular junction. Vesicles of acetylcholine are released into the synaptic gap. The acetylcholine binds to receptors on the muscle fibre's post-synaptic membrane. Acetylcholinesterase catalyses the breakdown of acetylcholine from the synaptic junction.

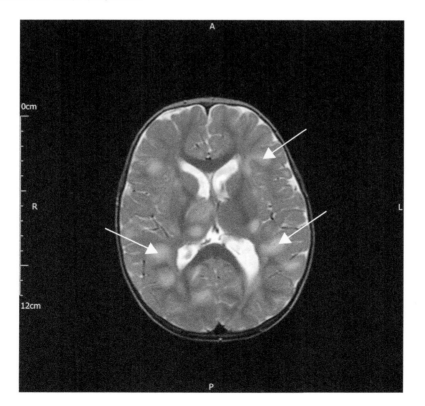

Figure 8.4.5 Magnetic resonance imaging of the brain showing multiple, large, randomly scattered, ill-defined T2 hyperintense lesions in the basal ganglia and white matter (three examples illustrated by white arrows). Appearances are characteristic for acute demyelinating encephalomyelitis.

Diagnoses to Consider

1. **Vascular: Anterior Spinal Artery Occlusion**
   - Caused by interruption of blood flow to the anterior spinal artery (ASA) causing ischaemia to the anterior two-thirds of the cord
   - There is sudden flaccid paralysis of the legs. If the cervical cord is involved, then the arms may be involved
   - Loss of pain and sensation is usually noted two levels below the injury. Often vibration, proprioception and touch are preserved
   - Risk factors for ASA occlusion include coarctation of the aorta, underlying connective tissue disorders (Ehlers–Danlos and Marfan syndromes), recent scoliosis surgery and umbilical artery catheterisation

When to consider: when there is rapid progression of symptoms over minutes to hours with normal CSF results and a vascular distribution on neuroimaging. This can be clinically difficult to distinguish from transverse myelitis; however, a rapid onset favours a diagnosis of ASA infarct

2. **Botulism**
   - Rare but serious condition resulting from botulinum toxin, from *Clostridium botulinum* bacteria, with 5–10% mortality
   - Symptoms begin 1–2 days after ingesting the botulism spores. The spores reproduce in the gut and form a toxin that is absorbed into the bloodstream
   - The toxin blocks the release of acetylcholine from motor neurons at the neuromuscular junction, causing neuromuscular blockade
   - Exposure is often food-borne, resulting in a descending flaccid paralysis. Commonest in infancy due to ingestion of food such as honey, but can be due to other improperly processed foods, or dirt. Rarely, older children are affected by wound contamination
   - Symptoms include muscle weakness, floppiness, constipation, bulbar weakness and respiratory failure in severe cases

When to consider: in children with weakness that starts on the face and progresses to the lower limbs

8.4.5 KEY HISTORY FEATURES

Dangerous Diagnosis 1

Diagnosis: Spinal cord compression

Questions

1. **Is there back pain?** The child may complain of pain or refuse to weight bear due to back pain. Quite often children can point to the exact location, which correlates well with the site of the tumour. Back pain can radiate to other parts of the body
2. **Is there any bowel or bladder involvement?** There may be a mixed picture of urinary retention or incontinence and constipation or faecal incontinence
3. **Has there been a change in gait or refusal to weight bear?** Gait disturbances can be a feature of slowly progressive disorders such as spinal tumours. Refusal to weight bear may indicate an acute underlying process, such as intense pain from a fracture site
4. **Is there a history of malignancy?** Spinal cord compression is commonly due to neoplasm, which may be primary or metastatic. A history of previous or current malignancy is extremely concerning for metastatic disease
5. **Is there a history of fever and being unwell?** Spikes of fever coupled with symptoms of symmetrical lower-limb weakness and unwillingness to weight bear are associated with underlying spinal abscess
6. **Is there a history of trauma?** Regardless of the age of the child, always consider spinal trauma as a possible cause for presentation

Dangerous Diagnosis 2

Diagnosis: Transverse myelitis

Questions

1. **Is there abrupt onset of spinal cord dysfunction?** Neurological symptoms develop very suddenly, progress rapidly over 1–2 days and then plateau
2. **Is there any back pain?** Sudden-onset back pain at a segmental level is classic. There may be shooting pains down the arms, chest, abdomen or legs, depending on the location of the lesion
3. **Is there history of acute progressive weakness and paraesthesia in the legs?** Child may complain of progressive weakness, associated with sensory symptoms of numbness, tingling, burning or a cold sensation
4. **Is there a history of previous optic neuritis?** Transverse myelitis may be associated with optic neuritis, which might precede the transverse myelitis
5. **Is there any bowel or bladder involvement?**
   Early loss of bowel and bladder control distinguishes this from Guillain–Barré

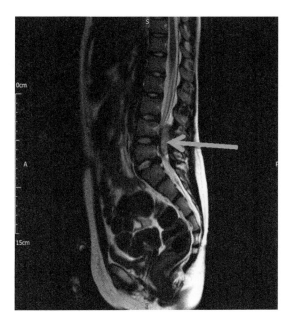

Figure 8.4.6 Magnetic resonance imaging of the spine showing cauda equina compression caused by an extradural mass (orange arrow), due to an Ewing's sarcoma.

Dangerous Diagnosis 3
Diagnosis: Guillain–Barré syndrome

Questions
1. **Did the weakness start in the legs?** Ascending symmetrical weakness is a classic presentation of GBS. Weakness often starts in the legs, then progresses upwards to involve the trunk, arms and facial muscles
2. **Have there been any preceding illnesses in the last 1 week to 1 month?** Many infections are associated with GBS, including Epstein–Barr virus, cytomegalovirus, herpes simplex virus, campylobacter, hepatitis B, human immunodeficiency virus and influenza
3. **Does the history suggest cranial nerve involvement?** Facial, oculomotor and oropharyngeal weakness frequently develop, leading to problems with talking and swallowing

Dangerous Diagnosis 4
Diagnosis: Myasthenic crisis

Questions
1. **Is there a history of ineffective cough?** This can be due to a combination of bulbar weakness altering the cough and swallowing reflex, as well as severe muscle weakness of the respiratory muscles
2. **Are there excess secretions and inability to clear them?** This can either be a sign of a myasthenic crisis or a cholinergic crisis and is due to a combination of bulbar weakness and oropharyngeal muscle weakness
3. **Is there a history of fatiguable weakness?** There is usually a long history of muscle weakness that is worse at the end of a day, or after activity. This can sometimes present with progressive swallowing difficulties or droopy eyes

Dangerous Diagnosis 5
Diagnosis: Acute disseminated encephalomyelitis

Questions
1. **Is there behavioural change?** Encephalopathy is a common presentation with lethargy, confusion and drowsiness
2. **Is there a history of preceding illness?** A viral illness preceding onset of neurological dysfunction is common. Symptoms can start 7–21 days from the initial illness
3. **What is the duration of symptoms?** There is an abrupt onset of neurological deficit and symptoms, mainly due to myelopathy and optic neuritis. There may also be focal neurological deficit
4. **Has the child had a seizure?** Seizures may be the presenting feature in children with severe ADEM

Box 8.4.5   Differentiating Guillain–Barré Syndrome and Transverse Myelitis

Features	Guillain–Barré syndrome	Transverse myelitis
Onset of paralysis	Acute, gradual progression (days to weeks)	Acute, rapid progression (1–2 days)
Lower motor neuron signs	Symmetrical, lower limbs (distal initially, then ascending)	May or may not be symmetrical, lower limbs, often no upper extremity involvement
Weakness	Begins distally and ascends	Static weakness of lower limbs
Hypotonia	Hypotonia ascends	Static hypotonia
Deep tendon reflexes	Absent, extends cranially	Absent
Sensation	Paraesthesia with numbness and tingling of hands and feet	Sensory level, with loss of sensation below
Cranial nerve involvement	Likely involvement of 7th, 9th, 10th, 11th and 12th cranial nerves	Absent
Autonomic signs and symptoms (labile blood pressure/temperature/sweating)	Likely	Present
Respiratory compromise	Likely, depends on ascension	Unlikely, depends on level
Bladder involvement	Possible	Present
Lumbar puncture	High protein, normal cell count	Normal

8.4.6 KEY EXAMINATION FEATURES

Varying levels of consciousness may accompany most of these diagnoses, which can be accurately assessed using the Glasgow Coma Scale (GCS; see Chapter 12.2, *Assessment of Consciousness*). See Chapter 8.3, *Acute Hemiparesis*, Box 8.3.8, *Medical Research Council Grading Scale for Muscle Strength* for grading scale for muscle strength

Dangerous Diagnosis 1
Diagnosis: Spinal cord compression

Examination Findings
1. **Symmetrical pattern of motor weakness.** Paraplegia or quadriplegia is seen, depending on the level of cord compression
2. **Hypotonia then hypertonia.** In the acute phase of spinal shock, reduced tone, absent reflexes and downgoing plantars are seen. Initial hypotonia can last up to 4 weeks, after which there is progression to increased tone, brisk reflexes and upgoing plantars
3. **Paraesthesia.** Intramedullary tumours could present with insidious onset of paraesthesia
4. **Dermatomal level of sensory loss.** Examine the spinothalamic (pain and temperature) and dorsal columns (light touch, proprioception and two-point discrimination). There may be loss of pain and temperature perception in a 'saddle' distribution, loss of pin-prick sensation in legs or loss of proprioception and vibration sense in feet. Even if these signs are demonstrated, there is poor correlation with the precise level of the cord compression
5. **Late signs of cord compression.** Check for bladder/bowel dysfunction. Loss of the abdominal reflex and loss of anal tone indicate late signs of cord compression

Dangerous Diagnosis 2
Diagnosis: Transverse myelitis

Examination Findings
1. **Identify segmental level.** A spinal cord sensory level is usually located in the thoracic region (80%). Cervical (10%) or lumbar (10%) involvement is less common. Pain, temperature and light touch are affected. Joint proprioception and vibration sense may be preserved
2. **Loss of sweating below the segmental level.** Disturbances in autonomic function include fluctuations in blood pressure (BP), temperature instability and loss of sweating
3. **Signs of flaccid paralysis.** Weakness may be asymmetrical, with decreased tone and depressed deep tendon reflexes
4. **Evidence of urinary/faecal retention or incontinence.** Early loss of bowel and bladder control distinguishes this from GBS

Dangerous Diagnosis 3

Diagnosis: Guillain–Barré syndrome

Examination Findings

1. **Bilateral, symmetrical lower-limb motor weakness.** Typical involvement of both lower limbs initially, with predominant motor weakness and associated areflexia
2. **Progressive ascending weakness.** The polyradiculopathy leads to progressive bilateral symmetrical weakness that goes on to involve the truncal muscles, muscles of respiration, arms and cranial nerves
3. **Bilateral sensory loss.** Mild sensory symptoms and signs can occur, such as numbness and paraesthesia involving the toes and fingertips
4. **Autonomic dysfunction.** Labile BP, orthostatic hypotension, sinus tachycardia/bradycardia, anhidrosis, swallowing difficulties and temperature instability can all be seen

Dangerous Diagnosis 4

Diagnosis: Myasthenic crisis

Examination Findings

1. **Fatiguability.** Fatiguability can be demonstrated by asking the child to sustain an upward gaze (progressive ptosis) or hold their arms outstretched (deltoid fatigues). Alternatively, a repetitive action, such as opening and closing of the fist, will not be able to be sustained
2. **Drooling.** A sign of muscle weakness and inability to clear secretions causing compromise of the airway
3. **Nasal speech.** This is due to involvement of muscles of the jaw, throat, palate, tongue and vocal tract. Muscular weakness stops the vocal folds from moving normally
4. **Reduced air entry, crackles.** Clinical signs of pneumonia with hypoxia may develop, due to both bulbar weakness and weakness of the respiratory muscles

Dangerous Diagnosis 5

Diagnosis: Acute disseminated encephalomyelitis

Examination Findings

1. **Signs of irritability or reduced consciousness.** Inconsolable crying with poor feeding, vomiting, lethargy, behavioural changes and alterations in conscious level may be present
2. **Visual loss.** Involvement of the optic nerve with optic neuritis commonly leads to visual loss, which may contribute to delirium
3. **Unsteadiness or inability to walk.** This is a sign of cerebellar or spinal involvement, although it may not be easily demonstrated if there is encephalopathy
4. **Abnormal movements.** Infiltration of basal ganglia can occur in ADEM, causing extrapyramidal movements including tremor, dystonia (uncontrolled muscle contractions), akathisia (restlessness) and tardive dyskinesia (jerky involuntary movements)
5. **Cranial nerve involvement.** Multiple cranial nerve palsies are possible, with the facial nerve most commonly affected

8.4.7 KEY INVESTIGATIONS

Bedside

Table 8.4.1 Bedside tests of use in patients presenting with acute lower-limb weakness

Test	When to perform	Potential result
Blood gas (capillary or venous)	• All children with acute lower-limb weakness • Any respiratory compromise guides need for respiratory support	• ↓ pH and ↑ CO_2 indicates respiratory acidosis • ↓ pH, ↓ HCO_3, ↑ lactate indicate metabolic acidosis, suggestive of poor perfusion, e.g. sepsis • ↑/↓ Glucose may occur in sepsis
ECG	• Monitoring cardiac dysfunction in GBS	• May determine need for temporary cardiac pacemaker

CO_2, carbon dioxide; ECG, electrocardiogram; GBS, Guillain–Barré syndrome; HCO_3, bicarbonate

Blood Tests

Table 8.4.2 Blood tests of use in patients presenting with acute lower-limb weakness

Test	When to perform	Potential result
FBC	• All children with acute lower-limb weakness	• ↑ WCC, ↑ neutrophils: bacterial infection • ↑ WCC, ↑ lymphocytes: viral infection
CRP	• All children with acute lower-limb weakness	• Significant ↑ in bacterial infections • Less marked ↑ in viral infections and inflammation
Coagulation screen	• All children with acute lower-limb weakness	• APTT, INR may be deranged after thrombotic event
Thrombophilia screen (seek advice)	• Suspected ASA occlusion to screen for hypercoagulable states	• Deficiency in specific factors

APTT, activated partial thromboplastin time; ASA, anterior spinal artery; CRP, C-reactive protein; FBC, full blood count; INR, international normalised ratio; WCC, white cell count

Imaging

Table 8.4.3 Imaging modalities of use in patients presenting with acute lower-limb weakness

Test	When to perform	Potential result
MRI brain and spine	• All children with acute lower-limb weakness	• Brain tumour • White matter changes in inflammatory conditions, e.g. ADEM • Spinal cord tumour, abscess, infarct, haemorrhage
CT head	• When rapid result is required and MRI is not available	• Acute subarachnoid haemorrhage • Other space-occupying lesions

ADEM, acute demyelinating encephalomyelitis; CT, computed tomography; MRI, magnetic resonance imaging

Special

Lumbar puncture should only be performed once raised intracranial pressure has been excluded.

Table 8.4.4 Additional tests in patients presenting with acute lower-limb weakness

Test	When to perform	Potential result
CSF MC&S, viral PCR, protein, glucose	Suspected: • Meningitis • GBS • Transverse myelitis	• Bacterial meningitis: ↑ WCC (neutrophils), ↑ protein, ↓ glucose, positive bacterial culture • Viral meningitis: ↑ WCC (lymphocytes), mildly ↑ protein, ↔ glucose, positive viral PCR • GBS: normal cell count, ↑ protein • Transverse myelitis: ↑ WCC (lymphocytes), ↔ protein
Nerve conduction studies	• To confirm sensory deficit	• GBS and transverse myelitis: reduced response in peripheral nerves
FVC	Suspected: • GBS • Myasthenic crisis	• FVC <12–15 mL/kg indicates need for respiratory support and mechanical ventilation should be considered

CSF, cerebrospinal fluid; FVC, forced vital capacity; GBS, Guillain–Barré syndrome; MC&S, microscopy, culture and sensitivity; PCR, polymerase chain reaction; WCC, white cell count

8.4.8 KEY MANAGEMENT PRINCIPLES

Diagnosis-specific management strategies are outlined here. It is expected that an 'ABCDE' approach to assessment and management is always undertaken (see Chapter 12.1, *The A to E Assessment*).

Box 8.4.6   Supportive Measures in the Management of Spinal Pathology

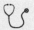

- Deep vein thrombosis risk is significant, therefore prophylaxis is mandatory (if spinal surgery is likely, discuss this with surgical team and consider mechanical thromboprophylaxis)
- Urinary bladder catheterisation – urinary retention is a common complication

- Laxatives for constipation
- Gastroprotection as risk of stress ulcer
- Nutritional support
- Psychological support

Dangerous Diagnosis 1
Diagnosis: Spinal cord compression

Management Principles
1. **Analgesia.** Pain is a significant symptom and analgesia should be prioritised. Opioids may be required
2. **High-dose steroids.** Dexamethasone 0.25 mg/kg intravenous (IV; max. 10 mg) is given to relieve spinal cord oedema
3. **Urgent neurosurgical evaluation.** Surgical decompression and stabilisation of the spine may be required, and all cases should be discussed urgently with neurosurgeons. A time-critical transfer may be needed
4. **In traumatic spinal cord injury, treat spinal shock.** Give IV methylprednisolone 30 mg/kg as a loading dose, followed by a continuous infusion 5 mg/kg/hr for 15hours
5. **Tertiary oncology.** If the cord compression is due to a neoplasm, oncology specialists will guide further treatment, which may include chemotherapy or radiotherapy
6. **Supportive measures.** These are described in Box 8.4.6

Dangerous Diagnosis 2
Diagnosis: Transverse myelitis

Management Principles
1. **IV steroids and IV immunoglobulin (Ig).** Discuss with paediatric neurology. High-dose IV steroids are the mainstay of treatment and significantly improve outcome. IVIg and plasmapheresis are also given for non-responders
2. **Supportive measures.** These are described in Box 8.4.6

Dangerous Diagnosis 3
Diagnosis: Guillain–Barré syndrome

Management Principles
1. **Respiratory support.** Discuss with paediatric neurology. There may be respiratory compromise, which is a complication of GBS due to respiratory muscle paralysis. If you are concerned, urgent anaesthetic assessment and admission to paediatric intensive care unit (PICU) are warranted. Intubation is required if vital capacity is less than 50% of normal or below 12–15 mL/kg
2. **IVIg.** 2 g/kg total dose. Plasmapheresis can be considered for non-responders
3. **Supportive measures.** These are described in Box 8.4.6

Dangerous Diagnosis 4
Diagnosis: Myasthenic crisis

Management Principles
1. **Respiratory support.** Discuss with paediatric neurology. If diagnosis is a myasthenic exacerbation but the patient is not in crisis, closely monitor vital capacity every 4–6 hours. If the forced vital capacity is less than 12–15 mL/kg, intubate and ventilate. If in established myasthenic crisis, do not delay intubation and ventilation. Call an anaesthetist/PICU early
2. **Pharyngeal suction.** Copious amounts of secretions will be present, obstructing the airway. Frequent regular suctioning is required
3. **IVIg and/or plasma exchange.** These provide significant and rapid improvement in the degree of weakness

4. **Temporary withdrawal of regular medication.** MG is treated with anticholinesterase inhibitors, such as pyridostigmine. During the acute phase of a myasthenic crisis, these are often withdrawn in patients who are intubated and ventilated, in order to reduce airway secretions, and can be restarted during recovery

Dangerous Diagnosis 5

Diagnosis: Acute disseminated encephalomyelitis

Management Principles

1. **Administer IV steroids.** The mainstay of treatment is with pulsed IV methylprednisolone (30 mg/kg, maximum 1 g daily for 3 days). Discuss with paediatric neurology early to guide management and for further treatment options, including plasmapheresis and/or IVIg
2. **Antibiotics, antiviral.** Do not delay empirical antibiotic and antiviral administration in suspected encephalitis. Further treatment will be determined once a micro-organism is isolated, according to local guidelines

8.5 Delirium and Agitation

Dannika Buckley

Department of Paediatrics, University Hospitals Sussex NHS Foundation Trust, Worthing, West Sussex, UK

CONTENTS

8.5.1 CHAPTER AT A GLANCE

> **Box 8.5.1   Chapter at a Glance**
>
> - Delirium is also known as an 'acute confusional state', and can be divided into two main types, hyperactive and hypoactive
> - Hyperactive delirium results in agitation, restlessness and labile mood
> - Hypoactive delirium, often used synonymously with encephalopathy, results in depressed sensorium, with inactivity, lethargy and drowsiness
>
> - Some diagnoses, such as hypoglycaemia, hyperglycaemia and metabolic disorders, rely almost solely on biochemical investigation. Others rely more on history and examination
> - Hypoactive delirium is covered in detail in Chapter 8.6, *Decreased Level of Consciousness* and will not be explored in this chapter

8.5.2 DEFINITION

- Delirium is an acute mental disturbance, secondary to an underlying medical illness, characterised by behavioural change, confusion, and altered environmental awareness
- Agitation is a state of psychomotor hyperactivity

Clinical Guide to Paediatrics, First Edition. Edited by Rachel Varughese and Anna Mathew. Series Editor: Christian Fielder Camm.
© 2022 John Wiley & Sons Ltd. Published 2022 by John Wiley & Sons Ltd.
Companion website: www.wiley.com/go/varughese/paediatrics

8.5.3 DIAGNOSTIC ALGORITHM

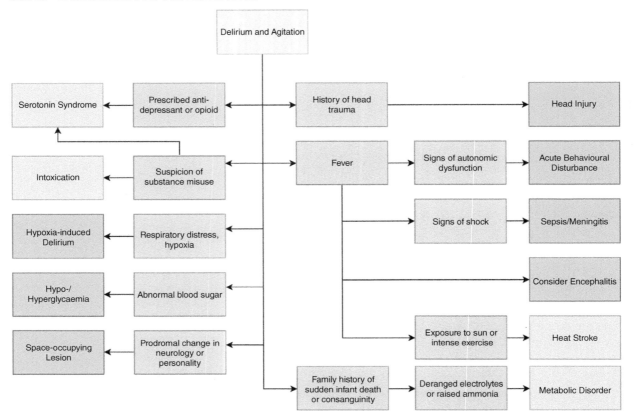

Figure 8.5.1 Diagnostic algorithm for the presentation of delirium and agitation.

8.5.4 DIFFERENTIALS LIST

Dangerous Diagnoses

1. **Hypoxia-Induced Delirium**
   - Hypoxia refers to decreased oxygenation at tissue level
   - Hypoxia can rapidly result in brain damage and cardiac arrest, and therefore needs to be treated as an emergency
   - High-flow oxygen should be considered for any child with altered mental state, titrated according to oxygen saturation readings
2. **Acute Behavioural Disturbance (ABD)**
   - Triad of acute delirium, aggression or severe agitation, and hyper-adrenergic autonomic dysfunction, e.g. hyperthermia
   - The diagnosis can be challenging, since behaviours and signs overlap with many other diagnoses
   - Most commonly associated with acute on chronic substance misuse or withdrawal
   - Organic causes include hypoglycaemia and sepsis
   - 10–20% of cases are due to an underlying psychiatric disturbance
   - Complications include metabolic acidosis, rhabdomyolysis, multi-organ failure and even death
3. **Encephalitis**
   - Encephalitis is an inflammation of the brain and is a rare but serious condition
   - Viral causes predominate, with herpes simplex being the most common. It can however occur as a consequence of bacterial, fungal and parasitic infections, as well as systemic conditions such as autoimmune diseases
   - The clinical presentation is highly variable, but personality change and behavioural disturbance are common features
4. **Head Injury**
   - Head injury can cause a wide range of symptoms, ranging from mild confusion to agitation to coma
   - This may be a manifestation of a concussion, or a secondary consequence of head injury, e.g. a bleed

- Always consider non-accidental injury (NAI), if there are inconsistencies with the history or any other concerning features
- Features to prompt consideration of NAI are discussed in Chapter 12.5, *Safeguarding*

5. **Hypoglycaemia and Hyperglycaemia**
   - A glucose reading is the first investigation that should be carried out in a child with delirium or agitation and should be remembered as part of any emergency 'ABCDE' assessment
   - The underlying cause for the abnormal glucose will need to be sought
   - Causes of hypoglycaemia include starvation, prolonged vomiting and diarrhoea, ketotic hypoglycaemia, and rarer metabolic causes
   - Causes of hyperglycaemia include diabetic ketoacidosis, sepsis and rarer metabolic causes
   - Hypoglycaemia and hyperglycaemia are covered in detail in Chapters 7.1 and 7.2 and will not be discussed further in this chapter

6. **Sepsis-Related Delirium**
   - Sepsis is the systemic response to severe infection. It can rapidly lead to multi-organ damage and even death
   - An altered mental state ranging from hyperactive delirium to hypoactive encephalopathy can be seen, in part due to reduced cerebral perfusion
   - Sepsis is covered in detail in Chapter 3.1, *Fever*, and will not be discussed further in this chapter

7. **Space-Occupying Lesion**
   - Space-occupying lesions can cause a change in personality. As the lesion increases in size it can cause agitation, progressing to a reduced level of consciousness
   - Tumours can be benign or malignant. Malignant brain tumours in children are most commonly primary (originating from the brain itself), rather than metastatic
   - Less common causes of a space-occupying lesion include infection, e.g. abscess, vascular, e.g. haematoma, or large aneurysm
   - Space-occupying lesions are covered in detail in Chapters 8.1, *Headache*, 8.2, *Suspected Seizures* and 8.3, *Acute Hemiparesis* and will not be discussed further in this chapter

---

Box 8.5.2   Neuroleptic Malignant Syndrome (NMS)

What is NMS?

- NMS is a rare but life-threatening iatrogenic disorder, characterised by fever, altered mental status, muscle rigidity and autonomic dysfunction
- Features overlap significantly with serotonin syndrome, but muscle rigidity is a feature unique to NMS (as opposed to hyperreflexia and clonus in serotonin syndrome)

What causes NMS?

- The reaction is usually triggered by medications with dopamine-receptor antagonist action (or, less commonly, by rapid withdrawal of dopaminergic medications)
- These medications are often used in psychiatry, e.g. typical (haloperidol, prochlorperazine) and atypical (risperidone, quetiapine, olanzapine) antipsychotics

Who should NMS be considered in?

- NMS usually develops within hours or days after exposure to a causative drug
- NMS should be considered in all patients with the relevant medication history

How can NMS be treated?

- Rapid treatment is essential to avoid multi-organ failure and death
- Treatment involves stopping the causative drug, correcting metabolic abnormalities and intensive care support
- In severe cases, dopaminergic medications are used

Common Diagnoses
1. Substance Misuse
- This includes intoxication or withdrawal from alcohol, prescribed medications, illicit drugs or other substances, e.g. glue
- Different substances have different effects on the mental state and the same substance could have varying manifestations, depending on person, dose, environment and concurrent ingestions

Diagnoses to Consider
1. Serotonin Syndrome
- This typically occurs when using two or more serotonergic medications or drugs, including prescribed medications, herbal remedies and some foods
- Symptoms include tremors, raised temperature, agitation, increased reflexes, dilated pupils and diarrhoea
- A detailed medication history, including past and current medications and recent changes, is very important
- Serotonin syndrome can be divided into mild, moderate and severe – see Box 8.5.8 for description of differentiating examination features

When to consider: if the child is on any serotonin-enhancing medications

Box 8.5.3   Serotonergic Agents

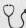

Group	Agents
Antidepressants	• Selective serotonin reuptake inhibitors (SSRIs) • Serotonin and noradrenaline reuptake inhibitors (SNRIs) • Monoamine oxidase inhibitors (MAOIs) • Tricyclic antidepressants (TCAs)
Opioids	• Tramadol • Pethidine • Fentanyl
Central nervous system stimulants	• MDMA • Amphetamines • Cocaine
Anti-emetics	• Ondansetron • Metoclopramide
Herbal	• St John's Wort • Nutmeg

Box 8.5.4   Serotonin Syndrome Risk Factors

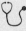

Several clinical scenarios predispose to development of serotonin syndrome:

- Introduction of single serotonergic drug
- Increase in dose of single serotonergic drug
- Switching from one serotonergic drug to another without adequate interval
- Concurrent use of two serotonergic agents (including prescribed medicines, illicit drugs or herbal remedies)
- Deliberate/accidental overdose of serotonergic drugs

2. Metabolic or Electrolyte Derangement
- This is an extremely broad differential that will typically be identified by blood tests
- The list of possible underlying causes is extensive, including some of those mentioned already
- It could also be secondary to an isolated organ dysfunction, e.g. thyroid, liver, kidney or an inborn error of metabolism
- Consanguineous parents are at an increased risk of both carrying the same gene for an inherited condition, such as those for inborn errors of metabolism

When to consider: Altered mental state in the absence of another explanation, with supporting blood tests

Box 8.5.5   Heat Stroke

- Heat stroke is a condition caused by heat exhaustion, when exposed to prolonged or significant high temperatures, exacerbated by dehydration. History is key to the diagnosis
- The result is an acute confusional state, accompanied by headache, nausea, tachypnoea, muscle cramps and a temperature of 38 °C or above
- Heat exhaustion is associated with excessive sweating, whereas those with heat stroke experience decreased sweating
- Although agitation can be present, more commonly children present floppy and sleepy
- Heat stroke is an emergency and requires urgent treatment

8.5.5 KEY HISTORY FEATURES

Dangerous Diagnosis 1
Diagnosis: Hypoxia-induced delirium

Questions
1. **Is there a background of respiratory illness?** The most common cause of hypoxia outside of the neonatal period is primary respiratory, e.g. an obstructed airway. This can be acute but may be acute on chronic, e.g. in asthma
2. **Is there a history consistent with foreign body aspiration?** Foreign body aspiration is more common between 6 months and 4 years and can rapidly cause hypoxia
3. **Has there been any colour change?** There may be episodes of pallor or cyanosis, for example in cardiovascular causes of hypoxia. The child could have been cyanotic prior to being given oxygen by emergency practitioners, before arriving in hospital

Dangerous Diagnosis 2
Diagnosis: Acute behavioural disturbance

Questions
1. **How quickly have the symptoms developed?** As the name suggests, there is an acute change in mental state that typically develops over hours to days after a trigger
2. **Is there a history of substance misuse?** The most common cause is acute on chronic substance misuse or withdrawal
3. **Is there a personal or family history of psychiatric illness?** Psychiatric disturbance accounts for up to 20% of cases. This could be the first presentation of psychiatric illness
4. **Have there been any recent illnesses?** ABD may be triggered by intercurrent illnesses, particularly in hypoglycaemia or sepsis

Dangerous Diagnosis 3
Diagnosis: Encephalitis

Questions
1. **Was there any preceding illness?** Encephalitis often occurs several days after symptoms of a non-specific viral infection
2. **Is there any history of herpetic lesions or suspected contact with herpes simplex?** Ask about vesicular lesions in the recent history or exposure to herpetic lesions elsewhere, e.g. from kissing a parent affected with a cold sore
3. **Is there any history of progressively worsening confusion, headache or seizures?** These symptoms are associated with encephalitis. Discuss baseline cognitive function with parents and whether they have noticed any deviation

Dangerous Diagnosis 4
Diagnosis: Head injury

Questions
1. **Does the parent or child report a head injury?** A witness account will confirm the diagnosis. However, the child could have sustained a head injury while unsupervised
2. **How old is the child?** Head injury in a pre-mobile child should always raise the possibility of NAI. This type of injury can be seen in children at any age
3. **Is the child on the Child Protection Register?** NAI should be considered in children with altered mental state with an unclear history, or if there are concerning features. Checks should be made to determine whether safeguarding concerns have been noted previously
4. **Has there been loss of consciousness, and for how long did this last?** Loss of consciousness is one of several concerning features, along with amnesia, recurrent vomiting, seizures and high-impact mechanism of injury, for which an urgent computed tomography (CT) scan should be considered

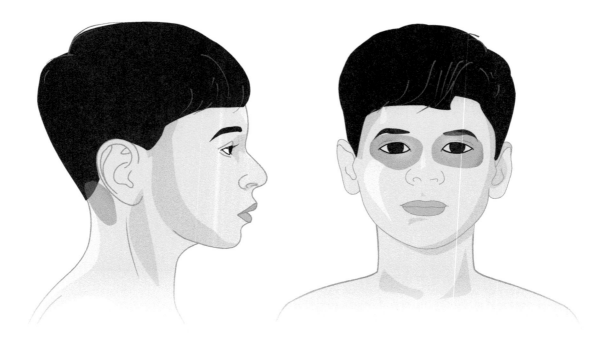

Figure 8.5.2 Signs of basal skull fracture: mastoid ecchymosis, known as 'battle sign' and periorbital bruising known as 'panda eyes'.

Box 8.5.6   Indications for Computed Tomography Head Scan in Children

Any one of	OR	More than one of
• Suspicion of non-accidental injury • Post-traumatic seizure, but no history of epilepsy • At initial assessment: Glasgow Coma Scale (GCS) <14, under 1 year GCS <15 • At 2 hours post injury GCS <15 • Suspected open or depressed skull fracture, or tense fontanelle • Any signs of basal skull fracture • Focal neurological deficit • Under 1 year: bruise, swelling or laceration >5 cm on the head		• Witnessed loss of consciousness >5 minutes • Abnormal drowsiness • 3 or more discrete episodes of vomiting • Amnesia (antegrade or retrograde) >5 minutes • Dangerous mechanism of injury (road traffic accident, fall from height >3 m, high-speed injury from an object)

Source: Adapted from National Institute for Health and Care Excellence (2019). Head injury: assessment and early management. Clinical guideline [CG176]. London: NICE.

Common Diagnosis 1
Diagnosis: Substance misuse

Questions
1. **Does the parent or child report the child taking anything?** Has the child been unsupervised with access to medications? Does the older child have the means to obtain drugs? In adolescents, alcohol is the most common substance misused
2. **What is the timeline for the change in mental state?** Any change in mental state would be expected in the period soon after taking the substance or during the period of withdrawing from it. In cases of chronic substance misuse, carers may report a gradual change in personality or behaviour, with episodic acute on chronic changes
3. **Have there been any previous admissions for similar presentations?** Previous admissions may suggest potential toxins or give information relating to wider social issues impacting on the child

8.5.6 KEY EXAMINATION FEATURES

Safety of both medical staff and child is paramount. Observation will play a key part when examining the child if they are particularly distressed or aggressive, in which case physical examination may worsen their condition.

Varying levels of consciousness may accompany some of these diagnoses, which can be accurately assessed using the Glasgow Coma Scale (GCS; see Chapter 12.2, *Assessment of Consciousness*).

Dangerous Diagnosis 1
Diagnosis: Hypoxia-induced delirium

Examination Findings
1. **Reduced oxygen saturations**. Hypoxia is essential for this diagnosis. Children will respond differently to hypoxia, but in general a sustained reduction of 5% from baseline can provoke delirium
2. **Respiratory distress.** There may be added airway sounds, such as stridor or wheeze. Signs of increased work of breathing include head bobbing, nasal flare, accessory muscle use and recessions
3. **Agitation or reduced consciousness.** Hypoxia can cause either one or both of agitation and reduced consciousness. For example, a child may initially become agitated secondary to hypoxia, before becoming quiet prior to decompensating to a respiratory arrest
4. **Cyanosis.** For cyanosis to be evident, hypoxia is likely to be marked, with saturations <85%

Dangerous Diagnosis 2
Diagnosis: Acute behavioural disturbance

Examination Findings
1. **Extreme distress.** Agitation can be extremely marked, including extreme distress, with threatening or aggressive behaviour that may put the patient or others at risk of serious harm
2. **Hyperthermia.** Behavioural problems are accompanied by autonomic dysfunction. Raised temperature is extremely common, along with profuse sweating, tachypnoea and tachycardia
3. **Increased activity.** The patient will usually display increased activity such as pacing, or excessive struggling to restraint. They may exhibit decreased pain sensitivity and can cause themselves harm as a result
4. **Signs suggestive of substance misuse.** A change in pupil size (constriction with opiates or dilatation with LSD/cocaine/ MDMA), characteristic odour (alcohol or marijuana), or evidence of administration (track marks, bruising, or a red, runny nose with glue sniffing) should be looked for

Dangerous Diagnosis 3
Diagnosis: Encephalitis

Examination Findings
1. **Fever and features of meningitis.** Fever may overlap with features of meningitis, such as headache and photophobia, which may lead to uncertainty about the diagnosis
2. **Focal neurology.** Examine limbs and cranial nerves carefully for focal neurological deficit. The child may also have seizures
3. **Altered mental state.** Alongside impaired consciousness, there may be confusion and personality change
4. **Herpetic skin lesions or evidence of other viral infections.** Assess for herpetic lesions – groups of vesicular lesions on an erythematous base. Other causes of encephalitis should also be considered, including searching for insect bites, chicken-pox or features of systemic disease

Dangerous Diagnosis 4
Diagnosis: Head injury

Examination Findings
1. **Bruising or laceration to the face or scalp.** Bruising, laceration or swelling more than 5 cm in a child less than 1 year of age warrants a CT head scan within 1 hour
2. **Abnormal pupil size.** Unequal or fixed dilated pupils are concerning features of significant intracranial pathology with raised intracranial pressure (ICP)
3. **Signs of basal skull fracture.** These should be looked for in any child with head injury

Box 8.5.7   Signs of Basal Skull Fracture

Sign	Explanation
Panda eyes (periorbital bruising)	Anterior skull base fracture
Cerebrospinal fluid (CSF) rhinorrhea	
CSF otorrhea	Middle skull base fracture
Haemotympanum	
Battle sign (mastoid bruising)	
Hypotension, tachycardia, altered respiration	Posterior skull base fracture

Common Diagnosis 1

Diagnosis: Substance misuse

Examination Findings

1. **Abnormal pupil size.** Many illicit drugs are associated with a change in pupil size (constriction with opiates or dilatation with LSD/cocaine/MDMA)
2. **Signs of substance administration.** There may be a characteristic odour (alcohol or marijuana use), or evidence of intravenous (IV) administration (track marks or bruising), or a red, runny nose with glue sniffing
3. **Other physical signs will vary according to the particular substance.** There may be tachycardia in cocaine use or raised temperature with MDMA. Signs of substance withdrawal can include tremor, tachycardia, fever, hypertension and confusion

Box 8.5.8   Signs of Mild, Moderate and Severe Serotonin Syndrome

Mild	Moderate	Severe
• Anxiety	• Agitation	• Hyperthermia
• Nausea	• Muscle rigidity	• Rhabdomyolysis
• Vomiting	• Clonus	• Seizures
• Tremor	• Brisk reflexes	• Respiratory failure
• Sweating		• Renal failure

8.5.7 KEY INVESTIGATIONS

Bedside

Table 8.5.1 Bedside tests of use in patients presenting with delirium and agitation

Test	When to perform	Potential result
Blood gas (capillary or venous)	• All children with delirium and agitation	• ↓ pH, ↓ HCO_3, ↑ lactate indicate metabolic acidosis, suggestive of circulatory compromise • ↓ pH and ↑ CO_2 indicates respiratory acidosis, suggestive of respiratory failure
Blood glucose	• All children with delirium and agitation	• ↑/↓ Glucose may be the cause for agitation and may occur in sepsis or in underlying metabolic/endocrine problems
ECG	• Suspected electrolyte disturbance	• ↑ K: peaked T wave, prolonged PR, ST depression, widened QRS, arrhythmia

CO_2, carbon dioxide; ECG, electrocardiogram; HCO_3, bicarbonate; K, potassium

Blood Tests

Table 8.5.2 Blood tests of use in patients presenting with delirium and agitation

Test	When to perform	Potential result
FBC	• All children with delirium and agitation • Normal platelet count should be confirmed before performing a lumbar puncture in an *unwell* child (not routinely necessary in a well child)	• ↑ WCC, ↑ neutrophils: bacterial infection • ↓ Platelets: DIC in meningitis/sepsis • ↓ Hb: in intracranial haemorrhage, may be falsely reassuring in acute haemorrhage • Pancytopenia: malignancy with bone marrow involvement
CRP	• All children with delirium and agitation	• Significant ↑ in bacterial infections
U&E, Ca, Mg, ammonia, LFTs	• All children with delirium and agitation	• ↑/↓ Na/K/Ca: may be cause of delirium • ↑ Ammonia, ↑ GGT: metabolic/liver disease • ↑ Urea, ↑ creatinine: renal disease
Clotting	• Systemically unwell children • Normal coagulation should be confirmed before lumbar puncture in an *unwell* child	• Severely septic patients may be coagulopathic, with derangements varying from mild coagulopathy to fulminant DIC
Blood culture	• Suspected sepsis	• Positive culture confirms bacterial infection and helps guide treatment
TFTs, morning cortisol	• Suspected endocrine disturbance	• Both hyperthyroidism and hypothyroidism should be excluded • Both Addison disease (hypocortisolism) and Cushing syndrome (hypercortisolism) should be excluded

Ca, calcium; CRP, C-reactive protein; DIC, disseminated intravascular coagulation; FBC, full blood count; GGT, gamma-glutamyltransferase; Hb, haemoglobin; LFTs, liver function tests; Mg, magnesium; Na, sodium; TFTs, thyroid function tests; U&E, urea and electrolytes; WCC, white cell count

Imaging

Table 8.5.3 Imaging modalities of use in patients presenting with delirium and agitation

Test	When to perform	Potential result
CT/MRI/MRA head (needs discussion with a paediatric radiologist)	• MRI head in suspected encephalitis • In head trauma or when non-traumatic intracranial pathology suspected	• MRI signs of encephalitis vary depending on the stage of disease. There may be signs of oedema, enhancement and hyperintensity of affected white matter • Haemorrhage, space-occupying lesion, features of raised intracranial pressure

CT, computed tomography; MRA, magnetic resonance angiography; MRI, magnetic resonance imaging

Special

Caution should be exercised when undertaking a lumbar puncture and every effort should be taken to rule out raised ICP. Senior advice should be sought.

Table 8.5.4 Special tests of use in patients presenting with delirium and agitation

Test	When to perform	Potential result
CSF MC&S and viral PCR	• Suspected encephalitis	• Viral encephalitis: ↑ WCC (lymphocytes), mildly ↑ protein, ↔ glucose • Viral PCR positive for causative organism, e.g. HSV
Urine toxicology	Suspected: • Substance misuse • Acute behavioural disturbance	• Presence of benzodiazepines, barbiturates, heroin, LSD, MDMA, cocaine, prescribed and over-the-counter medications
Hypoglycaemia screen	• If the initial blood glucose is low and the immediate cause is uncertain	• See Chapter 7.1, *Hypoglycaemia* for details

CSF, cerebrospinal fluid; HSV, herpes simplex virus; MC&S, microscopy, culture and sensitivity; PCR, polymerase chain reaction; WCC, white cell count

8.5.8 KEY MANAGEMENT PRINCIPLES

Diagnosis-specific management strategies are outlined here. It is expected that an 'ABCDE' approach to assessment and management is always undertaken (see Chapter 12.1, *The A to E Assessment*).

Box 8.5.9   General Considerations in the Management of the Agitated Patient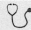

• Delirium and agitation can represent medical emergencies
• Should there be suspicion of an underlying non-organic cause, assistance should be sought from Child and Adolescent Mental Health Services (CAMHS)

• Note that using any form of restraint (including physical or chemical) places the patient at risk of deprivation of liberty

---

Dangerous Diagnosis 1
Diagnosis: Hypoxia-induced delirium

Management Principles
1. **Oxygen.** The primary treatment is provision of high-flow oxygen, titrated to saturations
2. **Treat cause.** Treatment of underlying causes is required for definitive management. Often, delirium resolves once hypoxia is corrected

Dangerous Diagnosis 2
Diagnosis: Acute behavioural disturbance

Management Principles
1. **Control of behaviour using verbal de-escalation.** Controlling the behaviour to reduce the risk of harm is the priority. Verbal de-escalation should be used in the first instance, utilising the help of parent(s)/carer(s) and any existing management plans. If this is not the first presentation, it is useful to know what has worked in the past
2. **Medical management.** Lorazepam, using an age- and weight-adjusted dose, is first line for rapid tranquillisation in a child or young person. A second dose should be considered if there is an inadequate response and a second opinion sought. Refer to local rapid tranquillisation guidelines
3. **Physical restraint as a last resort.** Physical restraint has been associated with patient injury, and even as a contributor to death. If used at all it should be for the shortest possible time to facilitate chemical restraint
4. **Investigations to seek the underlying cause of behaviour.** Once behaviour is controlled, a blood sugar test should be done once safe to do so, followed by further investigations to exclude organic causes

Dangerous Diagnosis 3
Diagnosis: Encephalitis

Management Principles
1. **IV aciclovir.** IV aciclovir is indicated if encephalitis is suspected, as herpes is the most common cause.
2. **Consider empirical meningitis treatment.** Given the overlap of clinical symptoms, it is often sensible to treat empirically with broad-spectrum antibiotics to cover for bacterial meningitis, until the diagnosis is confirmed
3. **Alert public health authorities.** Viral encephalitis is a notifiable disease.
4. **Treatment of complications.** Treatment of seizures should be managed with anticonvulsant medication (see Chapter 13.4, *Prolonged Seizure Management*)

Dangerous Diagnosis 4
Diagnosis: Head injury

Management Principles
1. **Early involvement of anaesthetics and paediatric intensive care unit (PICU).** A child with altered mental state and head injury may need intubation. This should be done without delay if GCS ≤8 or they appear agitated or combative.
2. **Neuroprotective measures for raised ICP.** In general, management of raised ICP focuses on 'neuroprotection', which encompasses strategies to avoid secondary brain injury after an acute insult. These optimise intracranial pressure and cerebral perfusion pressure to ensure adequate blood flow and oxygenation to the brain (see Chapter 13.5, *Raised Intracranial Pressure Management*)
3. **Neurosurgical referral.** The underlying injury or lesion may require a time-critical transfer to a neurosurgical centre. CT head scan should be done within 30 minutes, with images urgently sent to the neurosurgical team. Departure to neurosurgical unit should occur within a maximum of 60 minutes from end of CT scan
4. **Escalate safeguarding concerns.** In any presentation, consider whether non-accidental injury could be a cause. This is particularly true in young infants with injuries incompatible with their mobility

Common Diagnosis 1
Diagnosis: Substance misuse

Management Principles
1. **Treat for multiple possible substances.** Results from drug tests can take some time, therefore management may need to cover a number of potential toxins, especially if history is unclear
2. **An antidote may be indicated.** Several antidotes are available for specific toxins, including naloxone for opiates and N-acetylcysteine for paracetamol
3. **Poisons database for guidance on individual toxins.** All hospitals will have access to a poisons database, such as TOXBASE (**www.toxbase.org**), which provides detailed assessment and management advice for various toxin ingestions

8.6 Decreased Level of Consciousness

Karim Noordally

Department of Paediatrics, Oxford University Hospitals NHS Foundation Trust, Oxford, UK

CONTENTS

8.6.1 CHAPTER AT A GLANCE

> **Box 8.6.1   Chapter at a Glance**
>
> - A decreased conscious level is a medical emergency
> - It suggests significant brain impairment, which requires prompt assessment in order to identify the primary insult and instigate treatment, although some causes will result in permanent damage
> - Delay in treatment may result in secondary, irreversible brain injury
>
> - Encephalopathy is often used interchangeably with decreased level of consciousness, but actually also encompasses loss of memory, loss of cognitive ability, personality changes and an altered mental state
> - Inflicted injury must always be considered

8.6.2 DEFINITION

- Consciousness is a state of wakefulness with a responsiveness to the external environment
- A decreased conscious level is defined as only responsive to voice, pain or unresponsive on the AVPU (Alert, Voice, Pain, Unresponsive) Scale, or a Glasgow Coma Score (GCS) of 14 or less

Clinical Guide to Paediatrics, First Edition. Edited by Rachel Varughese and Anna Mathew. Series Editor: Christian Fielder Camm.
© 2022 John Wiley & Sons Ltd. Published 2022 by John Wiley & Sons Ltd.
Companion website: www.wiley.com/go/varughese/paediatrics

8.6.3 DIAGNOSTIC ALGORITHM

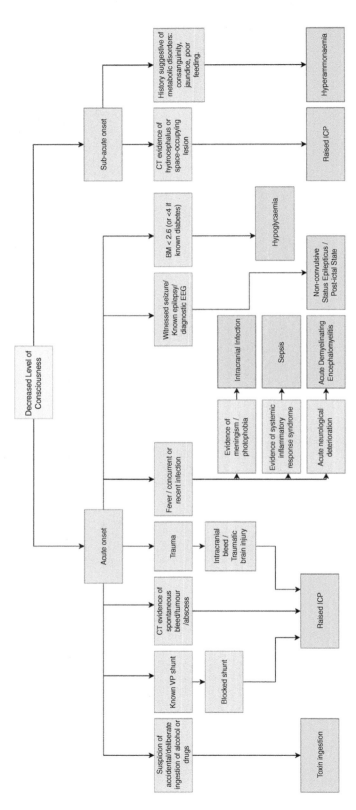

Figure 8.6.1 Diagnostic algorithm for the presentation of a decreased level of consciousness. In this instance, acute suggests onset over minutes to hours, whereas sub-acute onset suggests >24 hours of gradual decline.

8.6.4 DIFFERENTIALS LIST

Dangerous Diagnoses

All causes of a decreased level of consciousness are dangerous.

1. Raised Intracranial Pressure (ICP)

- Under normal circumstances, the volumes of the brain, blood and cerebrospinal fluid (CSF) are finely balanced. An increase in volume in one of these three variables, within the fixed space of the skull, increases the ICP
- In children with a ventriculo-peritoneal (VP) shunt, decreased conscious level is due to a blocked shunt until proven otherwise
- In infants, when the fontanelle is open, ICP is unlikely to rise unless there is a very rapidly expanding mass
- Always consider inflicted injury in traumatic head injury. History of trauma may not be forthcoming if it is being concealed

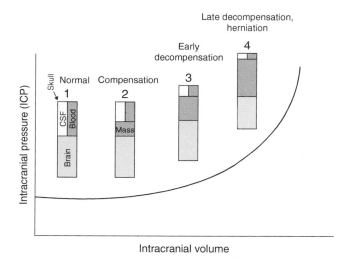

Figure 8.6.2 The Monroe–Kellie hypothesis explains that brain tissue, blood and cerebrospinal fluid (CSF) exist in equilibrium, within the fixed volume of the cranium. An increase in volume of one component forces the others to decrease. In practice, brain tissue is virtually incompressible. CSF and venous blood are compromised first. (1) Brain, blood and CSF are contained within the fixed volume of the skull. (2) A small mass causes some decrease in CSF and venous blood volume, without major increase in ICP (compensation). (3) A large mass dramatically reduces CSF and blood volume, leading to elevated ICP (decompensation). (4) Once in a decompensated state, small further increases in mass size cause a large increase in ICP, which will cause brain herniation. There are many types of herniation, the most serious being tonsillar herniation, where the cerebellar tonsils are forced down through the foramen magnum, compressing the brainstem.

Box 8.6.2   Mechanisms Contributing to Raised Intracranial Pressure (ICP)

Mechanism	Details
Increased brain volume	• Usually due to tumour or abscess • Also seen in traumatic brain injury due to cerebral oedema
Increased blood volume	• Most commonly due to haemorrhage, which may be secondary to trauma or vascular accident • Occasionally, increased intravascular blood volume without haemorrhage can result in raised ICP, for example in venous sinus thrombosis or aneurysms
Increased cerebrospinal fluid volume	• Generally divided into decreased reabsorption or increased production • Decreased reabsorption is seen in meningeal inflammation or obstructive hydrocephalus, which is often secondary to intraventricular haemorrhage (neonates) or tumour (older children) • Increased production is less common, sometimes seen with a choroid plexus tumour

2. Toxin Ingestion
- Drugs and alcohol may be ingested in combination or in isolation, either deliberately or accidentally
- Severity of presentation depends on the type and quantity of the ingested substance
- Alcohol intoxication can cause hypoglycaemia

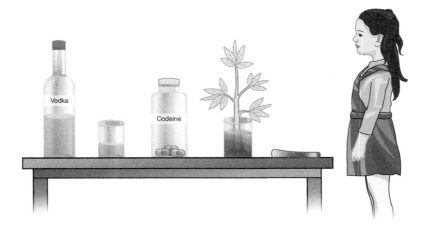

Figure 8.6.3 Drugs and alcohol may be ingested in combination or in isolation. Inappropriate ease of access for a child raises safeguarding concerns.

3. Hyperammonaemia
- A metabolic state characterised by elevated levels of ammonia in the blood
- There is a wide differential diagnosis of underlying conditions, including inborn errors of metabolism affecting the urea cycle, hepatic failure or drug ingestion
- Urea cycle defects may present throughout childhood. Early-onset urea cycle defects can involve rapid neurological deterioration with early seizures, neurological posturing and encephalopathy. Late-onset disorders may be more subtle, with eventual decompensation

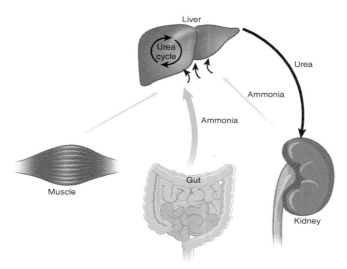

Figure 8.6.4 Ammonia is primarily derived from ingested nitrogenous compounds from the diet, metabolised by proteases and colonic flora. It is absorbed into the hepatic portal circulation and transported to the liver. A small amount comes from muscles and kidneys via the systemic circulation. In the liver, ammonia enters the urea cycle and is metabolised to urea, which is then excreted through the kidneys. A small amount of ammonia is 'detoxified' by hepatocytes using glutamine synthetase to convert ammonia to glutamine.

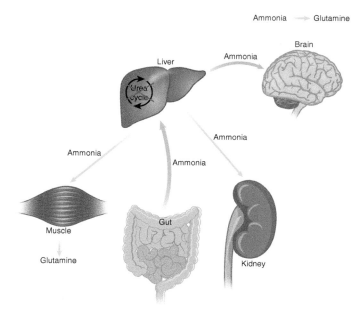

Figure 8.6.5 If there is a failure of this pathway, extrahepatic organs, such as muscles, kidneys and the brain, are relied upon to metabolise ammonia. The brain converts ammonia to glutamine in astrocytes. However, the accumulation of glutamine within brain cells causes osmotic stress, leading to oedema and ammonia encephalopathy.

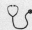

Box 8.6.3 Differential Diagnoses of Hyperammonaemia

Hyperammonaemia carries a wide differential diagnosis, many of which are rare. In general, disorders can be divided into four categories

Aetiology	Type of defect	Example
Congenital	Urea cycle enzyme defects	Carbamyl phosphate synthetase deficiency Ornithine carbamyl transferase deficiency Argininosuccinate synthetase deficiency
	Transport defects of urea cycle intermediates	Lysinuric protein intolerance Propionic acidaemia Methylmalonic acidaemia Isovaleric acidaemia and other organic acidaemias
	Miscellaneous inherited disorders (usually mild to moderate)	Fatty acid oxidation disorders Pyruvate carboxylase deficiency
Acquired	Acquired disorders	Transient hyperammonaemia of the newborn Reye syndrome Liver failure Infection with urease positive bacteria

4. Non-convulsive Status Epilepticus (NCSE)

- NCSE is a state of ongoing or intermittent epileptic activity without convulsions. It is likely more common than appreciated due to under-recognition
- NCSE is a highly heterogenous condition, making diagnosis difficult. Conditions range from manageable to fatal (often due to a fatal underlying condition)
- It is helpful to consider NCSE in three main groups: those following convulsive status epilepticus, those who have subtle clinical signs of seizure activity and those with no clinical signs
- NCSE may be seen in children with other neurological insults, such as hypoxic injury, which often indicates widespread cortical damage and carries a poor prognosis
- An urgent continuous electroencephalogram (EEG) will be an essential diagnostic tool

> **Box 8.6.4 Post-ictal State**
>
> - Children in a post-ictal state, following an epileptic seizure, will have an altered mental state with confusion, abnormal behaviour and decreased level of consciousness
>
> - This is self-limiting and transient, ending when the child returns to neurological baseline, although they may continue to be tired for several hours

5. Hypertensive Encephalopathy
- Hypertension is rare in children and is almost always secondary to an underlying condition
- Hypertension is defined by a blood pressure greater than the 95th centile for age, sex and height on two separate readings
- Even when hypertension is evident, all other causes of decreased conscious level must be ruled out
- Hypertensive encephalopathy is most commonly secondary to acute or chronic renal pathology. It might be the first manifestation of renal disease. Less commonly, it may be due to a cardiovascular or endocrine pathology
- It is essential to distinguish between hypertensive encephalopathy and hypertension secondary to raised ICP. In the latter, measures to reduce systemic blood pressure will precipitate a clinical deterioration due to a concomitant drop in cerebral perfusion pressure

6. Hypoglycaemia
- Defined as blood sugar level <2.6 mmol/L (or <4 mmol/L if known hyperinsulinism or diabetes)
- Hypoglycaemia can have detrimental effects on cerebral function and the state of consciousness
- Profound hypoglycaemia may trigger seizures and if prolonged or repeated can lead to long-lasting damage
- Hypoglycaemia is covered in detail in Chapter 7.1, *Hypoglycaemia*, and will not be discussed further in this chapter

7. Intracranial Infection/Sepsis
- Always consider sepsis of any infectious source. Intracranial infection should be highest on this list until proven otherwise
- In newborns, antenatal risk factors for sepsis help guide suspicions
- Older infants may have non-specific symptoms such as irritability or sleepiness
- Older children should be asked about symptoms of meningism
- Meningitis, encephalitis and sepsis are covered in detail in Chapters 3.1, *Fever*, 8.1, *Headache* and 8.5, *Delirium and Agitation*, and will not be discussed further in this chapter

8. Acute Demyelinating Encephalomyelitis (ADEM)
- ADEM is an immune-mediated disease of the central nervous system that usually presents following an infectious illness, with an acute and rapidly progressive neurological deterioration
- Neurological symptoms are multi-focal, and include paraparesis, encephalopathy, psychosis, brainstem deficits (dysarthria, cranial nerve dysfunction), seizures and elevated ICP
- ADEM is covered in detail in Chapter 8.4, *Acute Lower!Limb Weakness* and will not be discussed further in this chapter

9. Systemic Shock
- Circulatory shock of any cause results in reduced cerebral perfusion and will often cause a decreased conscious level
- This is covered in detail in Chapter 2.2, *Circulatory Collapse* and will not be discussed further in this chapter

8.6.5 KEY HISTORY FEATURES

Dangerous Diagnosis 1
Diagnosis: Raised intracranial pressure

Questions
1. **Has there been a headache?** Headache is the most common sign of raised ICP. Red-flag signs include early-morning headaches, progressive worsening and headache waking the child at night
2. **Is there a history of trauma?** Following trauma, always suspect intracranial bleed. Cerebral oedema occurs in traumatic brain injury, where the trauma is usually very significant
3. **What was the onset – sudden or progressive?** Aneurysmal bleed may be spontaneous, without any preceding symptoms. Space-occupying lesions can present subtly and in retrospect there is often an insidious onset of symptoms, such as headaches, vomiting, visual disturbance, behavioural change and clumsiness
4. **Has there been weight loss, night sweats or fever?** These are systemic symptoms suspicious of an underlying malignancy
5. **Is there a known VP shunt?** In patients with VP shunts, a blocked shunt should be suspected until proven otherwise

6. **Are there inconsistencies in the history?** Always remember to consider non-accidental injury in traumatic head injury. Does the history fit the presenting complaint and the age of the child? Is the story consistent or changing?

Dangerous Diagnosis 2
Diagnosis: Toxin ingestion

Questions
1. **Could the child have access to alcohol?** Adolescent patients may have easier access to alcohol, but always consider accidental ingestion by a younger patient. Even if alcohol is suspected, do not dismiss the possibility of other diagnoses
2. **Could the child have access to medications in the household?** History is vital here and directs investigations. Tricyclic antidepressants, insulin and other anti-diabetic medications may cause hypoglycaemia
3. **How did the child obtain the substance?** Inappropriate ease of access to substances raises safeguarding concerns

Dangerous Diagnosis 3
Diagnosis: Hyperammonaemia

Questions
1. **Is there a past medical history of liver or metabolic disease?** Ammonia processing occurs primarily in the liver through the urea cycle. Hepatic failure disrupts this cycle, leading to raised ammonia. Many metabolic diseases are associated with hyperammonaemia
2. **Is there a family history of infant death?** Previous infant death in the family raises the suspicion of inborn errors of metabolism
3. **Is there a history of consanguinity?** Although rare, most inborn errors of metabolism are autosomal recessive. Consanguinity significantly increases the chance of inheriting two affected alleles
4. **If a newborn, has there been difficulty with feeding?** Specifically ask about irritability, poor weight gain, difficulty feeding, recurrent vomiting, jaundice or family history of previous unexplained neonatal death
5. **If older, is there a history of behavioural problems?** There may be behavioural or psychiatric issues. There may even be a history of previous seizures

Dangerous Diagnosis 4
Diagnosis: Non-convulsive status epilepticus

Questions
1. **Is there a known seizure disorder?** NCSE can present in any child, but is more common in children with known epilepsy, particularly those with complex epilepsy syndromes. Other children at risk include those with learning difficulties and other neurological conditions
2. **How is the child's behaviour compared to baseline?** In a child with a known history of epilepsy, suspicion of NCSE may be raised by inexplicable alterations in behaviour with fluctuating lack of response or confusion. In any child, acute changes in speech, memory or school performance are suspicious
3. **Has there been a prolonged 'post-ictal' phase following a short seizure?** NCSE may start with a brief convulsive episode, followed by a period of reduced responsiveness, which might be wrongly dismissed as a post-ictal phase

Dangerous Diagnosis 5
Diagnosis: Hypertensive encephalopathy

Questions
1. **Has there been a headache, vomiting or blurred vision?** Severe headache, vomiting and blurred vision are signs of diffuse brain dysfunction from hypertensive encephalopathy
2. **Is there a known renal condition?** Hypertensive encephalopathy is most commonly due to an underlying renal condition. It is useful to ask about recurrent urine infections, which may have led to renal scarring
3. **Was the child very unwell in the neonatal period?** Invasive central umbilical lines inserted in the newborn period carry the risk of damaging the large vessels and affecting renal blood flow
4. **What is the medication/drug history?** Common drugs associated with hypertension include steroids and oestrogen-containing oral contraceptive pills. If age appropriate, ask about illicit drug use such as cocaine and amphetamines

8.6.6 KEY EXAMINATION FEATURES

Varying levels of consciousness may accompany most of these diagnoses, which can be accurately assessed using the GCS (see Chapter 12.2, *Assessment of Consciousness*).

Dangerous Diagnosis 1
Diagnosis: Raised intracranial pressure

Examination Findings
1. **Focal neurological signs.** Any focal peripheral neurology points towards a space-occupying lesion. 6th cranial nerve palsy is the classic example of a false localising sign (reflecting remote dysfunction), vulnerable to stretch by brainstem displacement. 3rd nerve palsy often manifests as dilated pupils, due to external pupilloconstrictor fibres being compromised first. 4th, 5th and 7th nerve palsies may also be seen
2. **Papilloedema.** This is swelling of the optic nerve head due to raised ICP. It requires a skilled practitioner to appreciate (often an ophthalmologist), which is difficult without pupillary dilatation
3. **Cushing's triad.** A triad of hypertension, bradycardia and bradypnoea is a late feature of raised ICP, indicating progressive brainstem compression

Dangerous Diagnosis 2
Diagnosis: Toxin ingestion

Examination Findings
1. **Alcohol smell.** Alcohol intoxication is often evident from the smell on the breath
2. **Variable findings.** Features depend on ingested substance – see Box 8.6.5

Box 8.6.5   Examination Findings with Ingestion of Different Substances   △△

Toxidrome	Mental state	Pupils	Observations	Other findings
Anticholinergic, e.g. antihistamine, TCA	Hypervigilant, hallucinating	Dilated	Temp ↑ HR ↑ BP ↑ RR ↑	Dry skin, urinary retention
Cholinergic, e.g. organophosphate pesticides, physostigmine	Confused, CNS depression	Constricted	Muscarinic: HR ↓ — Nicotinic: HR ↑ BP ↑	Salivation, lacrimation, urination, diarrhoea, GI upset, emesis
Hallucinogenic, e.g. PCP, LSD	Hallucination, agitated	Dilated	Temp ↑ HR ↑ BP ↑	Nystagmus
Opioid, e.g. morphine, heroin	CNS depression	Constricted	Temp ↓ HR ↓ BP ↓ RR ↓	Hyporeflexia, pulmonary oedema
Sedative, e.g. alcohol, benzodiazepine, barbiturates	Confused, CNS depression	Constricted	Temp ↓ HR ↓ BP ↓ RR ↓	Hyporeflexia
Serotonin syndrome, e.g. MAOI, SSRI	Confused, agitated, coma	Dilated	Temp ↑ HR ↑ BP ↑ RR ↑	Tremors, myoclonus, hyperreflexia, trismus, rigidity
Sympathomimetic, e.g. cocaine, amphetamine	Agitated, hyperalert	Dilated	Temp ↑ HR ↑ RR ↑	Tremors, seizures, hyperreflexia

BP, blood pressure; CNS, central nervous system; GI, gastrointestinal; HR, heart rate; MAOI, monoamine oxidase inhibitor; RR, respiratory rate; SSRI, selective serotonin reuptake inhibitor; TCA, tricyclic antidepressant

Dangerous Diagnosis 3
Diagnosis: Hyperammonaemia

Examination Findings
1. **Developmental delay.** Developmental delay is common
2. **Absence of specific findings.** There are no specific examination features in hyperammonaemia. The fact that specific findings are lacking makes it extremely important to remember to investigate ammonia levels

Dangerous Diagnosis 4
Diagnosis: Non-convulsive status epilepticus

Examination Findings
1. **Features of an atypical post-ictal state.** Cognitive defects in the post-ictal state are specific to each individual and in children with epilepsy, parents can often describe their typical post-ictal state. Alterations or prolongation of this is suspicious for NCSE
2. **Post-ictal delirium.** Delirium might manifest as agitated confusion or as hypoactivity, with withdrawn behaviour
3. **Abnormal movements.** NCSE is heterogenous and there are no defining specific clinical features besides the lack of convulsions. There may be other movements such as myoclonic jerks, nystagmus and lip smacking

Dangerous Diagnosis 5
Diagnosis: Hypertensive encephalopathy

Examination Findings
1. **Hypertension.** Hypertension is the mainstay of this diagnosis. Stage 1 hypertension is defined as blood pressure between 95th and 99th centiles + 5 mmHg. Stage 2 hypertension is that over 99th centile + 5 mmHg
2. **Papilloedema**. Examination for papilloedema is important, as its presence indicates malignant hypertension
3. **Seizures**. Seizures are the most common presenting sign in infants and small children with hypertensive encephalopathy.

8.6.7 KEY INVESTIGATIONS
Bedside

Table 8.6.1 Bedside tests of use in patients presenting with decreased level of consciousness

Test	When to perform	Potential result
Blood glucose	• All children with decreased level of consciousness	• Blood glucose <2.6 mmol/L is significant (<4 mmol/L if known diabetes)
Blood gas (capillary or venous)	• All children with decreased level of consciousness	• Acidosis: pH <7.35, alkalosis pH >7.45 • Respiratory acidosis – there is a reduced respiratory drive in all causes of decreased consciousness • Metabolic acidosis – consider infection, post-ictal or hyperammonaemia* • Alkalosis – consider toxin ingestion or hyperammonaemia* • Beware of artificially raised lactate in squeezed samples

* Metabolic conditions underlying hyperammonaemia can cause varied pH disturbance from alkalosis to acidosis

Blood Tests

Table 8.6.2 Blood tests of use in patients presenting with decreased level of consciousness

Test	When to perform	Potential result
FBC	• All children with decreased level of consciousness	• ↑ WCC, ↑ neutrophils suggest bacterial infection • ↓ Hb in intracranial bleed – beware of falsely reassuring Hb in acute haemorrhage
U&E, Ca, Mg	• All children with decreased level of consciousness • Electrolyte abnormalities may be the cause or consequence of intracranial pathology	• ↓ Na/Ca/Mg can cause seizures • Space-occupying lesions may cause diabetes insipidus (↑ Na) or SIADH (↓ Na) • ↑ Urea, ↑ creatinine may indicate reason for hypertensive encephalopathy, or may be a consequence of circulatory shock • Rapid correction of electrolytes (Na) may cause seizures
CRP	• All children with decreased level of consciousness	• ↑ CRP supports infection and is useful for monitoring trends
LFTs	• All children with decreased level of consciousness	• ↑ ALT, ↑ GGT, ↑ ALP, ↑ bilirubin: liver failure can cause hyperammonaemia
Ammonia	• All children with decreased level of consciousness • Must be a venous sample as capillary samples are poor quality	• Normal is <50 μmol/L, but up to 80 μmol/L is common • >100 μmol/L requires urgent specialist advice • >200 μmol/L requires urgent attention
Blood culture	• All children with suspected sepsis	• Significant growth of causative organism confirms infection • Sensitivities guide antimicrobial choice

ALP, alkaline phosphatase; ALT, alanine aminotransferase; Ca, calcium; CRP, C-reactive protein; FBC, full blood count; GGT, gamma-glutamyl-transferase; Hb, haemoglobin; LFTs, liver function tests; Mg, magnesium; Na, sodium; SIADH, syndrome of inappropriate antidiuretic hormone secretion; U&E, urea and electrolytes

Imaging

Table 8.6.3 Imaging modalities of use in patients presenting with decreased level of consciousness

Test	When to perform	Potential result
CT head	• All children with decreased level of consciousness • Quicker and better tolerated than MRI for initial screening	• Intracranial bleed (e.g. subarachnoid – often spontaneous; extradural/subdural – trauma) • Acute hydrocephalus (e.g. in blocked shunt) • Tumour • Abscess
MRI head	• Usually performed to confirm/expand upon CT findings • May require sedation as less well tolerated awake	• As above • Improved accuracy at identifying tumours • Evidence of viral encephalitis

CT, computed tomography; MRI, magnetic resonance imaging

Special

Table 8.6.4 Special tests of use in patients presenting with decreased level of consciousness

Test	When to perform	Potential result
CSF culture + viral PCR	• Suspected intracranial infection • A saved sample of CSF can be taken in case neuro-metabolic tests need to be added on • Only after CT/MRI head has excluded space-occupying lesion • Do not attempt lumbar puncture when critically unwell	• Bacterial/viral PCR can give rapid result to suggest meningitis/encephalitis • Positive culture of bacterial organism in meningitis confirms infection • ↑ Neutrophils, ↓ glucose, ↑ protein: bacterial cause • ↑ Lymphocyte, normal glucose and mildly ↑ protein: viral cause
EEG	• Suspected NCSE/epilepsy • Diagnosis may be limited if sedation given during stabilisation	• Needs specialist interpretation • Essential for diagnosis in NCSE, which may have limited or variable clinical features
Urine toxicology screen	• Suspected toxin ingestion (although diagnostic potential limited if on antiseizure medication)	• Presence of benzodiazepines, barbiturates, heroin, LSD, MDMA, cocaine, prescribed and over-the-counter medications
Hypoglycaemia screen	• If unexplained hypoglycaemia, to determine underlying cause • Involves blood and urine tests	• May reveal underlying metabolic condition predisposing to hypoglycaemia • Details are found in Chapter 7.1, *Hypoglycaemia*

CSF, cerebrospinal fluid; CT, computed tomography; EEG, electroencephalogram; MRI, magnetic resonance imaging; NCSE, non-convulsive status epilepticus; PCR, polymerase chain reaction

---

Box 8.6.6 Tips for Collection and Interpretation of Ammonia Levels

• Ammonia needs to be analysed urgently for interpretable results
• It is highly susceptible to haemolysis and needs a free-flowing sample
• Ideally, the sample should be transported rapidly to the laboratory on ice
• If ice is not quickly available, the sample should be transported rapidly at room temperature
• Delays in this process may cause an artefactual rise in ammonia. However, these samples should still be analysed with a comment about artefact

• Concentrations >100 µmol/L need discussion with a metabolic specialist, with immediate repeat if concerns about artefact. Concentrations >200 µmol/L are significantly raised and need prompt treatment
• There is great risk in rejecting a sample because of transport conditions due to delay in recognition of possible hyperammonaemia

---

8.6.8 KEY MANAGEMENT PRINCIPLES

Diagnosis-specific management strategies are outlined here. It is expected that an 'ABCDE' approach to assessment and management is always undertaken (see Chapter 12.1, *The A to E Assessment*).

All children with a decreased level of consciousness need to be urgently discussed with the Paediatric Intensive Care Unit

---

Box 8.6.7 C-spine and Airway Considerations in a Child with Decreased Level of Consciousness

	Reason for concern	Management
C-spine	• Unless otherwise known, assume any child presenting with a reduced level of consciousness has suffered a traumatic head injury with an associated cervical spine injury	• Control C-spine with manual inline stabilisation • This should not impede acute management of the airway
Airway	• GCS <9 or responding to pain on AVPU scale • Unable to maintain saturations or at risk of tiring • Possibility of delayed airway swelling following smoke inhalation or facial trauma • Potential for loss of airway maintenance during investigations and/or transfer	• 100% O_2 via non-rebreathe mask • Jaw thrust – *avoid head tilt and chin lift* • Airway adjuncts (oropharyngeal airway, laryngeal mask airway) – *avoid nasopharyngeal airway in potential head injury* • Low threshold for intubation

AVPU, Alert, Voice, Pain, Unresponsive; GCS, Glasgow Coma Scale; O_2, oxygen

Dangerous Diagnosis 1

Diagnosis: Raised intracranial pressure

Management Principles

1. **Neuroprotection.** In general, management of raised ICP focuses on 'neuroprotection', which encompasses strategies to avoid secondary brain injury after an acute insult. These optimise intracranial pressure and cerebral perfusion pressure to ensure adequate blood flow and oxygenation to the brain (see Chapter 13.5, *Raised Intracranial Pressure Management*)
2. **Safeguarding.** If there is any suspicion of non-accidental injury, discuss with a senior colleague and instigate safeguarding procedures

Dangerous Diagnosis 2

Diagnosis: Toxin ingestion

Management Principles

Management of different ingested substances is highly variable.

1. **Treat for multiple possible substances.** Results from drug tests can take some time, therefore management may need to cover a number of potential toxins, especially if history is unclear'
2. **An antidote may be indicated.** Several antidotes are available for specific toxins, including naloxone for opiates and N-acetylcysteine for paracetamol
3. **Poisons database for guidance on individual toxins.** All hospitals will have access to a poisons database such as TOXBASE **(www.toxbase.org),** which provides detailed assessment and management advice for various toxin ingestions

Dangerous Diagnosis 3

Diagnosis: Hyperammonaemia

Management Principles

1. **Discuss with metabolic centre.** Treatment of decompensated hyperammonaemia is urgent and requires highly specialised advice. If ammonia >200 µmol/L, urgent transfer is required, while instigating the following
2. **Nil by mouth.** Oral feeds should be stopped until diagnosis is known and patient is stable, to minimise further ammonia production
3. **Intravenous (IV) bolus.** An immediate bolus of 2 mL/kg 10% dextrose should be given
   - If peripheral circulation adequate → 10 mL/kg 0.9% sodium chloride should follow, *or*
   - If peripheral circulation is poor → 20 mL/kg 0.9% sodium chloride should be given instead, and repeated until perfusion improves
4. **IV maintenance fluids.** Estimate fluid deficit and calculate 24-hour volume as per routine paediatric prescribing. Deduct bolus fluid from the first 24-hour infusion volume. Give one-third of the 24-hour volume over the next 6 hours, and the remainder over the following 18 hours
5. **Medications.** Specific medications will be advised by a metabolic specialist and commonly include sodium benzoate, sodium phenylbutyrate, arginine and carnitine. All involve a loading dose over 90 minutes, followed by maintenance doses. There is a British Inherited Metabolic Diseases Group (BIMDG) online calculator for doses, volumes and rates of infusions. Carnitine should not be given if there is evidence of cardiomyopathy, cardiac arrhythmia or suspected long-chain fatty acid oxidation disorder
6. **Treat constipation.** If the patient is constipated, ammonia may be absorbed from the gut. Lactulose is recommended, although evidence is lacking
7. **Monitor glucose and potassium.** Hyperglycaemia after treatment is common – this may require an insulin infusion. Hypokalaemia is also common, and potassium can be added to fluids
8. **Recheck ammonia after 3 hours.** Re-discuss level with specialist centre. If the level is rising, urgent transfer to a metabolic centre to consider haemofiltration should be arranged

Dangerous Diagnosis 4

Diagnosis: Non-convulsive status epilepticus

Management Principles

1. **Seek urgent specialist advice.** Specialist opinion is vital. Even with electrographical evidence, there may be debate about whether the findings represent status epilepticus or widespread cortical damage. The presence of an underlying condition is important. Since NCSE encompasses a variety of heterogenous conditions, each individual case will be treated differently. Those with suspected poor prognoses will be treated aggressively with benzodiazepines, phenytoin and deep anaesthesia, where possible benefit outweighs the risk

Dangerous Diagnosis 5
Diagnosis: Hypertensive encephalopathy

Management Principles
1. **Anti-hypertensive therapy.** There is limited general consensus on management. The Royal College of Paediatrics and Child Health (RCPCH) recommends urgent advice from a paediatric nephrologist, cardiologist and paediatric intensive care unit (PICU) in guiding pharmacological treatment
2. **Rule out all other causes.** Remember that hypertension in children is rare. Ensure all other causes are ruled out, particularly raised ICP, which can itself be a cause of hypertension

8.7 Dizziness

Katie Mckinnon

Department of Paediatrics, North Middlesex University Hospital, London, UK

CONTENTS

8.7.1 CHAPTER AT A GLANCE

> **Box 8.7.1 Chapter at a Glance**
>
> - Dizziness is a fairly non-specific term, which encompasses a number of sensations
> - Can be used to describe pre-syncope, light-headedness, imbalance, ataxia, visual disturbance, weakness and true vertigo
>
> - Children can struggle to describe the characteristics of their symptoms, which may hamper diagnosis
> - Assessment is likely to reveal other features that will guide further investigations and management, whether that is neurological, ear, nose and throat, or cardiac

8.7.2 DEFINITION

- Dizziness is a feeling of loss of focus or balance
- Vertigo is an abnormal sensation of motion, where either the individual or environment is felt to be spinning

Clinical Guide to Paediatrics, First Edition. Edited by Rachel Varughese and Anna Mathew. Series Editor: Christian Fielder Camm.
© 2022 John Wiley & Sons Ltd. Published 2022 by John Wiley & Sons Ltd.
Companion website: www.wiley.com/go/varughese/paediatrics

8.7.3 DIAGNOSTIC ALGORITHM

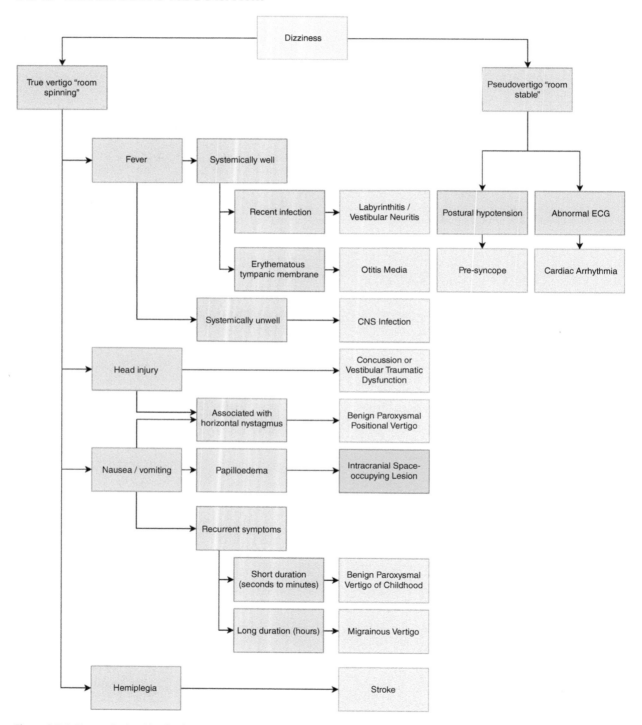

Figure 8.7.1 Diagnostic algorithm for the presentation of dizziness.

8.7.4 DIFFERENTIALS LIST

Dangerous Diagnoses

1. Infratentorial Tumour
- Infratentorial tumours can cause dizziness, particularly those affecting the cerebellum and brainstem
- The three most common types of infratentorial tumours are pilocytic astrocytomas (35%), medulloblastomas (30%) and ependymomas (15%)
- In children over 1 year old, over two-thirds of intracranial tumours arise from the brainstem or cerebellum
- Medulloblastoma is a primitive neuroectodermal tumour (PNET) occurring in the cerebellum. It is the most common malignant brain tumour in children

---

Box 8.7.2   Brainstem Strokes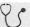

- Vertigo is a well-described early symptom of brainstem strokes
- However, as a whole, stroke is a rare cause of dizziness
- Isolated vertigo or dizziness strongly predicts a non-cerebrovascular cause

- Most brainstem strokes involve ischaemia in the distribution of the basilar or vertebral arteries, and may be associated with diplopia, blurred vision, an occipital headache and altered conscious level – Stroke is covered in detail in Chapter 8.3

Box 8.7.3   Medications Associated with Dizziness

Group	Examples
Anticonvulsants	Lamotrigine, carbamazepine, oxcarbazepine, gabapentin, pregabalin, benzodiazepines
Antipsychotic medications/antidepressants	Fluoxetine, sertraline
Antihypertensives	Beta blockers, lisinopril, amlodipine
Diuretics	Furosemide, hydrochlorothiazide
Analgesics	Codeine, ibuprofen, naproxen
Antibiotics	Ciprofloxacin, co-amoxiclav
Others	Barbiturates, ethanol, ketamine, carbon monoxide

Common Diagnoses

1. Concussion
- The vast majority of dizziness due to head trauma is as a result of concussion, with signs usually appearing within minutes to hours of a head injury
- A concussion is a temporary brain injury, which is self-limiting and self-resolving
- In children with head trauma, it is important to consider mechanical causes for dizziness. Blunt or penetrating injuries to the temporal or parietal areas may cause vestibular dysfunction, from inner ear or ossicular disruption ± tympanic membrane perforation

2. Vestibular Migraine
- The most common cause of dizziness in children, accounting for almost 25% of presentations
- Dizziness is known as migrainous vertigo
- Affected children are usually over 10 years of age
- Episodic vertigo can occur before, during, after or even without the headache

3. Benign Paroxysmal Vertigo of Childhood (BPVC)
- BPVC is one of the most common causes of dizziness in children, thought to be a variant of paediatric migraine
- It is seen in otherwise well children, mostly occurring in those less than 10 years of age. Girls are more commonly affected
- Vertigo is typically of sudden onset, lasting minutes with spontaneous resolution, and may occur in clusters
- It is distinct from benign paroxysmal positional vertigo (BPPV), which is uncommon in childhood. Some controversy exists around this

4. Otitis Media
- Common infection in children, accounting for 10% of children with dizziness
- Acute serous or suppurative otitis media causes vestibular disturbance and vertigo
- Chronic otitis media can lead to mastoiditis or cholesteatoma

5. Vestibular Neuritis
- Vestibular neuritis accounts for 8.5% of children with dizziness
- It is characterised by acute vertigo following a recent infection, such as mumps, measles, Epstein–Barr virus or herpes virus
- Labyrinthitis is a specific type of vestibular neuritis, associated with hearing loss

Diagnoses to Consider
1. Initial Orthostatic Hypotension (IOH)
- Pre-syncopal (feeling of impending loss of consciousness) symptoms including blurred vision and dizziness develop when changing posture from the lying position to sitting or standing
- IOH is not the same as orthostatic hypotension (OH), as symptoms are brief and short-lived. OH is associated with autonomic dysfunction, whereas IOH is not
- The blood pressure fall in IOH is transient, with quick recovery, unlike in OH where hypotension is more significant and prolonged
- If dizziness occurs immediately after posture change, it is likely to be IOH, which could lead to syncope. If it occurs minutes after posture change, consider an alternative diagnosis of OH
- Symptoms can be more prominent with intercurrent illnesses or dehydration

When to consider: in children with symptoms following postural change, without loss of consciousness

2. Benign Paroxysmal Positional Vertigo (BPPV)
- BPPV is uncommon in children and, when present, is often associated with previous head injury
- Dizziness is triggered by changing head position, and is associated with nausea, vomiting and horizontal nystagmus. Unidirectional, horizontal nystagmus is commonly noted during an episode
- Episodes tend to last less than a minute, but can be intense

When to consider: in children with a personal or family history of migraine or recent concussion

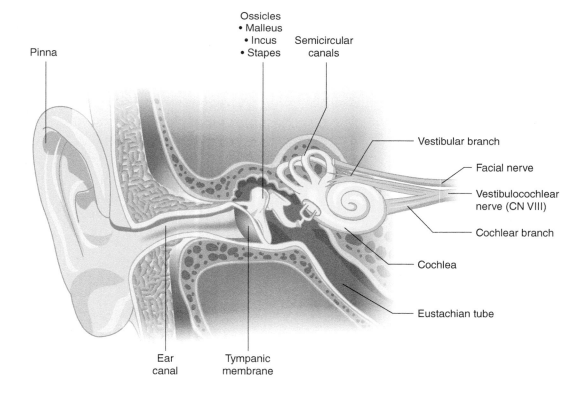

Figure 8.7.2 Anatomical diagram of the ear, showing some of the structures that can be affected in dizziness.

3. Cardiac Arrhythmia
- Various arrhythmias may be associated with pre-syncope or syncope
- Palpitations or chest pain are strong indicators of underlying cardiac disease
- There may be a family history of cardiac conditions or previous sudden death
- Cardiac arrhythmias are covered in detail in Chapters 2.3 and 2.5

When to consider: in those with palpitations, chest pain or family history of these

8.7.5 KEY HISTORY FEATURES

Dangerous Diagnosis 1
Diagnosis: Infratentorial tumour

Questions
1. **Are there symptoms suggesting raised intracranial pressure (ICP)?** The most common presentation of posterior fossa tumours in children is raised ICP. Symptoms include unexplained vomiting, visual disturbance or headache, particularly if it is progressive, worse on bending down/straining or on waking
2. **Has there been a change in vision or coordination?** Infratentorial tumours will cause diplopia, poor balance, ataxia and dysmetria
3. **Has there been a change in personality or behaviour?** There may be a general change in behaviour such as lethargy, irritability or decreased performance at school

Common Diagnosis 1
Diagnosis: Concussion

Questions
1. **Is there a history of recent head injury?** Head injuries are common in children, so determining the mechanism, location and severity is important
2. **After the injury, how has the child's behaviour been?** Common symptoms of a concussion include sleepiness, poor concentration, easy distraction and emotional lability. Post-traumatic amnesia may last up to 24 hours
3. **Any hearing loss?** Hearing loss would make a temporal bone fracture and consequent vestibular dysfunction more likely. If there is no hearing loss, dizziness may be due to concussion, whiplash syndrome or be non-specific
4. **Are there inconsistencies in the history?** Always remember to consider non-accidental injury in traumatic head injury. Does the history fit the presenting complaint and the age of the child? Is the story consistent or changing?

Common Diagnosis 2
Diagnosis: Vestibular migraine

Questions
1. **How old is the child?** Vestibular migraine is a disease of the older child, usually over 10 years of age
2. **How long does the dizziness last?** Duration has a wide range from minutes to up to 72 hours, which can precede or occur during or even after the migrainous episode
3. **Is the child photosensitive during these episodes?** Sensitivity to light and noise is often described
4. **Is there a family history of headaches?** A family history of migraine is frequently present

Common Diagnosis 3
Diagnosis: Benign paroxysmal vertigo of childhood

Questions
1. **How long does the dizziness last?** The dizziness and instability have a sudden onset and last for less than a minute at a time, often occurring in clusters
2. **What other symptoms manifest at the same time?** Autonomic symptoms such as sweating, pallor, expressions of fear, nausea and vomiting may also be present
3. **Any hearing loss?** As a peripheral vestibular disorder, there is no hearing loss
4. **How old is the child?** The age range is usually 2–12 years, with most presentations under 4 years
5. **Does the child or anyone in the family have headaches?** As a form of migraine syndrome, a personal or family history can also be present

Common Diagnosis 4
Diagnosis: Otitis media

Questions
1. **Is there any ear pain?** Inflammation and fluid collection behind the tympanic membrane can lead to significant pain. In younger patients, this could be evident by the child pulling at their ears
2. **Is there any change to hearing?** Fluid in the middle ear can cause acute conductive hearing loss
3. **Have they had ear infections in the past?** Otitis media is common in children, and recurrence can cause further complications

Common Diagnosis 5
Diagnosis: Vestibular neuritis

Questions
1. **Have there been any recent coughs and colds?** Recent viral upper respiratory tract infections can precede vestibular neuritis
2. **How long does the dizziness last?** The dizziness can be quite protracted, lasting hours to days
3. **How does the child describe the dizziness?** The child will often complain of the room spinning around, quite often with nausea and vomiting
4. **Has there been chickenpox in the past?** Ramsay Hunt syndrome is a specific type of vestibular neuritis with reactivation of varicella zoster virus. Facial nerve paralysis and hearing loss often accompany the painful shingles rash
5. **Is there any loss of hearing?** This would make labyrinthitis more likely than other types of vestibular neuritis. Hearing loss resolves over a few weeks, but there is a risk of permanent hearing loss with labyrinthitis.

8.7.6 KEY EXAMINATION FEATURES

Varying levels of consciousness may accompany many of these diagnoses, which can be accurately assessed using the Glasgow Coma Scale (see Chapter 12.2).

Dangerous Diagnosis 1
Diagnosis: Infratentorial tumour

Examination Findings
1. **Signs of raised ICP.** Signs of raised ICP are the most common presentation. Altered mental state includes irritability, lethargy and drowsiness. Hypertension with tachycardia can be a sign of raised ICP, with bradycardia and respiratory depression a late feature
2. **Focal neurological abnormality.** A focal abnormality could localise a lesion. Alternatively, there may be false localising signs, due to indirect nerve compression from raised ICP – 6th nerve is most commonly affected
3. **Cerebellar signs.** Cerebellar tumours may cause ataxia, nystagmus, dysmetria and poor coordination (see Chapter 8.1, *Headache*, Box 8.1.8, *Clinical Signs of Cerebellar Dysfunction, Using the Acronym DANISH*)
4. **Head tilt.** Head tilt may reflect tonsillar herniation or a 4th nerve palsy related to diffuse brainstem tumour

Common Diagnosis 1
Diagnosis: Head trauma

Examination Findings
1. **Wounds.** Look for visible injuries, whether lacerations, bruising or swelling, to explain the dizziness
2. **Abnormal ear examination.** Haemotympanum, otorrhoea and tympanic membrane perforation could all suggest a focal middle ear injury such as a temporal bone fracture
3. **Neck pain.** Whiplash injuries are associated with neck pain due to muscle and ligamentous sprains. The cervical spine should be assessed and immobilised if cervical spinal injury is suspected
4. **Normal examination.** Neurological examination tends to be normal in children with concussion, and any abnormalities should prompt investigation for an alternative diagnosis

Common Diagnosis 2

Diagnosis: Vestibular migraine

Examination Findings

1. **Spontaneous or positional nystagmus during episodes.** Nystagmus can be present during an attack
2. **Normal neurology in interim.** Between episodes, neurological examination is usually normal

Common Diagnosis 3

Diagnosis: Benign paroxysmal vertigo of children

Examination Findings

1. **Normal neurology in interim.** Between the short episodes of dizziness, neurological examination will be normal
2. **Holding on to furniture.** During episodes, children will feel acutely unsteady and hold on to nearby people or objects

Common Diagnosis 4

Diagnosis: Otitis media

Examination Findings

1. **Abnormal ear examination.** Erythema and bulging of the tympanic membrane are indicative of otitis media
2. **Changes to the mastoid process.** Swelling and erythema of the mastoid, with anterior displacement of the pinna, could suggest mastoiditis as a complication of otitis media
3. **Impaired hearing.** Conductive hearing loss can be caused by the infection, either acutely or as a more chronic change

Common Diagnosis 5

Diagnosis: Vestibular neuritis

Examination findings

1. **Vesicular rash.** Vesicles along the auditory canal could suggest a shingles outbreak and Ramsay Hunt syndrome. Unilateral facial nerve palsy will also be present
2. **Impaired hearing.** Viral infection of the auditory nerve causes hearing loss and is a feature of labyrinthitis

8.7.7 KEY INVESTIGATIONS

Not all children will require invasive investigations; often diagnoses are made on clinical evidence from history and examination. Consider carefully which investigations are required for which patient.

Bedside

Table 8.7.1 Bedside tests of use in patients presenting with dizziness

Test	When to perform	Potential result
Blood sugar	• All children with dizziness	• Blood sugar <2.6 mmol/L – hypoglycaemia*
Electrocardiogram (ECG)	• Suspected cardiac arrhythmia	• Variety of arrhythmias or evidence of structural heart disease

*2.6 is not an absolute cut-off, with variable evidence in different settings.

Blood Tests

Table 8.7.2 Blood tests of use in patients presenting with dizziness

Test	When to perform	Potential result
FBC	Suspected otitis media with complications	• ↑ WCC, ↑ neutrophils: bacterial infection
CRP	Suspected otitis media with complications	• ↑ CRP in infection

CRP, C-reactive protein; FBC, full blood count; WCC, white cell count

Imaging

Table 8.7.3 Imaging modalities of use in patients presenting with dizziness

Test	When to perform	Potential result
CT head	• In suspected infratentorial tumour where MRI not possible	• Tumour
MRI head	• In a more stable situation with central neurological concerns, an MRI will give more detailed information	• Accurate assessment of tumours and vestibular abnormalities

Note: Children with suspected concussion should not require any imaging. However, following head injury, always remember to consider a CT head if there is suspicion of intracranial injury. See Chapter 8.5, Box 8.5.6

CT, computed tomography; MRI, magnetic resonance imaging

Special

Table 8.7.4 Special tests of use in patients presenting with dizziness

Test	When to perform	Potential result
Pure tone audiogram	• In any child with suspected hearing impairment due to benign paroxysmal vertigo of childhood (BPVC), vestibular neuritis, complicated otitis media, trauma or Ramsay Hunt syndrome	• Normal hearing: BPVC • Reduced hearing: vestibular neuritis, otitis media, trauma and Ramsay Hunt
Specialised vestibular testing	• If vertigo symptoms persist without clear diagnosis, specialist further tests may be required, such as electronystagmography and audiometry	• Helps to identify serious and rare vestibular abnormalities

8.7.8 KEY MANAGEMENT PRINCIPLES

Diagnosis-specific management strategies are outlined here. It is expected that an 'ABCDE' approach to assessment and management is always undertaken (see Chapter 12.1).

Dangerous Diagnosis 1
Diagnosis: Infratentorial tumour

Management Principles
1. **Urgent neurosurgical specialist input.** Time-critical transfer to a neurosurgical unit may need to be arranged. Hydrocephalus/raised ICP will require emergency procedures such as ventriculostomy/external ventricular drain and shunt placement
2. **Manage raised ICP.** Medical treatment of raised ICP may be required prior to surgical management. Involvement of intensive care colleagues is essential, as children may require intubation and ventilation (see Chapter 13.5, *Raised Intracranial Pressure Management*)
3. **Tertiary oncology.** Management of paediatric brain tumours is complex and often involves surgery, radiotherapy (conventional or proton beam) and chemotherapy. Many children have lasting impairments of physical or cognitive ability, behaviour, hearing or vision, and will need long-term multi-disciplinary support

Common Diagnosis 1
Diagnosis: Concussion

Management Principles
1. **Reassurance and safety net.** After a minor head injury, children and parents may be concerned about intracranial bleed. It is important to reassure them that there is no clinical evidence of bleed, and that symptoms are in keeping with concussion. Importantly, offer safety-net advice to return if neurological red-flag symptoms emerge
2. **Simple analgesia.** Simple analgesia such as paracetamol can be taken for headaches
3. **Avoidance of contact sports.** Contact sports should be avoided for at least 3 weeks

4. **Advise children and parents of post-concussion syndrome.** Post-concussion syndrome is an essential part of the discussion. This can last for days to weeks and can be distressing for the patient. The syndrome is characterised by three main aspects: cognitive (memory, attention, concentration), physical (headache, sleep, dizziness, fatigue) and emotional (irritability, anger, depression, anxiety) difficulties

---

Box 8.7.4   Red Flags to Discuss When Safety Netting for Concussion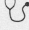

Patients should be counselled that any of the following red flags in a child with a concussion should prompt urgent medical review:

- Loss of consciousness or inability to be woken
- Any fits (collapsing or passing out suddenly)
- Clear fluid coming out of ears or nose
- Increasing disorientation
- Impairment of understanding or speaking

- Severe headache
- Weakness in one or more limbs
- Blurred or double vision
- Vomiting

Common Diagnosis 2
Diagnosis: Vestibular migraine

Management Principles
1. **Headache diary.** Monitoring of headache frequency, triggers and response to any treatments is beneficial, particularly if certain triggers can be avoided. Information about headache disorders and support organisations is also useful to aid understanding of the illness
2. **Acute treatment.** In children aged 12 years and older, treatment for migraine episodes can include a triptan with a non-steroidal anti-inflammatory drug (NSAID) or paracetamol, plus an anti-emetic. Symptomatic treatment for the vertigo is usually with antihistamines such as promethazine
3. **Prophylactic treatment.** Options can include topiramate, propranolol, amitriptyline or acupuncture

Common Diagnosis 3
Diagnosis: Benign paroxysmal vertigo in children

Management Principles
1. **Reassurance.** As the episodes are of short duration, most do not require treatment acutely
2. **Prophylactic treatment.** If episodes are sufficiently frequent to impair quality of life, preventative medications such as those used in other migraine disorders may be suitable

Common Diagnosis 4
Diagnosis: Otitis media

Management Principles
1. **Self-care.** In most children, antibiotics are not required. Paracetamol and ibuprofen as anti-pyretics and analgesics are beneficial, along with advice regarding the infection and usual self-limiting natural history of the illness
2. **Antibiotics.** Immediate antibiotics should be given in children who are systemically unwell, with evidence of mastoiditis, or with a comorbidity making them at higher risk of complications. They should also be considered in children less than 2 years old with infection in both ears, and children of any age with otorrhoea following tympanic membrane perforation. 'Delayed' antibiotic prescriptions could be considered, for use if symptoms worsen or are not improving within 3 days. Antibiotic choice should be based on local guidance

Common Diagnosis 5
Diagnosis: Vestibular neuritis

Management Principles
1. **Symptomatic treatment.** Antiemetics, antihistamines and anticholinergics can all be used in the management of symptoms. This should only be for the first 3 days of the presentation, as they can delay long-term recovery if continued
2. **Steroids.** A short course of an oral steroid can be considered in the absence of contraindications, with some improvement in short-term recovery
3. **Anti-viral therapy.** If Ramsay Hunt syndrome is present, with herpes zoster infection, then an anti-viral medication can be considered in addition to a steroid

9.1 Urticaria

Gary Foley

Department of Paediatrics, Centre for Genomics and Child Health, London, UK

CONTENTS

9.1.1 CHAPTER AT A GLANCE

> **Box 9.1.1   Chapter at a Glance**
>
> - Urticaria is a common skin rash, which can be present in benign or emergency conditions
> - Differentiating between acute and chronic urticaria is important to guide investigations

9.1.2 DEFINITION

Colloquially known as *wheals* (also spelled 'weals'), urticaria is raised erythematous patches with pale centres, pruritic in nature and lasting anywhere from a few minutes to 24 hours.

9.1.3 DIAGNOSTIC ALGORITHM

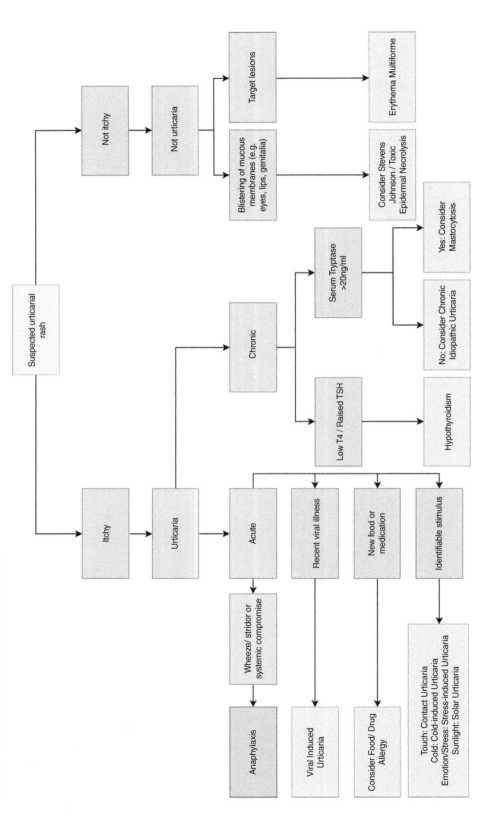

Figure 9.1.1 Diagnostic algorithm for the presentation of urticaria.

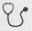

Box 9.1.2   Urticaria – Acute versus Chronic

- **Acute:** urticaria with complete resolution, usually within 6 weeks (generally within 48 hours)
- **Chronic:** urticaria that appears regularly and persists beyond 6 weeks

9.1.4 DIFFERENTIALS LIST

Dangerous Diagnoses

1. Anaphylaxis

- Widespread type 1 hypersensitivity immunoglobulin (Ig) E–mediated mast cell degranulation leading to systemic shock
- The most common cause in childhood is a reaction to a food allergen
- Anaphylaxis presents with urticaria, cough/stridor/wheeze ± hypotension
- Can evolve into cardiac (due to profound hypotension as a result of vasodilatation and increased vascular permeability) or respiratory (obstructive airways) arrest
- 20% may have a secondary (biphasic) anaphylactic reaction 2–6 hours after treatment

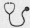

Box 9.1.3   Stevens–Johnson Syndrome (SJS) and Toxic Epidermal Necrolysis (TEN)

SJS and TEN are variants of the same condition and are dermatological emergencies, caused by a type 4 hypersensitivity reaction. SJS and TEN do not actually cause urticaria, but are very important differentials to consider due to their high morbidity and potential mortality

Prodrome	• Fever, sore throat, coryza, conjunctivitis, myalgia
Rash	• Sudden onset of macular erythematous rash, often starting on the face, neck and trunk, rapidly spreading over hours to days, and may become confluent • Painful blistering of skin with separation of the epidermis and dermis • Mucous membrane involvement is a defining feature, with involvement of conjunctivae, mouth, throat, anus and genitalia
Distribution	• SJS: <10% of body surface area affected • TEN: >30% of body surface area affected • Involvement of 10–30% is considered to be an overlap of the two
Triggers	• Most commonly related to an infection (herpes simplex virus) in children • Less commonly related to medications (sulphonamides and penicillin-based antibiotics)
Examination	• Mucosal involvement • Non-specific skin tenderness upon palpation • Nikolsky sign: gentle rubbing of the skin causes the epidermis to peel away • Flat, purpuric lesions precede desquamation • Blistering and desquamation can be as severe as third-degree burns
Complications	• Dehydration • Infection of skin and mucous membranes – sepsis • Acute respiratory distress syndrome • Acute kidney injury • Shock • Disseminated intravascular coagulopathy
Management	• ABCDE approach • Referral to burns unit or paediatric intensive care required • Stop medications identified as triggers • Analgesia: topical and parenteral • Supportive hydration: intravenous (IV) fluid maintenance, including replacement of insensible losses • Skin and wound dressing: non-adhesive dressings • Oral / Eye care: anaesthetic ± antibacterial mouth wash, conjunctival lubrication • Steroids: topical, oral or IV • Immunomodulation: seek specialist advice

Common Diagnoses
1. Viral-Induced Urticaria
- Presents 3–5 days into a viral illness
- Waxing and waning urticarial rash that resolves over a 24–48-hour period without treatment
- Often leads to a misdiagnosis of drug allergy
2. Food Allergy
- An IgE-mediated type 1 hypersensitivity reaction
- Urticaria appears 0–2 hours after ingestion or exposure
- Affects 6–8% of the paediatric population in the UK
- Most common food allergens in children are cow's milk, hen's eggs, soya, peanuts, tree nuts, wheat, fish and shellfish
- Other symptoms can include vomiting, diarrhoea or respiratory symptoms

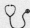

Box 9.1.4   Prevalence of Food Allergy in Children in the UK

Allergenic food	% of UK paediatric population affected
Cow's milk	2–3%
Hen's eggs	1.5–2.5%
Peanuts	1–2%
Tree nuts*	1–2%
Fish	0.2–0.5%
Wheat**	0.2–0.4%

*Includes hazelnut, cashew, pistachio, almond, brazil nut
**This is an immunoglobulin E–mediated allergy; coeliac disease is not an allergy and is categorised differently

3. Idiopathic Chronic Urticaria
- Chronic urticaria is defined as urticaria lasting for more than 6 weeks, or recurrent episodic urticaria over months
- Affects 1 in 200 children
- No cause is found in 50% of cases of chronic urticaria
- Self-limiting and usually resolves by adolescence/early adulthood
- Some will have an underlying autoimmune disease such as systemic lupus erythematosus (SLE)

Box 9.1.5   Types of Hypersensitivity Reactions

	Type 1: Immediate	Type 2: Cytotoxic	Type 3: Immune complex reaction	Type 4: Delayed hypersensitivity
Immune reactant	IgE	IgG or IgM	IgG and IgM	T cells
Time of onset	Within 1 hour	Minutes to hours	3–8 hours	48–72 hours (or longer)
Examples	<ul><li>Local and systemic</li><li>Anaphylaxis</li><li>Seasonal hay fever</li><li>Food allergy</li><li>Drug allergy</li></ul>	<ul><li>Transfusion reactions</li><li>Haemolytic disease of the newborn</li><li>Autoimmune haemolytic anaemia</li><li>Goodpasture's syndrome</li></ul>	<ul><li>Post-streptococcal glomerulonephritis</li><li>Rheumatoid arthritis</li><li>Systemic lupus erythematosus</li></ul>	<ul><li>Contact dermatitis</li><li>SJS/TEN</li><li>Type 1 diabetes mellitus</li><li>Hashimoto's thyroiditis</li></ul>

Ig, immunoglobulin; SJS, Stevens–Johnson syndrome; TEN, toxic epidermal necrolysis

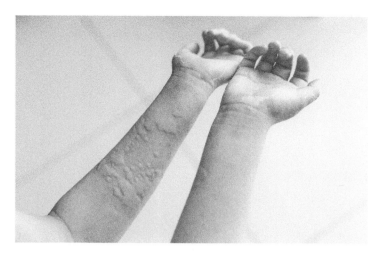

Figure 9.1.2 Urticaria is characterised by a raised, itchy erythematous rash. It can either be localised, as in this picture, or more generalised, which can give clues as to the aetiology. Source: Reproduced with permission from Shutterstock.

Diagnoses to Consider

1. Drug Allergy
- An IgE-mediated type 1 hypersensitivity reaction
- Not common in childhood
- Antibiotics (penicillin) and non-steroidal anti-inflammatory drugs (NSAIDs) are the most common triggers
- In chronic conditions requiring repeated courses of antibiotics, such as cystic fibrosis, drug allergy can develop over time; otherwise if the child has tolerated the medication previously, it is less likely to be the cause
- Viral-induced urticaria often leads to a misdiagnosis of drug allergy. A thorough clinical history can help prevent this

When to consider: if there is a clear history of ingestion/administration and immediate reaction

2. Hypothyroidism
- About 10% of those with chronic spontaneous urticaria are found to have autoimmune thyroid disease, such as Hashimoto's thyroiditis
- Hashimoto's thyroiditis is more common in females and often presents late in adolescence or adulthood

When to consider: in chronic urticaria with no identifiable trigger, particularly if there is a goitre or family history of thyroid/autoimmune disease

3. Mastocytosis
- Rare disease – can be localised (cutaneous) or cause systemic symptoms
- Involves pathological mast cell proliferation, which may be associated with other myeloproliferative or myelodysplastic disorders
- The elevated mast cell level results in inappropriate release of histamine, heparin and tryptase
- Skin changes include urticaria and angioedema, and may be triggered by temperature change, fever or exercise
- Systemic symptoms include weight loss, night sweats, appetite loss, nausea, vomiting or diarrhoea

When to consider: in those with chronic urticaria, particularly if organomegaly is present

---

Box 9.1.6   Erythema Multiforme (EM) Minor: An Urticaria Mimic

- EM minor is a benign rash caused by infections, e.g. herpes simplex virus, *Mycoplasma pneumoniae* or less commonly medications
- It is often mistaken for an urticarial rash, but unlike urticaria it is not pruritic
- The rash is typically erythematous, papular and non-tender. 'Target' or 'bull's-eye' lesions are pathognomonic

- Lesions usually start on the hands and feet. Arms, legs and torso are the most common areas affected in children
- Lesions spontaneously resolve over a 2–4-week period, leaving discoloured patches (brownish/blueish in nature) that also resolve over time

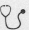

Box 9.1.7   Environmental Causes of Urticaria

- Urticaria can have a variety of external triggers, which often become apparent after several episodes following exposure
- These include contact (physical), solar (light), stress (hormonal), cold (temperature), water (aquagenic) and vibration (vibratory)
- It is possible to have more than one trigger
- Physical pressure causes histamine release and subsequent urticarial lesions

- Stress may trigger a hormonal-driven reaction leading to urticarial-type lesions
- Dermatographism (literally meaning 'writing on skin') is a separate entity where contact causes linear wheals to form

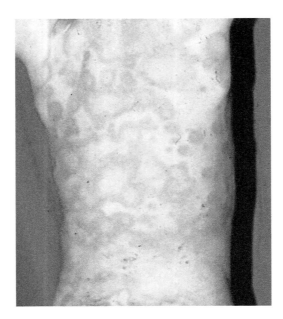

Figure 9.1.3 Erythema multiforme: an urticaria mimic. Source: Reproduced with permission from Newell, S.J., and Darling, J.C. (2014). *Paediatrics lecture notes*. Chichester: Wiley Blackwell.

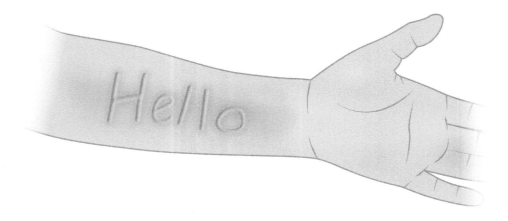

Figure 9.1.4 Dermatographism is a benign skin disorder in which urticaria appears where firm pressure is applied to the skin, allowing children to write and draw on their skin

9.1.5 KEY HISTORY FEATURES

Dangerous Diagnosis 1
Diagnosis: *Anaphylaxis*
Anaphylaxis is a clinical diagnosis that should lead to emergency treatment being initiated without waiting for a detailed history (see Chapter 13.2).

Questions
1. **Does the child have a known food/drug allergy?** In children, food will be the most common cause of anaphylaxis. In severe allergy, minimal exposure, even inhalation (e.g. through cooking), can cause anaphylaxis
2. **How soon after ingestion did the symptoms begin?** Symptoms usually begin within minutes of exposure, progress rapidly, and can lead to shock and death if not managed appropriately
3. **Did the child experience any tightness in the throat, abdominal pain, 'feeling of doom', dizziness or fainting?** These are just few of the symptoms of anaphylaxis that children may complain of soon after ingesting an allergen. Delayed reactions are also possible

---

Box 9.1.8   Symptoms of Anaphylaxis in Children

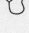

- Urticarial rash
- Swelling of lips/tongue/face
- Difficulty in breathing, with cough/wheeze/stridor
- Feeling of 'doom'
- Abdominal pain

- Nausea and vomiting
- Dizziness/fainting
- Disorientation/confusion (concerning for shock, impending cardiac arrest)

Common Diagnosis 1
Diagnosis: Viral-induced urticaria

Questions
1. **Was there evidence of a viral illness?** This is a non-specific reaction to viral antigens, which is not allergenic in nature. Cough, coryza and fevers will often precede the onset
2. **What are the pattern and timing of the rash?** The urticaria migrates around the body and leaves no marks once resolved

Common Diagnosis 2
Diagnosis: Food allergy

Questions
1. **Is this a new or accidental exposure?** If new, it is essential to try to identify the trigger. If an accidental exposure has occurred, re-education is essential (though most happen outside the home)
2. **When was the suspected food ingested?** Food allergy typically presents within 2 hours of exposure to the allergen (usually within the first 15 minutes)
3. **Is there a history of asthma?** Children with peanut allergy have a higher likelihood of severe asthma. Both conditions will need early intensive management

Common Diagnosis 3
Diagnosis: Idiopathic chronic urticaria
1. **Are there features of any other diagnoses?** Idiopathic chronic urticaria is a diagnosis of exclusion, and can only be considered when other potential causes have been ruled out

---

Box 9.1.9   Symptoms of Acquired Hypothyroidism in Children

- Faltering growth
- Delayed puberty
- Delayed tooth development
- Goitre
- Fatigue

- Constipation
- Coarse hair
- Dry skin
- Weight gain
- Intolerance to cold

Note that congenital hypothyroidism, which is present from birth, has different symptoms, with a significant impact on intellectual ability if untreated

9.1.6 KEY EXAMINATION FEATURES

Dangerous Diagnosis 1
Diagnosis: Anaphylaxis

Examination findings
1. **Swollen eyes/face.** Angioedema can occur, leading to swelling of the face, genitals and extremities
2. **Stridor and wheeze.** Due to laryngeal oedema and bronchoconstriction, stridor, wheeze and cough may be present, which can sometimes be confused with acute asthma
3. **Hypotension.** Anaphylaxis causes a distributive shock due to capillary leak and vasodilation, and hypotension can be profound

Common Diagnosis 1
Diagnosis: Viral-induced urticaria

Examination Findings
1. **Inflamed and injected pharynx and tympanic membranes.** The most common illness associated is a viral upper respiratory tract infection (URTI)
2. **Moveable rash.** The urticaria arises 1–7 days after the onset of the viral illness, and may come and go in various parts of the body

Common Diagnosis 2
Diagnosis: Food allergy

Examination Findings
1. **Facial and lip swelling.** Often when the food allergen has been in contact with the lips, angioedema will occur
2. **Widespread urticaria.** If ingested, the food allergen will cause a systemic reaction leading to widespread urticaria
3. **Isolated area of urticaria.** If the food allergen has only been in contact with a certain region of skin, isolated urticaria may be noted

Common Diagnosis 3
Diagnosis: Idiopathic chronic urticaria

Examination Findings
1. **Butterfly rash (malar rash).** Erythematous rash of the face that is associated with SLE, which can in some cases follow a history of idiopathic chronic urticaria
2. **Otherwise well child.** In most cases, the child is otherwise well

9.1.7 KEY INVESTIGATIONS

The majority of diagnoses are clinical. Any investigations need to be targeted to specific triggers or suspected underlying conditions.

Blood Tests

Table 9.1.1 Blood tests of use in patients presenting with urticaria

Test	When to perform	Potential result
TFTs	• Suspected hypothyroidism	• ↓ T_4 level, ↑ TSH level are diagnostic of hypothyroidism
Tryptase level	• Suspected mastocytosis • Although will be elevated after anaphylaxis, of limited diagnostic value	• ↑ Tryptase level: mastocytosis (highly elevated) • Not always useful in children
Total IgE	• Recurrent or chronic urticaria	• Provides supporting information for atopic status
Allergen-specific RAST	• Urticaria with suspected trigger	• Confirmation of allergy to suspected trigger

Ig, immunoglobulin; RAST, radioallergosorbent test; TFTs, thyroid function tests; TSH, thyroid-stimulating hormone

Imaging

Table 9.1.2 Imaging modalities of use in patients presenting with urticaria

Test	When to perform	Potential result
Ultrasound thyroid	• Suspected hypothyroidism if serum thyroid function tests are abnormal	• Enlarged, lobulated thyroid is a feature of Hashimoto's thyroiditis
Ultrasound abdomen	• Suspected mastocytosis to evaluate liver and spleen size	• Organomegaly consistent with mastocytosis

Special

Table 9.1.3 Special tests of use in patients presenting with urticaria

Test	When to perform	Potential result
Skin prick testing	• Urticaria with suspected trigger	• Confirmation of sensitisation

---

Box 9.1.10   Skin Prick Testing

- Skin prick testing involves placing an aliquot of the suspected allergen on the skin and introducing it into the epidermis using a small lancet
- A positive control (histamine) is used to ensure the child can react if allergic and a negative control (saline) is used to ensure they do not have contact urticaria, which would skew the results

- A positive result is when the sample produces a wheal that measures more than 3 mm in diameter. This only infers that the child is 'sensitised' to the allergen
- Some children who are sensitised to food allergens never have a reaction, which is why a clinical history is paramount – never skin prick test children for foods they do not react to, as this will only lead to anxiety and a possible mislabelling of allergy

---

9.1.8 KEY MANAGEMENT PRINCIPLES

Diagnosis-specific management strategies are outlined here. It is expected that an 'ABCDE' approach to assessment and management is always undertaken (see Chapter 12.1).

Dangerous Diagnosis 1
Diagnosis: Anaphylaxis

Management Principles
1. See Chapter 13.2

Common Diagnosis 1
Diagnosis: Viral-induced urticaria

Management Principles
1. **Symptomatic relief.** Paracetamol for pyrexia or antihistamines to combat the associated itch may be used

Common Diagnosis 2
Diagnosis: Food allergy

Management Principles
1. **Antihistamines.** Second-generation antihistamines such as cetirizine can be given. If vomiting, can use intravenous (IV) or intramuscular (IM) chlorpheniramine
2. **Observation.** Observe for 2–6 hours to ensure the reaction is subsiding

3. **Allergy management plan.** Arrange a review by the allergy team or make a referral. The patient should have an emergency management plan in place upon discharge

Common Diagnosis 3
Diagnosis: Idiopathic chronic urticaria

Management Principles
1. **Antihistamines.** A combination of non-sedating antihistamines during the day and sedating antihistamines at night can provide symptomatic relief
2. **Topical treatment**. Soothing agents such as calamine lotion and aqueous cream can be tried.
3. **Specialist options**. Persistent distressing symptoms require specialist allergy advice. Other options include tricyclic antidepressants, leukotriene receptor antagonists, glucocorticoids, anti-IgE monoclonal antibodies and immunosuppressive therapy

9.2 Non-blanching Rash

Nicola J. Smith

Department of Paediatrics, Oxford University NHS Foundation Trust, Oxford, UK

CONTENTS

9.2.1 CHAPTER AT A GLANCE

> **Box 9.2.1   Chapter at a Glance**
>
> - Rashes are common in children
> - Widespread public health education with the 'glass test' has made parents aware of the association between a non-blanching rash and meningococcal sepsis – a cause for significant anxiety
>
> - Non-blanching rash can be a sign of life-threatening illness, although commonly there may be a benign underlying cause
> - It is important to be able to quickly diagnose, treat and reassure if appropriate

9.2.2 DEFINITION

Red-to-purple macular skin lesions, which do not fade under pressure, caused by intradermal capillary bleeding.

> **Box 9.2.2   Definitions**
>
> - **Non-blanching**: does not disappear when pressure applied
> - **Petechiae**: smaller than 2 mm. Often like pinpricks or speckles. Can appear red-purple-near black
> - **Purpura**: larger than 2 mm, blotches of red-purple non-blanching rash
> - **Ecchymosis**: bruises. Cover larger areas. Often more diverse colour palette. Consequence of capillary and venular bleeding
>
> - **Purpura fulminans**: a haematological emergency with skin necrosis and disseminated intravascular coagulation, which may progress rapidly to multi-organ failure. Can be a complication of severe sepsis or may occur as an autoimmune response to infection

Clinical Guide to Paediatrics, First Edition. Edited by Rachel Varughese and Anna Mathew. Series Editor: Christian Fielder Camm.
© 2022 John Wiley & Sons Ltd. Published 2022 by John Wiley & Sons Ltd.
Companion website: www.wiley.com/go/varughese/paediatrics

9.2.3 DIAGNOSTIC ALGORITHM

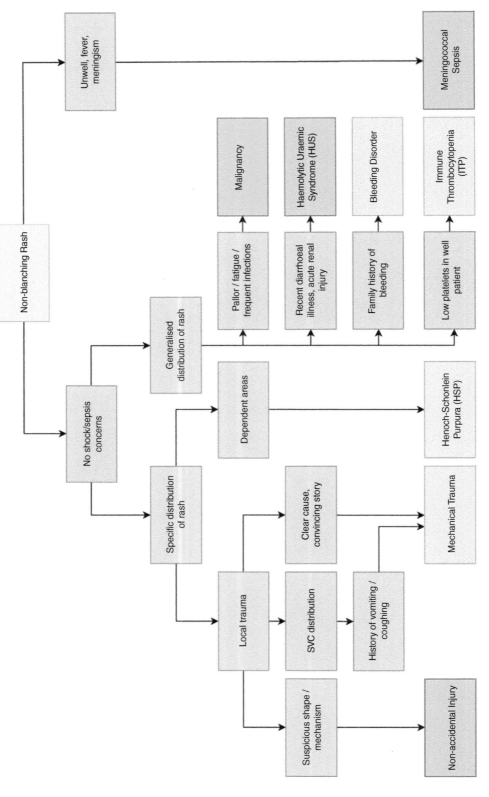

Figure 9.2.1 Diagnostic algorithm for the presentation of non-blanching rash.

9.2.4 DIFFERENTIALS LIST

Dangerous Diagnoses

1. Meningococcal Sepsis

- Caused by *Neisseria meningitidis,* of which there are currently 13 recognised serogroups
- Transmission is via respiratory secretions, but most infections lead to harmless colonisation
- Susceptible individuals develop invasive disease within 4 days of exposure
- An outer membrane endotoxin (lipopolysaccharide) causes the inflammatory response, leading to capillary leak syndrome and intravascular thrombosis, which may result in extensive organ damage. This is known as disseminated intravascular coagulation and can cause purpura fulminans
- Following the inclusion of routine immunisation against several meningococcal subtypes in the UK, the incidence of invasive meningococcal disease has significantly reduced.

Box 9.2.3   Infectious Causes of Thrombocytopaenia   △△

Sepsis itself can lower platelet counts through disseminated intravascular coagulation. Besides sepsis, other infections can directly cause thrombocytopenia

Bacteria	Viruses	Parasites
• *Meningococcus* • *Streptococcus pneumoniae* • *Haemophilus influenzae* species • Diphtheria • Leptospirosis	• Epstein–Barr • Parvovirus B19 • Human herpesvirus 6 and 7 • Enteroviruses • Measles • Varicella • Human immunodeficiency virus • Congenital cytomegalovirus • Dengue • Haemorrhagic fevers: Ebola virus, Rift Valley virus and Lassa fever	• Malaria • Leishmaniasis

---

2. Malignancy

- Many types of malignancy cause a reduction in platelet number due to bone marrow infiltration. Petechiae/purpura/bruising is a result of this thrombocytopenia
- The most common malignancy of childhood is acute lymphoblastic leukaemia (ALL), but other haematological and solid malignancies can also infiltrate the bone marrow
- Other consequences of bone marrow failure are anaemia and immunosuppression due to reduction in red and white blood cells
- Malignancy is discussed in several other chapters: Chapters 3.3, *Lymphadenopathy*, 4.1, *Bruising*, 4.2, *Pallor* and 5.2, *Abdominal Mass*. It will not be discussed further in this chapter

3. Haemolytic Uraemic Syndrome (HUS)

- The triad of haemolytic anaemia, thrombocytopenia and acute kidney injury, often preceded by a diarrhoeal illness that is bloody
- Major type is diarrhoea associated, due to *Escherichia coli* O157, which produces verocytotoxin (Shiga toxin), which in turn causes endothelial damage
- Despite thrombocytopenia, non-blanching rash is rarely a predominant symptom
- HUS is covered in detail in Chapters 4.2, *Pallor* and 5.4, *Diarrhoea*, and will not be discussed further in this chapter

Common Diagnoses

1. Mechanical Trauma

- Capillaries damaged by mechanical forces can cause a non-blanching rash
- Minor local trauma, such as the pressure of a tightened seatbelt, tightly laced shoes or a heavy school rucksack, can cause petechiae to appear over the various pressure points
- Petechiae may form in the distribution of the superior vena cava (above the nipple line) when there have been episodes of vomiting or coughing. These are caused by transient increased intrathoracic pressure

Box 9.2.4 Non-accidental Injury (NAI)

- When considering causes for mechanical trauma, always consider NAI
- Any injury purposefully inflicted on a child may result in petechiae or bruising

- Injuries caused by hands, implements, squeezing or ligatures can leave marks similar in appearance to purpuric rashes. See Chapters 4.1, *Bruising* and 12.5, *Safeguarding*

2. Immune Thrombocytopenia (ITP)
- Previously described as idiopathic thrombocytopenic purpura, this is the most common acquired disorder of coagulation
- An immune-mediated thrombocytopenia, involving an inappropriate immunoglobulin (Ig) G autoantibody response, leading to opsonisation and destruction of platelets
- ITP may be primary or secondary
- Typically seen in young (2–5 years), previously healthy children, with another peak during adolescence
- Often referred to as idiopathic, but many children present following a viral illness

3. Henoch–Schönlein Purpura (HSP)
- HSP is a systemic IgA vasculitis affecting the skin, mucosal membranes, joints and kidneys
- Palpable purpura are a key aspect of diagnosis, which may be associated with petechiae and ecchymoses. These are usually symmetrical, typically affecting gravity-dependent areas such as the lower limbs and buttocks
- Purpura is accompanied by arthritis in 50–75%, abdominal pain in 50% and renal involvement in 25–50% of children
- May be precipitated by infection, classically haemolytic streptococci
- Painful scrotal oedema is noted occasionally in affected boys

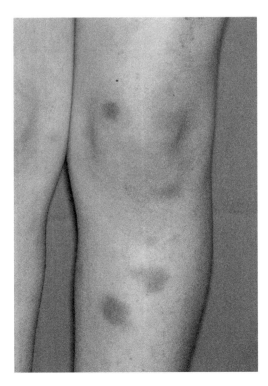

Figure 9.2.2 Immune thrombocytopenic purpura. Source: Reproduced with permission from Newell, S.J., and Darling, J.C. (2014). *Paediatrics lecture notes*. Chichester: Wiley Blackwell.

Diagnoses to Consider

Bleeding Disorders

- Bleeding disorders may be inherited or acquired
- There are three broad categories: coagulation disorders, fibrinogen disorders and platelet disorders. Some are very rare. These are addressed in Chapter 4.1, *Bruising*, Box 4.1.11, *Rare Bleeding Disorders*

When to consider: in those with significant purpura or ecchymoses following minor pressure/trauma, or those with prolonged bleeding following minor procedures

---

Box 9.2.5   Bleeding Disorders in Children

Hereditary disorders	Acquired defects
• Haemophilia A (factor VIII deficiency)	• Vitamin K deficiency
• Haemophilia B (factor IX deficiency)	• Liver disease
• Von Willebrand's disease	• Disseminated intravascular coagulation
• Other coagulation factor defects	• Antibody-generated coagulation disorders
• Platelet defects: Bernard–Soulier syndrome, Glanzmann thrombasthenia	

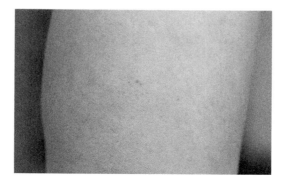

Figure 9.2.3 Typical appearance of a petechial rash with lesions <2 mm. Source: Reproduced with permission of Shutterstock.

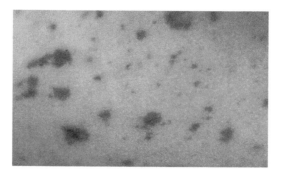

Figure 9.2.4 Typical appearance of a purpuric rash with lesions >2 mm. Source: Reproduced with permission from Newell, S.J., and Darling, J.C. (2014). *Paediatrics lecture notes*. Chichester: Wiley Blackwell.

9.2.5 KEY HISTORY FEATURES

Dangerous Diagnosis 1

Diagnosis: Meningococcal septicaemia

Questions

1. **Has the child been febrile?** Fever and malaise are invariably present. It is often abrupt in onset, with the child deteriorating very rapidly and becoming severely unwell
2. **How unwell is the child?** Parents will typically describe their child becoming suddenly very unwell, listless and lethargic, with varying degrees of disorientation
3. **Are there any symptoms indicative of meningitis?** Specifically ask about headache, photophobia, neck stiffness, decreased/altered consciousness and seizures. Meningococcal septicaemia can present in isolation and be fatal even in the absence of meningitis. However, neurology must always be evaluated, as the presence of meningitis will alter management

Common Diagnosis 1

Diagnosis: Mechanical causes

Questions

1. **Is there a history of coughing or vomiting?** Repeated coughing or vomiting causes increased intrathoracic pressure, which in turn can causes capillary damage in the distribution of the superior vena cava (SVC)
2. **Has there been any local trauma to the area?** Often the cause can seem quite innocuous, and so probing for any changes in habits or different activities may be required. This could extend to clothing, jewellery, carrying heavy items, recreational activities and school activities
3. **Is the child otherwise well?** Mechanical petechiae are not a result of generalised illness, apart from any preceding coughing/vomiting. As a result, children should be well

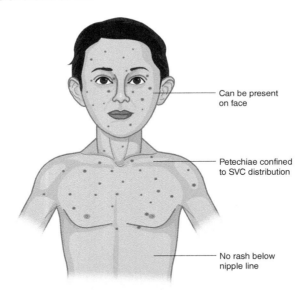

Can be present on face

Petechiae confined to SVC distribution

No rash below nipple line

Figure 9.2.5 Distribution of petechial rash caused by increased pressure in the superior vena cava (SVC).

Common Diagnosis 2

Diagnosis: Immune thrombocytopenia

Questions

1. **What was the onset of the bruising?** ITP tends to cause the sudden appearance of bruising or mucocutaneous bleeding
2. **Does the child have any other symptoms?** Children with ITP are typically otherwise well, with no other significant symptoms

3. Is there a history of a recent viral illness? ITP is frequently preceded by a viral illness about 10–14 days before the onset of the purpura

Common Diagnosis 3
Diagnosis: Henoch–Schönlein purpura

Questions
1. **Has the nature and distribution of the rash evolved over time?** The rash of HSP often appears as raised urticarial-type lesions, before morphing into purpura. The rash typically begins in a symmetrical distribution on the lower legs and then spreads to involve the back of the legs up to the bottom, and over time involves the extensor surfaces of the upper limbs
2. **Is there any joint pain?** Transient arthritis of multiple joints, especially knees and ankles, is common. Children are sometimes unable to bear weight
3. **Are there any abdominal symptoms?** HSP is often accompanied by abdominal pain, vomiting and gastrointestinal bleeding, all precipitated by bowel wall haemorrhages. Children are at risk of developing intussusception
4. **Haematuria.** 25–50% of children have renal involvement, and there may be macroscopic haematuria

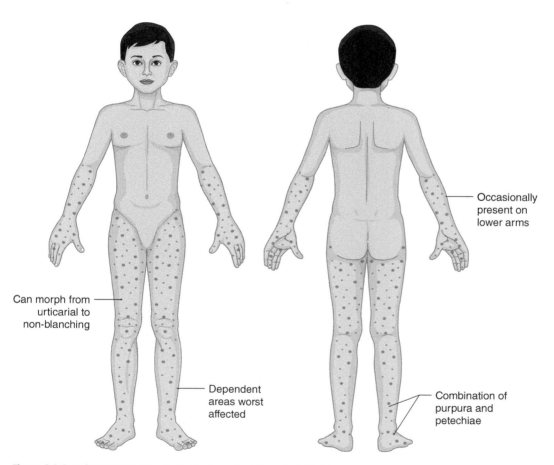

Figure 9.2.6 Body areas typically affected by the rash of Henoch–Schönlein purpura.

9.2.6 KEY EXAMINATION FEATURES

See Chapter 12.2 for assessment of consciousness using the Glasgow Coma Scale (GCS).

Dangerous Diagnosis 1

Diagnosis: Meningococcal septicaemia

Examination Findings

1. **Features of meningism.** There may be neck stiffness, photophobia and headache. Kernig's and Brudzinski's signs may be positive (see Chapter 8.1, *Headache*, Figure 8.1.4, *Detecting meningism on clinical examination*)
2. **Progressive rash.** Meningococcal sepsis can progress rapidly, so the rate of progression is important. A child may go from having a few petechiae in the morning to a fulminant rash by the afternoon
3. **Altered mental status.** Children may be drowsy, lethargic, confused or irritable. In addition, lack of response to social cues and a weak, high-pitched or continuous cry are all concerning.
4. **Signs of shock.** Capillary leak can cause distributive shock. Signs include tachycardia, poor peripheral perfusion, tachypnoea, oliguria and hypotension

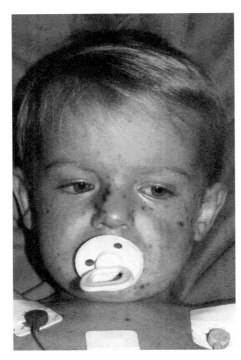

Figure 9.2.7 Petechial rash on the face and trunk in a child with meningococcal septicaemia. Source: Reproduced with permission from Newell, S.J., and Darling, J.C. (2014). *Paediatrics lecture notes*. Chichester: Wiley Blackwell.

Common Diagnosis 1

Diagnosis: Mechanical causes

Examination Findings

1. **Clinically well child.** The child looks well, is playful, running around, behaving normally. If vomiting or coughing has been present, the child may be recovering from a minor illness
2. **Petechial rash in the distribution of the superior vena cava.** No purpura, only petechiae. With a history of cough/vomiting, the rash is only present above the nipple line, typically involving the face, upper chest and back
3. **Petechial rash in the distribution of mechanical trauma.** Rash may be present over bony prominences, or areas consistent with history of trauma, e.g. sporting injury or carrying a school bag

Common Diagnosis 2

Diagnosis: Immune thrombocytopenia

Examination Findings

1. **Macular petechial or purpuric lesions.** Isolated purpura or petechiae may be the only examination finding. Serious bleeding is uncommon (1–3%)
2. **Clinically well child.** The child looks well, is playful, running around, behaving normally

Common Diagnosis 3
Diagnosis: Henoch–Schönlein purpura

Examination Findings
1. **Palpable rash.** Rash may begin as urticaria and progress to palpable purpura, preceding other symptoms by ~4 days. The distribution of the rash is typically initially over the lower legs, which then extends up the back of the legs to involve the bottom. Over time, the rash can also develop over the upper limbs
2. **Abdominal tenderness.** Non-specific abdominal tenderness is typical, but must be monitored closely, as children can develop several gastrointestinal complications, including intussusception
3. **Joint swelling and pain.** Arthritis/arthralgia affects up to 75% of those with HSP, predominantly affecting the knees and ankles. Usually resolves within a week
4. **Scrotal swelling/tenderness.** Boys may have a painful, swollen scrotum

9.2.7 KEY INVESTIGATIONS

Most children will require some baseline investigations, unless there is strong clinical evidence of a benign cause. Consider carefully which investigations are required for which patient.

Bedside

Table 9.2.1 Bedside tests of use in patients presenting with non-blanching rash

Test	When to perform	Potential result
Urine dipstick	• Suspected HSP	• + Blood, + protein: renal involvement in HSP and dictates management
Blood gas (capillary or venous)	• Suspected meningococcal septicaemia	• ↓ pH, ↓ HCO_3, ↑ lactate: metabolic acidosis, suggestive of sepsis • ↑/↓ Glucose may occur in sepsis

HCO_3, bicarbonate; HSP, Henoch–Schönlein purpura;

Blood Tests

Table 9.2.2 Blood tests of use in patients presenting with non-blanching rash

Test	When to perform	Potential result
FBC	• All children with a non-blanching rash unless strong clinical evidence of a benign cause	• ↓ Platelets: in ITP may be <20 × 10^9/L, in DIC secondary to sepsis • ↑ WCC, ↑ neutrophils: bacterial infection
Blood film	• All children with a non-blanching rash	• Left shift of neutrophils in infection • Platelet count might be falsely low on FBC due to platelet aggregation, but clumps are obvious on examination of film • Peripheral blasts indicate malignancy
U&E	• All children with a non-blanching rash unless strong clinical evidence of a benign cause	• ↑ Urea, ↑ creatinine in acute kidney injury as a result of sepsis, or rarely HSP
CRP	• Suspected meningococcal septicaemia	• Significant ↑ in bacterial infections
Clotting screen	• All children with a non-blanching rash unless strong clinical evidence of a benign cause	• ↑ PT and APTT time, ↓ fibrinogen: DIC
Whole-blood PCR for *Neisseria meningitidis*	• Suspected meningococcal septicaemia	• Confirm meningococcal disease in absence of positive blood culture
Blood cultures	• Suspected meningococcal septicaemia	• Positive culture confirms bacterial infection • Sensitivities will guide antibiotic treatment

APTT, activated partial thromboplastin time; CRP, C-reactive protein; DIC, disseminated intravascular coagulation; FBC, full blood count; HSP, Henoch–Schönlein purpura; ITP, immune thrombocytopenia; PCR, polymerase chain reaction; PT, prothombin time; U&E, urea and electrolytes

Box 9.2.6   Platelet count interpretation

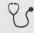

Platelet count	Interpretation
>80 × 10⁹/L	Normal haemostasis as long as platelet function is not altered
50–80 × 10⁹/L	Increased bleeding with trauma is likely, but spontaneous bleeding would be unusual
20–50 × 10⁹/L	A mild bleeding diathesis is expected
<20 × 10⁹/L	Spontaneous mucosal bleeding can occur
<10 × 10⁹/L	Spontaneous severe bleeding can occur

Box 9.2.7   Investigations in Henoch–Schönlein Purpura (HSP)

- HSP initially only requires blood pressure and urine dipstick
- If evidence of renal involvement, other than isolated microscopic haematuria, urea and electrolytes, liver function tests, bone profile, full blood count and clotting should be performed, with consideration given to anti-streptolysin O titre, antiDNAse B, complements, antineutrophil cytoplasmic antibody and immunoglobulins
- Persistent dipstick proteinuria warrants measurement of urine protein:creatinine ratio

9.2.8 KEY MANAGEMENT PRINCIPLES

Diagnosis-specific management strategies are outlined here. It is expected that an 'ABCDE' approach to assessment and management is always undertaken (see Chapter 12.1, *The A to E Assessment*).

Dangerous Diagnosis 1
Diagnosis: Meningococcal septicaemia

Management Principles
1. **Fluid resuscitation**. Intravenous (IV) fluids are part of the A to E assessment, and they are particularly important in the management of meningococcal sepsis, where fluid-refractory shock can occur
2. **Urgent broad-spectrum antibiotics**. This is the most important aspect of the management of sepsis. Antibiotics, typically an IV high-dose cephalosporin, should be given as soon as meningococcal septicaemia is suspected
3. **Early paediatric intensive care involvement**. Very close monitoring for signs of deterioration is required, with respiration, pulse, blood pressure, oxygen saturations and Glasgow Coma Scale score. Rapid deterioration is likely, regardless of initial severity, and may require intensive resuscitation
4. **Alert public health authorities.** Confirmed bacterial meningitis is a public health concern and the appropriate authorities should be informed. Contact tracing might be required, with prophylactic antibiotics provided to high-risk contacts.

See Chapter 13.1, *Sepsis Management*, and Chapter 13.5, *Raised Intracranial Pressure Management*.

Common Diagnosis 1
Diagnosis: Mechanical causes

Management Principles
1. **Reassurance and education.** Reassure parents that no serious illness is present, explain the mechanism of the rash, and inform them that it will fade with no complications
2. **Adjustments to contributing factors.** If a specific cause is found, adjustments should be made to avoid recurrence

Common Diagnosis 2
Diagnosis: Immune thrombocytopenia

Management Principles
1. **Activity restriction and education.** Children should be advised to restrict activities that carry a risk of bleeding from traumatic injury, e.g. contact sports. These decisions are collaborative with the family and there is no strict guidance. Protective helmets should be used when cycling. Education of risks and safety net advice for excessive bleeding should be discussed

2. **Avoidance of antiplatelet medications.** Non-steroidal anti-inflammatory drugs (NSAIDs) including ibuprofen should be avoided, although clinically significant bleeding with these drugs is unlikely

3. **Menstrual control.** Females who menstruate can consider hormonal therapy to inhibit menses and prevent severe menorrhagia

4. **Watchful waiting.** Most children will remain clinically stable, without dangerous bleeding. In the absence of significant bleeding, there is no strict numerical threshold for platelet count, and even $<10^9$/L can be tolerated

5. **Tranexamic acid.** Although this has no effect on platelets, it is helpful in stabilising clots with mucosal bleeding (e.g. gum or nose) or heavy periods

6. **IV immunoglobulin.** IVIg infusion is effective in 75% of patients, by halting the immune destruction of platelets. It is indicated in significant bleeding. Effects last up to 6 weeks

7. **Platelet transfusion.** The effect of a platelet transfusion is very short-lived, lasting only 24 hours. It is indicated as an emergency treatment in severe or life-threatening bleeding

8. **Steroids.** Occasionally, steroids can be used to increase platelet count, but this decreases as soon as steroids are stopped. Side effects are common

9. **Splenectomy.** In ITP, most platelets are destroyed in the spleen. However, splenectomy is a major operation, leaving children vulnerable to lifelong risk of infection by encapsulated organisms. It may be considered in chronic ITP, with recurrent severe bleeding

10. **Monitor platelet count.** Monitoring of platelet counts should be regular. This varies between units, but might initially be weekly, with spacing when improvement is seen. The majority of children recover spontaneously within 3–6 months

Common Diagnosis 3

Diagnosis: Henoch–Schönlein purpura

Management Principles

1. **Analgesia.** Regular paracetamol and a short course of NSAIDs can be used if not otherwise contraindicated

2. **Education.** HSP generally self-resolves within 6 weeks, but there is a recurrence rate of 33%. The rash is usually the last symptom to disappear

3. **Urinalysis and blood pressure (BP) follow-up.** Regular repetition of urinalysis and BP is required, either through an ambulatory care unit or the GP. This starts weekly for the first month, 2-weekly for the next 2 months and then single visits at 3, 6 and 12 months. Any macroscopic haematuria, 2+ proteinuria or BP >95th centile should prompt paediatric review

4. **Corticosteroids.** Prednisolone can be used to reduce the duration and severity of abdominal pain and joint pain, but does not impact renal complications. Always rule out an evolving intussusception before prescribing steroids

5. **Renal support.** Long-term morbidity is usually related to renal complications, which tend to present in the first 6 months, but occasionally take up to 12 months. 1% of children with HSP will progress to end-stage renal failure. Persistent purpura, severe abdominal pain or bloody stools are risk factors for significant renal involvement. Renal specialist review is required for hypertension, abnormal renal function, persistent macroscopic haematuria and persistent proteinuria

9.3 Other Childhood Rashes

Gary Foley

Department of Paediatrics, Centre for Genomics and Child Health, London, UK

CONTENTS

9.3.1 CHAPTER AT A GLANCE

Box 9.3.1 Chapter at a Glance

- Rash is an extremely common presenting complaint in children
- Many rashes should not cause concern and can be managed conservatively, but they can be difficult to distinguish from each other

- Occasionally, investigation and treatment are required

9.3.2 DEFINITION

Rashes are disruptions in the skin barrier, which can be caused by a range of triggers, including, but not limited to, infection, allergies, irritants, autoimmunity and genetics.

Clinical Guide to Paediatrics, First Edition. Edited by Rachel Varughese and Anna Mathew. Series Editor: Christian Fielder Camm.
© 2022 John Wiley & Sons Ltd. Published 2022 by John Wiley & Sons Ltd.
Companion website: www.wiley.com/go/varughese/paediatrics

9.3.3 DIAGNOSTIC ALGORITHM

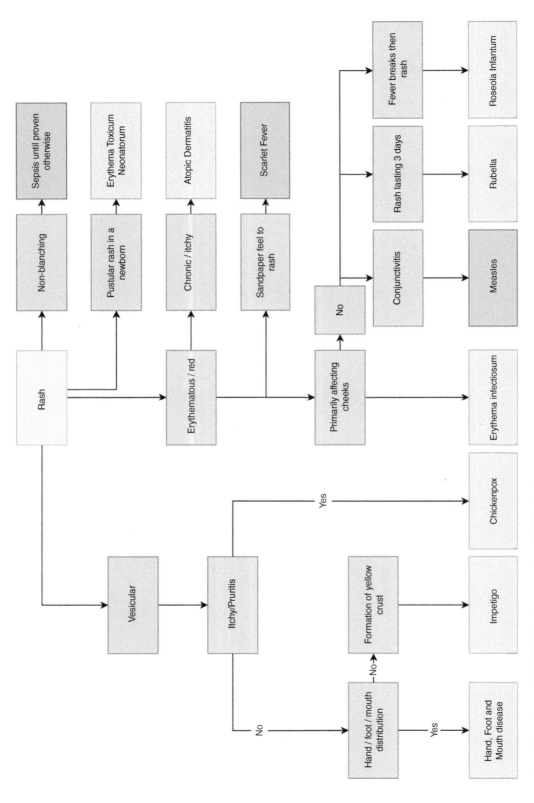

Figure 9.3.1 Diagnostic algorithm for the presentation of childhood rash.

9.3.4 DIFFERENTIALS LIST

Dangerous Diagnoses

1. Measles

- Highly contagious RNA virus spread through droplets – notifiable disease
- Associated with high fever, conjunctivitis and upper respiratory symptoms
- Recent outbreaks in the UK and Europe have been due to drop in vaccination rates, reducing herd immunity
- Up to 40% of those infected can experience secondary complications

Box 9.3.2 Complications of Measles Infection

System	Details
Ear, nose and throat	Otitis media
Respiratory tract	Interstitial pneumonia (measles virus) Bacterial superinfection (*Pneumococcus*, *Staphylococcus aureus*, *Haemophilus influenzae*) Laryngitis Bronchitis Tracheitis
Heart	Myocarditis
Central nervous system	Encephalomyelitis: acute phase Subacute sclerosing panencephalitis: late onset (8–10 years after primary infection)

2. Scarlet Fever

- Caused by exotoxins released by *Streptococcus pyogenes* (group A *Streptococcus*, GAS) during a throat infection – it is a notifiable disease
- Small, red, papular (sandpaper) rash starting on torso, with general malaise and pyrexia
- Treatment is aimed at preventing spread and prevention of rheumatic fever

Common Diagnoses

1. Atopic Dermatitis

- Pruritic, scaling and inflammatory skin condition linked to type 2 helper T cells
- In babies, most common on cheeks, body and extensor surfaces
- In older children, most common in the folds of elbows, wrists, knees and ankles
- A relapsing and remitting course is common even with treatment
- 30% of children will have a defect in the Filaggrin gene – a specialised cell protein that prevents water loss from the epidermis

2. Chickenpox

- Caused by varicella zoster virus (VZV), incubation period is 1–3 weeks
- High fever, coryza and cough are prodromal symptoms
- Children are infectious 2 days before the rash develops and until all the vesicles are crusted over
- A vaccine is available, but is not currently on the routine UK immunisation schedule
- Can cause a host of sequelae, including fulminant sepsis from secondary bacterial infection

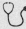

Box 9.3.3 Complications of Chickenpox Infection

System	Details
Secondary bacterial infection (group A *Streptococcus*, *Staphylococcus*)	• Impetigo • Cellulitis • Subcutaneous abscess • Lymphadenitis • Septicaemia • Pneumonia • Necrotising fasciitis • Osteomyelitis
Central nervous system	• Encephalitis • Meningoencephalitis • Cerebellar ataxia
Renal	• Glomerulonephritis • Nephrotic syndrome • Haemolytic uraemic syndrome
Cardiac	• Pericarditis • Myocarditis
Other systems	• Pancreatitis • Orchitis

3. **Hand, Foot and Mouth Disease**
   - Caused by Coxsackie virus A16 or enterovirus 71
   - Blister-like lesions appear on the hands (including palms), soles of the feet and oral mucosa. The buttocks can sometimes be involved
   - Treatment is symptomatic only, as the disease runs a benign course but has on rare occasions caused encephalitis
   - Good hand hygiene is essential, as it is spread via the faeco-oral route
4. **Impetigo**
   - Most common skin infection in children, with peak incidence at 2–5 years
   - Lesions can develop anywhere, but are most common on the head and face
   - Caused by members of the staphylococcal and streptococcal species
   - Highly contagious – children need to avoid creche, nursery and school for at least 48 hours into the treatment course
5. **Erythema Toxicum Neonatorum (ETN)**
   - Most common pustular rash in the newborn period
   - Caused by eosinophilic infiltration into the epidermis
   - Resolution occurs over the following 10–14 days
   - No treatment is necessary
6. **Erythema Infectiosum (Fifth Disease)**
   - Caused by parvovirus B19
   - Nearly 95% of children are seroconverted by 2 years of age
   - The rash tends to primarily affect the face and is colloquially termed 'slapped cheek syndrome'
7. **Roseola Infantum**
   - Caused by human herpesvirus 6 (HHV-6)
   - Most commonly seen in those 6 months–3 years
   - Initially very high fevers for around 3 days, after which the rash appears
8. **Rubella**
   - Also known as German measles; vaccination is available
   - Infection during pregnancy to non-immune women can be devastating to the foetus

Box 9.3.4   Distinguishing Measles versus Rubella   △△

Feature	Measles	Rubella
Incubation period	10–14 days	12–21 days
Prodromal stage	Yes	No (in adults yes)
Disease severity	More severe	Mild
Koplik spots	Yes	No
Posterior chain lymph nodes	Generally no	Yes
Rash persists for	4+ days	3 days
Vaccine available	Yes	Yes

9.3.5 KEY HISTORY FEATURES

A full immunisation history is important in every child with a rash, as any omissions in uptake can provide an alert to a potential diagnosis.

Dangerous Diagnosis 1
Diagnosis: Measles

Questions
1. **How did the illness begin? Was there evidence of an upper respiratory illness with conjunctivitis?** Measles typically begins with a dry cough, coryza and conjunctivitis. The child usually looks very unwell, much more so than one would expect with a simple upper respiratory tract infection (URTI)
2. **Did the child have a fever before the rash appeared?** Fever typically accompanies the URTI symptoms, and continues to rise until the rash appears. After this, in uncomplicated cases, the fever usually settles over the next 48 hours
3. **Where did the rash appear first and what did it look like?** The rash typically starts behind the ears and around the upper neck as erythematous macules. It rapidly spreads to involve the whole face, neck, chest and upper arms over a 24-hour period, becoming maculopapular as it spreads. Over time the whole body is covered and as the rash spreads to the lower limbs, the fever gradually settles. When the rash fades, it does so in the order in which it presented
4. **Has the child been immunised against measles?** Vaccination against measles is part of the MMR vaccine (measles, mumps and rubella), given in two doses, at 1 year and pre-school
5. **How old is the child?** Young children (under 3 years) are more likely to suffer from the complications associated with measles, especially pneumonia and croup. Those under 2 years are more likely to suffer from subacute sclerosing panencephalitis (SSPE) in later life

Box 9.3.5   Subacute Sclerosing Panencephalitis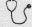

- This is a post-infective neurological disorder that is due to reactivation of the measles virus in the brain
- It occurs 8–10 years post the primary infection, and most commonly affects those who were aged 2 years or younger when infected
- It results in progressive and debilitating neurological deterioration secondary to inflammation
- This results in symptoms such as personality change, seizures, coma and even death

Dangerous Diagnosis 2
Diagnosis: Scarlet fever

Questions
1. **How old is the child?** Scarlet fever is most frequently seen in the 5–15 year age bracket. Can occur in younger children, but alternative diagnoses should be considered
2. **Has there been a recent sore throat associated with fever?** The illness usually has a sudden onset, with a high fever associated with a sore throat

3. **Any other symptoms such as headache or any swellings noted in the neck?** Headache and lymphadenopathy are frequently associated symptoms

4. **Where did the rash appear first and how has it changed?** A diffuse, finely papular, erythematous rash begins around the neck, before spreading to involve the cheeks, trunk and limbs. The skin develops a bright red discoloration, and the rash is described as having a 'sandpaper' feel. Additional stigmata are described as circumoral pallor and a strawberry tongue. When the rash fades, it does so in the order in which it presented

Common Diagnosis 1
Diagnosis: Atopic dermatitis

Questions
1. **When did the rash first start?** 50% of children will present with the rash in their first year of life, and most of the rest before their 5th birthday. There is often a genetic predisposition, frequently with a personal or family history of atopy. Parents will usually report that the rash waxes and wanes, frequently with no obvious explanation
2. **Is the rash itchy and which areas of the body are affected?** The rash is intensely itchy, and in infants has a predilection for the face and extensor surfaces. As the child grows older, the distribution changes and the flexors of the knees, ankles, elbows and wrists are more commonly affected
3. **Are there identifiable triggers?** Under 6 months, cow's milk, hen's eggs and soya are the most common triggers. In older children, dust mite faeces (which contain proteases), skin infection from commensals, environmental factors (cold, dry weather), fabrics and hormonal changes are more common

Common Diagnosis 2
Diagnosis: Chickenpox

Questions
1. **How did the illness begin? Has there been a fever?** The illness usually begins with a fever, malaise, lethargy and occasionally headache
2. **Where did the rash appear first and what did it look like?** The rash appears 24–48 hours after the initial symptoms. It is intensely itchy, usually beginning on the scalp, and then spreading to involve the face, trunk and extremities. Lesions can also appear on the mucous membranes of the mouth, the genitalia and the conjunctiva. The rash progresses from initial erythematous macules, to papules, to fluid-filled vesicles. These become umbilicated around 24 hours later, before crusting and healing begins. As the initial crop begins to heal, fresh crops appear, this is typical of chickenpox
3. **Are there any underlying immunodeficiencies or malignancy?** Children with immunodeficiencies, including those undergoing chemotherapy for treatment of malignancy, are at higher risk of complications from varicella and so need intravenous (IV) varicella zoster immunoglobulin (VZIg) treatment within 7 days of exposure
4. **How many children are in the family?** The incubation period is around 2–3 weeks, and siblings often pick up the infection from the index case. Frequently the infection worsens as it passes from one sibling to the next, due to close contact with a sibling with a high viral load

Common Diagnosis 3
Diagnosis: Impetigo

Questions
1. **Where did the rash appear first?** Impetigo typically appears initially over the site where the integrity of the skin has been breached, such as over an abrasion, an insect bite, laceration or eczematous patch. It usually starts as a tiny pustule, which rapidly develops into a honey-coloured crusted plaque
2. **Has the rash spread from its point of origin?** The rash can spread through clothing, bedding or fingernails to affect other parts of the body and is highly contagious
3. **Has there been a fever, or any other signs of being unwell?** Children usually appear well, with no fever and no pain associated with the rash. The rash is not typically itchy. This superficial bacterial infection is usually caused by *Staphylococcus aureus* or *Streptococcus pyogenes*

Common Diagnosis 4
Diagnosis: Hand, foot and mouth disease

Questions
1. **Where did the rash appear first?** As the name of the condition implies, lesions are seen over the hands, feet and mouth. Blister-like lesions appear on the hands (including palms), soles of the feet and oral mucosa. The buttocks can sometimes be involved. The lesions may also appear over eczematous areas. These take about a week to resolve

2. **How unwell has the child been?** This is usually a mild disease, associated with a low-grade fever
3. **Is the child tolerating fluids?** Ulcers/lesions of the mouth can sometimes be painful and if the child is not tolerating fluids enterally, they may need admission for nasogastric tube or IV fluids

Common Diagnosis 5
Diagnosis: Erythema toxicum neonatorum (ETN)

Questions
1. **Has the newborn had any fevers?** If the newborn has had a confirmed fever of ≥38 °C, a full septic screen is advisable and an alternative diagnosis is needed until infection is ruled out
2. **Was there meconium around the time of delivery?** Meconium can sometimes increase the severity of the pustular outbreak, but it remains a benign process
3. **Is the rash progressing in one area or moving around?** Classically, ETN moves around different areas of the body, but usually resolves spontaneously within 10–14 days

Common Diagnosis 6
Diagnosis: Erythema infectiosum (fifth disease)

Questions
1. **Where did the rash appear first?** The rash tends to primarily affect the face and is colloquially termed 'slapped cheek syndrome'
2. **Has the rash spread from its point of origin?** The rash can spread to involve the trunk anteriorly and posteriorly, as well as the limbs. It tends to be itchy, especially if the soles of the feet are affected. Rash usually resolves within 10 days, but can also wax and wane for a few weeks. As it resolves, it is said to develop a lacy pattern over affected areas
3. **How unwell has the child been?** Presenting symptoms are usually coryza, cough and malaise. Arthralgia of the wrist can occur over the next 2 weeks, more commonly seen in older children and teenagers
4. **Is there a history of haemoglobinopathy?** Children with sickle cell disease or hereditary spherocytosis will often be more severely affected during an intercurrent illness. Parvovirus B19 causes a drop in erythropoiesis in most individuals, but in those with decreased haemoglobin reserve a dangerous aplastic crisis can occur

Common Diagnosis 7
Diagnosis: Roseola infantum

Questions
1. **How unwell has the child been?** Prodrome of 3 days of very high fevers, often >40 °C and a runny nose, cough and sore throat. When the fever breaks, the rash appears. Associated with febrile convulsions
2. **Where did the rash appear first?** The rash typically starts on the trunk, anteriorly and posteriorly, before spreading to the face, neck and limbs. It is pinkish-red and maculopapular. It is not usually itchy. It tends to resolve in a couple of days from first eruption

Common Diagnosis 8
Diagnosis: Rubella

Questions
1. **How unwell has the child been?** Rubella is most often a very mild disease, with presentation possibly as innocuous as a a runny nose. Posterior auricular lymphadenopathy associated with posterior cervical/occipital lymphadenopathy is often the first inkling of the disease
2. **Where did the rash appear first?** A maculopapular rash begins on the face and spreads rapidly to the trunk. It may be mildly itchy. The rash typically lasts 3 days (the old term was 3-day measles) and is not as prominent as measles

Box 9.3.6   Viral Rashes: Route of Spread

Virus	Disease	Route of spread
Herpes zoster virus	Chickenpox	Respiratory droplets
Parvovirus B19	Erythema infectiosum	Respiratory droplets
Human herpesvirus 6	Roseola infantum	Respiratory droplets
Enterovirus/Coxsackie virus	Hand, foot and mouth	Stool shedding

9.3.6 KEY EXAMINATION FEATURES

Box 9.3.7 Defining a Skin Rash: How to Describe What You See

Visually	Medical term
Flat patch (<5 mm)	Macule
Raised lump (<5 mm)	Papule
Raised lump (>5 mm)	Nodule
Clear fluid-filled blister	Vesicle
Yellow fluid-filled blister	Pustule
Red + blanching	Erythematous
Large (>2 mm) purple + non-blanching	Purpura
Pinpoint, purple + non-blanching	Petechia

Box 9.3.8 Is the Rash Blanching or Non-blanching?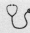

- Most infective maculopapular rashes will blanch when pressure is applied to the rash
- Meningococcaemia may initially present as a blanching rash, which then transitions into non-blanching lesions

Dangerous Diagnosis 1
Diagnosis: Measles

Examination Findings
1. **Conjunctivitis.** A bilateral, painful conjunctivitis appears in the prodromal phase along with cough and coryza
2. **Did the parents notice any spots in the mouth?** Koplik spots, described as whitish dots on a red base, are usually seen on the insides of the mouth over the buccal mucosa, and are a pathognomonic sign of measles. The distribution can be quite widespread and include the palate. Found in around 60% of patients, they develop before the rash appears and disappear as it spreads, meaning they are easily missed
3. **Maculopapular rash.** Widespread pronounced erythematous maculopapular rash, starting on the forehead and spreading to the face, body and limbs. The rash can coalesce into patches

Dangerous Diagnosis 2
Diagnosis: Scarlet fever

Examination Findings
1. **Sandpaper rash**. Typically described as small, red / pink pinprick-like rash (resembling sandpaper). This starts on the torso and spreads to the limbs and sometimes face.
2. **Strawberry tongue/fur tongue**. A bright red and papular tongue can develop as well as a white furry tongue as part of the disease
3. **Red skin creases**. Skin creases of the axilla, groin and antecubital fossa will often appear redder than the rest of the body. These are also known as Pastia lines
4. **Skin peeling**. Peeling of the palms of the hands, fingertips and soles of the feet can occur during disease resolution (remember, peeling in Kawasaki's disease is periungual). Peeling of the groin has also been noted

Common Diagnosis 1
Diagnosis: Atopic dermatitis

Examination Findings
1. **Pruritic, papular rash.** Presents as papular, intensely pruritic erythematous patches, which can appear anywhere on the body, but most prominently in the flexures of the elbow, wrists, knees and ankles. There are often signs of excoriation, with exudates where the skin's integrity has been breached
2. **Skin thickening.** Can often have areas of lichenification – skin thickening – secondary to inflammation and excoriation from persistent scratching
3. **Punched-out lesions.** Superimposed herpes simplex virus (HSV) infections can complicate severe eczema. This presents as red, punched-out lesions that spread along the eczematous skin. Fever is a common feature

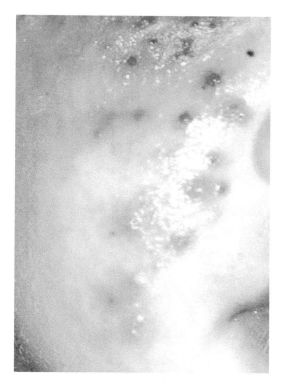

Figure 9.3.2 Eczema herpeticum on the face. Source: Reproduced with permission from Newell, S.J., and Darling, J.C. (2014). *Paediatrics lecture notes*. Chichester: Wiley Blackwell.

Common Diagnosis 2
Diagnosis: Chickenpox

Examination Findings
1. **Vesicular rash.** Depending on the time of presentation, the rash can be very variable. The rash is intensely itchy and evolves from initial erythematous macules, to papules, to fluid-filled vesicles. These become umbilicated around 24 hours later, before crusting and healing begins. As the initial crop begins to heal, fresh crops appear. Lesions are seen on the scalp, the face, trunk and extremities, and can also appear on the mucous membranes of the mouth, the genitalia and the conjunctiva
2. **Red, warm, well-demarcated areas of skin.** Secondary streptococcal skin infection can lead to a severe septicaemia. Lesions should be regularly reviewed with this in mind

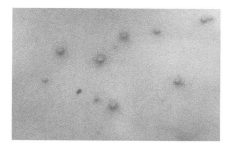

Figure 9.3.3 The classic rash of chickenpox involves pruritic, fluid-filled vesicles on an erythematous base. Source: Reproduced with permission of Shutterstock.

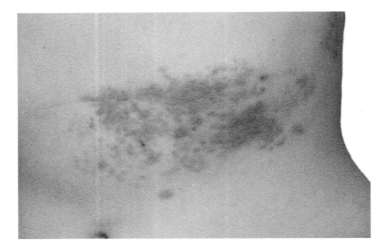

Figure 9.3.4 Reactivation of herpes zoster infection leads to shingles, which is characterised by a vesicular rash in a dermatomal distribution. Source: Reproduced with permission of John Wiley & Sons Ltd.

Common Diagnosis 3
Diagnosis: Impetigo

Examination Findings
1. **Golden crusted lesions.** Start as red, erythematous blisters, which develop into golden/yellow crusted lesions (resembling cornflakes)
2. **How unwell has the child been?** Children usually appear well, with no fever or pain associated with the rash. The rash is not usually itchy

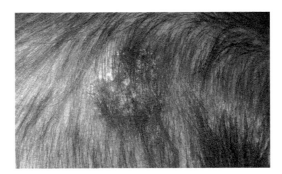

Figure 9.3.5 Impetigo on the scalp, characterised by the golden crusted lesion. Source: Reproduced with permission from Newell, S.J., and Darling, J.C. (2014). *Paediatrics lecture notes*. Chichester: Wiley Blackwell.

Common Diagnosis 4
Diagnosis: Hand, foot and mouth disease

Examination Findings
1. **Vesicular rash on hands, feet and oral mucosa.** Fluid-filled vesicles can appear on the hands, palms and soles of the feet, and sometimes buttocks. Ulcerative lesions appear on the oral mucosa and pharynx
2. **How unwell has the child been?** This is usually a mild disease, associated with a low-grade fever

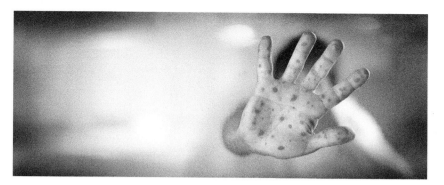

Figure 9.3.6 Vesicles on the palm in hand, food and mouth disease, usually caused by an enterovirus infection, most commonly Coxsackie A16. Source: Reproduced with permission of John Wiley & Sons Ltd.

Common Diagnosis 5
Diagnosis: Erythema toxicum neonatorum (ETN)

Examination Findings
1. **White pustules on erythematous base.** Crops of white/yellow-headed pustules seen in a newborn, with a surrounding ring of erythema
2. **How unwell has the baby been?** Babies are otherwise well, with no signs of sepsis

Common Diagnosis 6
Diagnosis: Erythema infectiosum (fifth disease)

Examination Findings
1. **Red cheeks with circumoral pallor.** Typical rash shows bilateral macular erythematous patches of the cheeks, with sparing/pallor of the nasolabial folds, forehead and mouth. A lacy red rash can also appear on the body when the facial rash subsides
2. **Wrist swelling.** This usually occurs 1–2 weeks into the disease and occurs in older children and teenagers. It can last for a few weeks and does not lead to autoimmune arthritis in later life

Common Diagnosis 7
Diagnosis: Roseola infantum

Examination Findings
1. **Papular pink rash.** When the fever has broken (defervesced), a fine, papular, red/pink rash appears on the body and spreads to the limbs, sparing the face

Common Diagnosis 8
Diagnosis: Rubella

Examination Findings
1. **Faint maculopapular rash.** A maculopapular erythematous rash begins behind the ears and spreads towards the face and then torso and limbs. It does not coalesce and is fainter than that of measles
2. **Red spots on the soft palate.** Petechiae or small haemorrhages of the soft palate can be seen, also called Forchheimer sign. (Similar features can be seen in scarlet fever and measles)

9.3.7 KEY INVESTIGATIONS

Most skin rashes in this chapter are self-limiting illnesses with spontaneous resolution, and investigations are generally not necessary. Confirmation is, however, required where any notifiable diseases are considered, or where complications develop, and as such investigations are important in this subgroup.

Blood Tests

Table 9.3.1 Blood tests of use in patients presenting with childhood rashes

Test	When to perform	Potential result
FBC	Suspected: • Secondary bacterial infection • Parvovirus-induced aplastic anaemia	• ↑ WCC, ↑ neutrophils could indicate secondary bacterial infection • ↓ Hb, (± ↓ WCC, ↓ platelets): parvovirus-induced aplastic anaemia
Anti-measles IgM	• Suspected measles	• ↑ IgM confirms an acute infection
Anti-rubella IgM	• Suspected rubella	• ↑ IgM confirms an acute infection
ASOT	Suspected: • Secondary bacterial infection of chickenpox • Scarlet fever	• ↑ ASOT indicates GAS infection, as seen in scarlet fever and secondary bacterial infections of chickenpox

ASOT, anti-streptolysin O titre; FBC, full blood count; GAS, group A *Streptococcus*; Hb, haemoglobin; Ig, immunoglobulin

Imaging

Table 9.3.2 Imaging modalities of use in patients presenting with childhood rashes

Test	When to perform	Potential result
Chest X-ray	• Suspected respiratory complications	• Consolidation may suggest viral pneumonia in measles or chickenpox
MRI Head	• Suspected varicella-induced cerebellar ataxia	• Cerebellitis: post VZV infection

MRI, magnetic resonance imaging; VZV, varicella zoster virus

Special

Table 9.3.3 Special tests of use in patients presenting with childhood rashes

Test	When to perform	Potential result
Bacterial throat swab	• Suspected scarlet fever	• Isolating GAS will guide antibiotic choice
Bacterial skin swab	Suspected: • Secondary bacterial infections • Impetigo	• Isolating GAS or *Staphylococcus* species will guide antibiotic choice
Viral PCR skin swab	• Suspected secondary HSV infection of eczema, eczema herpeticum	• A positive result for HSV will guide antiviral treatment, e.g. aciclovir

GAS, group A *Streptococcus*; HSV, herpes simplex virus; PCR, polymerase chain reaction

9.3.8 KEY MANAGEMENT PRINCIPLES

Diagnosis-specific management strategies are outlined here. It is expected that an 'ABCDE' approach to assessment and management is always undertaken (see Chapter 12.1).

Dangerous Diagnosis 1
Diagnosis: Measles

Management Principles
1. **Notify Public Health authorities.** Measles is a notifiable disease
2. **Conservative management.** Management of fever, with attention to fluid and dietary intake, is often all that is required. Vigilance is necessary to detect complications such as pneumonia or secondary bacterial infection
3. **Vitamin A.** Malnourished children tend to be severely affected by measles. Although uncommon in the UK, measles is particularly associated with vitamin A deficiency. If this is suspected, supplementation is recommended to help prevent severe disease
4. **Post-exposure prophylaxis.** Blood products such as intravenous immunoglobulin (IVIg) or human normal immunoglobulin (HNIg) may be indicated for those with immunodeficiencies or non-immune pregnant women who have been exposed to the measles virus

Dangerous Diagnosis 2
Diagnosis: Scarlet fever

Management Principles
1. **Notify Public Health authorities.** Scarlet fever is a notifiable disease
2. **Antibiotics.** A 10-day course of an oral penicillin-based antibiotic usually suffices. Phenoxymethylpenicillin is generally a reasonable choice. If the patient is allergic to beta lactam antibiotics, a macrolide is a good alternative; refer to local guidelines

Common Diagnosis 1
Diagnosis: Atopic dermatitis

Management Principles
1. **Emollient treatment.** This is the mainstay of treatment. Oil-based (greasy) emollients keep moisture locked into the skin better. Creams will be absorbed faster, but have a shorter action. They should be generously applied several times a day. If used correctly, these can reduce the need for steroid creams by 40–60%
2. **Steroid creams.** The potency of steroid creams ranges from mild, moderate to very potent. In children older than 6 months, mild steroid (hydrocortisone) for the face and if necessary moderate steroid (clobetasone butyrate) for the body are generally advised. Higher-potency steroids should only be used on the advice of paediatric dermatologists
3. **Soap substitutes.** There are many soap/bath substitutes available such as Dermol 600 or Oilatum. These are used instead of shampoos and soaps
4. **Antihistamines.** Eczema is intensely pruritic and sleep disturbance is therefore extremely common. Non-sedating antihistamines, such as cetirizine, can offer some relief
5. **Avoidance of triggers.** In children under 12 months with moderate to severe eczema not responding to treatment, dietary exclusion of milk, egg and soya is an appropriate management step. In older children, education around house dust mite eradication is important, including a non-carpeted house, regular dusting/hoovering and washing bed linen at 60 °C (neutralises dust mites)

Box 9.3.9   Atopic Dermatitis Treatments

Treatment	Examples
Emollients	50:50 paraffin Epaderm® ointment
Bath/soap substitutes	Dermol 600 Oilatum®
Mild steroid	Hydrocortisone 1% Fluocinolone acetonide 0.0025% (Synalar®)
Moderately potent steroid	Clobetasone butyrate 0.05% (Eumovate) Betamethasone valerate 0.025% (Betnovate®)
Potent steroid	Mometasone furoate 0.1% (Elocon®)
Immune modulator	Tacrolimus (Protopic®)

Common Diagnosis 2
Diagnosis: Chickenpox

Management Principles
1. **Antipyretics.** Paracetamol is the preferred antipyretic. An association between non-steroidal anti-inflammatory drugs (NSAIDs), such as ibuprofen, and severe secondary skin infections such as necrotising fasciitis has been described
2. **Antipruritics**. Camomile lotion is widely used, but may cause the spread of secondary bacterial infection due to the 'smearing' in its application. Chlorpheniramine or cetirizine may be useful to help reduce itch in some children

Common Diagnosis 3
Diagnosis: Impetigo

Management Principles
1. **Avoid school/nursery.** As this is a highly contagious infection, parents should be advised to keep their child away from school/nursery for at least 48 hours after starting antibiotics, or till the rash subsides
2. **Antibiotics.** A course of oral flucloxacillin or topical fusidic acid can help if the bacterium is methicillin-sensitive *Staphylococcus aureus* (MSSA). Check local guidelines

Common Diagnosis 4
Diagnosis: Hand, foot and mouth disease

Management Principles
1. **Hydration**. Children may have poor fluid intake due to the oral lesions, so it is important to ensure they are not dehydrated and in need of nasogastric tube feeding or IV hydration

Common Diagnosis 5
Diagnosis: Erythema toxicum neonatorum (ETN)

Management Principles
1. **Reassurance**. Parents will often be very worried about this rash, especially first-time parents. After a thorough examination, reassure them that it will resolve over the next few weeks

Common Diagnosis 6
Diagnosis: Erythema infectiosum (fifth disease)

Management Principles
1. **Conservative management.** Most children recover from this self-limiting illness without additional support or treatment. As children are no longer contagious once the rash erupts, it is not necessary to keep them away from nursery/school
2. **Ask about and advise regarding contact with pregnant women.** This is due to the risk of severe anaemia to the developing foetus
3. **Haematology advice for those at risk of severe anaemia.** In children with blood dyscrasias such as sickle cell disease or hereditary spherocytosis, parvovirus serology should be sent as part of the initial investigations. Advice regarding subsequent management including blood transfusions should be sought from a specialist team

Common Diagnosis 7
Diagnosis: Roseola infantum

Management Principles
1. **Conservative management.** Antipyretics and fluid intake are important treatment steps. Antipyretics are not thought to prevent febrile seizures from occurring, and families at risk should be made aware of this

Common Diagnosis 8
Diagnosis: Rubella

Management Principles
1. **Notify Public Health authorities.** Rubella is a notifiable disease
2. **Conservative management**. Management of fever, with attention to fluid and dietary intake, is often all that is required

Box 9.3.10   Ask about Pregnancy

Due to the risk of adverse effects to the foetus, it is important to ask about contact with pregnant women in the following suspected infections/rashes:

- **Rubella:** can cause cataracts, microcephaly, heart defects (such as pulmonary stenosis and patent ductus arteriosus) and sensorineural deafness
- **Parvovirus B19:** can cause bone marrow failure in the foetus, leading to anaemia and hydrops fetalis (cardiac failure, peripheral oedema and effusions)
- **VZV:** can cause skin scarring, limb defects and central nervous system abnormalities such as cortical atrophy and microcephaly

10.1 Limp

Benjamin Carter

Department of Paediatrics, University Hospitals Sussex NHS Foundation Trust, Chichester, UK

CONTENTS

10.1.1 CHAPTER AT A GLANCE

> **Box 10.1.1   Chapter at a Glance**
>
> - A child with a limp can have a wide range of pathologies that range from very mild disorders to acute emergencies
> - The type of limp varies depending on the site and nature of pathology
> - Causes of limp are not just limited to orthopaedic pathology
> - Infection in either a joint or bone tissue should be considered a limb- (and sometimes life-) threatening emergency
> - Similarly, injuries that cause swelling in a joint compartment can have life-changing consequences if not promptly recognised
>
> - With any potential injury, child safeguarding must always be considered, as a missed diagnosis could lead to further injury
> - If in doubt about the diagnosis, discuss with other specialities – in particular orthopaedics, surgery and radiology
> - This chapter should be used in conjunction with Chapter 10.2, Swollen Joint, as there is significant overlap, and differentials are divided into the most relevant chapter

10.1.2 DEFINITION

The impediment of normal gait, by way of painful or restricted movement.

Clinical Guide to Paediatrics, First Edition. Edited by Rachel Varughese and Anna Mathew. Series Editor: Christian Fielder Camm.
© 2022 John Wiley & Sons Ltd. Published 2022 by John Wiley & Sons Ltd.
Companion website: www.wiley.com/go/varughese/paediatrics

10.1.3 DIAGNOSTIC ALGORITHM

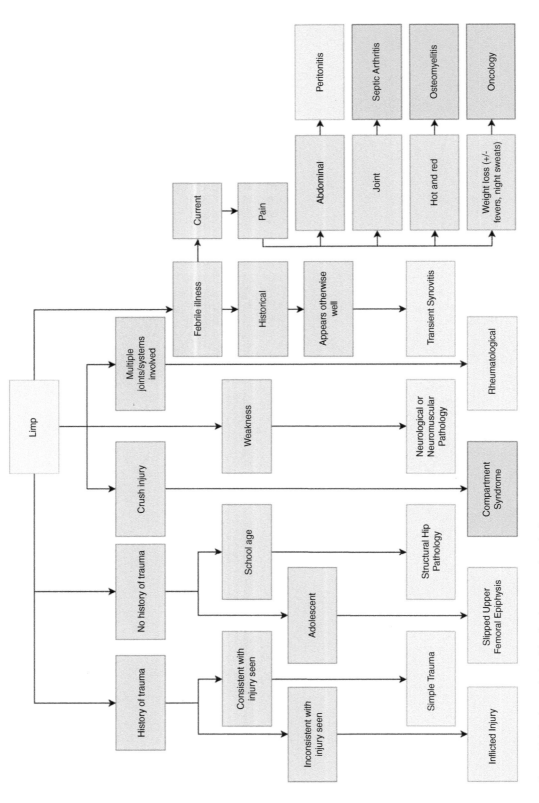

Figure 10.1.1 Diagnostic algorithm for the presentation of a limp.

10.1.4 DIFFERENTIALS LIST

Dangerous Diagnoses

1. Septic Arthritis
- Caused by bacterial infection infiltrating the joint capsule
- The joint capsule and surrounding tissue become acutely inflamed and synovial fluid becomes purulent
- It can be highly destructive and lead to significant disability if not managed promptly
- Septic arthritis is potentially life-threatening if it progresses to systemic sepsis
- Discitis in the spine has a similar aetiology, and must be considered where there is fever, limp and inflammatory symptoms in/around the spine
- Boys are twice as likely as girls to develop a septic arthritis

2. Osteomyelitis
- Bacterial infection of bone, typically with *Staphylococcus*, *Streptococcus* or *Enterobacter* species
- Lower-limb bones are the site of infection in >50% of cases of osteomyelitis
- Can lead to abscess formation, which is a risk for severe sepsis and can be difficult to treat with antibiotics due to poor penetration. Prolonged courses are routinely required
- Without prompt treatment, chronic osteomyelitis can develop and cause sclerosis and deformity of the affected bone
- If there is inadequate response to antibiotics, surgical debridement may be warranted
- Many features of osteomyelitis overlap with septic arthritis. If it is difficult to ascertain whether the infection is in the joint or bone from clinical examination, urgent imaging is required

3. Compartment Syndrome
- Pain and neurological deficit associated with compression of soft tissues, vasculature and nerves
- Typically associated with crush injuries, but can be seen after all trauma, especially when an injury requires a rigid support such as plaster of Paris
- Can cause permanent injury to nerves and consequent sensorimotor compromise
- Secondary pathology can be caused by rhabdomyolysis, which increases the risk of renal failure and cardiac arrhythmia

4. Malignancy
- Malignancy should always be considered in the context of a new-onset limp
- Most commonly, these will either be a primary bony tumour or haematological malignancy

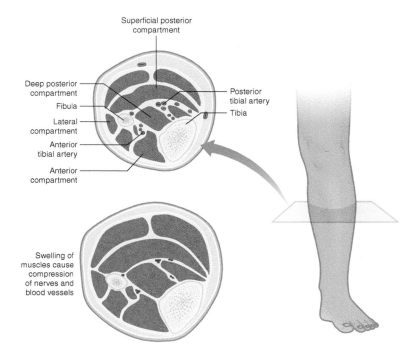

Figure 10.1.2 Compartment syndrome occurs when swelling of injured muscles compresses blood vessels and nerves.

- Osteosarcoma and Ewing's sarcoma are the commonest malignant bone tumours in children, with osteosarcoma frequently affecting the distal femur, and Ewing's sarcoma affecting the pelvis, femur, humerus or ribs
- Red-flag features include bone pain, bony swellings, weight loss, unexplained fever, night sweats or generalised lymphadenopathy
- Bone pain waking the child from sleep is particularly concerning
- Malignancy is covered in detail in several chapters, including Chapters 3.3 (Fever), 4.1 (Bruising), 4.2 (Pallor), and will not be discussed further in this chapter

---

Box 10.1.2   Inflicted Injury   △△

- Missing inflicted injury can have devastating and sometimes fatal consequences for the child
- If there are any doubts as to the consistency of the history given, or if there is a description of an injury that does not fit with what is seen, seek senior review
- The discomfort and personal unease associated with addressing a safeguarding concern should not delay initiating appropriate child protection measures
- Seek senior advice. See Chapter 12.5, Figures 12.5.2 and 12.5.3 for body maps depicting suspicious areas for bruising.

Common Diagnoses
1. Transient Synovitis
- Very common, but remains a diagnosis largely of exclusion
- Specific cause not fully understood, but pain is related to inflammation and hypertrophy of the synovial membrane within a joint
- Typically affects younger children, who present as being generally well with a mild to moderate limp shortly after a viral illness
- Low-grade fever may be present

2. Simple Trauma
- Injuries are a direct, but surprisingly frequently overlooked, source of limp
- A careful history will most likely identify events leading to trauma
- Trauma may cause soft tissue bruising, ligamental injury, tendon injury or bone fracture
- With fractures, the degree of involvement of the growth plate affects the management strategy, as growth arrest is sometimes a risk.

3. Slipped Upper Femoral Epiphysis (SUFE)
- Defined as slippage of the femoral metaphysis, where it moves out of alignment with the epiphysis of the femoral head, due to weakness in the proximal growth plate
- Risk factors for growth plate weakening include obesity, rapid adolescent growth spurt, hypothyroidism and renal osteodystrophy
- SUFE is typically seen in adolescent males with a raised Body Mass Index (BMI) and is the most common hip disorder in this age group
- Can result in avascular necrosis of the femoral head

Diagnoses to Consider
1. Perthe's Disease
- Perthe's disease is a rare condition, involving avascular necrosis of the femoral head, usually occurring in children between 4 and 10 years old, with males four times as likely to be affected
- Disease is bilateral in 20% of children
- The cause of Perthe's disease is not well understood, although thrombophilia and trauma are known to increase risk
- Perthe's disease is classically described as a painless limp. However, often there is associated pain in the hip, thigh or knee, particularly after physical activity
- There is stiffness and reduced range of motion in the hip joint, particularly in internal rotation or abduction. The affected leg may be shorter, with smaller muscle bulk
- Perthe's disease may last for a few years, with intermittent symptoms during this time. About 60% of children recover without any treatment. Surgical treatment is considered for severe cases
  When to consider: in a young boy presenting with a painless or mildly painful limp

2. Rheumatological Cause
- Limp in the presence of multiple joint swellings, rashes and other autoimmune-associated symptoms may be due to an inflammatory cause such as juvenile idiopathic arthritis (JIA), systemic lupus erythematosus (SLE) or dermatomyositis

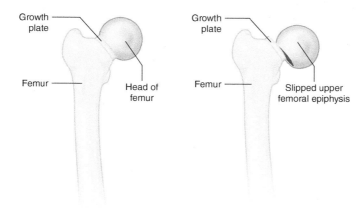

Figure 10.1.3 Although named 'slipped upper femoral epiphysis', this is actually a misnomer. In SUFE the femoral head remains within the acetabulum, and it is actually the metaphysis that displaces in a superior, anterior direction.

- These causes are explored in Chapter 10.2, Swollen Joint

When to consider: in a child with diurnal symptoms, worse in the morning and better in the evening

3. Neurological/Neuromuscular Cause

- Neurological and neuromuscular conditions can all manifest as a limp
- The cause may be related to any part of the motor pathway, including neurological (e.g. cerebral palsy) or muscular (e.g. muscular dystrophy)
- Presentation is insidious, with delayed walking a prominent feature. These children do not usually present to acute paediatrics, and are instead managed within outpatient services
- Acute causes are explored in Chapter 8.3

When to consider: in children who have suffered neonatal hypoxic injury or with developmental delay

---

Box 10.1.3 Peritonitis △△

- Limp may not always be related to lower-limb pathology and may instead be a result of the patient attempting not to irritate an inflamed peritoneum

- Occurs secondary to the characteristic guarding and rigidity seen on abdominal examination
- Causes of intra-abdominal sepsis should be considered

Box 10.1.4 Developmental Dysplasia of the Hip (DDH) △△

- DDH is a spectrum of joint disease, where a shallow or underdeveloped acetabulum predisposes to joint subluxation or dislocation
- Most cases are identified from antenatal risk factors (breech, family history) or at the newborn check

- Delayed presentation beyond this, and certainly by the time the child starts walking, increases the risk of permanent damage with progressive deformities of the joint, and children can therefore present with a limp
- Consider DDH in toddlers who are delayed in standing and walking

Dangerous Diagnosis 3
Diagnosis: Compartment syndrome

Questions
1. **Has the patient sustained a fracture or 'crush'-type injury?** Fractures and crush injuries are the most common events associated with the development of compartment syndrome
2. **Does the patient have a closed rigid support for an injury?** Compartment syndrome can be caused by inflammation restricted by an external factor, such as a plaster cast
3. **Has the child started complaining of 'new' pain and tingling in the affected limb, even intermittently?** Be mindful of the 5 Ps of compartment syndrome

---

Box 10.1.6   The 5 Ps of Compartment Syndrome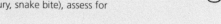

If the history suggests a risk of compartment syndrome (acute trauma, burns, crush injury, snake bite), assess for the five signs that indicate arterial compromise:

- Pain
- Paraesthesiae
- Paralysis
- Pallor
- Pulselessness

Common Diagnosis 1
Diagnosis: Transient synovitis

Questions
1. **Has the child had a recent illness?** The typical history of a transient synovitis is that it follows a mild, usually viral illness
2. **Is the child otherwise generally well?** Transient synovitis is a mild condition that causes a limp in an otherwise well child
3. **Does simple analgesia improve the symptoms?** Non-steroidal anti-inflammatory drugs (NSAIDs) and rest are the mainstays of treatment and parents may have already noticed this prior to consultation

Common Diagnosis 2
Diagnosis: Simple trauma

Questions
1. **Was there a clear precipitating event?** Slips, trips, falls and rough activities are all likely to cause traumatic injuries. However, at times an incident may have seemed harmless or even been unwitnessed, so close questioning is always required
2. **Was the onset abrupt?** Bony, ligamentous or tendon injuries typically have an abrupt onset following a certain movement or accident. This may then be followed by a more gradual manifestation of inflammation, which will worsen pain and disability
3. **Is the mechanism of injury consistent with the presentation?** A clear, consistent history of an injury that fits with the clinical presentation is important. Any inconsistencies should raise concern about inflicted injury

---

Box 10.1.7   Childhood Fractures Commonly Associated with Non-accidental Injury

- Spiral femoral fractures in a non-mobile child
- Non-supracondylar fractures of the humerus in a non-mobile child
- Posterior rib fractures
- Scapula fractures
- Sternal fractures
- Vertebral body or spinous process fractures
- Complex skull fractures
- Digit fractures
- Multiple fractures at different stages of healing

Common Diagnosis 3
Diagnosis: Slipped upper femoral epiphysis

Questions
1. **How old is the child and are they a boy?** SUFE is the most common hip pathology in adolescent children. Males are twice as likely as females to be affected
2. **Does the patient have a large body habitus?** Increased BMI is associated with higher incidence of SUFE
3. **Is there a history of an endocrine disorder?** Children with hypothyroidism and pituitary disorders, particularly panhypopituitarism, are more likely to develop SUFE

10.1.6 KEY EXAMINATION FEATURES

A key examination feature for any limp is noting exactly what the limp looks like, as this can help diagnosis. Most diagnoses in this chapter will present with some form of antalgic gait unless otherwise specified. See Chapter 10.2, Box 10.2.8 for details on joint examination.

Box 10.1.8   Types of Limp

Gait type	Details
Antalgic gait	• Shortened stance time on affected side caused by pain on weight bearing • Short swing phase on the contralateral side
Trendelenburg gait	• Can result from any hip pathology • If unilateral, the hip girdle drops on the affected side and the trunk moves over the affected side to maintain balance • If bilateral, the trunk swings from side to side
Circumduction (vaulting) gait	• Straight-legged walking where affected side is swung out to overcome inability to lift • May result from hemiplegia • Can also occur where there is unilateral restricted joint movement
Steppage equinus gait	• Foot drop caused by peroneal nerve injury and weakness of tibialis anterior muscle
Toe-walking	• May be a normal variant or habit • Can result from upper motor neurone disorders, e.g. cerebral palsy
Waddling gait	• Wide-based stance to maintain balance • May result from myopathy, e.g. muscular dystrophy
Ataxic gait	• Unsteady, wide-based and uncoordinated gait • Related to neurological dysfunction of the cerebellum

Dangerous Diagnosis 1
Diagnosis: Septic arthritis

Examination Findings
1. **Child appears unwell.** In septic arthritis the child will typically appear miserable, unwell and have a high fever
2. **Red, hot, swollen and tender joint.** These are the salient features of a joint affected by septic arthritis
3. **Limited range of movement.** Both the joint effusion and the pain associated with the inflammation will significantly limit movement of the joint, on both active and passive motion. The child is highly unlikely to tolerate weight bearing

Box 10.1.9   Kocher Criteria in Septic Arthritis

There are four criteria:

1. Non-weight-bearing
2. Erythrocyte sedimentation rate >40 mm/hr
3. White cell count >12 × 10^9/L
4. Temperature >38.5 °C

Score:
- 1: likelihood of septic arthritis is 3%
- 2: likelihood of septic arthritis is 40%
- 3: likelihood of septic arthritis is 93%
- 4: likelihood of septic arthritis is 99%

Dangerous Diagnosis 2
Diagnosis: Osteomyelitis

Examination Findings
1. **Child appears unwell.** In osteomyelitis the child will typically appear miserable, unwell and have a high fever
2. **Swelling, redness and pain.** There may not always be appreciable soft tissue signs associated with osteomyelitis. When these are present, they are usually along the length of the bone, rather than affecting the joint, as in septic arthritis
3. **Local inoculation point.** A wound or lesion near the symptomatic site may represent the source of inoculation and should heighten suspicion of a deeper-seated infection

10.1.5 KEY HISTORY FEATURES

Dangerous Diagnosis 1
Diagnosis: Septic arthritis

Questions
1. **Has there been a fever?** A history of fever is strongly suspicious of septic arthritis (or osteomyelitis)
2. **Is there evidence of a swollen and painful joint?** Septic arthritis should be considered where there is an acute onset of a swollen, red and painful joint, associated with fever and an antalgic gait
3. **Which joint seems to be affected?** The joints of the lower limbs, hips, knees and ankles are most often affected
4. **Is there any preexisting joint or systemic disease?** A septic arthritis will typically be 'seeded' from bacteraemia in an already unwell child. Immunosuppressed individuals or those who have existing joint pathology or prostheses are at higher risk
5. **Is the child fully vaccinated?** Before introduction of the HiB vaccination, *Haemophilus Influenzae* was a frequently isolated causative organism in septic arthritides

Dangerous Diagnosis 2
Diagnosis: Osteomyelitis

Questions
1. **Has there been a fever?** A history of fever is strongly suspicious of osteomyelitis (or septic arthritis)
2. **Is there a route of introduction for infection?** Osteomyelitis may follow introduction of bacteria by way of localised infection (cellulitis), trauma or iatrogenic means such as frequent venepuncture/cannulation
3. **Is there a risk of immunosuppression or another underlying disorder?** Children undergoing chemotherapy, or those with conditions such as type 1 diabetes mellitus, are at greater risk of osteomyelitis. Children with haemoglobinopathy are also specifically at greater risk
4. **Is the child still growing?** Growth plates are at higher risk of bacterial seeding due to their richer blood supply but sluggish flow. Therefore, children who still have active growth are at higher risk of osteomyelitis. A third of cases present by 2 years, and half by 5 years

---

Box 10.1.5   Organisms in Septic Arthritis and Osteomyelitis   ΔΔ

Septic arthritis	Osteomyelitis
Staphylococcus aureus • Most common organism across paediatric age groups >2 years • Some strains of community-acquired methicillin-resistant *Staphylococcus aureus* (MRSA) have the genotype for Panton–Valentine leukocidin (PVL) cytotoxin production • PVL-positive strains are more associated with complex infections and complications such as systemic sepsis and deep vein thrombosis	
Group B *Streptococcus* (GBS) • Most common organism in neonates • Usually acquired from birth canal in GBS-positive mothers	
HACEK organisms • Fastidious Gram-negative organisms • *Haemophilus, Aggregatibacter, Cardiobacterium, Eikenella, Kingella* species	
Group A beta-haemolytic *Streptococcus* • Greater risk following varicella infection	Pseudomonas • Usually associated with direct puncture wounds
Neisseria gonorrhoeae • Common organism in adolescent septic arthritis (more so in USA than Europe) • Commonly associated with maculopapular rash on trunk • High-dose penicillin alone sometimes sufficient	*Mycobacteria* tuberculosis • Paediatric patients are more likely to have extra-pulmonary disease • Positive culture for acid-fast bacilli is diagnostic
	Salmonella • More common in sickle cell patients

Dangerous Diagnosis 3
Diagnosis: Compartment syndrome

Examination Findings
1. **Affected limb feels firm and is tender to palpation.** Swelling is the salient pathophysiological process in compartment syndrome and will lead to a firm/tense feeling over the affected limb. The pain felt is described as being severe and out of proportion with that normally expected for the injury
2. **Neurovascular compromise.** Sluggish capillary return or a cool periphery indicates vascular compromise and pulselessness is the end stage of this process. This, along with parasthesiae, loss of sensation or loss of motor function, heralds potentially catastrophic limb compromise and must be definitively managed as an emergency
3. **Pallor.** Lack of effective blood supply will cause a pallid appearance of the limb

Common Diagnosis 1
Diagnosis: Transient synovitis

Examination Findings
1. **Well-looking child.** Transient synovitis is typically a 'post-viral' phenomenon. Children usually appear generally well besides the limp
2. **Unilateral.** Transient synovitis is nearly always a unilateral complaint
3. **Mild to moderate pain with limitation of motion.** The hip joint is typically affected and is uncomfortable on active/passive movement. Pain is responsive to simple analgesia

Common Diagnosis 2
Diagnosis: Simple trauma

Examination Findings
1. **Specific injury site.** Knees, ankles and feet are all common sites of injuries precipitating a limp. Pain can, however, be referred, so always examine the joints above and below the suspected injury site
2. **Tenderness.** This is usually the salient feature. If there is a point of tenderness over bony areas, consider imaging
3. **Swelling.** This may vary depending on the time of presentation from injury
4. **Limitation of motion.** Often related to pain, and usually limited to the specific injury site. Be wary of pseudo-paralysis in anxious children

Common Diagnosis 3
Diagnosis: Slipped upper femoral epiphysis

Examination Findings
1. **Pain on affected side.** SUFE may only present with vague pain in the groin, thigh or sometimes knee on the affected side. Gait is typically antalgic, sometimes so much so that the patient cannot bear weight
2. **Obligatory external rotation during hip flexion.** Considered a very sensitive sign of SUFE, even in milder cases
3. **Limb length discrepancy.** The affected leg may be shorter than the unaffected side

10.1.7 KEY INVESTIGATIONS

Most children with a new limp will require some baseline investigations, unless there is strong clinical evidence of a benign cause.

Bedside

Table 10.1.1 Bedside tests of use in patients presenting with a limp

Test	When to perform	Potential result
Blood gas (capillary or venous)	• Systemically unwell children	• ↓ pH, ↓ HCO_3, ↑lactate indicate metabolic acidosis, suggestive of poor perfusion in sepsis • ↑/↓ Glucose may occur in sepsis

HCO_3, bicarbonate

Blood Tests

Table 10.1.2 Blood tests of use in patients presenting with a limp

Test	When to perform	Potential result
FBC	Suspected: • Septic arthritis • Osteomyelitis • Compartment syndrome • Malignancy • Rheumatological/inflammatory cause	• ↓ Hb, normal MCV: anaemia of chronic disease, acute bleeding in compartment syndrome • ↑ WCC: infection (usually neutrophilia if bacterial, lymphocytosis if viral), leukaemia • ↑ Platelets: chronic inflammation • Pancytopenia: leukaemia, solid malignancy with bone marrow involvement – blood film required to further evaluate
ESR	Suspected: • Septic arthritis • Rheumatological/inflammatory cause	• ↑ ESR: Kocher criteria for septic arthritis • May be seen in rheumatological pathology, e.g. JIA or SLE
CRP	Suspected: • Septic arthritis • Osteomyelitis • Transient synovitis	• Significantly ↑ CRP: septic arthritis or osteomyelitis • Normal or mildly ↑ CRP supportive of transient synovitis
Blood culture	Suspected: • Septic arthritis • Osteomyelitis	• Positive cultures confirm infective pathology • Sensitivities guide antibiotic choice
Rheumatoid factor and ANA	• Markers of rheumatological disease	• Positive rheumatoid factor may be found in JIA • Positive ANA supportive for SLE

ANA, anti-nuclear antibodies; CRP, C-reactive protein; ESR, erythrocyte sedimentation rate; FBC, full blood count; Hb, haemoglobin; JIA, juvenile idiopathic arthritis; MCV, mean corpuscular volume; SLE, systemic lupus erythematosus; WCC, white cell count

Imaging

Injuries and bone/joint pathology can be very subtle and in cases of inflicted injury, the interpretation of imaging may need to be defended in a court of law at some point. If in doubt, consult with the on-call radiologist or relevant specialty team.

Table 10.1.3 Imaging modalities of use in patients presenting with a limp

Test	When to perform	Potential result
Limb X-ray	• All children presenting with a limp • Frog-leg views essential if assessing for SUFE	• Joint changes: septic arthritis, rheumatological, SUFE, Perthe's disease • Bone changes: osteomyelitis, tumour, fractures
Joint ultrasound	• Suspected septic arthritis, for diagnosis and to help guide aspiration	• Can identify effusions that may require drainage, which can also be guided by USS
MRI	Suspected: • Osteomyelitis and septic arthritis – more sensitive and specific for early damage • Bone malignancy	• Increased signal (contrast enhanced or T2 sequence) in joints may indicate effusion, in bone may indicate osteomyelitis • May identify malignancy, e.g. osteosarcoma
Bone scintigraphy	• Suspected osteomyelitis	• Increased radiotracer uptake in surrounding bone

MRI, magnetic resonance imaging; SUFE, slipped upper femoral epiphysis; USS, ultrasound scan

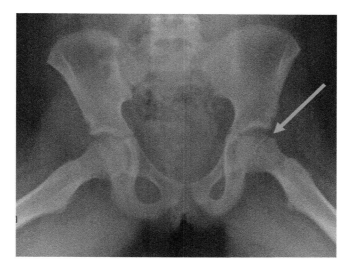

Figure 10.1.4 Anteroposterior view of a left slipped upper femoral epiphysis. Because the slip is posteromedial, it can be seen better on a lateral view.

Special

Table 10.1.4 Special tests of use in patients presenting with a limp

Test	When to perform	Potential result
Joint aspiration and culture	• Can lead to definitive diagnosis if septic arthritis suspected • If immediately available, ideally taken prior to antibiotics, but antibiotics should not be delayed for this	• Positive cultures confirm causative organism • Sensitivities guide antibiotic choice

---

Box 10.1.10   Radiological Findings in Septic Arthritis

X-ray
- X-ray may be normal in early disease
- Joint effusion
- Juxta-articular osteoporosis
- Narrowing of joint space (due to cartilage destruction)
- Destruction of subchondral bone
- If advanced: juxta-articular sclerosis

Ultrasound
- Joint effusion
- Echogenic debris
- Increased peri-synovial vascularity on Doppler

Box 10.1.11   X-Ray Findings in Osteomyelitis

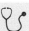

X-ray may be normal in early disease. Changes in osteomyelitis rely on at least 1 cm of infection, with 30–50% bone compromise. The later in the disease course, the more likely changes will be seen

- Swelling of adjacent soft tissues
- Blurring or loss of normal fat planes
- Effusion in adjacent joint
- Osteopaenia

- Periosteal thickening
- Loss of trabecular architecture
- Lytic lesions or cortical loss
- New bone apposition

10.1.8 KEY MANAGEMENT PRINCIPLES

Diagnosis-specific management strategies are outlined here. It is expected that an 'ABCDE' approach to assessment and management is always undertaken (see Chapter 12.1).

Dangerous Diagnosis 1
Diagnosis: Septic arthritis

Management Principles
See Chapter 13.1, Sepsis Management.
1. **Antibiotics**. Early intervention with broad-spectrum intravenous antibiotics is essential to eradicate causative organisms. Seek microbiology advice and refer to local antibiotic guidelines. Adjustments can be made following sensitivities from blood culture or culture of joint aspiration
2. **Analgesia.** Septic arthritis is exquisitely painful, so providing regular analgesia is essential. Opiates such as oramorph may be required
3. **Orthopaedic referral for debridement and washout.** Keep the patient nil by mouth if surgery is anticipated. Most cases of confirmed septic arthritis will require joint washout to prevent further damage to the synovial membranes and bone, and microbiology samples can be taken at the same time
4. **Peripherally inserted central catheter (PICC) line.** Antibiotics are likely to be required for several weeks and a PICC line may be necessary
5. **Avoid weight bearing.** Avoiding stress to the affected joint can help minimise subsequent damage and deformity

Dangerous Diagnosis 2
Diagnosis: Osteomyelitis

Management Principles
See Chapter 13.1, Sepsis Management.
1. **Antibiotics.** Antibiotics should be administered early, guided by local antibiotic guidelines or advice from microbiology. The choice will frequently involve a cephalosporin, with additional staphylococcal cover such as vancomycin or clindamycin
2. **Orthopaedic referral for surgical debridement.** May be required if there is formation of sub-periosteal abscess, for debridement of necrosed tissue in severe cases or if there is a failure to respond to antibiotics. The child will need to be placed nil by mouth if surgery is planned
3. **PICC line.** Antibiotics are likely to be required for several weeks and a PICC line may be necessary
4. **Analgesia.** Osteomyelitis is exquisitely painful and analgesia with opiates is essential.

Dangerous Diagnosis 3
Diagnosis: Compartment syndrome

Management Principles
1. **Orthopaedic referral for fasciotomy.** Confirmed compartment syndrome is an orthopaedic emergency and is treated by surgically opening the fascial compartments to release pressure. Liaise urgently with the orthopaedic team to arrange this, and ensure the child is nil by mouth
2. **Analgesia.** Compartment syndrome is exquisitely painful and analgesia with opiates is essential

Common Diagnosis 1
Diagnosis: Transient synovitis

Management Principles
1. **Analgesia**. Simple analgesia is frequently sufficient to manage the pain. Non-steroidal anti-inflammatory drugs (NSAIDs) will provide anti-inflammatory relief
2. **Conservative management.** Transient synovitis is self-limiting, and management is symptomatic
3. **Encourage mobilisation.** Encouraging the child to mobilise facilitates recovery of function

Common Diagnosis 2
Diagnosis: Simple trauma

Management Principles
1. **RICE.** The initial management of a swollen joint secondary to a sprain is Rest for 48–72 hours with Ice, Compression and Elevation. If there is ligamentous injury, initial management will additionally comprise protected weight bearing and bracing

2. **Analgesia**. The level of analgesia required will vary from injury to injury. Use a validated pain score and escalate from simple paracetamol/NSAIDs, to opiates, nitrous oxide mixes and local anaesthesia
3. **Orthopaedic referral for fixation.** This is a broad management principle and varies from splinting sprain injuries for support, casting fractures that are not significantly displaced, and surgical fixation of severe or significantly unstable or displaced fractures
4. **Bed rest and physiotherapy.** Total bed rest is likely to be required initially. During rehabilitation for a sprain, ligamentous injury or fracture, physiotherapy focuses on restoring range of motion and strength

Common Diagnosis 3
Diagnosis: Slipped upper femoral epiphysis

Management Principles
1. **Limit/stop weight bearing.** SUFEs are classed as stable or unstable depending on the degree of slippage. Unstable SUFEs should remain non-weight bearing to minimise risk of further slippage and subsequent compromise of the blood supply to the femoral head. Even stable SUFEs should be minimally weight bearing due to this same risk
2. **Orthopaedic referral for fixation.** SUFE is an orthopaedic emergency and should be stabilised as soon as is practical. The orthopaedic team will determine whether internal or external fixation is required
3. **Analgesia.** The patient is likely to be in discomfort, so analgesia may be required

10.2 Swollen Joint

Emily Operto[1] and Rachel Varughese[2]
[1] Department of Paediatrics, The Royal Brompton Hospital, London, UK
[2] Department of Paediatrics, Oxford University Hospitals NHS Foundation Trust, Oxford, UK

CONTENTS

10.2.1 CHAPTER AT A GLANCE

> **Box 10.2.1   Chapter at a Glance**
>
> - An acutely swollen joint may represent local or systemic pathology
> - Diagnosis can be difficult and often symptomatic treatment is all that is required in the first instance
> - It is frequently, but not always, associated with pain
> - This chapter should be used in conjunction with Chapter 10.1, Limp, as there is significant overlap, and as differentials are divided into the most relevant chapter

10.2.2 DEFINITION

Localised enlargement of a joint.

Clinical Guide to Paediatrics, First Edition. Edited by Rachel Varughese and Anna Mathew. Series Editor: Christian Fielder Camm.
© 2022 John Wiley & Sons Ltd. Published 2022 by John Wiley & Sons Ltd.
Companion website: www.wiley.com/go/varughese/paediatrics

10.2.3 DIAGNOSTIC ALGORITHM

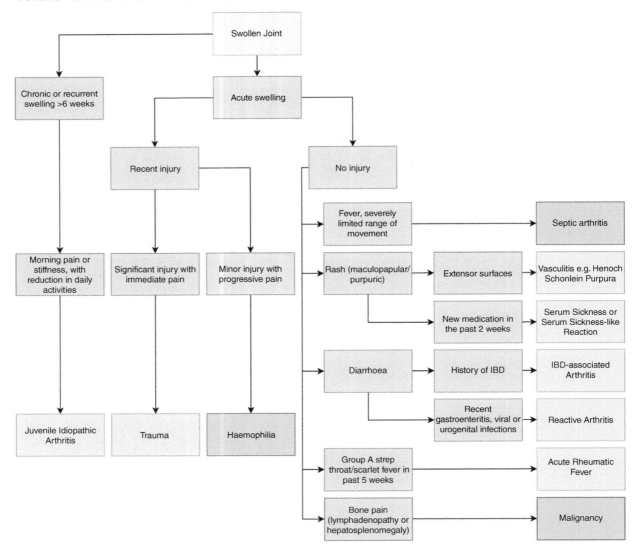

Figure 10.2.1 Diagnostic algorithm for the presentation of a swollen joint.

10.2.4 DIFFERENTIALS LIST

Dangerous Diagnoses

1. Haemophilia

- Haemophilia is inherited as an X-linked recessive bleeding disorder, seen in males
- Haemophilia A, B and C are caused by deficiencies of clotting factor VIII and IX and XI, respectively
- Haemarthrosis following minor trauma may be the first presentation
- Commonly affects elbows, knees and ankles in ambulatory children
- Spontaneous haemarthrosis is characterised by joint stiffness, pain and swelling

2. Septic Arthritis
- Septic arthritis is a bacterial or occasionally fungal infection of any synovial joint, most commonly the hip, knee, shoulder or ankle
- This is an orthopaedic emergency
- Bacterial infection may arise from haematogenous spread, local osteomyelitis or direct penetrating injury
- Children are more affected than adults, particularly those under 4 years old
- Common organisms include *Staphylococcus aureus* (most common), group A *Streptococcus*, *Enterobacter* and *Kingella Kingae*
- Delayed diagnosis and treatment can lead to serious complications, including systemic sepsis, cartilage destruction, growth plate damage and avascular necrosis of the femoral head
- Septic arthritis is covered in detail in Chapter 10.1 and will not be discussed further in this chapter.

3. Malignancy
- Joint pain or swelling can be due to an underlying haematological malignancy, primary bone tumour or bone metastases
- Bone pain is a red flag for malignancy
- Acute lymphoblastic leukaemia is the most common haematological malignancy of childhood causing joint swelling. Small or large joints may be affected
- Neuroblastoma can also cause joint swelling due to bony metastases
- The most common bone malignancies in children are osteosarcoma (usually long bones in legs or arms) and Ewing's sarcoma (predominantly affecting the pelvis, femur, humerus or ribs). Both tend to affect children over the age of 10
- Malignancy is covered in several chapters, such as Chapters 3.3 (Fever), 4.1 (Bruising), 4.2 (Pallor), and will not be discussed further in this chapter

---

Box 10.2.2 Inflammatory Bowel Disease (IBD)–Associated Arthropathy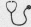

- IBD is associated with various extra-intestinal manifestations, of which arthritis is the most common. This is a subtype of seronegative spondyloarthropathy
- Arthritis tends to be non-deforming and non-erosive
- Arthropathy in IBD can be classified as axial or peripheral (subdivided into oligoarticular or polyarticular)
- Axial arthropathy includes sacroiliitis, ankylosing spondylitis and inflammatory back pain
- Peripheral arthritis is usually symmetrical and tends to flare in parallel with bowel disease. In contrast, there is poor correlation between axial arthropathy and disease activity

Type 1 oligoarticular arthritis	Type 2 polyarticular arthritis
• Involves 5 or fewer joints	• Affects more than 5 joints
• Mostly affects large lower-limb joints (knees)	• Mostly affects upper-limb joints (metacarpophalangeal)
• Acute and self-limiting, correlates with disease activity	• Symmetrical involvement
• Arthritis tends to be non-deforming and non-erosive	• Chronic, less correlation with disease activity

---

Common Diagnoses
1. Henoch–Schönlein Purpura (HSP)
- HSP is a systemic immunoglobulin (Ig) A vasculitis affecting the joints, skin, mucosal membranes and kidneys
- Typical presentation is with a purpuric rash on extensor surfaces of the lower half of the body
- Purpura is accompanied by arthritis in 50–75%, abdominal pain in 50% and renal involvement in 25–50% of children
- Arthritis and arthralgia usually affect large joints, most commonly the knees

2. Post-infectious Arthritis
- Post-infectious arthritis is a broad term, which refers to joint swelling and pain that develops 7–14 days after an infection
- It usually presents as monoarthritis of large joints
- In children, infectious agents are most commonly viral (parvovirus/rubella/Epstein–Barr virus) or gastrointestinal (*Salmonella*, *Shigella*, *Campylobacter*)
- Reactive arthritis is a term often used synonymously with post-infectious arthritis, but this is in fact incorrect. Reactive arthritis, formerly known as Reiter's syndrome, is characterised by the triad of joint inflammation, conjunctivitis and a urogenital infection

3. Trauma

- Traumatic injury most commonly involves a single joint
- The joint cartilage, ligaments or bones may be affected
- The onset of joint pain and swelling will immediately follow the precipitating event
- Trauma is covered in detail in Chapter 10.1. This focuses on lower-limb trauma, however the principles discussed are generally applicable to all joints. Trauma will therefore not be discussed further in this chapter

Diagnoses to Consider

1. Juvenile Idiopathic Arthritis (JIA)

- JIA is a chronic condition (>6 weeks), but is included here as it may occasionally present with acute flare-ups
- Joint swelling is typically associated with stiffness, which is worse in the early morning
- The peak age of incidence is 1–5 years and girls are more affected than boys
- JIA is a term that encompasses all forms of chronic arthritis that start before 16 years of age
- There may be a 'quotidian' fever, rising daily to >39 °C then returning to <37 °C between peaks, with a 'salmon pink' rash often coinciding with fever
- This includes oligoarthritis (involvement of four or fewer joints), systemic-onset JIA, psoriatic arthritis, polyarthritis – rheumatoid factor (RhF) +ve or –ve – and enthesitis-related arthritis

When to consider: in a patient who has had arthritis for >6 weeks, with diurnal variation

---

Box 10.2.3   Systemic Juvenile Idiopathic Arthritis (JIA)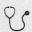

- Systemic JIA is characterised by arthritis in one or more joints, preceded by fever of at least 2 weeks' duration
- It should be accompanied by one or more of the following: a salmon-coloured rash, generalised lymphadenopathy, hepatosplenomegaly, pericarditis and serositis

- Signs and symptoms must be documented for at least 3 consecutive days

---

2. Lyme Disease

- Joint swelling and pain are late symptoms of this tick-borne illness
- As the early stages of the disease may be asymptomatic, a swollen joint may be the presenting feature
- The knee is most commonly affected (90% of cases), and symptoms wax and wane over years
- Diagnosis is by a positive serology for *Borrelia burgdorferi* or polymerase chain reaction (PCR) testing of synovial fluid
- Many of the initial symptoms are reminiscent of flu, with headache, fatigue, myalgia and fevers, and are so non-specific that the infection may go unrecognised. Erythema migrans, red lesions with central clearing in a classic 'bull's-eye' pattern, is pathognomonic

When to consider: in a patient with a history of recent rural travel or known tick bites

3. Acute Rheumatic Fever (ARF)

- Triggered by group A beta-haemolytic streptococcal pharyngitis
- Post-streptococcal reactive arthritis (PSRA) is diagnosed when arthritis does not satisfy other systemic features for diagnosis of ARF
- Presents with migratory, polyarticular joint involvement
- Onset is usually 1–5 weeks after a throat infection or scarlet fever
- ARF is covered in Chapter 3.1, Fever

When to consider: in those with a recent tonsillopharyngitis

Box 10.2.4   Serum Sickness   ΔΔ

- Self-limiting immune complex–mediated hypersensitivity reaction to medications containing heterologous (non-human) proteins, 1–2 weeks after exposure
- Symptoms include fever, a variable rash that may be maculopapular, urticarial or purpuric, and arthritis affecting multiple joints. There is no mucous membrane involvement, which is important as Stevens–Johnson syndrome may be a differential

- Medications that are implicated include monoclonal antibodies, e.g. infliximab, and some vaccinations, e.g. rabies
- Be aware that there is also a 'serum sickness–like reaction' that results in a similar clinical presentation, without immune complex deposition. Medication triggers include antibiotics such as the penicillins, cephalosporins and sulphonamides
- Infections such as hepatitis B and streptococcus may also be a trigger

> **Box 10.2.5   Baker's Cyst** △△
>
> - This is an idiopathic, painless, synovial fluid-filled swelling behind the knee in the popliteal fossa
> - Although Baker's cysts are common in adults, they are relatively rare in children
> - When present, boys aged 4–8 years are most commonly affected
> - They resolve spontaneously, but 40% recur

10.2.5 KEY HISTORY FEATURES

Dangerous Diagnosis 1
Diagnosis: Haemophilia

Questions
1. **Was there a preceding event?** There is often a minor injury, with symptoms out of proportion to the mechanism
2. **How quickly did the symptoms evolve?** Significant pain of the joint frequently precedes joint swelling. Depending on the trigger, bruising of soft tissue may also be evident
3. **Is there a history of easy bruising?** There might be a history of previous unrecognised significance. Ask about easy bruising, muscle haematomas or bleeding from the oropharynx
4. **Is there a family history of haemophilia or another bleeding disorder?** As this is an X-linked recessive disorder, a positive family history with affected males is likely
5. **Which joint is affected, and has it been affected before?** The joints of the knees, ankles and elbows are most frequently affected and repeated bleeding into the same joint can lead to chronic joint problems

> **Box 10.2.6   Consequences of Repeated Haemarthrosis**
>
> - Chronic synovitis
> - Degenerative arthritis
> - Limb length discrepancy (bony growth affected)
> - Osteoporosis (reduced mobility due to acute bleeds and chronic joint changes)

Common Diagnosis 1
Diagnosis: Henoch–Schönlein purpura (HSP)

Questions
1. **Did the illness begin with a rash, and has that evolved over time?** Children usually present with an urticarial rash over their lower legs that evolves over days to become purpuric, and to extend over the back of the legs, up to the buttocks and then over both arms
2. **What is the pattern of joint involvement?** There is transient joint swelling and pain that most commonly affect the knees, ankles or wrists and typically last for 7–10 days
3. **Has there been any abdominal pain?** It is not uncommon to get a history of abdominal pain due to the generalised IgA vasculitis causing oedema and haemorrhage of the bowel wall

Common Diagnosis 2
Diagnosis: Post-infectious arthritis

Questions
1. **Has there been a recent infection?** Post-infectious arthritis is very often attributed to a non-specific viral upper respiratory tract infection. Gastrointestinal infections (particularly those causing bloody diarrhoea) are also a common trigger. Rubella and parvovirus can cause arthritides in older children and adolescents
2. **Is there a family history of spondyloarthropathy?** There is a strong association between human leucocyte antigen (HLA) B27 and reactive arthritis/'Reiter's syndrome'
3. **If an adolescent, is the patient sexually active?** *Chlamydia trachomatis* infection of the genitourinary tract should be considered, especially if there is concurrent conjunctivitis (reactive arthritis/Reiter's syndrome)

Box 10.2.7 The Three Stages of Lyme Disease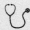

Stage 1: Localised erythema migrans	Stage 2: Disseminated infection	Stage 3: Persistent infection
Initial phase of the infection may be asymptomatic or unrecognised • Erythematous macule/papule appears at site of tick bite • Flu-like symptoms with fever, rigors, headache, myalgia, fatigue • Lesions progress from erythematous → indurated → vesicular → necrotic • Multiple secondary lesions can develop, 'erythema chronicum migrans', predominantly over the thigh, groin and axilla	Central nervous system (CNS), cardiac or joint symptoms may appear, weeks to months later, in untreated children CNS • Cranial nerves: most commonly unilateral or bilateral facial palsy • Peripheral neuropathy: asymmetrical motor and/or sensory neuropathy • Other neurological manifestations: meningitis, Guillain–Barré syndrome, idiopathic intracranial hypertension, cerebellar ataxia, chorea, demyelinating encephalopathy, memory impairment, depression Cardiac • Atrioventricular block, pericarditis, myocarditis Joint • Initial arthralgias evolve to arthritis, involving large joints, especially the knee	Rarely seen in children, may last years • Progressive arthritis leading to permanent disability • Demyelinating disease • Mental health difficulties, depression and memory impairment

10.2.6 KEY EXAMINATION FEATURES

Box 10.2.8 Joint Examination

Inspection

- Inspect both limbs and joints for shape and comparative size
- Look for colour change, swelling, bony change, wasting and deformity
- Assess whether any change is limited to the joint or involves surrounding structures

Palpation

- Assess joints for tenderness, warmth and fluid
- Assess muscles for bulk, tone, strength, tenderness and fasciculation
- Note any wasting or hypertrophy

Manipulation

- Assess range of movement: active (child's ability to independently move their joint) and passive (doctor's ability to move the child's joint)
- Note limitation, tenderness, presence of crepitus and stability of the joint

Dangerous Diagnosis 1
Diagnosis: Haemophilia

Examination Findings
1. **Systemically well.** In spite of the pain and limitation of movement, the child is not pyrexial and does not look systemically unwell. This is helpful when differentiating haemarthrosis from septic arthritis
2. **Limited range of motion.** The range of movement of the joint may already be reduced due to chronic damage from recurrent bleeds. This will be further affected with fresh bleeding
3. **Antalgic gait.** With each episode the child may display an antalgic gait or be unable to bear weight on the affected limb
4. **Soft tissue haematomas, bruising.** In addition to the haemarthrosis, bruising and bleeding into soft tissues may also be evident

Common Diagnosis 1
Diagnosis: Henoch–Schönlein purpura

Examination Findings
1. **Joint swelling without overlying skin changes.** The affected joints (predominantly knees and ankles) are swollen and painful, with reduced range of motion. There is no overlying erythema or warmth
2. **Rash.** Rash begins as urticaria and progresses to palpable purpura, preceding other symptoms by 4 days. The distribution of the rash is typically initially over the lower legs, which then extends up the back of the legs to involve the bottom. Over time, the rash can also develop over the upper limbs
3. **Abdominal tenderness.** Non-specific abdominal tenderness is typical, but must be monitored closely, as children can develop several gastrointestinal complications including intussusception
4. **Scrotal swelling/tenderness.** Boys may have a painful, swollen scrotum
5. **Haematuria.** 25–50% of children have renal involvement, and there may be macroscopic haematuria

Common Diagnosis 2
Diagnosis: Post-infectious arthritis

Examination Findings
1. **Joint inflammation.** Affected joints are swollen and painful, with overlying skin erythema and warmth
2. **Signs of precipitating infection.** There may be signs of an upper respiratory tract infection. If gastroenteritis is the suspected trigger, examine for hydration status
3. **Systemically well.** Compared to those with septic arthritis, children with post-infectious arthritis are generally well
4. **Conjunctivitis.** If conjunctivitis is present, this might point to a diagnosis of reactive arthritis/Reiter's syndrome

10.2.7 KEY INVESTIGATIONS

Not all children will require invasive investigations; often diagnoses are made on clinical evidence from history and examination. Consider carefully which investigations are required for which patient.

Bedside

Table 10.2.1 Bedside tests of use in patients presenting with swollen joints

Test	When to perform	Potential result
Urinalysis	Suspected: • HSP to determine renal involvement • Reactive arthritis with suspected UTI	• Haematuria, proteinuria: HSP • Leukocytes, nitrites: UTI
Urine culture	• Suspected reactive arthritis with possible UTI	• Positive culture confirms causative organism • Sensitivities guide antibiotic choice
Stool culture	• Suspected post-infectious arthritis with concurrent diarrhoea	• Positive culture confirms causative organism
Throat culture	• Suspected ARF	• Group A streptococcus infection supports ARF
ECG	• Suspected ARF to look for signs of carditis	• Prolonged PR interval: indicative of carditis, supports diagnosis of ARF

ARF, acute rheumatic fever; ECG, electrocardiogram; HSP, Henoch–Schönlein purpura; UTI, urinary tract infection

Blood Tests

Table 10.2.2 Blood tests of use in patients presenting with swollen joints

Test	When to perform	Potential result
FBC	Suspected: • Haemophilia • Septic arthritis • Malignancy • HSP • JIA	• ↓ Hb, normal MCV: anaemia of chronic disease, acute bleeding in haemophilia • ↑ WCC: infection (usually neutrophilia if bacterial, lymphocytosis in viral), leukaemia • ↑ Platelets: chronic inflammation • Pancytopenia: leukaemia, solid malignancy with bone marrow involvement – blood film required to further evaluate
Blood film	• Suspected malignancy	• Blast cells, pancytopenia indicate malignancy
ESR and CRP	Suspected: • Septic arthritis • ARF	• ↑ Indicate infection or inflammation • Specific levels could meet criteria for ARF
Coagulation profile	• Suspected haemarthrosis due to a bleeding disorder	• ↑ APTT, normal PT and normal bleeding time seen in haemophilia
Coagulation factors	• Factor 8, factor 9 and VWF	• Identifies haemophilia A, B or von Willebrand disease, and also indicates severity of disorder
Blood culture	• Suspected septic arthritis	• Positive result confirms bacterial infection • Sensitivities guide antibiotic choice
Anti-streptolysin O titre	• Suspected ARF	• ↑ Titres confirm group A streptococcal infection
Anti-DNaseB serology	• Suspected ARF	• ↑ Titres support group A streptococcal infection
Lyme serology	• Suspected Lyme disease	• ↑ Titres support Lyme disease • However, high false positive and false negative results, so unreliable – diagnosis should be clinical

APTT, activated partial thromboplastin time; ARF, acute rheumatic fever; CRP, C-reactive protein; ESR, erythrocyte sedimentation rate; FBC, full blood count; Hb, haemoglobin; HSP, Henoch–Schönlein purpura; JIA, juvenile idiopathic arthritis; MCV, mean corpuscular volume; PT, prothrombin time; VWF, von Willebrand factor; WCC, white cell count

Imaging

Table 10.2.3 Imaging modalities of use in patients presenting with swollen joints

Test	When to perform	Potential result
X-ray of joint ± limb	• All children with a swollen joint	• Changes consistent with chronic arthritis, septic arthritis, tumour, fracture or enthesitis
Ultrasound of affected joint	• All children with a swollen joint • Useful for diagnosis and guiding joint aspiration	• Joint effusion in reactive arthritis, septic arthritis, Henoch–Schönlein purpura • Extent of bleeding, cartilage damage in haemophilia
Computed tomography (CT)	Suspected: • Trauma • Haemophilia	• Fracture in trauma • Extent of bleeding, cartilage damage in haemophilia
Magnetic resonance imaging (MRI)	Suspected: • Children where greater detail is required	• Ligamentous injury, fracture or enthesitis • Extent of bleeding, cartilage damage in haemophilia

...se in patients presenting with swollen joints

Table 10.2.4 Special test...

	When to perform	Potential result
	• Suspected reactive arthritis	• Positive result supports reactive arthritis • Negative result does not exclude reactive arthritis
	• Suspected septic arthritis	• Positive result confirms bacterial infection • Sensitivities guide antibiotic choice
	• Suspected Lyme disease, microscopy may identify spirochete	• *Borrelia burgdorferi* spirochete seen

...osteosarcoma in the femur (accounts for 40% of osteosarcomas).

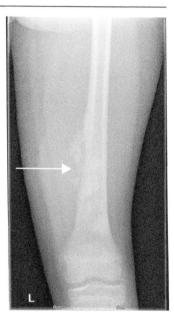

Figure 10.2.3 X-ray of osteosarcoma in the humerus (accounts for 15% of osteosarcomas).

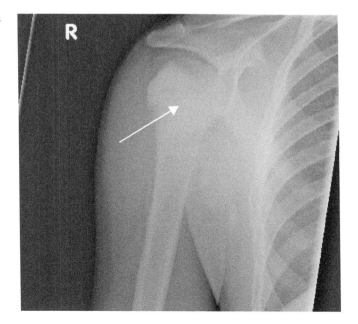

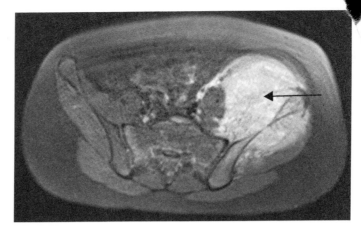

Figure 10.2.4 Magnetic resonance imaging of pelvic Ewing's sarcoma.

10.2.8 KEY MANAGEMENT PRINCIPLES

Diagnosis-specific management strategies are outlined here. It is expected that an 'ABCDE' approach to assessment and management is always undertaken (see Chapter 12.1, *The A to E Assessment*).

Dangerous Diagnosis 1
Diagnosis: Haemophilia

Management Principles
1. **Haemophilia specialist service.** Most regions will have a haemophilia specialist service and should be referred there for tertiary oversight. This is essential in coordinating a multidisciplinary team approach to counselling, education, chronic care and managing complications
2. **Factor replacement therapy.** Decisions regarding treatment are individualised, and involve weighing up long-term prophylaxis, short-term prophylaxis and on-demand treatment. Factor replacement also carries the risk of inhibitor development, where neutralising antibodies are formed to exogenous factor, which is recognised as foreign. Following a bleed into a joint, factor 8 (haemophilia A) or factor 9 (haemophilia B) can be given as an infusion
3. **Immobilisation.** Patients should avoid weight bearing and rest the affected joint
4. **Analgesia.** Manage pain with paracetamol or opioids if necessary

Common Diagnosis 1
Diagnosis: Henoch–Schönlein purpura

Management Principles
1. **Analgesia.** The joint pain should be managed with paracetamol or a non-steroidal anti-inflammatory drug (NSAID)
2. **Education.** HSP generally self-resolves within 6 weeks, but there is a recurrence rate of 33%. The rash is usually the last symptom to disappear
3. **Urinalysis and blood pressure (BP) follow-up.** Regular repetition of urinalysis and BP is required, either through an ambulatory care unit or the GP. This starts weekly for the first month, 2-weekly for the next 2 months and then single visits at 3, 6 and 12 months. Any macroscopic haematuria, 2+ proteinuria or BP >95th centile should prompt paediatric review
4. **Corticosteroids.** Steroids can be used to reduce the duration and severity of abdominal pain and joint pain, but do not impact renal complications. Caution should be exercised in the acute phase, as steroids can mask the signs of an acute abdomen
5. **Renal support.** Long-term morbidity is usually related to renal complications. Renal specialist review is required for hypertension, abnormal renal function, persistent macroscopic haematuria and persistent proteinuria

Common Diagnosis 2
Diagnosis: Post-infectious arthritis

Management Principles
1. **NSAIDs.** Post-infectious arthritis is self-resolving and management centres on symptomatic relief. NSAIDs, e.g. ibuprofen, are very effective
2. **Treatment of underlying infection.** If there is an identified urogenital or gastrointestinal infection, this should be treated

11.1 Neonatal Jaundice

Rebecca Puddifoot

Oxford University Hospitals NHS Foundation Trust, Oxford, UK

CONTENTS

11.1.1 CHAPTER AT A GLANCE

> **Box 11.1.1   Chapter at a Glance**
>
> - Neonatal jaundice is a common problem encountered on the post-natal and paediatric wards
> - The mainstay of treatment is monitoring the bilirubin levels, ensuring adequate feeding through support and phototherapy when indicated
>
> - It is important to be mindful of the less common and potentially serious causes that may need further urgent management

11.1.2 DEFINITION

The yellow colouring of the skin and the sclera caused by an elevated level of bilirubin in babies of less than 28 days of age.

Clinical Guide to Paediatrics, First Edition. Edited by Rachel Varughese and Anna Mathew. Series Editor: Christian Fielder Camm.
© 2022 John Wiley & Sons Ltd. Published 2022 by John Wiley & Sons Ltd.
Companion website: www.wiley.com/go/varughese/paediatrics

11.1.3 DIAGNOSTIC ALGORITHM

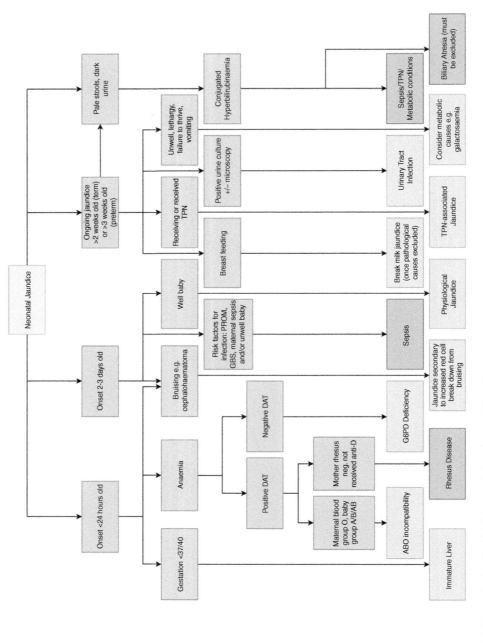

Figure 11.1.1 Diagnostic algorithm for the presentation of neonatal jaundice.

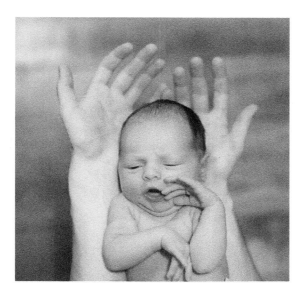

Figure 11.1.2 Baby with jaundiced skin. Source: Reproduced with permission of Shutterstock.

11.1.4 DIFFERENTIALS LIST

Dangerous Diagnoses
1. Rhesus Disease of the Newborn

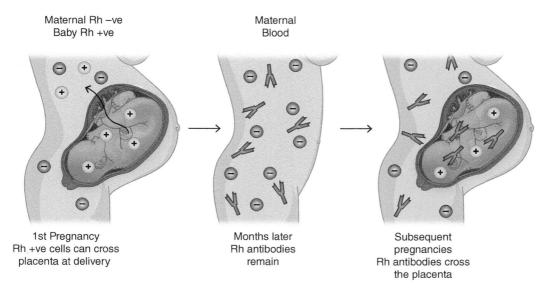

Figure 11.1.3 Rhesus Disease. Formation of rhesus antibodies occurs during delivery when rhesus-positive red blood cells (RBCs) cross the placenta. In subsequent pregnancies, rhesus antibodies cross the placenta, causing haemolysis of foetal RBCs (if the foetus is rhesus positive).

- Rhesus D (RhD) is an antigen found on the surface of red blood cells
- Rhesus disease happens when the mother is rhesus negative and the baby is rhesus positive

- A 'sensitising' event is required, where the mother is exposed to the baby's blood, stimulating the production of antibodies. This may happen as a result of a miscarriage, antepartum haemorrhage or birth
- Rapid-onset jaundice, often starting antenatally, which can lead to still birth, neonatal death and kernicterus
- Very rare in developed countries due to screening and administration of anti-D antibodies where indicated

2. Sepsis
- Neonatal sepsis can present non-specifically; jaundice may be the first warning sign, especially if within the first 24 hours of life

3. Biliary Atresia
- Congenital obstruction of the bile ducts, either completely or partially impairing bile flow into the small intestine
- Jaundice is due to conjugated hyperbilirubinemia, and classic symptoms include pale stools and dark urine
- The accumulation of bile in the liver causes progressive cirrhosis
- Early intervention is critical to prevent irreversible liver damage or death

Common Diagnoses
1. Physiological Jaundice
- The most common cause of jaundice in neonates, presenting on days 2–3 of life
- Secondary to foetal haemoglobin (HbF) breakdown (to be replaced with adult Hb), combined with the immaturity of the liver's metabolic pathways in processing bilirubin

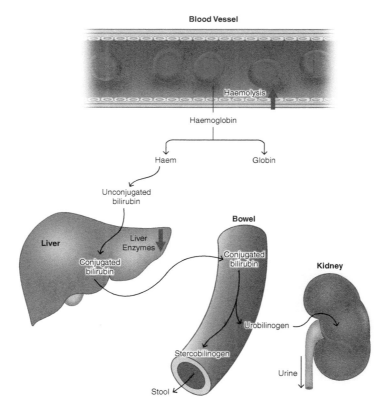

Figure 11.1.4 Physiological jaundice: the process of metabolism of bilirubin. In physiological jaundice, there is increased red blood cell breakdown and reduced metabolism of bilirubin in the liver. This leads to the build-up of bilirubin and the onset of jaundice.

2. Breast Milk Jaundice
- The most common cause for prolonged jaundice (persistent jaundice beyond 2 weeks of age in a term neonate and beyond 3 weeks of age in a preterm neonate)
- The exact mechanism behind why breastfeeding causes jaundice is not clearly understood. It is thought that a substance in the breast milk inhibits the metabolism of bilirubin

3. ABO Incompatibility
- Incompatibility between neonatal and maternal blood groups can lead to autoimmune haemolysis, which is generally milder than in RhD disease
- Although ABO incompatibility is due to an autoimmune process, the direct antiglobulin test (DAT) is sometimes negative

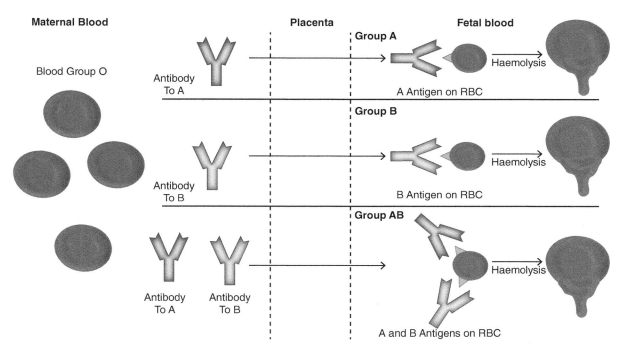

Figure 11.1.5 ABO Incompatibility. Maternal antibodies (immunoglobulin G) to A and/or B in a mother who is blood group O can cross the placenta and bind to A and/or B antigens in foetal blood groups A, B and AB, causing haemolysis and subsequent jaundice.

Diagnoses to Consider
1. Urinary Tract Infection (UTI)
- The signs and symptoms of a UTI in a neonate can be non-specific and therefore jaundice is sometimes the only feature. Consider this in prolonged jaundice

When to consider: in cases of prolonged jaundice or failure to gain weight as expected. UTI is not common in the first 2 weeks of life

2. Congenital Hypothyroidism
- Hypothyroidism can lead to the development of prolonged jaundice and if unrecognised can potentially lead to severe neurodisability
- Congenital hypothyroidism is usually identified on the day 5 routine neonatal blood spot screening done in the UK

When to consider: in cases of prolonged jaundice, particularly if newborn blood spot has not been done

3. Total Parenteral Nutrition (TPN)
- Diagnosis of exclusion
- Conjugated hyperbilirubinemia may develop after starting TPN, most commonly after 2 weeks of TPN

When to consider: if the raised bilirubin is conjugated and the baby has received at least 2 weeks of TPN

4. Metabolic Conditions

- Metabolic causes are rare, but should be considered as a potential cause in cases of prolonged jaundice and/or conjugated hyperbilirubinaemia
- Metabolic conditions that cause jaundice include glucose-6-phosphate dehydrogenase (G6PD) deficiency, galactosaemia, alpha-1-antitrypsin deficiency, aminoacidurias and organoacidaemias

When to consider: in cases of prolonged jaundice with family history of consanguinity or issues with hypoglycaemia

---

Box 11.1.2   Relationship between Onset of Jaundice and Diagnosis   ΔΔ

	<24 hours old	2–3 days	>2 weeks*
Dangerous	• Rhesus disease • Sepsis	• Sepsis	• Biliary atresia
Common	• ABO incompatibility • Prematurity • Extensive bruising from delivery	• ABO incompatibility • Physiological jaundice • Prematurity • Extensive bruising from delivery	• Breast milk jaundice
To consider in 'prolonged jaundice'			• Hypothyroidism • Urinary tract infection • Metabolic problems, e.g. galactosaemia • Total parenteral nutrition–associated jaundice

*Prolonged jaundice is defined as >2 weeks in a term baby, or >3 weeks in a preterm baby.

11.1.5 KEY HISTORY FEATURES

Box 11.1.3   General Approach to History Taking in Neonatal Jaundice

Is the baby feeding well?

- Jaundice can make the infant very sleepy, resulting in reduced feeding and not waking for feeds
- This will lead to increased bilirubin levels
- Therefore, it is important to address this in the history to ensure it is managed correctly alongside other treatments

Are there risk factors for jaundice?

- Gestational age <38 weeks
- Jaundice commencing at <24 hours of age
- Previous sibling requiring phototherapy for jaundice
- Exclusive breastfeeding

Are there features that suggest a pathological underlying cause requiring further investigation?

- Onset of jaundice at less than 24 hours of age
- Conjugated hyperbilirubinemia (defined as conjugated bilirubin >25 µmol/L or >25% of total bilirubin)
- Dark urine/pale stool (indicating conjugated hyperbilirubinemia)
- Systemically unwell – fever, respiratory distress, shock
- Anaemia

Dangerous Diagnosis 1

Diagnosis: Rhesus disease of the newborn

Questions

1. **Did the jaundice start within the first 24 hours of life?** Bilirubin levels rise very rapidly in rhesus disease and therefore jaundice starts early and may cross exchange transfusion thresholds. Haemolysis often starts in utero
2. **What is the mother's blood group?** In rhesus disease, the mother's blood group is RhD negative and the baby's blood group is RhD positive
3. **Is this the mother's first baby?** Rhesus disease normally occurs in the second pregnancy, unless there has been a sensitising event such as an early antepartum haemorrhage
4. **Did the mother receive anti-D post-partum during her other pregnancies?** Strongly consider this diagnosis if anti-D was not received in the post-partum period in previous pregnancies and/or was not given during this pregnancy. Anti-D is given at 28 weeks' gestation and after delivery to rhesus-negative mothers

Dangerous Diagnosis 2

Diagnosis: Sepsis

Questions

1. **Is the baby unwell?** Check for other features that may be present in neonatal sepsis. These include fever, hypoglycaemia, poor feeding and/or feed intolerance and seizures
2. **Are there any risk factors for sepsis?** See Box 11.1.4

Box 11.1.4   Risk Factors for Neonatal Sepsis

- Prolonged rupture of membranes for over 18 hours in a preterm baby
- Group B *Streptococcus* colonisation, bacteraemia or infection in this pregnancy
- Invasive group B *Streptococcus* infection in a previous baby
- Maternal fever in labour or suspected/confirmed chorioamnionitis

- Prematurity (born at <37 weeks' gestation) following spontaneous onset of labour
- Confirmed or suspected invasive infection in the mother requiring intravenous antibiotic therapy peri-partum
- Pre-labour rupture of membranes

Dangerous Diagnosis 3

Diagnosis: Biliary atresia

Questions

1. **Is the jaundice prolonged?** Biliary atresia generally presents with a history of prolonged jaundice. However, conjugated hyperbilirubinaemia at any age is always pathological and biliary atresia should be considered
2. **What colour are the stools and urine?** Pale stools and dark urine are classic due to the obstruction posed by the atretic bile ducts, preventing conjugated bilirubin from entering the intestines. This may also result in faltering growth due to malabsorption

Common Diagnosis 1

Diagnosis: Physiological jaundice

Questions

1. **When did you first notice the jaundice?** Physiological jaundice first appears on days 2–3 of life. This is when the bilirubin levels rise secondary to erythrocyte breakdown. Physiological jaundice resolves by 1–2 weeks of life
2. **Is the baby well?** In physiological jaundice, the baby generally remains well, although they may become sleepy as a result of the jaundice
3. **Is there significant bruising from delivery (e.g. a cephalohaematoma)?** Bruising from delivery increases the quantity of red blood cells that are broken down
4. **Has the baby been born preterm?** Babies born before 37 weeks' gestation have immature metabolism of bilirubin in the liver

Common Diagnosis 2

Diagnosis: Breast milk jaundice

Questions

1. **Is the baby being predominantly breastfed?** Breast milk jaundice only occurs in breastfed babies and is a diagnosis of exclusion in prolonged jaundice
2. **Is the baby well?** In breast milk jaundice the baby remains well, although they may become sleepy as a result of the jaundice

Common Diagnosis 3

Diagnosis: ABO incompatibility

Questions

1. **What are the blood groups for mother and baby?** The mother's blood group will be O and the baby's blood group A, B or AB. Consider this diagnosis when the mother's blood group is O until the baby's blood group is known
2. **When did the jaundice develop?** In ABO incompatibility, the jaundice often develops within the first 24 hours of life. However, it can also develop over the first few days

11.1.6 KEY EXAMINATION FEATURES

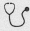

> **Box 11.1.5   General Examination Features in Neonatal Jaundice**
>
> - Yellowing of the skin (starting at the head and moving downwards)
> - Yellow sclera
> - Drowsiness
> - Reduced feeding

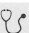

> **Box 11.1.6   Kernicterus**
>
> Kernicterus is a complication of severe neonatal jaundice. Elevated levels of unconjugated bilirubin cross the blood–brain barrier and damage the central nervous system. Features start to develop from the first week of life and result in long-term impairments. It is rare in the UK due to awareness and prompt treatment of jaundice. Features include the following.
>
> | Acute | Chronic |
> | --- | --- |
> | - Hypotonia | - Hearing loss |
> | - Poor suck | - Visual problems |
> | - Absent reflexes | - Seizures |
> | - High-pitched cry | - Learning impairment |
> | - Seizures | - Rigidity and movement disorders |

Dangerous Diagnosis 1
Diagnosis: Rhesus disease of the newborn

Examination Findings
1. **Pallor.** Pallor is a sign seen in significant haemolytic anaemia. Other signs include hepatosplenomegaly, tachycardia, systolic 'flow' murmur and haemodynamic instability
2. **Hydrops fetalis**. If the haemolytic disease is severe, the foetus may develop hydrops fetalis. Postnatal features include oedema, ascites, pleural effusions and pericardial effusions

Dangerous Diagnosis 2
Diagnosis: Sepsis

Examination Findings
1. **Signs of infection**. Generalised signs of infection include respiratory distress (subcostal recession, tracheal tug, head bobbing), apnoea, tachycardia and poor tone
2. **Signs of meningitis**. In neonates, these include irritability, seizures and a bulging fontanelle

Dangerous Diagnosis 3
Diagnosis: Biliary atresia

Examination Findings
1. **Normal examination.** Often, jaundice and pale stools are the sole findings, which can be falsely reassuring
2. **Hepatosplenomegaly.** In advanced disease, hepatomegaly or hepatosplenomegaly might be present
3. **Syndromic features.** Consider the possibility of an underlying syndrome, such as Alagille syndrome

> **Box 11.1.7   Features Seen in Alagille Syndrome**
>
> - Facial features: broad forehead, deep-set eyes, small pointed chin
> - Abnormal bile ducts: liver damage, jaundice, itchy skin, xanthomas
> - Congenital cardiac disease: pulmonary stenosis, ventricular septal defect, tetralogy of Fallot
> - Skeletal abnormalities: butterfly vertebrae
> - Vascular anomalies: intracranial bleeding
> - Central nervous system: mild developmental delay
> - Less commonly, there may be renal dysplasia and pancreatic insufficiency

Common Diagnosis 1
Diagnosis: Physiological jaundice

Examination Findings
1. **Normal examination.** Other than visible jaundice, examination is unremarkable
2. **Bruising from delivery, e.g. cephalohaematoma.** Bruising increases the risk of developing neonatal jaundice

Common Diagnosis 2
Diagnosis: Breast milk jaundice

Examination Findings
1. **Normal examination.** Other than visible jaundice, examination is unremarkable

Common Diagnosis 3
Diagnosis: ABO incompatibility

Examination Findings
1. **Signs of anaemia.** Pallor is a common sign of anaemia, but is not always obvious. Anaemia is often not severe enough in ABO incompatibility to display other clinical features
2. **Systemic features of haemolysis.** In unusual circumstances this could include hepatosplenomegaly, tachycardia, systolic murmur and haemodynamic instability

11.1.7 KEY INVESTIGATIONS

Neonatal jaundice is most often physiological, and other than monitoring transcutaneous/serum bilirubin levels, most of the investigations listed here are not necessary. Which investigations need to be undertaken will be directed by the time of onset of the jaundice, the bilirubin level and the presenting features on clinical examination.

Bedside

Table 11.1.1 Bedside tests of use in patients presenting with neonatal jaundice

Test	When to perform	Potential result
Transcutaneous bilirubin	• All babies with jaundice	• Reliable <250 µmol/L
SBR	• All babies with jaundice if transcutaneous bilirubin >250 µmol/L or if previously treated with phototherapy	• May be above treatment or exchange transfusion threshold
Spun HCT	• All babies having an SBR or in suspected polycythaemia	• ↑ HCT: polycythaemia predisposes to jaundice
Blood gas (capillary or venous)	Suspected: • Sepsis • Dehydration	• ↓ pH, ↓ HCO_3, ↑ lactate: metabolic acidosis in sepsis, severe dehydration
Blood glucose (mmol/L)	• Suspected sepsis	• <2: hypoglycaemia in the first 48 hours (ranges for concern depend on clinical symptoms) • After 48 hours, <2.6 constitutes hypoglycaemia
Urine MC&S	• Prolonged jaundice	• Positive urine culture directs antibiotic choice

HCO_3, bicarbonate; HCT, haematocrit; MC&S, microscopy, culture and sensitivity; SBR, serum bilirubin

Blood Tests

Table 11.1.2 Blood tests of use in patients presenting with neonatal jaundice

Test	When to perform	Potential result
FBC	• Suspected sepsis • Prolonged jaundice	• ↓ Hb, ↑reticulocytes: haemolysis • ↑ WCC, ↑neutrophils: sepsis
Blood group	• Suspected rhesus disease and ABO incompatibility • Prolonged jaundice	• Rhesus disease: maternal group will be RhD negative and foetal group RhD positive • ABO incompatibility: maternal blood group is usually O and foetal blood group is A, B or AB
DAT	• Suspected rhesus disease and ABO incompatibility • Prolonged jaundice	• Positive in ABO incompatibility and rhesus disease
Blood film	Suspected: • Rhesus disease • ABO incompatibility • Haemolysis of uncertain cause	• Red blood cell fragments (schistocytes) indicating haemolysis • Spherocytes may indicate alternative diagnosis of hereditary spherocytosis
Split bilirubin	• Prolonged jaundice	• Determine the percentage split of conjugated and unconjugated bilirubin • ↑ Conjugated bilirubin: biliary atresia must be excluded, TPN-associated jaundice
LFTs	• Prolonged jaundice	• ↑ AST/ALT indicates liver injury/disease
CRP	• Suspected sepsis	• ↑ CRP determines need for consideration of meningitis, lumbar puncture and escalation of antibiotics • Thresholds vary between hospitals – consult local guidelines
U&E	Suspected: • Sepsis • Dehydration	• ↑ Na/urea/creatinine: dehydration or acute kidney injury in sepsis
Blood culture	• Suspected sepsis	• Positive blood culture confirms bacterial infection • Sensitivities guide antibiotic choice

ALT, alanine aminotransferase; AST, aspartate aminotransferase; CRP, C-reactive protein; DAT, direct antibody test; FBC, full blood count; Hb, haemoglobin; LFTs, liver function tests; Na, sodium; TPN, total parenteral nutrition; U&E, urea and electrolytes; WCC, white cell count

Imaging

Table 11.1.3 Imaging modalities of use in patients presenting with neonatal jaundice

Test	When to perform	Potential result
Ultrasound abdomen	• Conjugated hyperbilirubinemia to investigate biliary atresia	• Absence of all or part of the biliary tree

Special

Table 11.1.4 Special tests of use in patients presenting with neonatal jaundice

Test	When to perform	Potential result
G6PD	• Consider in male babies of Mediterranean origin with prolonged jaundice	• ↓ Levels in G6PD deficiency
Urinary-reducing substances	• Screening test for galactosaemia • Indicated in prolonged jaundice with other features suggestive of galactosaemia	• Positive for galactose, lactose and/or fructose

Table 11.1.4 (Continued)

Test	When to perform	Potential result
GAL-1-PUT	• Screening test for galactosaemia • Indicated in prolonged jaundice with other features suggestive of galactosaemia	• Diminished levels of GAL-1-PUT indicate galactosemia
Lumbar puncture: CSF examination and culture	• Suspected meningitis (clinically or CRP)	• ↑ Neutrophils suggest bacterial meningitis • Positive culture confirms infection
TORCH screen	• Prolonged jaundice if suspicion of congenital infections	• Positive result confirms specific congenital infection

Ensure routine metabolic and thyroid screening has been performed in the routine neonatal blood spot

CRP, C-reactive protein; CSF, cerebrospinal fluid; G6PD, glucose-6-phosphate dehydrogenase; GAL-1-PUT, galactose-1-phosphate uridyl transferase

11.1.8 KEY MANAGEMENT PRINCIPLES

Diagnosis-specific management strategies are outlined here. It is expected that an 'ABCDE' approach to assessment and management is always undertaken (see Chapter 12.1).

Box 11.1.8   General Management of Neonatal Jaundice

Encourage regular feeding

• The baby may not wake spontaneously for feeds and may need waking 3-hourly to feed

Monitor bilirubin levels

• Transcutaneous bilirubinometer can be used to measure bilirubin for babies who are over 35 weeks' gestation and over 24 hours of age. A transcutaneous bilirubinometer measures the bilirubin levels using a light probe against the skin
• Serum bilirubin levels are required:
  • For babies <24 hours of age
  • For babies <35 weeks' gestation
  • If the transcutaneous bilirubin >250 µmol/L
  • If the measurement is at the treatment threshold line
  • For monitoring during phototherapy and for rebound bilirubin measurements (transcutaneous measurements are inaccurate after phototherapy)

Phototherapy

• If the bilirubin level exceeds the treatment threshold line, phototherapy should be commenced. A chart appropriate for the gestational age should be used, which plots the age of the baby against the level of bilirubin
• During phototherapy, as much of the baby as possible should be exposed to the lights, and protective eyewear is required

• Bilirubin levels should be monitored during phototherapy and regular feeds should be continued
• Regular adequate feeds are important to flush out the bilirubin. However, every attempt should be made to minimise time away from phototherapy for feeds and nappy changes
• Once the bilirubin levels fall to over 50 below the treatment threshold line, phototherapy can be discontinued, and a rebound bilirubin level checked at 12–18 hours after discontinuing phototherapy

Exchange transfusion

• Exchange transfusion is rarely required. It is indicated in cases of severe neonatal jaundice above the exchange transfusion threshold line and/or clinical signs of bilirubin encephalopathy
• Exchange transfusion is performed by removing aliquots of blood from the baby through a central line and replacing them with blood from packed red cells
• During exchange transfusion, intensive phototherapy should be continued

Intravenous immunoglobulin (IVIg)

• IVIg can be used in suspected or confirmed rhesus disease and ABO incompatibility while preparing for exchange transfusion

Box 11.1.9 How to Plot Bilirubin Levels

- The correct chart for gestational age should be selected. Charts run from 23 weeks' gestation weekly up to >38 weeks'
- 0 on the x-axis is the date and time of birth of the baby. For example, 5/7/2020 at 10:05 am
- 1 on the x-axis is the following day at the same time of birth. For example, 6/7/2020 at 10:05 am
- The lines between numbers normally indicate 6-hourly time intervals

- The y-axis is the bilirubin level
- If the level plots above the blue phototherapy line, but below the red exchange transfusion line, phototherapy should be commenced
- If the level plots above the exchange transfusion line, commence phototherapy, and prepare for exchange transfusion

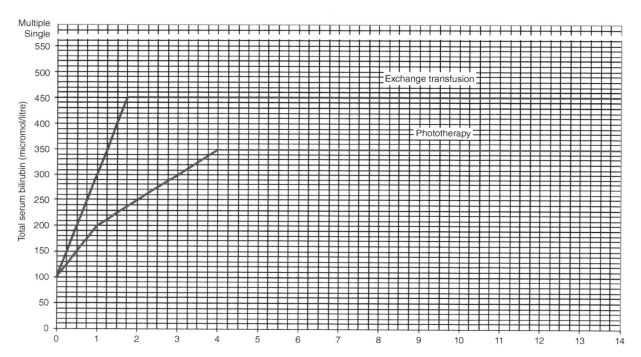

Figure 11.1.6 Treatment threshold chart for ≥38 weeks' gestation. Source: National Institute for Health and Care Excellence (2016). Jaundice in newborn babies under 28 days. Clinical guideline [CG98]. London: NICE.

Dangerous Diagnosis 1
Diagnosis: Rhesus disease of the newborn

Management Principles
1. **Antenatal management.** In the UK, mothers are screened for antibodies to RhD and circulating levels are measured. If a foetus is at risk of rhesus disease, they receive invasive monitoring during pregnancy and may receive intrauterine blood transfusions
2. **Red blood cell transfusion.** Anaemia may be severe and require emergency O-negative blood transfusion in the delivery room. Once stabilised, anaemia can be managed with crossmatched blood or exchange transfusion
3. **Management of hyperbilirubinemia.** Phototherapy and intravenous (IV) fluids should be commenced immediately. Jaundice is likely to require exchange transfusion. Intravenous immunoglobulin (IVIg) can be also given to help prevent further haemolysis
4. **Folic acid.** Folic acid is required in babies with positive DAT, with follow up after 6–8 weeks to assess Hb and determine duration of treatment

Dangerous Diagnosis 2
Diagnosis: Sepsis

Management Principles
1. **Commence IV antibiotics.** IV antibiotics should be commenced urgently, ideally after blood cultures. Antibiotics should not be delayed if obtaining blood cultures is difficult. Choice of antibiotic is determined by local neonatal microbiology guidelines
2. **Review perinatal risk factors for sepsis**. Particular care should be taken to note positive maternal microbiology, for example group B *Streptococcus* swabs or positive placental swabs. These may impact antibiotic escalation

Dangerous Diagnosis 3
Diagnosis: Biliary atresia

Management Principles
1. **Refer to a liver unit.** Prompt referral of any baby considered to have biliary atresia is of paramount importance, as prognosis is better the earlier the surgery is undertaken. Further imaging such as a hepatobiliary iminodiacetic acid (HIDA) scan will most likely be done at the tertiary unit prior to surgery, to confirm the diagnosis
2. **Surgery.** A Kasai procedure will be performed once the diagnosis is confirmed. The procedure uses small bowel to create a connection between the liver and small intestine to allow bile flow. Liver transplant is often required in the long term
3. **Medical management**. Supportive management includes ursodeoxycholic acid and supplementation of fat-soluble vitamins (A, D, E and K)

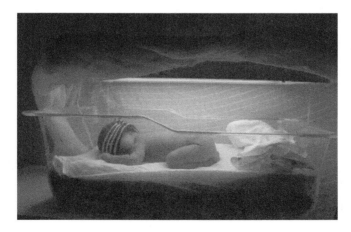

Figure 11.1.7 Baby being treated for jaundice under phototherapy lights. Source: Reproduced with permission of Shutterstock.

Common Diagnosis 1
Diagnosis: Physiological jaundice

Management Principle
1. **Feeding support.** Other than supporting feeding and following the general management principles outlined above, with phototherapy if necessary, there is no specific treatment.

Common Diagnosis 2
Diagnosis: Breast milk jaundice

Management Principle
1. **Reassurance**. Breast milk jaundice resolves spontaneously over the first few months of life. Mothers should not be discouraged from continuing with breastfeeding

Common Diagnosis 3

Diagnosis: ABO incompatibility

Management Principles

1. **Management of hyperbilirubinaemia.** Phototherapy is frequently required in ABO incompatibility. Exchange transfusion is rarely indicated
2. **IVIg.** IVIg can be used in severe hyperbilirubinemia caused by ABO incompatibility to reduce haemolysis
3. **Anaemia management.** A significant fall in haemoglobin may require packed red cell transfusion
4. **Folic acid.** Folic acid is required in babies with positive DAT, with follow up after 6–8 weeks to assess Hb and determine duration of treatment

11.2 The Unsettled Baby

Ilana Levene

National Perinatal Epidemiology Unit, University of Oxford, Oxford, UK

CONTENTS

11.2.1 CHAPTER AT A GLANCE

> **Box 11.2.1 Chapter at a Glance**
>
> - Fussing and crying are extremely common in the first weeks of a baby's life
> - Serious pathology is uncommon, and symptoms resolve with time
> - There can be significant negative effects on breastfeeding establishment, parental mental health and risk of non-accidental injury
>
> - Avoid investigation and treatment unless there are red flags for a serious underlying condition, or significant suspicion of cow's milk protein allergy

11.2.2 DEFINITION

- A young baby displaying crying, fussing or unsettled behaviour that parents report as problematic
- 'Excessive crying' is often defined as more than 3 hours a day for 3 or more days a week (the modified Wessel criteria)

11.2.3 DIAGNOSTIC ALGORITHM

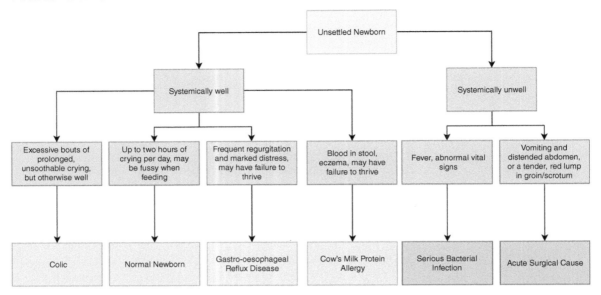

Figure 11.2.1 Diagnostic algorithm for the presentation of an unsettled baby.

11.2.4 DIFFERENTIALS LIST

Dangerous Diagnoses

1. Serious Bacterial Infection
- Common infections include sepsis (bacteraemia), meningitis and urinary tract infection
- Rare cause of infant crying and unsettled behaviour without other signs
- Will deteriorate progressively and likely to have a fever and abnormal vital signs (more than 80% of serious bacterial infections in infants present with fever)

2. Acute Surgical Cause
- Rare but time-critical cause of infant crying and unsettled behaviour
- Incarcerated inguinal hernia is the most common acute surgical cause of sudden excessive crying in a newborn, with up to 5% of term babies having an inguinal hernia and up to 16% of these presenting with incarceration in the first year of life
- Other surgical causes (torted testicle, intussusception and volvulus) are seen in less than 0.1% of infants

Common Diagnoses

1. Normal Newborn Behaviour
- On average, infants in the first 6 weeks of life cry for 2 hours a day, decreasing to 70 minutes a day by 12 weeks. 70% of this crying happens between noon and midnight
- Many mothers and babies need time to establish breastfeeding and find comfortable, effective methods of positioning and attachment
- First-time parents may need support with identifying simple causes for crying, such as discomfort, hunger, excessive heat/cold or itching due to eczema. They may also be surprised by the infant's intense need to be held in the first months of life

2. Colic
- Excessive infant crying, with prolonged and unsoothable bouts
- No underlying pathological cause
- 17–28% of babies fit diagnostic criteria for colic in the first 6 weeks of life, decreasing to 11% by 2 months of age and 0.6% by 3 months
- Associated with subsequent depression in parents, and risk of non-accidental injury

3. Gastro-oesophageal Reflux Disease (GORD)
- Reflux of stomach contents (also called 'posseting' or 'regurgitation') is a normal physiological event in infants, affecting 40% of all infants to a varying extent
- Physiological reflux tends to start before 8 weeks of age and peaks at 3–4 months. 90% have resolved by 1 year

- GORD is the presence of gastro-oesophageal reflux with evidence of harm to the baby, most commonly with marked distress or faltering growth
- Investigation and treatment are not usually indicated. GORD tends to be over-diagnosed and over-treated, because both crying and physiological reflux are common in babies

4. Cow's Milk Protein Allergy (CMPA)

- Immune-mediated allergic response to proteins found in cow's milk, commonly presenting in the first month of life, often with skin and gastrointestinal symptoms
- Either immunoglobulin (Ig) E mediated or non-IgE mediated, dependent on speed of reaction seen
- Occurs in 2–3% of babies who are partially or fully formula fed, often within days of first exposure to formula, and 0.5% of exclusively breastfed babies
- Up to 15% of infants have symptoms that could be consistent with CMPA, but most are not confirmed by dietary exclusion and re-challenge

Diagnoses to Consider

1. Supraventricular Tachycardia (SVT)

- Presents non-specifically in infants with crying, unsettled behaviour
- Usually well tolerated in infants, but can lead to congestive cardiac failure if prolonged
- Raised heart rate is the diagnostic clue

When to consider: Unusually high heart rate on initial observations

---

Box 11.2.2   Corneal Abrasion   △△

- Common in infants due to self-inflicted scratching (49% of babies under 3 months have corneal abrasions if examined with fluorescein)

- On examination, there may be excessive tearing and conjunctival redness. Other scratches on the face may be a clue
- Not necessarily associated with crying
- Heals rapidly without consequence

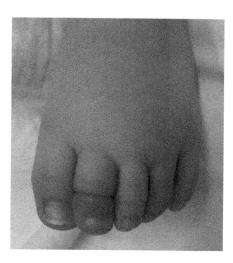

Figure 11.2.2 Hair tourniquet. Courtesy of James Heilman, MD, CC BY-SA 3.0.

Box 11.2.3   Hair Tourniquet   △△

- Occurs when a hair (or thread) becomes tightly wound around an infant's appendage, causing pain and potentially tissue necrosis if unrecognised
- These are usually not suspected by the parent and should be sought during examination

- Most commonly occurs on the toes, but also reported on fingers and genitalia. Ensure that you examine each digit and the genitalia in a child with unexplained crying to exclude this diagnosis
- First-line treatment is with depilatory cream

11.2.5 KEY HISTORY FEATURES

Dangerous Diagnosis 1

Diagnosis: Serious bacterial infection

Questions

1. **Is there any history of fever?** If the parent reports a fever in the baby, even if not measured by a thermometer, the infant should be managed as having sepsis, in accordance with the National Institute for Health and Care Excellence (NICE) guidelines, which state that any fever in a baby <3 months is considered a red flag for serious bacterial infection

2. **Is there known maternal carriage of group B *Streptococcus* (GBS)?** This increases the risk of late-onset GBS sepsis, even if the mother received antibiotics before/during labour, or the baby received intravenous (IV) antibiotics. This is no longer routinely tested for during pregnancy. Other risk factors include prematurity and black ethnic origin

3. **Have any apnoeas been noted?** Apnoeas are a worrying sign of possible infection. There may also be a history of increasingly poor feeding

4. **Do the parents report any focal signs of infection?** Respiratory infections may present with cyanosis and shortness of breath. Neurological infections may present with decreased level of consciousness or seizures

Dangerous Diagnosis 2

Diagnosis: Acute surgical cause

Questions

1. **Has there been any bilious vomiting, or abdominal distension?** Bilious (dark green) vomiting in an infant requires urgent paediatric surgical assessment. Vomiting with abdominal distension is also indicative of a surgical problem

2. **Was the baby born premature, or with low birth weight?** Low birth weight and preterm infants are at highest risk for an inguinal hernia, and are at higher risk for incarceration. Being male and having a family history of hernia are also risk factors

3. **Are there intermittent episodes of pallor associated with crying and drawing the legs up?** This is a classic history for intussusception, along with vomiting. Babies with colic may draw their legs up with crying, but are likely to be red in the face rather than pale. Bloody stool ('redcurrant jelly') is a late sign of intussusception. See Chapter 5.3, *Vomiting*, Box 5.3.2, *Causes of Intestinal Obstruction in Childhood*.

Box 11.2.4 Taking a Breastfeeding History – Signs That Breastfeeding Is Going Well

Weight gain
- Average time to regain birth weight is 8 days
- Weight should then stabilise on a centile and follow it. A drop of more than two centile lines is concerning

Nappies
- After the first week of life: at least 6 wet nappies per day
- After the first few days of life: at least 2 stools per day (at least the size of a £2 coin), changing from meconium to yellow stool by days 3–4
- After 4–6 weeks of age stool frequency can reduce to as little as one per week

How many feeds per day?
- At least 8 in 24 hours while solely breastfeeding

Length of feeds
- Generally between 5 and 40 minutes of active sucking

Nature of feeds
- Baby wakes for feeds
- Rhythmic sucking, audible swallowing
- Baby ends feed spontaneously and is content
- Breasts and nipples comfortable

Common Diagnosis 1

Diagnosis: Normal newborn behaviour

Questions

1. **What time of day does the baby cry, how long does each bout last?** The median time for crying in the first 6 weeks of life is 2 hours per day, the majority of which is in the afternoon and evening. Normal newborn crying will then start to decrease in intensity over the next few months

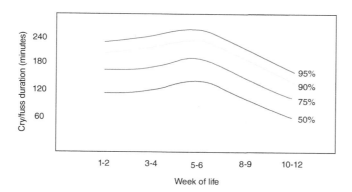

Figure 11.2.3 Centile chart of crying time in the first 12 weeks of life, as established during a meta-analysis by Dr Dieter Wolke and colleagues.

2. **Are there any feeding concerns?** Any difficulties with breastfeeding are likely to contribute to the unsettled behaviour of the baby. Parents who try to feed the baby on a schedule, for example 4-hourly, may not realise that the child is crying because they are hungry. Equally, if formula is being made up incorrectly, it may be too dilute or too concentrated, contributing to hunger, diarrhoea or constipation
3. **How often is the baby winded?** Folk wisdom says that wind can contribute to a baby being unsettled, although there is no objective evidence that winding babies decreases crying. Generic advice is for parents to wind or burp a baby after each feed, and they can also try to wind the baby in the middle of the feed if unsettled

Common Diagnosis 2
Diagnosis: Colic

Questions
1. **Does the mother have a history of migraine, anxiety disorder or have anxious personality traits?** Infantile colic is associated with maternal migraine and with a history of preexisting maternal anxiety
2. **What soothing techniques have the parents tried?** This will help to direct advice on management of colic and should be attempted. Babies suffering from colic, however, are often inconsolable
3. **Sensitively ask about the parents' mood and support network.** Depression is more likely to occur in parents of babies with colic. Most parents find prolonged and inconsolable crying extremely frustrating – 6% of parents of normal 6-month-old babies report having shaken, slapped or smothered their baby in response to excessive crying. There is a significant association of colic and serious non-accidental injury, although the absolute risk is very small

Common Diagnosis 3
Diagnosis: Gastro-oesophageal reflux disease (GORD)

Questions
1. **What is the growth pattern of the baby?** Symptoms of gastro-oesophageal reflux along with poor growth may be an indication for GORD treatment
2. **Is there any projectile, dark green (bilious) or bloodstained vomit?** These would be red flags that the baby does not have reflux, but rather has a more serious condition such as pyloric stenosis, a surgical abdomen or gastro-oesophageal abnormality
3. **Was the baby premature, or do they have a known neurological disorder?** These conditions make significant GORD more likely. Repaired diaphragmatic hernia and repaired oesophageal atresia are also associated with GORD

Common Diagnosis 4
Diagnosis: Cow's milk protein allergy (CMPA)

Questions
1. **Is there a parental or sibling history of atopy, including asthma, eczema, food allergy and allergic rhinitis?** CMPA is more likely in the context of an atopic family history

2. **Does the baby have significant eczema, blood and/or mucous in the stool, and/or diarrhoea?** These symptoms make a diagnosis of CMPA more likely, particularly if eczema is treatment resistant. Most babies will have symptoms in two organ systems (for example, cutaneous and gastrointestinal). A smaller proportion have respiratory symptoms such as recurrent cough and wheeze

3. **Has the baby ever had infant formula?** For non-exclusively breastfed babies, symptoms tend to occur within a few days of the first exposure to infant formula. Exclusively breastfed babies are less likely to have CMPA, although it is still possible. See Chapter 5.3, *Vomiting*, Box 5.3.4, *Signs and Symptoms of Immunoglobulin (Ig) E versus non-IgE Cow's Milk Protein Allergy*.

11.2.6 KEY EXAMINATION FEATURES

Dangerous Diagnosis 1
Diagnosis: Serious bacterial infection

Examination Findings
1. **Fever**. Serious bacterial infection usually presents with fever. A temperature above 38 °C is particularly concerning in a baby under 3 months
2. **Abnormal vital signs**. Signs such as tachycardia, tachypnoea, hypotension, prolonged capillary refill time, pale/mottled/ashen or blue skin colour, or generally looking unwell to a healthcare professional, are concerning
3. **Neurological abnormalities**. Meningitis does not always present with classic signs in the infant. They may have a bulging fontanelle, altered tone, altered responsiveness and a weak or high-pitched, continuous cry

Dangerous Diagnosis 2
Diagnosis: Acute surgical cause

Examination Findings
1. **Distended, tender abdomen.** Caused by obstruction secondary to intussusception, volvulus or incarcerated hernia
2. **Red, hard, tender lump in groin or scrotum**. Incarcerated inguinal hernia, which may be strangulated. 80% are on the right side or bilateral
3. **Tender, swollen testicle**. Postnatal testicular torsion. Tissue ischaemia can occur within 4–6 hours of onset of symptoms

Common Diagnosis 1
Diagnosis: Normal newborn behaviour

Examination Findings
1. **Normal infant examination and growth pattern**. No abnormalities should be found in the infant if the unsettled behaviour is a normal developmental stage. Look at previous records of weight gain on a growth chart
2. **Identifiable sources of discomfort**. Identify any source of discomfort – for example, severe nappy rash or clothing inappropriate for the weather

Common Diagnosis 2
Diagnosis: Colic

Examination Findings
1. **Normal infant examination and growth pattern**. No abnormalities should be found in the infant if the baby has colic. Look at previous records of weight gain on a growth chart
2. **Parent and infant interaction and handling**. Signs of rough handling or poor attachment may raise concerns around the risk of non-accidental injury
3. **Bruises, petechiae or other signs of trauma**. Bruising in a non-mobile child should trigger a full child protection assessment

Common Diagnosis 3
Diagnosis: Gastro-oesophageal reflux disease (GORD)

Examination Findings
1. **Faltering growth.** Plot weight on a centile chart appropriate for age. Faltering growth (for example, crossing down two centile lines) may be an indication for GORD treatment
2. **Normal systems examination.** A full clinical assessment should otherwise be normal in a child with no known medical problems
3. **Clinical features supporting known diagnoses.** Children with risk factors for GORD such as ex-premature babies, neurodisability or syndromic diagnoses will have signs related to these conditions

Common Diagnosis 4
Diagnosis: Cow's milk protein allergy (CMPA)

Examination Findings
1. **Significant eczema, erythematous or urticarial rash.** Common in CMPA. There may also be a nappy rash secondary to diarrhoea
2. **Wheeze, cough, angio-oedema.** Signs of IgE-mediated CMPA. If the baby has anaphylaxis, they should be given emergency treatment and admitted to hospital
3. **Faltering growth.** Plot weight on centile chart appropriate for age. Faltering growth automatically puts the infant in the severe category of CMPA

11.2.7 KEY INVESTIGATIONS

Not all children will require invasive investigations; often diagnoses are made on clinical evidence from history and examination. Consider carefully which investigations are required for which patient.

Bedside

Table 11.2.1 Bedside tests of use in infants presenting with unsettled behaviour

Test	When to perform	Potential result
Urine MC&S	• All babies with a fever • Significant vomiting or faltering growth	• Positive urine culture should be treated as UTI regardless of white cell count • Negative culture with pyuria should be treated as UTI if strong clinical suspicion
ECG	• Unexplained tachycardia	• Diagnosis of SVT
Fluorescein staining	• Suspected corneal abrasion	• Confirms presence of corneal abrasion

ECG, electrocardiogram; MC&S, microscopy, culture and sensitivity; SVT, supraventricular tachycardia; UTI, urinary tract infection

Blood Tests

Table 11.2.2 Blood tests of use in infants presenting with unsettled behaviour

Test	When to perform	Potential result
FBC	Suspected: • Serious bacterial infection • Severe, longstanding CMPA	• ↑ WCC, ↑ neutrophils: bacterial infection • ↓ Hb in severe, longstanding CMPA
CRP	• Suspected serious bacterial infection	• Significant ↑ in bacterial infections • Less marked ↑ in viral infections
Blood culture	• Suspected serious bacterial infection	• Positive culture confirms bacterial infection • Sensitivities guide antibiotic choice

CMPA, cow's milk protein allergy; CRP, C-reactive protein; FBC, full blood count; Hb, haemoglobin

Imaging

Table 11.2.3 Imaging modalities of use in infants presenting with unsettled behaviour

Test	When to perform	Potential result
Abdominal x-ray	• Suspected surgical abdomen	• Obstruction: dilated bowel loops, fluid levels • Perforation: free peritoneal air
Abdominal ultrasound	• Suspected intussusception	• Shows intussuscepted section of bowel

Special

Table 11.2.4 Special Tests Of Use In Infants Presenting With Unsettled Behaviour

Test	When to perform	Potential result
Lumbar puncture: cerebrospinal fluid examination and culture	• Suspected serious bacterial infection	• ↑ Neutrophils suggest bacterial meningitis • Positive culture confirms infection

11.2.8 KEY MANAGEMENT PRINCIPLES

Diagnosis-specific management strategies are outlined here. It is expected that an 'ABCDE' approach to assessment and management is always undertaken (see Chapter 12.1, *The A to E Assessment*).

Dangerous Diagnosis 1
Diagnosis: Serious bacterial infections

Management Principles
See Chapter 13.1, *Sepsis Management*
1. **Antibiotics.** Treat with broad-spectrum IV antibiotics if suspicion of serious bacterial infection, according to local guidelines. Be aware of perinatal risk factors for neonatal sepsis, such as known maternal GBS carriage, which may prompt escalation of antibiotics

Dangerous Diagnosis 2
Diagnosis: Acute surgical cause

Management Principles
1. **IV fluids and analgesia.** Make the baby nil by mouth and prescribe IV fluids and parenteral analgesia as required
2. **Nasogastric tube on free drainage.** Decompresses the stomach if there is suspicion of bowel obstruction
3. **Urgent surgical referral.** For definitive management, surgery will often be required. Intussusception may be successfully managed by air insufflation. Incarcerated hernia, torted testicle and volvulus require urgent surgery.
See Chapter 5.1, *Abdominal Pain*; Figure 5.1.2 *Intussusception*; Figure 5.1.3 *Volvulus*; Box 5.1.3 *Testicular and Ovarian Torsion*; Box 5.1.11 *Non-operative reduction of intussusception*

Common Diagnosis 1
Diagnosis: Normal newborn behaviour

Management Principles
1. **Parental reassurance and education.** Inform parents about the characteristics and extent of normal crying and emphasise that it will improve over time. Acknowledge that the crying may be stress inducing. If there is concern that crying in a breastfed baby signifies hunger due to poor milk supply, advise on true markers of milk supply (wet/dirty nappies and growth)
2. **Feeding support.** All breastfeeding mothers with unsettled babies should go to a breastfeeding clinic or breastfeeding support group for expert, face-to-face assessment. In formula-fed babies, there is no evidence that partially hydrolysed or lactose-free formula improves unsettled behaviour. There is also no compelling evidence for diet modification in a breastfeeding mother, unless there is a suspicion of CMPA
3. **Practical soothing measures.** When babies are carried by their parents, e.g. by using a sling, they cry less than those who have infrequent body contact. Breastfeeding mothers can be encouraged to feed responsively whenever the baby is

unsettled. Breastfeeding can provide comfort as well as nutrition, and mothers should not be worried about over-feeding. Other soothing measures are gentle motion, the use of 'white noise', reduction in excessive or exaggerated stimulation, and a warm bath

4. **Inform health visitor.** Presentation of an unsettled baby to acute paediatric services is an indication of the level of anxiety felt by the parents. The health visitor should be informed to provide further support at home. Direct parents to community support groups if these are available locally

Common Diagnosis 2
Diagnosis: Colic

Management Principles
1. **Parental reassurance and education.** These should follow the same pattern as described for normal newborn crying and are the cornerstone of management
2. **Recommend expert breastfeeding support. Consider recommending probiotics for breastfed babies.** Expert, face-to-face breastfeeding assessment is the first-line treatment for colic in breastfed babies. There is moderate evidence that the probiotic *Lactobacillus reuteri* reduces crying time in breastfed babies, although there is still some controversy in this area
3. **Do not recommend over-the-counter colic remedies or manual therapies.** There is insufficient good-quality evidence to advise simethicone (such as Infacol®) or lactase (such as Colief®) drops, or any herbal remedies. This is also true for manual therapies such as spinal manipulation or cranial osteopathy
4. **Self-care for parents.** Acknowledge that the crying may be stress inducing. Advise parents that if they feel they might hurt the baby, they should put the baby down in a safe place and give themselves some 'time out'. Advise them to ask friends and family for support, and meet other carers with babies of the same age, or a bit older, to access peer support
5. **Follow-up and referral.** Recommend further medical assessment if symptoms do not improve. Ensure health visitor follow-up is in place and inform the health visitor and/or GP of any specific concerns over parents' mental health or the interaction of parent and infant

Common Diagnosis 3
Diagnosis: Gastro-oesophageal reflux disease

Management Principles
1. **Treat babies only if there is frequent regurgitation and marked distress. Where treatment threshold is not reached, parents can be advised on positioning.** Basic positioning advice consists of keeping the baby upright during and for 30 minutes after feeds and lying the baby on a surface that is angled at 30° rather than completely flat. Safe sleep messages should not be compromised – babies should sleep on their backs on a firm, even surface
2. **Breastfed babies should receive expert breastfeeding support. Formula-fed babies should receive feeding modification advice.** First-line treatment for breastfed babies is a breastfeeding assessment by someone with appropriate expertise and training, e.g. an International Board Certified Lactation Consultant (IBCLC), infant feeding lead or breastfeeding counsellor. For formula-fed babies, advise parents to feed the baby with smaller, more frequent feeds. If this doesn't work then trial a thickened formula.
3. **Alginate treatment (for example infant Gaviscon).** Second-line treatment is alginate therapy for a trial period of 1–2 weeks (thickened formula must be stopped in order to use alginate. Breastfed babies can be given infant Gaviscon mixed with water before feeds). Parents should try to stop it at regular intervals to see if the infant has recovered
4. **Acid-suppressant treatment.** Histamine receptor antagonists (e.g. ranitidine) or proton pump inhibitors (e.g. omeprazole) should be used with caution as a third-line treatment. If they are used there should be a 4-week trial period to assess response

Common Diagnosis 4
Diagnosis: Cow's milk protein allergy

Management Principles
1. **Breastfed babies: maternal dietary exclusion of cow's milk protein.** When there is significant suspicion of CMPA, mothers should exclude cow's milk protein from their diet for 2–4 weeks, followed by a 1-week re-challenge. If symptoms resolve and then return on re-challenge, a diagnosis can be made and dietary exclusion restarted. The re-challenge is important, to avoid mothers unnecessarily modifying their diets, with the risks of calcium deficiency. However if symptoms are severe or IgE mediated, these babies should be referred to allergy services. Dietitian referral is required to check the mother's dietary calcium
2. **Formula-fed babies: hydrolysed formula.** In formula-fed babies an extensively hydrolysed formula is used for a 2–4-week trial, followed by a 1-week re-challenge. If symptoms are severe and non-IgE mediated, then amino acid formula should be used instead and re-challenge may not be appropriate

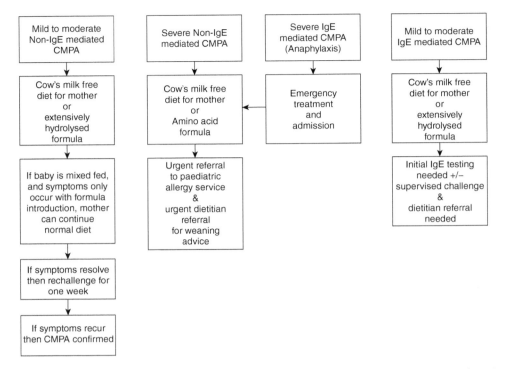

Figure 11.2.4 Diagnosis and management flowchart for cow's milk protein allergy. Source: Reproduced with permission from GP Infant Feeding Network (GPIFN) (2019). The milk allergy in primary care (MAP) guideline 2019. https://gpifn.org.uk/imap.

3. **Referral to paediatric allergy specialist and dietitian**. All babies with severe symptoms, significant eczema, faltering growth or IgE-mediated symptoms should have a referral to a paediatric allergy specialist and dietitian

4. **Continue dietary exclusion**. When CMPA is confirmed by exclusion and re-challenge, dietary exclusion should continue for at least 6 months, and until the baby is at least 9 months old. Introduction of complementary food at 6 months of age should exclude cow's milk protein

5. **Milk ladder.** After at least 6 months, and when the baby is at least 9 months old, parents can start to reintroduce cow's milk protein in the form of a milk ladder under the guidance of a dietitian and, if necessary, the paediatric allergy team. See Chapter 5.3, *Vomiting*, Box 5.3.11, *The 'Milk Ladder'*

Box 11.2.5   Resources for Parents

Condition	Resource	How to access
Excessive crying	Cry-sis: UK charity offering support with crying or sleeping problems	**www.cry-sis.org.uk** Telephone helpline 0845 122 8669
	The period of purple crying: informative website	**http://purplecrying.info**
Gastro-oesophageal reflux (GORD)	Living with Reflux: UK charity supporting families with children with GORD	**www.livingwithreflux.org**
Cow's milk protein allergy (CMPA)	CMPA Support: not-for-profit organisation run by volunteers for allergy support	**www.cmpasupport.org.uk**
	Allergy UK: UK charity supporting adults and children with allergies	**www.allergyuk.org** (parent section on CMPA)

11.3 Breastfeeding Advice

Ilana Levene

National Perinatal Epidemiology Unit, University of Oxford, Oxford, UK

CONTENTS

11.3.1 CHAPTER AT A GLANCE

Box 11.3.1 Chapter at a Glance

- The UK has some of the lowest breastfeeding rates in the world, with 8 out of 10 women stopping breastfeeding before they would have wanted
- There is plenty of evidence to support breastfeeding as the optimum way to feed a baby, with protective effects against common childhood illnesses, for example infections
- Supporting families to breastfeed is therefore one of the highest-impact public health interventions paediatricians are involved with

- Rates of exclusive breastfeeding drop below 50% by 1 week of age, despite over 80% of mothers initiating breastfeeding
- In order to offer opportunistic and consistent support, doctors must understand the common pitfalls encountered when establishing breastfeeding, and how to protect breastfeeding while treating other medical problems. This does not replace specialist breastfeeding support

11.3.2 BREASTFEEDING IN THE UK

- In the UK, and many other Westernised countries, infant formula is the dominant cultural mode of feeding
- Mothers have very little support to establish and continue breastfeeding and many therefore end up using infant formula despite their desire to continue breastfeeding, with consequent increased risk of postnatal depression in those who want to breastfeed and cannot
- Breastfeeding is a highly emotive subject, particularly with families who have tried breastfeeding without success
- UNICEF, together with the World Health Organisation (WHO), works to support breastfeeding through the Baby Friendly Initiative
- The Baby Friendly Initiative also supports parents who are formula feeding through provision of information on milk choice and advocating against inappropriate marketing of breastmilk substitutes, to support unbiased, informed choices

Box 11.3.2 Breastmilk Benefits

- Breastfeeding reduces the risk of childhood infections such as pneumonia, otitis media and gastroenteritis, including resulting hospitalisations
- Importantly, this is not simply a consequence of contaminated water used for formula; it is also due to the complex immune properties of breastmilk

- Breastfeeding also reduces the risk of sudden infant death syndrome, childhood leukaemia and maternal breast cancer, among a long list of other conditions

Clinical Guide to Paediatrics, First Edition. Edited by Rachel Varughese and Anna Mathew. Series Editor: Christian Fielder Camm.
© 2022 John Wiley & Sons Ltd. Published 2022 by John Wiley & Sons Ltd.
Companion website: www.wiley.com/go/varughese/paediatrics

11.3.3 BACKGROUND

WHO Recommendations
- Exclusive breastfeeding for 6 months, and then breastfeeding alongside complementary food for at least 2 years

UNICEF UK Recommendations
- Newborns should be fed responsively, which means 'a mother responding to her baby's cues, as well as her desire to feed her baby'
- Crucially, feeding responsively recognises that feeds are not just for nutrition, but also for love, comfort and reassurance between baby and mother
- Newborns are unlikely to feed at regular intervals or for a similar length of time at each feed, and doctors should not expect this when taking a history
- Bottle-fed babies should also be fed according to their hunger cues rather than to a schedule, and it is particularly important not to encourage or force babies to finish what is in the bottle to prevent overfeeding

---

Box 11.3.3   Establishing Milk Supply

- Milk supply is determined in the first few weeks of the baby's life
- If the breasts are frequently stimulated and emptied in that period a full supply will be established, which can then respond to the baby's needs on a supply-and-demand basis as the baby grows
- If the breasts are not frequently stimulated and emptied, either because the baby is feeding ineffectively or because they are

being fed infant formula as well, then a full supply may not be established, and the baby cannot be exclusively breastfed
- Expressing breast milk by hand or with the aid of a mechanical pump can provide stimulation and drainage if the baby is not able to do so

---

11.3.4 HOW TO APPROACH DIFFICULTIES IN THE FIRST TWO WEEKS OF LIFE

Modes of presentation
- Self-reported problems:
  - Difficulty in latching the baby to the breast
  - Nipple/breast pain
  - Feeling that they do not have enough milk
- Referral from midwife for jaundice or excessive weight loss

---

Box 11.3.4   Newborn Triad

Always assess the baby fully for signs that they might be unwell. This may involve a period of observation. It is essential to exclude serious conditions:

- Sepsis
- Congenital cardiac anomaly

- Inborn errors of metabolism

Assessment
- Full assessment for medical concerns
- If jaundiced, check the bilirubin
- If excessive weight loss (variously defined as more than 10–15% in different areas), or clinically dehydrated, then check glucose, lactate and sodium level
- Assess the efficacy of breastfeeding

Box 11.3.5   Markers of Effective Breastfeeding*

Facet of breastfeeding	Reassuring	Notes
How many feeds per day?	• 8 or more in 24 hours	• Gap between feeds matters less than number in 24 hours
How many wet nappies per day?	• Days 1–2: at least 2 • Days 3–4: at least 3 • Day 5+: at least 6	
How many stools per day?	• Days 1–2: at least 1 • Day 3+: at least 2 (changing from meconium to lighter, seedy stool)	• Stools count if they are as big as a £2 coin • Stool frequency may reduce significantly after about 6 weeks of age
Length of feeds	• Generally between 5 and 40 minutes	• Consistently longer than 45 minutes means baby is unlikely to be feeding effectively
Nature of feeds	• Baby wakes for feeds • Rhythmic sucking, audible swallowing (once milk has come in) • Baby ends feed spontaneously and is content • Breasts and nipples comfortable	• Brief pain at the beginning of a feed may be normal
Weight loss in the breastfed baby	• Average maximum weight loss is up to 9% • Average time to regain birth weight is 8 days	

*Based on the Unicef Baby Friendly Initiative Breastfeeding Assessment Tool

Management
- If there is any concern over the baby being unwell, treat this immediately
- Seek urgent specialist, face-to-face breastfeeding support with positioning and attachment
- Refer to National Institute for Health and Care Excellence (NICE) guidance on neonatal jaundice for management if required
- If there are concerns about breastfeeding efficacy:
  - Advise the mother to express breastmilk at least 4 times a day (8 times a day if significant concern) and give all the resultant milk to the baby
  - Advise that the baby must be fed at least 8 times per day (10–12 times a day if significant concern)
  - The family must then be assessed again within 24–72 hours depending on the level of concern to see if further escalation is required

Box 11.3.6   Breastfeeding Specialist Support

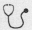

- This is a professional with a higher level of training than a standard midwife or health visitor – they may be called an infant feeding lead, breastfeeding counsellor or lactation consultant
- The hospital may provide this specialist support through a breastfeeding clinic, or community breastfeeding support groups
- The post-natal ward can provide a list of services, and they are usually listed in the mother's discharge pack

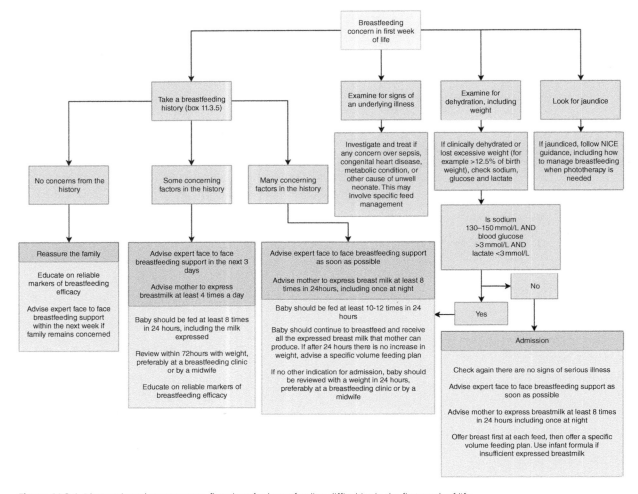

Figure 11.3.1 Diagnostic and management flowchart for breastfeeding difficulties in the first week of life.

11.3.5 HOW TO PROTECT BREASTFEEDING IN MEDICAL CONDITIONS

Gastroenteritis
- Breastfeeding should continue during gastroenteritis, unless triggering persistent vomiting
- Oral rehydration solution may be necessary in addition to breastfeeding if there is clinical dehydration. Intravenous (IV) fluid may be necessary if this fails, or if the child is shocked
- Do not disturb breastfeeding because of a desire to measure input. Use urine output and clinical markers of dehydration when monitoring fluid balance
- If a baby or young child is breastfeeding significantly less than usual, then the mother's breasts will feel uncomfortably full – this can be elicited in the history

Respiratory Distress
- If nasogastric feeds are required, for example in bronchiolitis, ensure the mother is provided with a breastmilk pump
- If the baby has been feeding poorly, the mother is likely to be able to immediately express a large volume
- If breastfeeding is well established (baby is more than 2 weeks old and there were no previous concerns about feeding or growth), then the mother can express enough to keep comfortable and provide whatever volume the baby requires
- If the baby is less than 2 weeks old or there have been concerns over milk supply or growth, then the mother should express at least 8 times a day to protect her milk supply

Prior to General Anaesthetic

- Breastfeeds are not equivalent to formula when fasting for a general anaesthetic
- Guidelines vary, but breastfeeding is allowed to continue 1–2 hours longer than infant formula

11.3.6 TOP TIPS

- **Parents can be desperate.** Validate their experience and make it clear you understand how difficult their experience has been
- **Emphasise that breastfeeding is a learned skill**. It will come with time and practice, under the guidance of lactation experts
- **Emotions run high around feeding decisions**. Mothers feel pressured and guilty however they feed their babies. Use sensitive language with those using infant formula, particularly when this was not their initial plan
- **Breastfeeding provides pain relief**. Babies and children are comforted during uncomfortable or painful procedures. Check if the mother would like to breastfeed during venepuncture, capillary blood sampling or other procedures
- **Breastfeeding is not all or nothing**. Breastfeeding is about more than just nutrition. When exclusive direct breastfeeding is not possible, giving expressed breastmilk by another route, or mixed feeding, are also very valuable and should be encouraged and supported
- **Problems may arise over weekends and public holidays**. This is when face-to-face breastfeeding support is not available urgently. In this situation parents can be directed to national telephone helplines, or informed that they can find a private lactation consultant via the Lactation Consultants of Great Britain (LCGB) website.

11.3.7 UNDERAPPRECIATED FACTS

- Most medications are safe to use when breastfeeding
  - The British National Formulary (BNF) provides some limited information, but this is often not enough
  - A ward pharmacist can assist with inpatient queries
  - Useful specialist resources include the UK Drugs in Lactation Advisory Service (UKDILAS) and the Breastfeeding Network factsheets
- Although it is unusual in the UK to breastfeed beyond infancy, it is biologically and anthropologically normal, and recommended by the WHO
  - There is no specific age at which a child should no longer be breastfeeding, although the majority would self-wean by the age of 5 years
  - Health professionals should avoid judgement of families whose breastfeeding experiences are outside the professional's own expectations of normality
- It is normal for breastfed babies (indeed, all babies) to wake and feed frequently during the night throughout the first year of life
  - Although continued night breastfeeds beyond this age may lead to broken sleep for parents, there is no medical need to advise parents to change their practice if the family is coping

Box 11.3.7   Resources for Parents and Doctors

	Resource	Contact
For parents	Association of Breastfeeding Mothers: for general information on breastfeeding problems	**https://abm.me.uk/breastfeeding-information**
	National Breastfeeding Helpline: live online webchat support	**http://www.nationalbreastfeedinghelpline.org.uk**, 0300 100 0212
	La Leche League Breastfeeding Helpline	0345 120 2918
	Lactation Consultants of Great Britain: to find a private lactation consultant	**https://lcgb.org/find-an-ibclc/**
For doctors	UK Drugs in Lactation Advisory Service	**https://www.sps.nhs.uk/articles/ukdilas**
	Breastfeeding Network: drug factsheets	**https://www.breastfeedingnetwork.org.uk/drugs-factsheets**
	Hospital Infant Feeding Network: support for simple medical problems relating to breastfeeding in mothers and babies (primary care-focused resource)	**www.hifn.org**

12.1 The A to E Assessment

Rachel Varughese

Department of Paediatrics, Oxford University Hospitals NHS Foundation Trust, Oxford, UK

CONTENTS

12.1.1 CHAPTER AT A GLANCE

> **Box 12.2.1 Chapter at a Glance**
>
> - An 'ABCDE' (or 'A to E') assessment is a useful structure for all clinical evaluation, but it is primarily used in emergency assessment
> - The key to an A to E assessment is that management takes place in parallel to examination
>
> - Many chapters will have referenced an A to E assessment as the mainstay of examination and management
> - This chapter provides an overview of how to conduct this evaluation

12.1.2 TOP TIPS

- Only move to the next part of the A to E assessment once the previous one is stable
- Continually reassess
- Escalate concerns early, with appropriate involvement of other specialist teams
- Assessment in the trauma patient is different: C-spine stabilisation and control of major haemorrhage are prioritised – this is not covered here
- In unwell children, assign a team member to support and update the family

Clinical Guide to Paediatrics, First Edition. Edited by Rachel Varughese and Anna Mathew. Series Editor: Christian Fielder Camm.
© 2022 John Wiley & Sons Ltd. Published 2022 by John Wiley & Sons Ltd.
Companion website: www.wiley.com/go/varughese/paediatrics

12.1.3 KEY ASPECTS OF ASSESSMENT AND MANAGEMENT

Airway
Purpose: Assess patency of airway

Table 12.1.1 Airway assessment

What to look for	Interpretation
• Vocalising • Crying • Breathing with no added sounds	• Signs of a patent airway
• Snoring • Stridor • Wheeze	• Signs of a partially obstructed airway
• No air movement despite effort of breathing	• Signs of a completely obstructed airway
• Secretions, blood, vomit • Decreased conscious level • Soft tissue neck swelling or mass • Known inhalation of foreign body • Anaphylaxis or severe exacerbation of asthma	• Risk factors for an airway at risk of obstruction

Table 12.1.2 Airway management options

Intervention	Details
• Call for help	• Seek immediate support from senior colleagues, particularly anaesthetics – ideally via an emergency or 'crash' call
• Inspect airway	• If there is a visible obstruction, a finger sweep can be attempted
• Suction	• Suction secretions/blood/vomit under direct vision
• Airway manoeuvres	• Neutral head position in infants/young children • Head tilt and chin lift: only to be used in older children and *never* in suspected C-spine injury • Jaw thrust
• Airway adjuncts	• Oropharyngeal airway • Nasopharyngeal airway • Laryngeal mask airway (LMA)/iGEL • Intubation
• Medications to consider	• Dexamethasone oral/intravenous: this is useful for airway swelling and is particularly useful in children with croup • Adrenaline nebuliser: this is useful for airway swelling and is particularly useful in children with croup

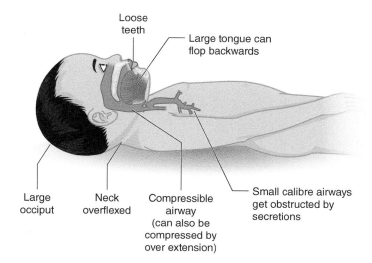

Figure 12.1.1 The airway assessment of children has fundamental differences from that of adults. (1) Large occiput predisposes to neck flexion – particularly significant up to 1 year of age, but remains relevant until 8 years of age. (2) Milk teeth may be loose and cause foreign body obstruction if dislodged. (3) Trachea supple and may compress if head over-extended. (4) Anterior larynx may make laryngoscopy view difficult. (5) Small-calibre airways increase risk of obstruction from secretions. (6) Large tongue relative to size of mouth that can fall backwards.

Breathing
Purpose: Assess effectiveness of respiration

Table 12.1.3 Breathing assessment

What to do	Interpretation
• Measure oxygen saturations	• Saturations <94% suggest need for supplemental oxygen
Inspection	
• Count respiratory rate	• A slow rate may be due to sedation, raised intracranial pressure or medication toxicity, e.g. opioids • A fast rate may be due to airway obstruction, pneumonia, pneumothorax, pulmonary oedema, asthma, pulmonary embolism
• Look for cyanosis	• This indicates hypoxia, usually with saturations <80%
• Observe the degree of respiratory effort	• Signs of respiratory distress include nasal flaring, use of accessory muscles, intercostal and subcostal muscle recession and the tripod position • In a verbal child, inability to form full sentences indicates severe respiratory distress
• Observe the pattern of respiration	• Normal breathing should be regular • Apnoeas or gasping breaths may indicate Cheyne–Stokes respiration, a pre-terminal sign • Deep sighing breaths may indicate Kussmaul's breathing, associated with metabolic acidosis, e.g. diabetic ketoacidosis

(Continued)

Table 12.1.3 (Continued)

What to do	Interpretation
• Observe the symmetry of chest expansion	• Suspicions of asymmetrical chest expansion should be confirmed with palpation • Asymmetrical: may suggest unilateral lung pathology, usually resulting in ipsilateral reduction in expansion, e.g. pneumothorax, pneumonia, pleural effusion • Paradoxical movement of a section of chest wall indicates flail chest and suggests rib trauma
Palpation	
• Assess tracheal position	• Normal position is central • Deviation can either be away from pathology (e.g. tension pneumothorax, large pleural effusions) or towards pathology (e.g. collapse)
Percussion	
• Percuss to assess resonance	• Dull percussion note may indicate effusion, haemothorax or consolidation • Unilateral hyperresonance indicates pneumothorax
Auscultation	
• Compare quality and equality of breath sounds	• Wheeze: asthma, viral-induced wheeze • Crackles: consolidation, bronchiolitis, pulmonary oedema, secretions • Decreased breath sounds: pneumothorax, life-threatening asthma • Absent breath sounds: pleural effusion, haemothorax

Table 12.1.4 Breathing management options

Intervention	Details
• Supplemental oxygen	• Nasal cannulae • Non-rebreathe face mask
• Ventilation	• Non-invasive ventilation: humidified nasal high-flow, continuous positive airway pressure (CPAP), bilevel positive airway pressure (BiPAP) • Bag-valve mask ventilation: if poor respiratory effort • Invasive mechanical ventilation: definitive management
• Procedures	• Needle thoracocentesis: first step for tension pneumothorax • Chest drain: definitive management of pneumothorax, or for haemothorax/large effusions
• Medications to consider	• Bronchodilators, e.g. nebulised salbutamol, ipratropium: to be used in wheeze or decreased air entry secondary to hyperactive airways
• Refer to paediatric intensive care	• Children with an unstable respiratory status, particularly those requiring invasive mechanical ventilation, will need to be cared for in paediatric intensive care

Circulation

Purpose: Assess adequacy of perfusion

Table 12.1.5 Circulation assessment

What to do	Interpretation
• Inspection	• Pink: normal • Pallor, mottled: compromised
• Estimate adequacy of perfusion	• Capillary refill: prolonged in shock • Core–periphery temperature gap: present in shock • Urine output: reduced in shock
• Measure heart rate	• Tachycardia: fever, dehydration, early compensatory mechanism in shock, tachyarrhythmia • Bradycardia: bradyarrhythmia, profound hypoxia, raised intracranial pressure
• Measure blood pressure	• Hypotension: sign of decompensation in shock • Hypertension: malignant hypertension, raised intracranial pressure
• Auscultation	• Murmur: consider congenital cardiac disease

Table 12.1.6 Circulation management options

Intervention	Details
• Procedures	• Gain intravenous access. If there are signs of circulatory compromise and intravenous access is not achieved quickly, move to intraosseous access • Take relevant bloods and blood gas
• Medications to consider	• Antibiotics: sepsis • Fluid bolus 20 mL/kg 0.9% saline (consider 10 mL/kg if concerns about congestive cardiac failure) • Inotropes and vasopressors for hypotension refractory to fluid resuscitation
• Refer to paediatric intensive care	• Children with signs of shock, particularly those requiring inotropes, will need to be cared for in paediatric intensive care

Disability

Purpose: Assess neurological compromise

Table 12.1.7 Disability assessment

What to do	Interpretation
• Assess conscious level	• This can be done using the Glasgow Coma Scale (GCS) or Alert, Voice, Pain, Unresponsive (AVPU) scale • A GCS <8 or a decreasing GCS may indicate the need for invasive airway support
• Measure glucose with a point of care test	• A blood sugar of <2.6 mmol/L is indicative of hypoglycaemia, for which there may be no other clinical signs • A blood sugar of >11 mmol/L may suggest diabetic ketoacidosis • Remember that children have limited glycogen liver stores, meaning hypoglycaemia is common in illness, particularly when oral intake is reduced
• Examine fontanelle	• Soft and flat: normal • Sunken: dehydration • Tense or bulging: increased intracranial pressure
• Assess pupils	• Responsive to light: normal • Pinpoint: opioid intoxication • Fixed and dilated: 3rd nerve palsy, raised intracranial pressure • Asymmetrical: consider focal intracranial pathology
• Assess tone	• Hypotonic: lower motor neuron injury/spinal shock • Hypertonic: upper motor neuron injury
• Grossly assess movement and power	• Spontaneous movement: normal • Asymmetrical, reduced, seizures: abnormal

Table 12.1.8 Disability management options

Intervention	Details
• Medications to consider	• Benzodiazepines: seizures • Glucose: hypoglycaemia. Options include glucose gel, intravenous (IV) 10% dextrose 2 mL/kg, or intramuscular glucagon (if drowsy but no IV access) • Naloxone: opioid toxicity • Insulin and IV fluids: diabetic ketoacidosis
• Referrals	• Depending on the nature of the assessment, referrals may be required to several tertiary teams, e.g. neurosurgery, neurology, paediatric intensive care • If referring to neurosurgery, consideration must be made as to whether referral is time critical

Exposure
Purpose: Everything else!

Table 12.1.9 Exposure assessment

What to do	Interpretation
• Measure temperature	• Temperature >38 °C indicates fever – consider sepsis • Temperature <36 °C indicates hypothermia – consider sepsis or cold exposure • Children have a large surface area:weight ratio, meaning rapid temperature loss
• Abdominal examination	• There may be evidence of peritonism, abdominal injury or masses
• Log-roll	• This allows examination of the flank and back while protecting the C-spine, in order to assess previously concealed signs
• Assess for injury	• Bruising or obvious fractures: are there consistent explanations or could this be non-accidental injury?
• Look for a rash	• Blanching rash: non-specific. If maculopapular, could indicate a viral infection. If urticarial, consider allergy and anaphylaxis. • Petechial or purpuric rash: consider sepsis with disseminated intravascular coagulation (e.g. meningococcal sepsis)

Table 12.1.10 Exposure management options

Intervention	Details
• Keep warm	• Once the patient is exposed and assessed, cover them up to keep them warm • If they are hypothermic, commence warming • Babies can be warmed with an overhead heater, e.g. a Rescuscitaire® • Babies and infants can be warmed with an infant warming mattress, e.g. a Transwarmer® • Children can be warmed with a forced air warmer, e.g. Bair-hugger® • In severe hypothermia, warmed fluids can be administered intravenously, as well as warmed irrigation fluids for rectal and gastric administration
• Medications to consider	• Antibiotics: sepsis (these may already have been given earlier) • Blood products: haemorrhage
• Referrals	• Depending on the nature of the assessment, referrals may be required to several teams, e.g. general surgery, trauma and orthopaedics, specialist surgery • Discuss with radiology about relevant imaging

12.2 Assessment of Consciousness

Rachel Varughese

Department of Paediatrics, Oxford University Hospitals NHS Foundation Trust, Oxford, UK

CONTENTS

12.2.1 CHAPTER AT A GLANCE

Box 12.2.1   Chapter at a Glance

- The assessment of a child with a decreased conscious level relies on the use of an approved score, in order to monitor progress across different users

- The two most commonly used scores are AVPU (basic overview) and the Glasgow Coma Scale (GCS, more comprehensive)

12.2.2 AVPU

The simplest form of assessment is the AVPU scale:
- **A**lert
- Responds to **V**oice
- Responds to **P**ain
- **U**nresponsive

12.2.3 GCS

- The Glasgow Coma Scale (GCS) is a widely approved scoring system for quantification of conscious level
- A GCS ≤8 signifies the patient is at high risk of airway compromise
- The GCS incorporates three components: eyes, verbal and motor
- The verbal component is particularly challenging in non-verbal children and requires modification

Table 12.2.1 Glasgow Coma Scale

Best eye response	
1	No eye opening
2	Eye opening to pain
3	Eye opening to verbal command
4	Eye opening spontaneously

Best verbal response		
	Verbal children	**Non-verbal children**
1	No vocal response	No response to pain
2	Non-specific sounds	Mild grimace/moans to pain
3	Inappropriate words	Vigorous grimace/cries to pain
4	Confused speech	Only response to touch stimuli
5	Alert and orientated	Spontaneous normal facial/oromotor activity

Best motor response	
1	No motor response to pain
2	Abnormal extension to pain
3	Abnormal flexion to pain
4	Withdrawal from painful stimuli
5	Localises to painful stimuli
6	Obeys commands or performs normal spontaneous movements

12.2.4 INTERPRETATION

- The GCS score has good clinical correlation with neurological status and is commonly used to make important management decisions
- Although basic, the AVPU scale can be used to provide an estimate of the GCS score

---

Box 12.2.2   AVPU and GCS Interpretation

AVPU

- Alert: GCS 15
- Voice responsive: GCS 12
- Pain responsive: GCS 8
- Unresponsive: GCS 3

GCS

- 13–15: Mild brain injury
- 9–12: Moderate brain injury
- 3–8: Severe brain injury

12.3 Tips for Fluid Prescribing

Rachel Atherton

Department of Paediatrics, Oxford University Hospitals NHS Foundation Trust, Oxford, UK

CONTENTS

12.3.1 CHAPTER AT A GLANCE

> **Box 12.3.1   Chapter at a Glance**
>
> - Fluid prescribing can be confusing in paediatrics and is guided by the weight of the child
> - This chapter will help guide decisions on choosing the right type of fluid and the volume required

12.3.2 GENERAL PRINCIPLES

Three questions should be taken into account when prescribing fluids for children and young people:

1. **What Is the *Purpose* of My Fluid Prescription?**
   There are three principal indications for prescribing fluids in children:
   - Resuscitation
   - Replacement
   - Maintenance
   The purpose of the fluid prescription is guided by the clinical assessment of the child.
2. **What Is the Most Appropriate *Route* to Administer Fluids?**
   The most common routes of administration are intravenous or enteral. Intraosseous fluid resuscitation can be used in emergency situations where intravenous access is not possible.
3. ***Which* Fluid Should I Use, and *How Much*?**
   The type and volume of fluid are guided by the clinical situation and intended outcome.

Box 12.3.2   Assessing Dehydration in Children

	No dehydration	Mild-moderate dehydration	Severe dehydration 'hypovolaemic shock'
Deficit	None	5%	>10%
General	Well	Unwell or deteriorating	Unwell or deteriorating
	Alert and responsive	Altered responsiveness (e.g. irritable, lethargic)	Decreased level of consciousness
Fontanelle	Soft	Flat	Sunken
Skin	Skin colour unchanged	Skin colour unchanged	Pale or mottled skin
	Normal skin turgor	Reduced skin turgor	Reduced skin turgor
Extremities	Warm extremities	Warm extremities	Cold extremities
	Normal capillary refill time	Normal capillary refill time	Prolonged capillary refill time
	Normal peripheral pulses	Normal peripheral pulses	Weak peripheral pulses
Face	Eyes not sunken	Sunken eyes	Sunken eyes
	Moist mucous membranes	Dry mucous membranes	Dry mucous membranes
Observations	Normal urine output	Decreased urine output	Decreased urine output
	Normal heart rate	Tachycardia	Tachycardia
	Normal breathing pattern	Normal breathing pattern	Tachypnoea
	Normal blood pressure	Normal blood pressure	Hypotension (decompensated shock)

12.3.3 RESUSCITATION

Severe Dehydration/Hypovolaemic Shock
Route of fluid
- Intravenous, given as a 'push', usually from a 50 mL syringe

Type of Fluid
- Isotonic crystalloid, e.g. 0.9% sodium chloride
- *Note:* Colloid solutions are not currently recommended for use in resuscitation of children

Volume of Fluid
- Boluses of 20 mL/kg
- After 40 mL/kg, consider high-dependency care
- After 60 mL/kg, consider paediatric intensive care input

12.3.4 REPLACEMENT

Mild to Moderate Dehydration
Route of Fluid
- Enteral: oral, naso/orogastric tube, or gastrostomy
- If enteral fluid administration is unsuccessful, use intravenous route

Type of Fluid
- Enteral: oral rehydration therapy
- Intravenous: isotonic crystalloid, e.g. 0.9% sodium chloride + 5% dextrose

Volume of Fluid
- Depending on estimated deficit

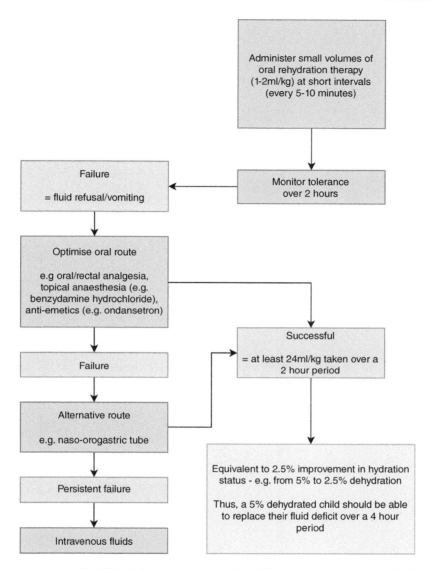

Figure 12.3.1 Enteral replacement and the 'fluid challenge'. In a non-shocked child, intravenous replacement of fluids is to be avoided where possible. The oral intake should be attempted with a 'fluid challenge'.

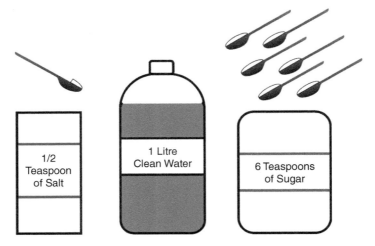

Figure 12.3.2 Instructions for making a simple oral rehydration solution (ORS).

Box 12.3.3 Hypokalaemia

- If serum K+ <4.5 mmol/L, add 10–20 mmol potassium chloride per 500 mL bag
- This should only be done in replacement or maintenance fluid prescribing

- Potassium should not be included in fluid boluses

- *Note:* Fluid should be replaced over a 24–48-hour period, with a maximum rate of sodium correction of 0.5 mmol/L/hr (12 mmol/L in 24hr). More rapid correction of sodium introduces a risk of cerebral oedema

12.3.5 MAINTENANCE

No Dehydration
Route of Fluid
- Enteral *or* intravenous

Type of Fluid
- Enteral: normal drink e.g. breastmilk, formula, water
- Intravenous: isotonic crystalloid, e.g. 0.9% sodium chloride + 5% dextrose

Volume of Fluid
- Traditionally calculated using the Holliday–Segar formula, according to the weight of the child

---

Box 12.3.4 Calculating Maintenance Volumes

Volume of maintenance fluids required over 24 hours =
  100 mL/kg for the first 10 kg
  50 mL/kg for the next 10 kg
  20 mL/kg for the subsequent weight above 20 kg
Example: Calculation of maintenance fluid for a 35 kg child:

  $(100 \times 10) + (50 \times 10) + (20 \times 15) = 1800$ mL in 24 hours
  Hourly rate = 1800 mL/24 hr = 75 mL/hr

12.3.6 MONITORING

Patients on intravenous fluid replacement should have regular monitoring:
- Fluid balance chart
- Daily body weight
- 12-hourly clinical reassessment of hydration status and fluid requirement
- Minimum once daily electrolyte monitoring (6-hourly in electrolyte derangement)

12.3.7 SPECIAL SITUATIONS

Na⁺/K⁺ Derangement
- If electrolytes within normal range, use 0.9% sodium chloride + 5% dextrose
- In children with electrolyte derangement, further calculation is required:
  - Daily sodium requirement: 2–3 mmol/kg/day
  - Daily potassium requirement: 1–2 mmol/kg/day

Unwell Children
- Must be resuscitated as appropriate
- For maintenance, note risk of developing syndrome of inappropriate antidiuretic hormone secretion (SIADH) in children with central nervous system or respiratory disease
- Limit fluids to two-thirds of the usual maintenance volume to avoid fluid overload

Neonates (<28 days)
- Fluid prescribing in neonates is complex and is not covered in detail here
- When intravenous fluid is required, the most common choice is 10% dextrose, with sodium and potassium supplementation from day 2 of life
- Volume of maintenance fluid is calculated according to age, as follows:
  - Day 0: 60 mL/kg/day
  - Day 1: 90 mL/kg/day
  - Day 2: 120 mL/kg/day
  - Days 3–28: 120–150 mL/kg/day

12.4 Childhood Immunisations

Rachel Atherton

Department of Paediatrics, Oxford University Hospitals NHS Foundation Trust, Oxford, UK

CONTENTS

12.4.1 CHAPTER AT A GLANCE

Box 12.4.1 Chapter at a Glance

- The opportunity to discuss immunisations should be taken at every opportunity and should be asked about in every history
- There is a lot of misinformation about vaccinations that can scare parents into avoiding them for their children

- Simple advice may help mitigate these fears and encourage immunisation

The UK childhood immunisation schedule is provided in the 'Green Book', a publication found at https://www.gov.uk/government/collections/immunisation-against-infectious-disease-the-green-book. It is advisable always to check the schedule prior to immunisation, since updates and improvements may occur. Countries outside the UK may use different schedules.

12.4.2 ROUTINE IMMUNISATIONS

Table 12.4.1 Routine immunisations in the UK

Age due	Vaccine given	Trade name	Diseases protected against	Site
8 weeks old	DTaP/IPV/Hib/HepB '6-in-one'	Infanrix Hexa	Diphtheria, tetanus, pertussis (whooping cough), polio, *Haemophilus influenzae* type B (Hib) and hepatitis B	Thigh
	MenB	Bexsero	Meningococcal group B	Left thigh
	Rotavirus	Rotarix	Rotavirus gastroenteritis	By mouth
12 weeks old	DTaP/IPV/Hib/HepB '6-in-one'	Infanrix Hexa	Diphtheria, tetanus, pertussis, polio, Hib and hepatitis B	Thigh
	Pneumococcal conjugate vaccine (PCV)	Prevenar 13	Pneumococcal (13 serotypes)	Thigh
	Rotavirus	Rotarix	Rotavirus	By mouth
16 weeks old	DTaP/IPV/Hib/HepB '6-in-one'	Infanrix Hexa	Diphtheria, tetanus, pertussis, polio, Hib and hepatitis B	Thigh
	MenB	Bexsero	MenB	Left thigh
1 year old (within a month of the 1st birthday)	Hib/MenC	Menitorix	Hib and MenC	Upper arm/thigh
	PCV	Prevenar 13	Pneumococcal	Upper arm/thigh
	MMR	MMR VaxPRO or Priorix	Measles, mumps and rubella (German measles)	Upper arm/thigh
	MenB	Bexsero	MenB	Left thigh
Eligible paediatric age groups[1]	Live attenuated influenza vaccine (LAIV)	Fluenz Tetra	Influenza, annually from September	Both nostrils
3 years 4 months old (or soon after)	DTaP/IPV or dTaP/IPV '4-in-one'	Infanrix IPV or Repevax	Diphtheria, tetanus, pertussis and polio	Upper arm
	MMR	MMR VaxPRO or Priorix	Measles, mumps and rubella	Upper arm
Girls aged 12–13 years old	HPV (two doses, 6–24 months apart)	Gardasil	Cervical cancer caused by human papillomavirus (HPV) types 16/18 (and genital warts caused by types 6/11)	Upper arm
14 years old (school year 9)	Td/IPV '3-in-one' (check MMR status)	Revaxis	Tetanus, diphtheria and polio	Upper arm
	MenACWY	Nimenrix or Menveo	Meningococcal groups A, C, W and Y disease	Upper arm

1. www.gov.uk/government/publications/influenza-the-green-book-chapter-19

12.4.3 SELECTIVE IMMUNISATIONS

Table 12.4.2 Selective immunisations in the UK

Age due	Vaccine given	Trade name	Diseases protected against	Site
At birth, 4 weeks and 12 months old	Hepatitis B	Engerix B/ HBvaxPRO	Hepatitis B	Thigh
Infants born to hepatitis B–infected mothers				
At birth	BCG	n/a	Tuberculosis	Left upper arm
At risk infants[1]				

12.4.5 COMMON QUESTIONS REGARDING IMMUNISATION

Is It Safe? I Heard That 'X' Vaccine Causes 'Y'

Parents/carers may raise concerns regarding the safety of vaccines. Those with general concerns can be advised:

- All vaccines are extensively tested prior to being included on the schedule
- Most adverse effects are mild and not dangerous
- The risk of rarer, more serious adverse effects is outweighed by the risk of natural infection

Concerns linking specific vaccines to specific diseases have variable bases in scientific fact. They are often exaggerated and distorted by both the media and online community

- Common fears include the association of the MMR vaccine with autism, and both the meningococcal conjugate vaccine and the influenza vaccine with Guillain–Barré. No evidence exists for either, despite large-scale assessment
- Intussusception is known to represent a rare but serious adverse effect of the rotavirus vaccination, occurring in between 1 in 20,000 and 1 in 100,000 recipients. Parents can be advised to monitor for symptoms, but reassured that the risk is far outweighed by the risk of severe rotavirus gastroenteritis in the unvaccinated infant

Is My Child Really at Risk of Dangerous Disease? I've Never Heard of a Child in This Country with Tetanus/Polio etc.

- Parents/carers may be unaware of the potentially devastating consequences of vaccine-preventable disease. The risks of infection should be emphasised, followed by signposting to other appropriate patient information resources
- Concerns may also be raised regarding the perceived benefit of natural infection versus vaccination. Again, the risks of natural infection should be highlighted

Isn't My Child Protected, as Long as Everyone Else Is Vaccinated?

- This is the concept of 'herd immunity', i.e. the indirect protection experienced by an individual within a predominantly immune community
- However, it should be emphasised that relying on herd immunity to protect individual children from a disease is unreliable:
  - Not every other child is vaccinated, some for medical reasons
  - Certain diseases may be contracted from the environment (e.g. tetanus)
  - Herd immunity is required to benefit those who cannot be vaccinated for medical reasons

Won't Having Lots of Vaccines at Once Overwhelm the Immune System?

- Explain to parents/carers that immunocompetent children are able to easily respond to multiple antigens simultaneously – their immune systems are naturally exposed to these every day
- Different immunisation schedules exist for immunocompromised children (see the Green Book, 'Immunisation of individuals with underlying medical conditions')

Should the Vaccination Be Delayed? My Child Isn't Well

- Vaccinations should be rescheduled in children with febrile illnesses; however, in children with mild illness and no accompanying fever (e.g. mild coryzal illness), they should be given

Can My Child Have the Different Components of the Vaccine Separately?

- Parents/carers may request MMR to be given as split components at separate appointments
- This is not available on the NHS, and is not recommended, due to the risk of natural infection between each visit

12.5 Safeguarding

Dannika Buckley[1] and Lottie Mount[2]

[1] Department of Paediatrics, University Hospitals Sussex NHS Foundation Trust, Worthing, UK
[2] Department of Community Paediatrics, Sussex Community NHS Foundation Trust, Worthing, UK

CONTENTS

12.5.1 CHAPTER AT A GLANCE

Box 12.5.1 Chapter at a Glance

- Child maltreatment is a global problem that affects children in every culture, race, religion and society
- Safeguarding children and young people is one of the most important parts of paediatric medicine. The purpose of this chapter is to give the reader a basic understanding of safeguarding procedures
- Each week in the UK, 1–2 children die as a direct consequence of child abuse. The majority of those who suffer abuse do so at the hands of their parents, relatives or someone they know well
- Abuse in childhood has significant long-lasting consequences on individuals' physical, mental and emotional health

- To be able to protect children from harm, doctors and health professionals must be prepared to question the information given to them. This requires them to be prepared to think the unthinkable
- In essence, safeguarding as a junior doctor is straightforward: *always* share and escalate any concerns, regardless of how minor they may initially appear to be
- Safeguarding is everyone's responsibility
- Serious case reviews of high-profile cases have highlighted common themes and weaknesses

12.5.2 DEFINITION

- Defined in Working Together to Safeguard Children 2018:
  - Protecting children from maltreatment and harm
  - Preventing the impairment of children's health or development
  - Ensuring that children grow up in circumstances consistent with the provision of safe and effective care
  - Taking action to enable all children to have the best outcomes
- In the context of safeguarding, a child is considered as someone who has not yet reached their 18th birthday

Clinical Guide to Paediatrics, First Edition. Edited by Rachel Varughese and Anna Mathew. Series Editor: Christian Fielder Camm.
© 2022 John Wiley & Sons Ltd. Published 2022 by John Wiley & Sons Ltd.
Companion website: www.wiley.com/go/varughese/paediatrics

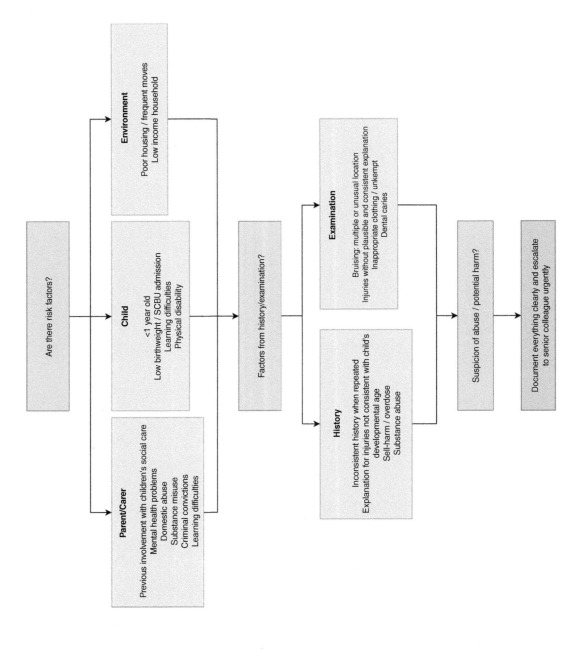

Figure 12.5.1 Factors to consider when assessing the probability of safeguarding issues.

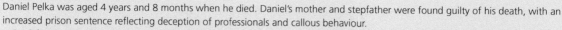

Box 12.5.2 A Case Example – Daniel

Daniel Pelka was aged 4 years and 8 months when he died. Daniel's mother and stepfather were found guilty of his death, with an increased prison sentence reflecting deception of professionals and callous behaviour.

Daniel was subjected to a period of prolonged physical abuse and neglect. At his post mortem, Daniel was found to have 40 injuries in total, including dehydration, gross malnourishment, acute subdural haematoma, with an older subdural haemorrhage. Daniel had presented to medical professionals many times with multiple injuries, including fractures, in the 18 months prior to his death. School had also raised concerns about Daniel.

False reassurances

- Daniel and his siblings appeared well cared for, wearing clean clothing

The voice of the child

- Daniel spoke Polish and very little English. No one ever asked Daniel how he was through a formal interpreting service

Multiagency working and communication

- Repeated domestic violence incidents occurred within the family home
- Referrals to social care were made, after which it was assumed that they were being actioned
- Information in hospital letters often did not allude to the concerns regarding the social situation. Missed opportunities to communicate effectively between multiple agencies occurred

12.5.3 TYPES OF CHILD ABUSE

Child abuse can be classified into several main categories. The types of abuse commonly overlap, with an element of emotional abuse with all types of maltreatment. Remember, identifying one type of abuse should encourage you to look for others.

Physical

- Physical abuse includes anything that causes physical harm to a child and includes hitting, biting, shaking, suffocating, drowning, burning or scalding
- Physical abuse can also include fabricated illness, where a parent or carer exaggerates symptoms or deliberately induces them

Neglect

- Neglect is a persistent failure to meet physical and/or psychological needs, sufficient to be detrimental to health or development
- It includes failure to attend appointments, provide food or clothing, and failure to access education for the child

Emotional

- Emotional abuse is the persistent maltreatment of a child, causing severe and persistent negative effects on the child's emotional development
- It can include ridiculing a child, placing inappropriate expectations on them for their developmental age, exposing them to domestic violence or not allowing them to express their views or participate socially

Sexual

- Sexual abuse involves forcing or enticing a child to engage in sexual activity
- This can involve physical contact, which includes penetrative (rape or oral sex), and non-penetrative (for example, kissing or touching)
- Non-contact activities that are examples of sexual abuse include children looking at or producing sexual images, encouraging sexualised behaviour and grooming a child

Other

- There are unfortunately many other ways that harm can be inflicted on children, including bullying, witnessing domestic violence (or, for older children, being in an abusive relationship themselves), trafficking, radicalisation, child sexual exploitation, forced marriage, female genital mutilation and internet abuse

Box 12.5.3   Definitions of Commonly Used Terms in Child Safeguarding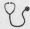

There are several terms used in safeguarding that may be completely unfamiliar. It is useful to have an understanding of what they mean when discussing child protection cases. They are listed here in alphabetical order.

- **Child in need**. A child that is unlikely to achieve or maintain a reasonable standard of health or development, or where health or development is likely to be significantly impaired or further impaired without the services of a local authority, or where the child is disabled (as defined by section 17 of the Children's Act 1989)
- **Child Protection Plan**. This is a record of recommendations to keep the named child safe or promote their welfare. It details actions including who needs to complete them and by when. The child will have a named social worker. The plan will be reviewed regularly either until the local authority is happy they are no longer at risk of harm, or they are taken into care, or they reach the age of 18
- **Discharge planning meeting**. This is a multi-agency meeting involving hospital and community teams to discuss any concerns and ensure there is a safe plan for discharge
- **Duty children's social worker**. This is the 'on call' or emergency social worker, available 24 hours a day
- **Emergency protection order**. This is obtained by application to the court, and gives authority to remove the child and place them under protection of the applicant, usually the local authority. It lasts for a maximum of 8 days. Further to this there are four different care orders that can be granted by the courts: interim care order, initially granted for 8 weeks; care order; placement order; adoption order
- **Gillick competent**. This is the term used if a person under the age of 16 has capacity to give consent. It originates from case law on providing contraception to patients under the age of

16 without parental consent. The Fraser Guidelines link in with this and can be found online (https://learning.nspcc.org.uk/child-protection-system/gillick-competence-fraser-guidelines)
- **Looked-after children**. Children and young people whose care is being overseen by social services. This includes children provided with accommodation for more than 24 hours, which may be for respite care or to protect them from harm
- **Named doctors and nurses**. These professionals have additional roles and responsibilities for child protection. They provide advice and expertise to fellow professionals, within either their organisation or their geographical location. They have a key role in promoting good professional practice, through training and governance
- **Parental responsibility**. This is who has legal responsibility for the child. In medicine, it is who can give consent on the child's behalf. The Children Act 1989, section 3, defines it as all the rights, duties, powers, responsibilities and authority that, by law, a parent of a child has in relation to the child and their property
- **Section 47 inquiry**. This refers to the section of the Children's Act 1989 that describes the local authority's duty to investigate when there is suspected actual/potential significant harm
- **Strategy meeting**. Held by social services and attended by all interested/involved parties when safeguarding concerns have been raised and an assessment suggests a child has been or is likely to be subject to significant harm. The outcome is to decide if there are grounds for a Section 47 inquiry

12.5.4   KEY HISTORY FEATURES

- **Inconsistent history.** For example, different mechanism of injury given by parent and child, or changing stories when told repeatedly
- **Explanation for injury unlikely**. For example, if not compatible with developmental age of the child
- **Risk factors identified.** These may be in the parent, child and/or environment, as outlined in Figure 12.5.1
- **Parent/carer unwilling to engage**. This may be apparent when with the healthcare worker or child
- **An older child with substance dependency.** This may be on tobacco, alcohol or any other substance. This makes them vulnerable to manipulation, including child sexual exploitation. Ask them who buys it for them or how they fund it
- **Overdose or self-harm**. The trigger could be underlying child abuse. There could also be concern around neglect, if the carer cannot keep the child safe

12.5.5   KEY EXAMINATION FEATURES

- A thorough 'top-to-toe' formal examination must be undertaken, with a body map and a chaperone
- Any visible marks and injuries should be marked, with photographs taken of any concerns
- Before and during the examination, always observe the child and carer carefully
- Does the carer–child dynamic seem normal?
- Does the carer comfort the child appropriately?
- Particular findings that may be associated with child abuse include:
  - Any bruise/other physical injury in a non-mobile child
  - Bruises within 'protected' regions, as shown in Figures 12.5.2 and 12.5.3, are more suspicious for non-accidental injury (NAI)
  - 'Frozen watchfulness', where the child appears terrified within the clinical interaction
  - Self-harm injuries
  - Vaginal discharge and/or bruising to thighs/abdomen should raise sexual abuse as a possible differential

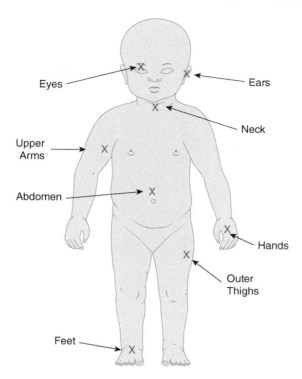

Eyes

Ears

Neck

Upper
Arms

Abdomen

Hands

Outer
Thighs

Feet

Figure 12.5.2 A body map with markings for suspicious areas for bruising from the front. In mobile children, some bruising is expected as part of daily life. However, it is important to be discerning about the location of bruises. Bruises on bony prominences are commonly accidental. Look for bruises in suspicious areas to help decide if they may be non-accidental.

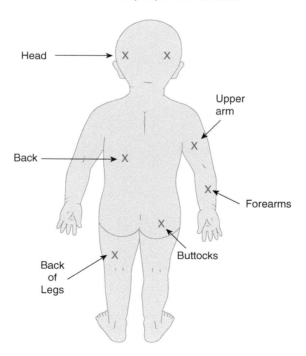

Head

Upper
arm

Back

Forearms

Buttocks

Back
of
Legs

Figure 12.5.3 Suspicious areas for bruising from the back.

12.5.6 KEY INVESTIGATIONS

Investigations will depend on the case and the particular concerns, but the following areas should be considered.

Table 12.5.1 Areas for investigation

Test	When to perform	Potential result
Growth parameters: height, weight and head circumference	• In all children with safeguarding concerns • Ask for the 'red book' (Personal Child Health Record) to monitor the growth trend	• Faltering growth from neglect • Rapid growth in head circumference prior to suture fusion may indicate intracranial problems
Skeletal survey	• In all children with suspicion of physical abuse • Chest and long bone x-rays	• May identify hidden acute fractures, or old healing injuries
Computed tomography (CT) head	• Consider in infants less than 1 year old	• Fractures or bleeds, particularly associated with shaking
Ophthalmology	• In infants who may have been shaken	• Retinal haemorrhages
Full blood count, clotting and clotting factors, Von Willebrand factor	• In children with bruising, to look for abnormalities with haemostasis • Remember, a child with a clotting abnormality can still suffer non-accidental injury	• Idiopathic thrombocytopenia • Von Willebrand disease • Clotting factor deficiencies • Rarer clotting disorders

---

Box 12.5.4   Information Sharing and Confidentiality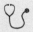

- The doctor–patient relationship is viewed as confidential
- Many may worry that information sharing with social care will be breaking this duty of confidence to their patients and families
- Disclosure of information is actually allowed in a number of cases. If it is thought that withholding information will result in harm of a child/young person, the information must be shared

---

Box 12.5.5   The Common Assessment Framework

The Common Assessment Framework (CAF) is a standardised tool used to assess children and young people (including unborn babies) who may need additional services from more than one agency.
A CAF should be completed if you are worried about the child's:

- Health
- Development
- Welfare
- Behaviour
- Progress in learning
- Any aspect of the well-being of a child or young person

Informed consent must be taken from parents, and the child if they have capacity, including consent to share information with other professionals. *It is not a referral to social care* and should not be used if there are concerns that the child may be at risk of harm. If there are concerns regarding a child's wellbeing, this should be discussed with social services.
Needs are assessed in the following areas:

- Development of the child or young person
- Parents and carers
- Family and environment

12.5.7 THE CHALLENGES OF CHILD PROTECTION WORK

- Thinking the unthinkable – always think non-accidental injury (even if the current presenting complaint is legitimate).
- Requirement for excellent communication with colleagues within multiple disciplines.
- The emotive nature of child protection work can make discussions with families uncomfortable. Keep it factual.
- There may be confrontation with families who act aggressively or who are manipulative. Equally, dealing with families who are polite and pleasant can also be challenging in a different way.
- Very detailed history and examination, looking for subtle clues – this takes time.

12.5.8 TWO CASES

Think about the two cases in Boxes 12.5.6 and 12.5.7. What is concerning? What would you do next?

Box 12.5.6   A Case Example – Asif

3-year-old Asif has an appointment at the GP surgery with his mother. Asif has had 24 hours of fever >38 °C, with an accompanying cough. He has not been wanting to eat much food, but has been drinking lots of fluid.

The GP takes off Asif's T-shirt to listen to his chest. On the lateral aspect of Asif's upper right thorax are three small, circular purple marks located close together in a line. On asking Asif's mother the medical history, she does not know how he has acquired them.

Asif's mother speaks very little English. She moved to the country 4 years ago, when she married her British husband and moved into his family home, where she lives with multiple members of her husband's family.

Concerning factors

- Injury located in an unusual location. Children sustain bruises obtained through play in a particular distribution, according to their developmental maturity
- Bruise pattern is consistent with fingertip marks
- No explanation available/given for the marks seen

- Mother's poor English language. She is living in a new country with her husband's family and is possibly socially isolated. Has a formal interpreting service previously been offered for health appointments when she attends?

What to do next

- Document everything clearly
- Write down contemporaneously the history given (very important if history subsequently changes)
- Inform and discuss with senior colleagues. A referral to social care is very likely

- Arrange for a formal child protection medical examination to be performed, including completion of a body map and photographs of areas of concern
- Find out whether Asif is already known to social care

Box 12.5.7   A Case Example – Ellie-May

7-year-old Ellie-May presents to A&E with a superficial burn to the dorsal aspect of her left hand and left wrist. It is her fourth attendance at A&E in the last 3 months. Ellie-May says that the burn happened when she was making instant noodles for her tea, and she spilt the water from the kettle. Ellie-May has attended the department with her 14-year-old brother. When questioned on the location of their parents, the siblings state that their mother and stepfather left for the pub last night and have not yet returned home 20 hours later.

Ellie-May is also noted to be wearing unkempt clothing, with evidence of lice seen in her hair.

Concerning factors

- Injury suggesting lack of adequate supervision
- Ellie-May has been seen regularly at A&E. What were the reasons for previous attendances?
- 7-year-old Ellie-May has been left in the care of her 14-year-old

brother for almost 24 hours. If this is a regular occurrence, this is even more concerning
- Ellie-May looks generally unkempt

What to do next

- Document everything clearly
- Write down contemporaneously, in the child's words, the history given
- Inform and discuss with senior colleagues
- Find out if the children and family are already known to social care. A social care referral must be made regarding this attendance at A&E

- Find out where the parents are. They need to be contacted to come to the hospital
- Find out if school, GP or any other agencies have concerns regarding the children and family

---

12.5.9 SUMMARY POINTS

- Document everything clearly and contemporaneously
- Have a child-centred approach: listen to the voice of the child and be patient
- Provide opportunities for parents and children to disclose separately
- Understand the impact of mental health within the family

- Recognise disguised compliance (family members covering up for each other)
- Maintain an enquiring mind: question what you are being told
- Inform and discuss *all* concerns with senior colleagues

12.5.10 ADDITIONAL REFERENCES

GMC guidance for protecting children and young people. https://www.gmc-uk.org/ethical-guidance/ethical-guidance-for-doctors/protecting-children-and-young-people

HM Government (2015). Working together to safeguard children. https://www.gov.uk/government/publications/working-together-to-safeguard-children--2

Royal College of Paediatrics and Child Health (2021). Child protection and safeguarding. https://www.rcpch.ac.uk/key-topics/child-protection. The RCPCH provides extensive resources on child protection: when to think about it, what to look out for and the evidence behind best practice.

13.1 Sepsis Management

Rachel Varughese[1] and Anna Mathew[2]

[1] Department of Paediatrics, Oxford University Hospitals NHS Foundation Trust, Oxford, UK

[2] Department of Paediatrics, University Hospitals Sussex NHS Foundation Trust, Worthing, UK

CONTENTS

13.1.1 KEY POINTS

- Paediatric sepsis is a time-critical medical emergency requiring a systematic approach
- All elements of initial assessment and management should be completed within 1 hour of the child presenting to paediatric services
- 'Sepsis Six', initially an adult initiative demonstrating improved survival, has been modified for the paediatric population, and has been widely adopted across the UK as best practice

13.1.2 ADDITIONAL REFERENCE

Tong J, Plunkett A, Daniels R (2014). G218(P) The paediatric Sepsis 6 initiative. Archives of Disease in Childhood 99:A93.

Clinical Guide to Paediatrics, First Edition. Edited by Rachel Varughese and Anna Mathew. Series Editor: Christian Fielder Camm.
© 2022 John Wiley & Sons Ltd. Published 2022 by John Wiley & Sons Ltd.
Companion website: www.wiley.com/go/varughese/paediatrics

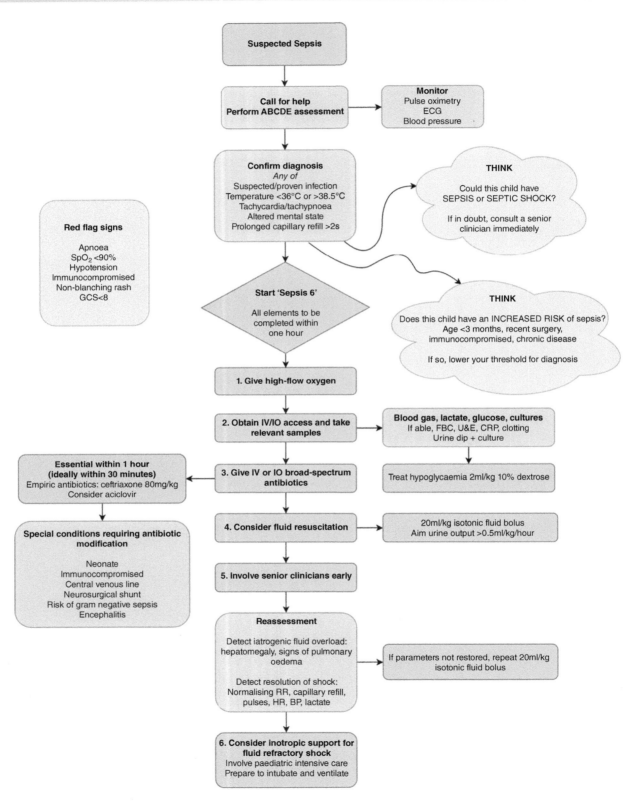

Figure 13.1.1 Algorithm for the approach to the management of sepsis.

13.2 Anaphylaxis Management

Rachel Varughese[1] and Anna Mathew[2]

[1] Department of Paediatrics, Oxford University Hospitals NHS Foundation Trust, Oxford, UK

[2] Department of Paediatrics, University Hospitals Sussex NHS Foundation Trust, Worthing, UK

CONTENTS

13.2.1 KEY POINTS

- Anaphylaxis is an immunoglobulin (Ig) E–mediated severe hypersensitivity reaction that can rapidly lead to cardiorespiratory arrest and death if not treated promptly
- Anaphylaxis should always be considered in those with acute airway, breathing and circulation problems, even without a clear history of exposure to an allergen or known allergy

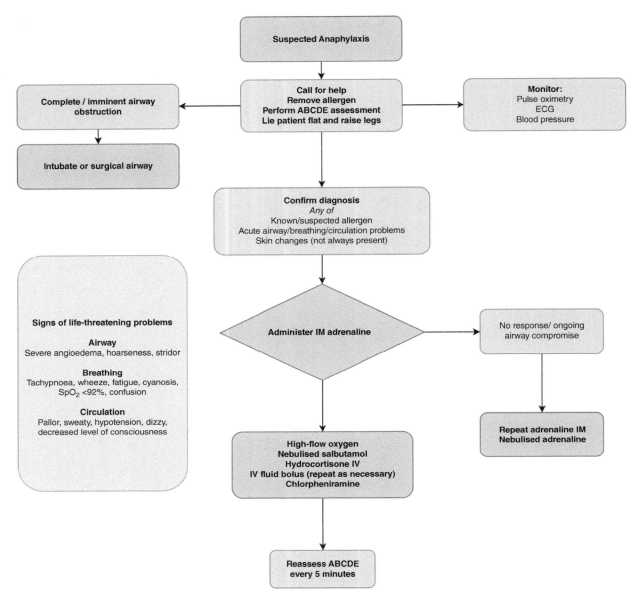

Figure 13.2.1 Algorithm for the approach to the management of anaphylaxis.

Table 13.2.1 Medications used in the management of anaphylaxis

Medications	Doses according to age			
	<6 months	6 months–6 years	6–12 years	>12 years
Adrenaline 1:1000 (IM)	150 μg (0.15 mL)		300 μg (0.3 mL)	500 μg (0.5 mL)
Salbutamol (nebulised)	2.5 mg		5 mg	
Hydrocortisone (IM or slow IV)	25 mg	50 mg	100 mg	200 mg
0.9% saline (IV)	20 mL/kg bolus			
Chlorpheniramine (IM or slow IV)	250 μg/kg	2.5 mg	5 mg	10 mg

IM, intramuscular; IV, intravenous

13.2.2 IMPORTANT NOTES ABOUT ADRENALINE

- In hospital, where adrenaline is drawn up rather than delivered through an auto-injector, a dose of 10 µg/kg intramuscular (IM) adrenaline can be used
- It is possible to use 1:10,000 strength adrenaline in infants and young children, for whom volumes are impractically small when using 1:1000
- In hospital, intravenous (IV) adrenaline of 1 µg/kg can be used for shock resistant to IM adrenaline, but is only to be used by experienced clinicians

13.2.3 ADDITIONAL REFERENCES

UK Resuscitation Council (2013). Emergency treatment of anaphylactic reactions. https://www.resus.org.uk/library/additional-guidance/guidance-anaphylaxis/emergency-treatment

13.3 Acute Asthma Management

Rachel Varughese[1] and Anna Mathew[2]

[1] Department of Paediatrics, Oxford University Hospitals NHS Foundation Trust, Oxford, UK
[2] Department of Paediatrics, University Hospitals Sussex NHS Foundation Trust, Worthing, UK

CONTENTS

13.3.1 KEY POINTS

- Asthma management has several facets: chronic control, management of acute mild to moderate asthma and management of acute severe to life-threatening asthma
- Management of acute mild to moderate asthma is found in Chapter 1.1
- This chapter focuses on the management of severe and life-threatening acute asthma exacerbations

13.3.2 ADDITIONAL REFERENCES

British Thoracic Society and NHS Scotland (2019). SIGN 158: British guideline on the management of asthma. https://www.sign.ac.uk/media/1773/sign158-updated.pdf

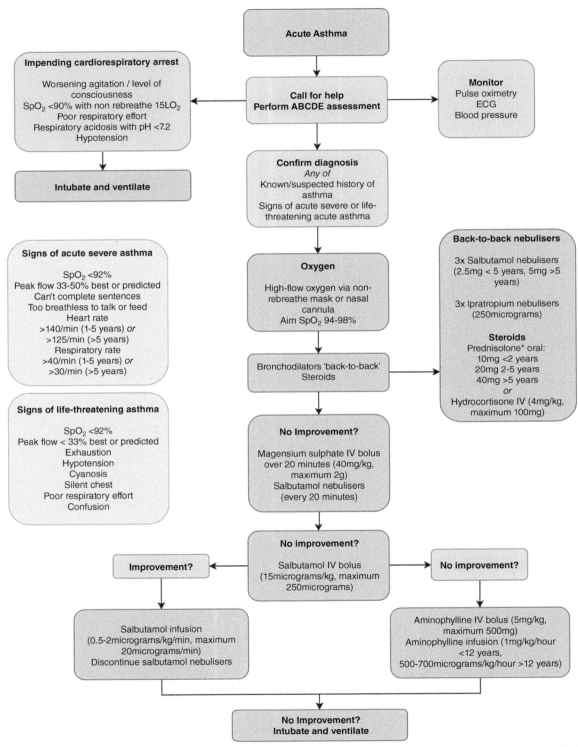

*There is a gradual change in clinical practice to accommodate dexamethasone as an option instead of prednisolone. Benefits include being more palatable and the need for only one dose.

Figure 13.3.1 Algorithm for the management of acute severe and life-threatening asthma.

13.4 Prolonged Seizure Management

Rachel Varughese[1] and Anna Mathew[2]

[1] Department of Paediatrics, Oxford University Hospitals NHS Foundation Trust, Oxford, UK
[2] Department of Paediatrics, University Hospitals Sussex NHS Foundation Trust, Worthing, UK

CONTENTS

13.4.1 KEY POINTS

- A prolonged seizure is defined as a generalised seizure ≥5 minutes
- Status epilepticus is defined as a generalised seizure ≥30 minutes or 2 or more seizures within a 30-minute period without full recovery in between
- Children with a seizure lasting more than 5 minutes are treated in the same way as those in established status epilepticus, in order to stop the seizure and prevent status epilepticus

13.4.2 ADDITIONAL REFERENCES

National Institute for Health and Care Excellence (2020). Epilepsy diagnosis and management. Clinical guideline [CG137]. London: NICE.

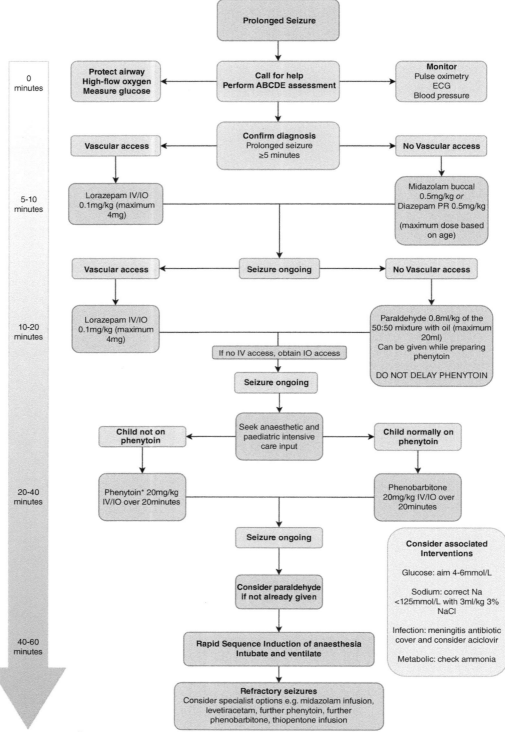

Prolonged Seizure

0 minutes

Protect airway
High-flow oxygen
Measure glucose

Call for help
Perform ABCDE assessment

Monitor
Pulse oximetry
ECG
Blood pressure

Confirm diagnosis
Prolonged seizure
≥5 minutes

Vascular access

No Vascular access

5-10 minutes

Lorazepam IV/IO
0.1mg/kg (maximum 4mg)

Midazolam buccal
0.5mg/kg *or*
Diazepam PR 0.5mg/kg

(maximum dose based on age)

Vascular access

Seizure ongoing

No Vascular access

10-20 minutes

Lorazepam IV/IO
0.1mg/kg (maximum 4mg)

Paraldehyde 0.8ml/kg of the 50:50 mixture with oil (maximum 20ml)
Can be given while preparing phenytoin

DO NOT DELAY PHENYTOIN

If no IV access, obtain IO access

Seizure ongoing

Seek anaesthetic and paediatric intensive care input

Child not on phenytoin

Child normally on phenytoin

20-40 minutes

Phenytoin* 20mg/kg IV/IO over 20minutes

Phenobarbitone 20mg/kg IV/IO over 20minutes

Seizure ongoing

Consider associated Interventions

Glucose: aim 4-6mmol/L

Sodium: correct Na <125mmol/L with 3ml/kg 3% NaCl

Infection: meningitis antibiotic cover and consider aciclovir

Metabolic: check ammonia

Consider paraldehyde
if not already given

40-60 minutes

Rapid Sequence Induction of anaesthesia
Intubate and ventilate

Refractory seizures
Consider specialist options e.g. midazolam infusion, levetiracetam, further phenytoin, further phenobarbitone, thiopentone infusion

*Evidence now suggests that the efficacy and safety of Levetiracetam and Phenytoin are comparable in the treatment of benzodiazepine-resistant CSE. Many UK centres now use Levetiracetam instead of Phenytoin in benzodiazepine-resistant CSE due to the advantages of ease of administration as an intravenous push, no requirement for ECG monitoring, minimal drug interactions, and few serious side effects.

Figure 13.4.1 Algorithm for the approach to the management of prolonged seizures and status epilepticus.

13.5 Raised Intracranial Pressure Management

Rachel Varughese[1] and Anna Mathew[2]

[1] Department of Paediatrics, Oxford University Hospitals NHS Foundation Trust, Oxford, UK
[2] Department of Paediatrics, University Hospitals Sussex NHS Foundation Trust, Worthing, UK

CONTENTS

13.5.1 KEY POINTS

- Raised intracranial pressure (ICP) can result from intracranial space-occupying lesions, disorders of cerebrospinal fluid (CSF) circulation and diffuse brain injury
- It should be considered in any child with a known CSF diversion device who presents with altered mental state
- Raised ICP is an important cause of secondary brain injury and emergency management is essential

13.5.2 SIGNS OF RAISED INTRACRANIAL PRESSURE

- Reduced/fluctuating level of consciousness (Glasgow Coma Scale <9 or drop of 3 or more)
- Relative bradycardia and hypertension
- Focal neurological signs
- Abnormal posture/posturing
- Unequal, dilated or poorly responsive pupils
- Papilloedema
- Abnormal 'doll's-eye' movements

Clinical Guide to Paediatrics, First Edition. Edited by Rachel Varughese and Anna Mathew. Series Editor: Christian Fielder Camm.
© 2022 John Wiley & Sons Ltd. Published 2022 by John Wiley & Sons Ltd.
Companion website: www.wiley.com/go/varughese/paediatrics

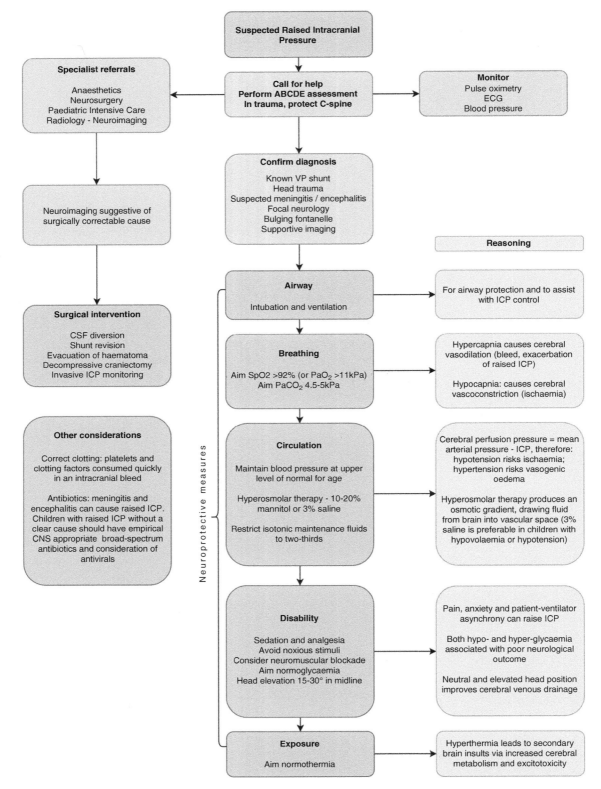

Figure 13.5.1 Algorithm for the emergency management of raised intracranial pressure.

Guidelines

Condition	Guideline title	Issuing agency	Publication date	Internet link
Adrenal insufficiency	Guidelines for the diagnosis and management of critical illness-related corticosteroid insufficiency (CIRCI) in critically ill patients, Part 1 & Part 2	Society of Critical Care Medicine; European Society of Intensive Care Medicine	2017	http://pure-oai.bham.ac.uk/ws/files/44483862/Corticosteroid_Guideline_Part_1_FINAL_08_08_17_docx_Revision.pdf
Anaphylaxis	CG 134 Anaphylaxis: assessment and referral after emergency treatment	National Institute for Health and Care Excellence (NICE)	2011	https://www.nice.org.uk/guidance/cg134
Anaphylaxis	Allergy care pathway for anaphylaxis	Royal College of Paediatrics and Child Health (RCPCH)	2011	https://www.rcpch.ac.uk/resources/allergy-care-pathway-anaphylaxis
Arrhythmias	Pharmacological and non-pharmacological therapy for arrhythmias in the pediatric population	European Heart Rhythm Association; Association for European Paediatric and Congenital Cardiology	2013	https://academic.oup.com/europace/article/15/9/1337/486169
Arrhythmias	Arrhythmias in congenital heart disease: a position paper	European Heart Rhythm Association, Association for European Paediatric and Congenital Cardiology and the European Society of Cardiology	2018	https://academic.oup.com/europace/article/20/11/1719/4944677
Asthma	NG 80 Asthma: diagnosis, monitoring and chronic asthma management	NICE	2017 (updated 2020)	https://www.nice.org.uk/guidance/ng80
Asthma	SIGN 158 British Guideline on the Management of Asthma	British Thoracic Society (BTS) and Scottish Intercollegiate Guidelines Network (SIGN)	2019	https://www.sign.ac.uk/sign-158-british-guideline-on-the-management-of-asthma
Asthma	TA 131 Inhaled corticosteroids for the treatment of chronic asthma in children under the age of 12 years	NICE	2007	https://www.nice.org.uk/guidance/ta131
Asthma	TA 138 Inhaled corticosteroids for the treatment of chronic asthma in adults and in children aged 12 years and over	NICE	2008	https://www.nice.org.uk/guidance/ta138

Clinical Guide to Paediatrics, First Edition. Edited by Rachel Varughese and Anna Mathew. Series Editor: Christian Fielder Camm.
© 2022 John Wiley & Sons Ltd. Published 2022 by John Wiley & Sons Ltd.
Companion website: www.wiley.com/go/varughese/paediatrics

Condition	Guideline title	Issuing agency	Publication date	Internet link
Atopic dermatitis (eczema)	CG 57 Atopic eczema in under 12s: diagnosis and management	NICE	2007 (updated 2019)	https://www.nice.org.uk/guidance/cg57
Atopic dermatitis (eczema)	QS 44 Atopic eczema in under 12s	NICE	2013	https://www.nice.org.uk/guidance/qs44
Atopic dermatitis (eczema)	Allergy care pathway for eczema	RCPCH	2005	https://www.rcpch.ac.uk/resources/allergy-care-pathway-eczema
Behavioural disturbance	NG10 Violence and aggression: short-term management in mental health, health and community settings	NICE	2015	https://www.nice.org.uk/guidance/NG10/chapter/1-recommendations
Behavioural disturbance	Guidelines for the management of excited delirium/acute behavioural disturbance (ABD)	Royal College of Emergency Medicine	2016	https://www.rcem.ac.uk/docs/College%20Guidelines/5p.%20RCEM%20guidelines%20for%20management%20of%20Acute%20Behavioural%20Disturbance%20(May%202016).pdf
Bleeding disorders	UKHCDO protocol for first line immune tolerance induction for children with severe haemophilia A	United Kingdom Haemophilia Centre Doctors' Organisation	2017	http://www.ukhcdo.org/wp-content/uploads/2017/01/ITI-protocol-2017.pdf
Brain tumours in childhood	Brain pathways guideline: a guideline to assist healthcare professionals in the assessment of children who may have a brain tumour	Headsmart (NICE and RCPCH accredited)	2017	https://www.headsmart.org.uk/clinical/clinical-guideline/
Bronchiolitis	QS 122 Bronchiolitis in children	NICE	2016	https://www.nice.org.uk/guidance/qs122
Bronchiolitis	NG 9 Bronchiolitis in children: diagnosis and management	NICE	2015	https://www.nice.org.uk/guidance/ng9
Coeliac disease	NG 20 Coeliac disease: recognition, assessment and management	NICE	2015	https://www.nice.org.uk/guidance/ng20
Colic	Colic – infantile	NICE	2017	https://cks.nice.org.uk/colic-infantile
Congenital heart disease	Guidelines for the management of congenital heart diseases in children and adolescents	German Society of Pediatric Cardiology	2017	https://www.cambridge.org/core/journals/cardiology-in-the-young/article/guidelines-for-the-management-of-congenital-heart-diseases-in-childhood-and-adolescence/FF22F05D3676503D12FEDCE1ADB2165D
Congenital hypothyroidism	Screening, diagnosis, and management of congenital hypothyroidism	European Society for Paediatric Endocrinology	2015	https://ep.bmj.com/content/100/5/260.long
Constipation	CG 99 Constipation in children and young people: diagnosis and management	NICE	2010 (updated 2017)	https://www.nice.org.uk/guidance/cg99

Condition	Guideline title	Issuing agency	Publication date	Internet link
Constipation	QS 62 Constipation in children and young people	NICE	2014	https://www.nice.org.uk/guidance/qs62
Cow's milk protein allergy	Cow's milk allergy in children	NICE	2019	https://cks.nice.org.uk/cows-milk-allergy-in-children
Cow's milk protein allergy	Cow's milk allergy	British Society for Allergy & Clinical Immunology	2014	https://www.bsaci.org/guidelines/bsaci-guidelines/cows-milk-allergy/
Cow's milk protein allergy	The milk allergy in primary care (MAP) guideline 2019	Allergy UK	2019	https://gpifn.org.uk/imap/
Croup	Croup	NICE	2019	https://cks.nice.org.uk/croup#!scenarioRecommendation
Cystic fibrosis	NG 78 Cystic fibrosis: diagnosis and management	NICE	2017	https://www.nice.org.uk/guidance/ng78
Cystic fibrosis	Guidelines for the performance of the sweat test for the investigation of cystic fibrosis in the UK	Cystic Fibrosis Trust (RCPCH endorsed)	2014	http://www.exeterlaboratory.com/images/sweat-guideline-v2-1.pdf
Decreased conscious level	Management of children and young people with an acute decrease in conscious level	RCPCH	2015	https://www.rcpch.ac.uk/resources/management-children-young-people-acute-decrease-conscious-level-clinical-guideline
Dehydration	NG 29 Intravenous fluid therapy in children and young people in hospital	NICE	2015 (updated 2020)	https://www.nice.org.uk/guidance/ng29
Diabetes	NG 18 Diabetes (type 1 and type 2) in children and young people: diagnosis and management	NICE	2015 (updated 2016)	https://www.nice.org.uk/guidance/ng18
Diabetes	QS 125 Diabetes in children and young people	NICE	2016	https://www.nice.org.uk/guidance/qs125
Diabetes	SIGN 116 Management of Diabetes	SIGN	2017	https://www.sign.ac.uk/assets/sign116.pdf
Diabetic ketoacidosis	DKA guideline	British Society for Paediatric Endocrinology and Diabetes	2018	https://www.bsped.org.uk/media/1798/bsped-dka-guideline-2020.pdf
Drug allergy	Allergy care pathway for drug allergy	RCPCH	2011	https://www.rcpch.ac.uk/resources/allergy-care-pathway-drug-allergy
Enteric fever	Public health operational guidelines for typhoid and paratyphoid (enteric fever)	Public Health England, Chartered Institute of Environmental Health	2017	https://assets.publishing.service.gov.uk/government/uploads/system/uploads/attachment_data/file/614875/Public_Health_Operational_Guidelines_for_Typhoid_and_Paratyphoid.pdf
Epilepsy	QS 27 Epilepsy in children and young people	NICE	2013	https://www.nice.org.uk/guidance/qs27
Epilepsy	CG 137 Epilepsies: diagnosis and management	NICE	2012 (updated 2020)	https://www.nice.org.uk/guidance/cg137

Condition	Guideline title	Issuing agency	Publication date	Internet link
Faltering growth	NG 75 Faltering growth: recognition and management of faltering growth in children	NICE	2017	https://www.nice.org.uk/guidance/ng75
Febrile neutropenia	CG 151 Neutropenic sepsis: prevention and management in people with cancer	NICE	2012	https://www.nice.org.uk/guidance/cg151
Fever	NG 143 Fever in under 5s: assessment and initial management	NICE	2019	https://www.nice.org.uk/guidance/ng14 3
Food allergy	Allergy care pathway for food allergy	RCPCH	2011	https://www.rcpch.ac.uk/resources/allergy-care-pathway-food-allerg y
Gastroenteritis	CG 84 Diarrhoea and vomiting caused by gastroenteritis in under 5s: diagnosis and management	NICE	2009	https://www.nice.org.uk/guidance/cg84
Gastroesophageal reflux	NG1 Gastro-oesophageal reflux disease in children and young people: diagnosis and management	NICE	2019	https://www.nice.org.uk/guidance/ng1
Gastroesophageal reflux	QS 112 Gastro-oesophageal reflux in children and young people	NICE	2016	https://www.nice.org.uk/guidance/qs11 2
Glomerulonephritis	KDIGO clinical practice guideline for glomerulonephritis	Kidney Disease Improving Global Outcomes	2012	https://kdigo.org/wp-content/uploads/2017/02/KDIGO-2012-GN-Guideline-English.pdf
Glycogen storage disorders	Consensus guidelines for management of glycogen storage disease type I (Von Gierke)	European Study on Glycogen Storage Disease Type I (ESGSD I)	2002	https://pubmed.ncbi.nlm.nih.gov/1237358 5
Glycogen storage disorders	Guideline on respiratory management of children with neuromuscular weakness type II (Pompe)	British Thoracic Society (BTS)	2012	https://pubmed.ncbi.nlm.nih.gov/2273042 8
Guillain–Barré syndrome	Evidence-based guideline update: plasmapheresis in neurologic disorders	American Academy of Neurology	2011	https://pubmed.ncbi.nlm.nih.gov/2124249 8
Guillain–Barré syndrome	Evidence-based guideline: intravenous immunoglobulin in the treatment of neuromuscular disorders	American Academy of Neurology	2012	https://pubmed.ncbi.nlm.nih.gov/2245426 8
Haemolytic diseases in childhood	Guideline for the use of anti-D immunoglobulin for the prevention of haemolytic disease of the fetus and newborn	British Committee for Standards in Haematology	2014	https://b-s-h.org.uk/guidelines/guidelines/use-of-anti-d-immuno globin-for-the-prevention-of-haemolytic-disease-of-the-fetus-and-newborn
Haemolytic uraemic syndrome	an international consensus approach to the management of atypical hemolytic uremic syndrome in children	HUS International	2016	https://pubmed.ncbi.nlm.nih.gov/2585975 2
Haemophilia	Guidelines for the management of hemophilia	World Federation of Hemophilia	2019	https://elearning.wfh.org/resource/treatment-guidelines

Condition	Guideline title	Issuing agency	Publication date	Internet link
Haemophilia	UKHCDO protocol for first line immune tolerance induction for children with severe haemophilia A: a protocol from the UKHCDO Inhibitor and Paediatric Working Parties	United Kingdom Haemophilia Centre Doctors' Organisation	2018	http://www.ukhcdo.org/wp-content/uploads/2015/12/UKHCDO_ITI_FINALfor_UKHCDO_website.pdf
Headaches	CG 150 Headaches in over 12s: diagnosis and management	NICE	2012 (updated 2015)	https://www.nice.org.uk/guidance/cg150
Headaches	QS 42 Headaches in over 12s	NICE	2013	https://www.nice.org.uk/guidance/qs42
Head injury	CG 176 Head injury: assessment and early management	NICE	2014 (updated 2019)	https://www.nice.org.uk/guidance/cg176
Head injury	QS 74 Head injury	NICE	2014	https://www.nice.org.uk/guidance/qs74
Head injury	Abusive head trauma and the eye in infancy	RCPCH/Royal College of Ophthalmologists	2013	https://www.rcophth.ac.uk/wp-content/uploads/2014/12/2013-SCI-292-ABUSIVE-HEAD-TRAUMA-AND-THE-EYE-FINAL-at-June-2013.pdf
Hereditary spherocytosis	Guidelines for the diagnosis and management of hereditary spherocytosis	British Committee for Standards in Haematology	2012	https://pubmed.ncbi.nlm.nih.gov/22055020
Hereditary spherocytosis	Guideline on prevention and treatment of infection in patients with absent or dysfunctional spleen	British Committee for Standards in Haematology	2011	https://pubmed.ncbi.nlm.nih.gov/21988145
Herpes encephalitis	Management of suspected viral encephalitis in children – Association of British Neurologists and British Paediatric Allergy, Immunology and Infection Group National Guidelines	Association of British Neurologists/ British Paediatric Allergy, Immunology and Infection Group (ABN/BPAIIG)	2011	https://pubmed.ncbi.nlm.nih.gov/22120594
HIV	HIV testing: encouraging uptake QS	NICE	2017	www.nice.org.uk/guidance/qs157
Hypoglycaemia	Recurrent hypoglycaemia	BIMDG	2008 (updated 2016)	http://www.bimdg.org.uk/store/guidelines/Hypoglycaemia_2016_189288_09092016.pdf
Hypoglycaemia	NG 18 Diabetes (type 1 and type 2) in children and young people: diagnosis and management	NICE	2015	https://www.nice.org.uk/guidance/ng18
Idiopathic intracranial hypertension	Idiopathic intracranial hypertension: consensus guidelines on management	Association of British Neurologists, British Association for the Study of Headache, the Society of British Neurological Surgeons and the Royal College of Ophthalmologists	2018	https://pubmed.ncbi.nlm.nih.gov/29903905

Condition	Guideline title	Issuing agency	Publication date	Internet link
Idiopathic thrombocytopaenic purpura	Eltrombopag for treating chronic immune (idiopathic) thrombocytopenic purpura. Technology appraisal guidance [TA293]	NICE	2011 (updated 2018)	https://www.nice.org.uk/guidance/TA293
Idiopathic thrombocytopaenic purpura	Romiplostim for the treatment of chronic immune (idiopathic) thrombocytopenic purpura. Technology appraisal guidance [TA221]	NICE	2011 (updated 2018)	https://www.nice.org.uk/guidance/TA221
Immunisations	The Green Book	UK government	2020	www.gov.uk/government/collections/immunisation-against-infectious-disease-the-green-book#the-green-book
Inborn errors of metabolism	Consensus statement: chromosomal microarray is a first-tier clinical diagnostic test for individuals with developmental disabilities or congenital anomalies	American Society of Human Genetics	2010	https://pubmed.ncbi.nlm.nih.gov/20466091
Infective endocarditis	Prophylaxis against infective endocarditis: antimicrobial prophylaxis against infective endocarditis in adults and children undergoing interventional procedures	NICE	2008 (updated 2016)	https://www.nice.org.uk/guidance/cg64
Inflammatory bowel disease	NG129 Crohn's disease: management	NICE	2019	https://www.nice.org.uk/guidance/ng129
Inflammatory bowel disease	Guidelines for the management of inflammatory bowel disease in children in the United Kingdom	IBD Working Group of the British Society of Paediatric Gastroenterology, Hepatology, and Nutrition	2010	https://pubmed.ncbi.nlm.nih.gov/20081543
Iron-deficiency anaemia	Anaemia – iron deficiency	NICE	2018	https:// cks.nice.org.uk/anaemia-iron-deficiency
Jaundice	CG98: Jaundice in newborn babies under 28 days	NICE	2010 (updated 2016)	https://www.nice.org.uk/Guidance/CG98
Jaundice	Guideline for the investigation of neonatal conjugated jaundice	British Society of Paediatric Gastroenterology, Hepatology and Nutrition	2016	https://old.bspghan.org.uk/sites/default/files/guidelines/2016_guideline_for_the_investigation_of_neonatal_conjugated_jaundice.pdf
Juvenile idiopathic arthritis	Guideline for the treatment of juvenile idiopathic arthritis: therapeutic approaches for non-systemic polyarthritis, sacroiliitis, and enthesitis	American College of Rheumatology/ Arthritis Foundation	2019	https://www.rheumatology.org/Portals/0/Files/JIA-Guideline-2019.pdf
Juvenile idiopathic arthritis	Standards of care for juvenile idiopathic arthritis	British Society for Paediatric and Adolescent Rheumatology	2017	https://academic.oup.com/rheumatology/article/49/7/1406/1785261
Juvenile idiopathic arthritis	TA 373 Technology appraisal on abatacept, adalimumab, etanercept and tocilizumab for treating juvenile idiopathic arthritis	NICE	2015	https://www.nice.org.uk/guidance/ta373

Condition	Guideline title	Issuing agency	Publication date	Internet link
Kawasaki disease	NG 143 Fever in under 5s: assessment and initial management	NICE	2019	https://www.nice.org.uk/guidance/ng14 3
Leukaemia	QS 150 Haematological cancers	NICE	2017	https://www.nice.org.uk/guidance/qs150
Leukaemia	Haematological cancers – recognition and referral	NICE	2016	https://cks.nice.org.uk/haematological-cancers-recognition-and-referral
Limp	Acute childhood limp	NICE	2015	https://cks.nice.org.uk/acute-childhood-limp#!scenario
Liver failure	Investigation and treatment of liver disease with acute onset	British Society of Paediatric Gastroenterology, Hepatology and Nutrition	2013	https://old.bspghan.org.uk/sites/default/files/guidelines/acute_liver_failure.pdf
Malaria	Guidelines for malaria prevention in travellers from the UK 2019	Public Health England	2019	https://assets.publishing.service.gov.uk/government/uploads/system/uploads/attachment_data/file/833506/ACMP_Guidelines.pdf
Malignancy	NG12 Suspected cancer: recognition and referral	NICE	2015 (updated 2017)	https://www.nice.org.uk/guidance/ng12/chapter/Recommendations-organised-by-symptom-and-findings-of-primary-care-investigations#symptoms-in-children-and-young-people
Meningitis	CG 102 Meningitis (bacterial) and meningococcal septicaemia in under 16s: recognition, diagnosis and management	NICE	2010 (updated 2015)	https://www.nice.org.uk/guidance/cg102
Meningitis	QS 19 Meningitis (bacterial) and meningococcal septicaemia in children and young people	NICE	2012	https://www.nice.org.uk/guidance/qs19
Nephrotic syndrome	Guidelines for the management of nephrotic syndrome in children	Children's Kidney Centre Wales	2017	http://www.wcnpn.wales.nhs.uk/sitesplus/documents/1216/Guidelines%20for%20the%20management%20of%20Nephrotic%20syndrome%20in%20children.pd f
Neuroblastoma	International neuroblastoma response criteria	International Neuroblastoma Risk Group	2011 (updated 2019)	https://link.springer.com/content/pdf/10.1007/s00247-019-04397-2.pd f
Non-accidental injury/safeguarding	Abusive head trauma and the eye in infancy	RCPCH/RCOphth	2013	https://www.rcophth.ac.uk/wp-content/uploads/2014/12/2013-SCI-292-ABUSIVE-HEAD-TRAUMA-AND-THE-EYE-FINAL-at-June-2013.pd f
Non-accidental injury/safeguarding	The radiological investigation of suspected physical abuse in children	Royal College of Radiologists	2017 (updated 2018)	https://www.rcr.ac.uk/publication/radiological-investigation-suspected-physical-abuse-children
Non-accidental injury/safeguarding	CG 89 Child maltreatment: when to suspect maltreatment in under 18s	NICE	2009 (updated 2017)	https://www.nice.org.uk/guidance/cg89

Condition	Guideline title	Issuing agency	Publication date	Internet link
Non-accidental injury/safeguarding	NG 76 Child abuse and neglect	NICE	2017	https://www.nice.org.uk/guidance/ng76
Otitis media	CG 60 Otitis media with effusion in under 12s: surgery	NICE	2008	https://www.nice.org.uk/guidance/cg60
Otitis media	NG 91 Otitis media (acute): antimicrobial prescribing	NICE	2018	https://www.nice.org.uk/guidance/ng91
Pneumonia	NG 138 Pneumonia (community-acquired): antimicrobial prescribing	NICE	2019	https://www.nice.org.uk/guidance/ng138
Pneumonia	CG 139 Healthcare-associated infections: prevention and control in primary and community care	NICE	2012 (updated 2017)	https://www.nice.org.uk/guidance/CG139
Pulmonary hypertension	BTS guidelines for home oxygen in children	British Thoracic Society (BTS)	2009	https://pubmed.ncbi.nlm.nih.gov/1958696 8
Rabies	WHO guide on rabies preexposure and postexposure prophylaxis	World Health Organisation	2010	https://www.who.int/rabies/PEP_prophylaxis_guidelines_June10.pdf
Renal and ureteric stones	NG 118 Renal and ureteric stones: assessment and management	NICE	2019	https://www.nice.org.uk/guidance/ng118
Rheumatic fever	Guidelines for the diagnosis of rheumatic fever. Jones criteria	American Heart Association	1992 (updated 2015)	https://www.ahajournals.org/doi/full/10.1161/CIR.0000000000000205
Sepsis	NG 51 Sepsis: recognition, diagnosis and early management	NICE	2016 (updated 2017)	https://www.nice.org.uk/guidance/ng5 1
Sepsis	QS 161 Sepsis	NICE	2017	https://www.nice.org.uk/guidance/qs161
Sepsis	CG 151 Neutropenic sepsis: prevention and management in people with cancer	NICE	2012	https://www.nice.org.uk/guidance/cg151
Sepsis	CG149 Neonatal infection (early onset): antibiotics for prevention and treatment	NICE	2012	https://www.nice.org.uk/guidance/cg149/chapter/1-Guidance#risk-factors-for-infection-and-clinical-indicators-of-possible-infection-2
Sickle cell disease	QS 58 Sickle cell disease	NICE	2014	https://www.nice.org.uk/guidance/qs58
Sickle cell disease	CG 143 Sickle cell disease: managing acute painful episodes in hospital	NICE	2012	https://www.nice.org.uk/guidance/cg143
Sickle cell disease	Management of acute chest syndrome in sickle cell disease	British Society for Haematology	2015	https://onlinelibrary.wiley.com/doi/full/10.1111/bjh.13348
Spinal injury	NG 41 Spinal injury: assessment and initial management	NICE	2016	https://www.nice.org.uk/guidance/ng41
Stroke	NG 128 Stroke and transient ischaemic attack in over 16s: diagnosis and initial management	NICE	2019	https://www.nice.org.uk/guidance/ng128

Condition	Guideline title	Issuing agency	Publication date	Internet link
Stroke	Stroke in childhood – clinical guideline for diagnosis, management and rehabilitation	RCPCH	2017	https://www.rcpch.ac.uk/ resources/stroke-childhood- clinical-guideline-diagnosis- management-rehabilitation
Syncope	Guidelines on diagnosis and management of syncope	European Society for Cardiology	2018	https://www.escardio.org/ Guidelines/Clinical-Practice- Guidelines/Syncope-Guidelines- on-Diagnosis-and-Management-of
Thalassaemia	Guidelines on red cell transfusion in sickle cell disease. Part I: Principles and laboratory aspects	British Society for Haematology	2017	https://pubmed.ncbi.nlm.nih. gov/2809210 9
Tuberculosis	NG33 Tuberculosis	NICE	2016	https://www.nice.org.uk/ guidance/ng3 3
Tuberculosis	QS 141 Tuberculosis	NICE	2017	https://www.nice.org.uk/ guidance/qs14 1
Ulcerative colitis	NG 130 Ulcerative colitis: management	NICE	2019	https://www.nice.org.uk/ guidance/ng130
Urinary tract infections	CG 54 Urinary tract infection in under 16s: diagnosis and management	NICE	2007 (updated 2018)	https://www.nice.org.uk/ guidance/cg5 4
Urinary tract infections	QS 36 Urinary tract infection in children and young people	NICE	2013 (updated 2017)	https://www.nice.org.uk/ guidance/qs3 6
Urinary tract infections	NG 113 Urinary tract infection (catheter-associated): antimicrobial prescribing	NICE	2018	https://www.nice.org.uk/ guidance/ng11 3
Urinary tract infections	NG 112 Urinary tract infection (recurrent): antimicrobial prescribing	NICE	2018	https://www.nice.org.uk/ guidance/ng11 2
Viral hepatitis	CG 165 Hepatitis B (chronic): diagnosis and management	NICE	2013	https://www.nice.org.uk/ guidance/cg16 5
Von Willebrand disease	The Diagnosis and management of Von Willebrand Disease: a United Kingdom Haemophilia Centre Doctors Organization guideline approved by the British Committee for Standards in Haematology	United Kingdom Haemophilia Centre Doctors Organization	2014	https://pubmed.ncbi.nlm.nih. gov/2511330 4
Von Willebrand disease	Diagnosis of inherited platelet function disorders	International Society on Thrombosis and Haemostasis	2015	http://pubmed.ncbi.nlm.nih. gov/25403439?dopt=Abstract
Wilms tumour	Scottish Intercollegiate Guidelines Network (SIGN) national clinical guideline on long-term follow-up of survivors of childhood cancer	SIGN	2013	https://www.sign.ac.uk/ media/1070/sign132.pdf
Wilms tumour	Long-term follow-up guideline on survivors of childhood, adolescent, and young adult cancers	Children's Oncology Group	2018	http://www.survivorship guidelines.org/pdf/2018/ COG_LTFU_Guidelines_v5.pdf

Index

Clinical Guide to Paediatrics, First Edition. Edited by Rachel Varughese and Anna Mathew. Series Editor: Christian Fielder Camm.
© 2022 John Wiley & Sons Ltd. Published 2022 by John Wiley & Sons Ltd.
Companion website: www.wiley.com/go/varughese/paediatrics